Child & Adolescent
Psychopharmacology

S. P. Kutcher, MD, FRCP(C)

Department of Psychiatry, Dalhousie University
Queen Elizabeth II Health Sciences Centre
Halifax, Nova Scotia
Canada

Child & Adolescent Psychopharmacology

W.B. SAUNDERS COMPANY

A Harcourt Health Sciences Company

Philadelphia   London   New York   St. Louis   Toronto   Sydney

W.B. SAUNDERS COMPANY
A Harcourt Health Sciences Company

The Curtis Center
Independence Square West
Philadelphia, Pennsylvania 19106

Library of Congress Cataloging-in-Publication Data

Kutcher, Stanley P.
    Child and adolescent psychopharmacology / S.P. Kutcher. — 1st ed.
      p. cm.
    ISBN 0–7216–5749–4
    1. Pediatric psychopharmacology.   I. Title.
    [DNLM: 1. Mental Disorders—in infancy & childhood.   2. Mental
Disorders—drug therapy.   3. Mental Disorders—in adolescence.   WS
350.2 K97c   1997]
RJ504.7.K88   1997
618.92'8918—dc20
DNLM/DLC
                                                          96-43068

NOTICE

Psychopharmacology is an ever-changing field. Standard safety precautions must be followed, but as new research and clinical experience broaden our knowledge, changes in treatment and drug therapy become necessary or appropriate. The editors of this work have carefully checked the generic and trade drug names and verified drug dosages to ensure that the dosage information in this work is accurate and in accord with the standards accepted at the time of publication. Readers are advised, however, to check the product information currently provided by the manufacturer of each drug to be administered to be certain that changes have not been made in the recommended dose or in the contraindications for administration. This is of particular importance in regard to new or infrequently used drugs. It is the responsibility of the treating physician, relying on experience and knowledge of the patient, to determine dosages and the best treatment for the patient. The editors cannot be responsible for misuse or misapplication of the material in this work.

THE PUBLISHER

For my father and my children

Foreword

All those concerned with the care of children owe this book and its author a debt of gratitude. It is the first to provide an overview of critical therapeutic issues in the management of children's and adolescents' mental disorders. It does not ignore the need for systematic diagnosis and quantitative assessments for optimal pharmacotherapy. This book gives guidance on how to derive clinical diagnoses, how to evaluate symptom severity for each diagnosis, how to decide on the first line of treatment, and if necessary, what alternatives are plausible, while communicating unfailing concern and care for children and families. It synthesizes an enormous amount of information that will be invaluable to the practitioner at every step of the clinical process.

This book will be a resource to experienced clinicians as well as to those in training. It presents the issues, some clearly controversial, with clarity and appreciation for the complexity of managing troubled lives in familial contexts. Dr. Kutcher is obviously an outstanding clinician who communicates fully that pharmacotherapy of children and adolescents encompasses far more than prescription writing. The nuances of treatment are dealt with head on, with complete respect for patients' and parents' autonomy.

There will be no confusion in the reader's mind regarding the source of the clinical recommendations made because the book is straightforward about the paucity of systematic research in child psychopharmacology. It states unequivocally when observations come from empirical research or simply clinical observations. When the latter are from a critically minded, astute observer, they must be considered respectfully. Dr. Kutcher is just such a clinician, and his voice is one of reasoned intelligence.

The publication of this book is a major event for the field of child psychiatry and represents a unique contribution to all mental health professionals. No one with an interest in the care of children should be without it, not only for the scope of its clinical content but also for its coverage of the history of the development of child psychopharmacology, which makes for informative and stimulating reading. We are fortunate indeed that an erudite clinician has shared his experience with us.

Rachel G. Klein, Ph.D.
New York State Psychiatric Institute

Preface

Any book, at least in part, must be a personal odyssey. This book is no exception and arose from my experiences as a learner, teacher, and provider of psychiatric medicine to children and adolescents. It is an attempt to synthesize the humanistic and caring demands of our discipline with its pragmatic and scientific needs. It is my contention that the proper practice of child and adolescent psychiatry is the provision of this synthesis by the clinician to the patient and his or her family.

Because there is little or nothing in the available child and adolescent psychiatric literature that can provide a guide for trainee and practitioner alike regarding this type of practice, this book attempts to do so. Taking to heart William Osler's famous dictum that "medicine is a science, the practice of which is an art," this book presents a synthesis of the science and art of child and adolescent psychopharmacology. It attempts not only to provide basic, practical scientific information about psychopharmacology in the context of the art of psychiatric practice in this population but also to construct a framework that molds humanism with neurochemistry in the delivery of therapeutics.

This book could not have been written without the assistance and support of many others. Dr. K. Shulman, Dr. P. Garfinkel, and my colleagues at the University of Toronto and the Sunnybrook Health Sciences Centre helped to support my sabbatical year, which was dedicated to the writing of this book. The Ontario Mental Health Foundation provided partial salary support and allowed me to use my Senior Research Fellowship funding for this project. Dr. J. McDermott of the University of Hawaii and Dr. Ian Goodyer of Cambridge University (Wolfson College) kindly provided me with an academic "home" for periods of the writing year.

Jill Green compiled and prepared the appendixes, a daunting task that she accomplished with expertise and wry perseverance.

A number of colleagues from the University of Toronto read and criticized various chapters of the book: Dr. J. Beitchman, Dr. S. Bradley, D. Gardner, Dr. G. Papatheodorou, and Dr. R. Schachar. Dr. B. Birmaher from the University of Pittsburgh, Dr. R. Klein from Columbia University, and Drs. J. Garland and D. Smith from the University of British Columbia read the entire manuscript and provided valuable feedback that enhanced and improved the final product. For their help I am grateful. The strengths of the book owe much to their input. The weaknesses are my responsibility.

Finally, I am particularly grateful for the technical assistance and constructive editing provided by Jan Sheppard-Kutcher, whose support and good humor helped make this task tolerable if not at times enjoyable.

S. P. Kutcher, M.D., FRCP(C)
Department of Psychiatry, Dalhousie University
Queen Elizabeth II Health Sciences Centre

Contents

Beginnings

CHAPTER 1

Read Me First: Why This Book?

"Medicine is a science, the practice of which is an art." Those words, written by William Osler, apply equally well to the practice of medicine today as they did over 100 years ago. The foundation of medical practice is the experimental and evaluative science that allows it to diagnose clearly, to treat well, and to predict outcome with confidence. This is the science of medicine. The practical application of knowledge thus derived, however, occurs within a framework that allows for the shaping of the human relationship between physician and patient in the joint pursuit of the common goal of alleviating suffering. That is the art of medicine.

The developing discipline of child and adolescent psychiatry illustrates well Osler's famous dictum. In this arena, experimentally derived and evaluated knowledge about developmental neurobiology, psychology, and pharmacology has recently been coupled with similar advances in the diagnostic and epidemiologic disciplines. Practitioners working in the field of child and adolescent psychiatry are now better able to identify and classify psychiatric disturbances in this population, to prescribe effective treatments, and to predict outcomes. Further naturalistic, experimental, and evaluative investigations are underway that may reasonably be expected to improve and direct clinical practice in the future.

Child and adolescent psychopharmacology has been an important part of this development. In adopting the experimental and evaluative paradigms of "adult" psychopharmacology and joining with the expanding scientifically based disciplines of developmental neurobiology and developmental psychology, child and adolescent psychopharmacology has, in large measure, helped bring the rigors of evaluative-based thinking and practice to child and adolescent psychiatry. For example, early investigations into pharmacologic interventions for seriously disturbed children led to the realization of the inadequacies of the then-current models of pathoetiology. This realization became one of the factors that led to a rethinking of diagnostic nomenclature in child and adolescent psychiatry. And the practical necessities of clinical pharmacologic investigations identified the need for empiric-based descriptive and evaluative tools. Many diagnostic and symptom-rating instruments owe their genesis to this necessity. The laboratory-learned lessons regarding measurement and outcome evaluation that empirical studies of pharmacotherapeutics demanded gradually began to influence the practice of child and adolescent psychiatry. This did not apply simply to the use of medication but also in a wider sense encouraged the application of an empiric evaluative-based paradigm in day-to-day clinical activity. These factors, evolving in part from child and adolescent psychopharmacology, played an important role in the further development of the scientific basis of child and adolescent psychiatry.

The face of child and adolescent psychiatry is changing, as the field evolves from a discipline that is primarily theory driven to one that is theory based and experimentally driven. This is an important change because these two paradigms (theory driven and theory based) are quite different. In the theory-driven paradigm, theories of understanding pathoetiology are developed and hypotheses are derived from them. These hypotheses are then used to drive clinical practice. In this paradigm, however, the hypotheses are not treated as such; that is, they are not usually understood as concepts in need of external validation but rather as driving principles. As such, they tend to stand outside any independent means of evaluation. What evaluation does occur is usually based on observations that operate largely within the framework of the model. These observations are then most often used to provide "information" to illustrate and support the hypothesis. This hypothesis evaluated in this manner is then used to validate or support the underlying theory.

Thus, in the theory-driven paradigm, the process of validation becomes circular. The same assumptions that underlie the theory are carried over into the hypotheses that arise from it. These hypotheses are then not examined critically outside of the assumptions from which they were derived. When these hypotheses are discussed, the assumptions that they are based on dictate what information is collected and used. This information is then applied to "prove" the hypothesis correct, and the "proven" hypothesis is used to justify the theory. Illustration, not critical evaluation, is the methodology used for "validation" in the theory-driven paradigm.

This type of theory-driven discipline is thus based essentially on tautologic reasoning and is characterized by "evidence" that is indistinguishable from the assumptions from which it arises. A discipline that is primarily theory driven is identifiable by the nature of the information that it uses as evidence. First, that information is by and large observational and is presented primarily to illustrate the underlying hypotheses. Second, that information uses data that are selected a priori as suitable for illustrative purposes. Information that does not fit into the model is either ignored or rejected on principle. Third, the information selected avoids independent evaluation using empirical experimental methods and instead chooses argument and discourse as its preferred evaluative tool. The classic identifier of a theory-driven discipline is one in which the supportive documentation is primarily observational, presented within the context of discussion and debate in the absence of experimental challenge. The classic documentation of a theory-driven discipline is the discursive essay. In child and adolescent psychiatry, this is identified as the "theoretical discourse" or the "illustrative case report."

A theory-based discipline differs substantially from a theory-driven discipline. A theory-based paradigm develops theories of understanding pathoetiology and creates hypotheses from them. These hypotheses are then subjected to critical review using an experimental evaluative framework that is not based on the same assumptions that underlie the hypothesis. Thus, the hypotheses are tested not to demonstrate that they are correct but to demonstrate that they may be indeed incorrect. Critical experimental evaluation, not illustration, is the model used for hypothesis evaluation. These hypotheses are then used to either reject or support the theory from which they arose.

The hypotheses that drive practice in a theory-based discipline are subjected to independent critical experimental evaluation. Accordingly, a theory-based discipline is identifiable by the nature of the information that is used as its evidence. First, that information is used in a way that allows for the rejection of the hypothesis. The information is not only observational but empirical as well. Second, data that are expected to lead to the invalidation of the hypothesis (the "null" hypothesis) are identified and collected. Third, that information is then subjected to the scientific methodologies of empirically sound experimental investigation. The classic identifier of a theory-based discipline is one in which the supportive documentation is primarily that of argument arising from experimental designs developed to test the null hypothesis. The classic documentation of the theory-based discipline is the experimental study. In child and adolescent psychiatry, this is known as the *experimental or hypothesis testing study,* the *empirical descriptive study* (such as an epidemiologic survey), or the *information case report* (a case report designed to provide new data about a particular topic, for example, a rare adverse effect of a treatment or a report that describes a clinically uncommon phenomenon).

As a review of the papers in journals and other publications and child and adolescent psychiatry of the last 40 years will demonstrate, the discipline of child and adolescent psychiatry is becoming increasingly a theory-based and experimentally driven one. Concurrent with this, the critical evaluation of the utility of pharmacologic interventions in the psychiatric disturbances of children and adolescents has increased substantially. Child and adolescent psychopharmacology has developed a core of knowledge founded on the theory-based and experimentally driven model. This information is expanding quickly and at the same time is being subjected to continued critical scrutiny.

Successful pharmacologic interventions in a wide variety of child and adolescent psychiatric illnesses have provided countless children and adolescents with a decrease in suffering and an improved quality of life. However, what we know about pharmacologic treatment of psychiatric conditions in this age group is still limited. There are still great gaps in our knowledge regarding what kind of pharmacologic treatment works best and for whom. Our medicines are still sometimes crude and problematic, and our practical use of them often flows from a model of clinical practice that still owes more to tradition and word of mouth than to a rationally derived application of therapeutics.

In part, this is because child and adolescent psychopharmacology is still a relatively young discipline, and enough time has not yet passed to allow the proper evaluation of various pharmacologic compounds across the many psychiatric conditions in which they might be indicated. However, this is in part because the results of controlled conditions in the laboratory or controlled experimental designs need to be themselves challenged in the "real world," at the interface between the physician and the patient. In addition, the successes of pharmacologic interventions have created a demand for their use in child and adolescent psychotherapeutics. This use, however, cannot be directed primarily by therapeutic methods that have arisen from nonpharmacologic models of clinical care. Rational pharmacotherapy *must* be driven by a therapeutic model that develops from and accounts for the specific features of pharmacologic interventions.

This is where the "art" of child and adolescent psychopharmacology enters, and this is what this book is about. Our rapidly expanding scientific knowledge about the "what" and "for whom" of medications must be paralleled by an equally expanding and sophisticated "what" and "for whom" of pharmacotherapeutics. Older, primarily unidimensional, psychologically derived and driven models of physician-patient interaction cannot simply be applied to the revolution in clinical practice that successful pharmacologic treatment brings to child and adolescent psychiatry. A new understanding, a new clinical model, is needed to allow for the rational and optimal application of psychopharmacology in everyday clinical practice. This new model is needed to provide the "art" of psychopharmacology, the application of the science of psychopharmacology.

How to Use This Book

The rational day-to-day clinical use of psychopharmacotropics depends on two things: its foundations in the science of pharmacology and the clinical art of its application. The purpose of this book is to provide practitioners with a clinically useful approach to using medications in the treatment of child and adolescent psychiatric disorders. To this end, this book is not a textbook that itemizes, lists, and describes much of what is known about potentially useful medications, often presented in such a manner as to isolate this knowledge from any rational application. Nor does this book attempt to give the practitioner a step-by-step, cookie-cutter approach to using medications, because real life rarely if ever fits into such a mold. Instead, this book provides the prac-

ticing physician and trainee with a clinically useful model that can be used to apply the science of psychopharmacology in treating the child or adolescent suffering from a psychiatric disorder.

This model—the art of psychopharmacology—has arisen from years of clinical psychiatric practice; clinical psychopharmacologic research into a variety of child and adolescent psychiatric disorders; and teaching to and learning from medical students, residents in psychiatry and medicine, nurses, allied mental health workers, physicians, patients, and their families. It owes much to principles taken from psychotherapeutic work with children, adolescents, and their families, and from individual, family, and group experiences. It also owes much to the study of interpersonal interactions by caring and knowledgeable clinicians with patients. These clinicians are not limited to psychiatrists but instead come from all fields of the practice of medicine, because no one group of clinicians has a monopoly on the understanding of people or physician-patient relationships. Finally, this model owes much to the rigors and demands of clinical research, particularly those parts that help the clinician evaluate the outcome of his interventions and the mind-set that not only demands this evaluation but compels the practitioner to question his intervention, and not the recipient of the intervention, if the outcome is not optimal.

This model is also practical. The responsible clinician no longer has the luxury of avoiding "difficult cases" or of practicing a unidimensional type of intervention of unproven efficacy. "Good psychotherapy candidates" should no longer be the criteria upon which treatment is offered. Children and adolescents with severe psychiatric symptomatology require the knowledge and application of multiple therapeutic techniques. In many, if not most, such cases, pharmacologic treatments are a necessary, albeit not sufficient, component of optimal intervention. Physicians need to know not only what and how to prescribe, but how to modify their clinical activities to take into account the exigencies of pharmacotherapeutics and how to integrate pharmacotherapy with other treatment modalities.

This model is also unabashedly empirical. It demands that the utility of all therapeutic interventions stand the test of critical empirical evaluation and argues that evidence-based care is the appropriate approach to psychiatric treatments. As such, this therapeutic model is outcome driven, evaluation based, and hypothesis testing. Concurrently, this model also, however, provides the practitioner with the tools with which to properly evaluate his or her therapeutic interventions.

While some of these methods are often specific to pharmacologic treatments, others may be used to better evaluate not only pharmacologic interventions but other psychiatric treatments as well.

Some practitioners may not be familiar with this type of approach to clinical practice. Others may not have had the background or training in pharmacology that current treatment paradigms demand. Still others may have deep-seated philosophical or personal views or biases about the use of pharmacotherapies in the treatment of children and adolescents. Others may have recognized the need to change traditional models of clinical practice to accommodate to the challenge of pharmacotherapeutics but have not yet been able to develop a new model that takes these issues into account. Some may at times feel overwhelmed as they struggle to separate the pharmacologic wheat from the pharmacologic chaff and come up with a useful approach to selecting what is best for whom and using it properly. This book is for all those practitioners, for it attempts to provide a rational way to do just that.

Section Two—Chapters 2 through 5—deals with the core conceptual framework and methodologies of this model of care. The chapters in this section describe and illustrate the practice of useful assessment, techniques, and the evaluation of symptoms and associated disturbances. Section Three—Chapters 6 and 7—describe a rational approach to the general principles of identification, selection, and implementation of pharmacotherapy for children and adolescents.

Section Four—Chapters 8 through 17—deals with individual psychiatric disorders and common psychiatric problems and their pharmacologic treatment using the principles outlined in Sections Two and Three. Each chapter in Section Four uses the concepts described in Section Two and Three and applies them to the real-life clinical care of a child or adolescent with a particular psychiatric disturbance. In each area of potentially pharmacologically treatable psychopathology, the reader is given a useful framework from which to approach the pharmacotherapy of a child or adolescent with a particular psychiatric problem, a framework that can readily be applied to all or most children or adolescents who present with such difficulties. The necessary scientific information that provides the foundation for that framework is included in each chapter and is woven into the narrative by the use of case examples that illustrate the application of the art.

Section Five provides an historical overview of child and adolescent psychopharmacology. It is included to provide a model by which to understand the development and use of this therapeutic area. Finally, the book ends with appendixes that provide a variety of clinically useful assessment and evaluation tools.

Given this approach, not every potential medication for every possible disorder or disturbance can be dealt with, and indeed this is not the purpose of the book. This book provides practical and useful information that covers most clinical scenarios and gives the practitioner the tools—both conceptual and practical—to go beyond the scientific information presented here. The book thus treads the middle road regarding medications. It acknowledges the recent advances in pharmacotherapy and gives due consideration to medications that are "tried and true." However, it also incorporates new information regarding pharmacologic treatments for children and adolescents without endorsing the use of compounds that may seem promising but remain largely untested. In this sense the book is up-to-date yet at the same time not ahead of itself.

Given the gaps in available scientific data, a number of criteria have been applied to provide direction in areas in which less than optimal information regarding the use of pharmacotropic agents in children and adolescents is available. Data from controlled studies in children and adolescents are always considered. Data from uncontrolled or naturalistic studies are also used, but their limitations are taken into account. Data from case reports and studies of adult populations with similar conditions are also used but are given less credibility because of their nature. Detailed information about most medicines that are useful in treating the psychiatric disorders of children and adolescents is available in this book. If the required information does not appear in a chapter that discusses a particular disorder, then the reader will be directed to that part of the book where more detailed information can be found. This approach parallels the practice of pharmacotherapy itself, because many medications are useful in treating a number of different disorders.

The chapters are written in a discursive style, and no references are included to break the flow. Individual cases are used to bring the "art" of pharmacotherapy alive. Each case is taken from clinical experience, and both mistakes (how not to do it) and successes (how to do it) are presented. This is because clinicians learn not only from their successes but also from their mistakes.

Each chapter is followed by a list of useful references for further reading that can take the interested clinician closer to the source. These references are usually excellent reviews of particular aspects of the subject, although in some cases seminal original research papers may also be included. Clinicians are encouraged to read these sources for further information.

The book concludes with appendixes of clinically useful assessment and evaluative tools. These have been selected using utilitarian principles because of their demonstrated value in the clinical practice of child and adolescent psychopharmacology. They include forms useful in the practical day-to-day function of the pediatric pharmacologic clinic or in the education of patients and their families. The appendixes also include instruments designed to measure treatment-emergent side effects of specific medications and measures of symptoms that may be the target of pharmacologic interventions. In those cases where copyright laws prohibit the publication of the entire instrument, examples of items from the identified scales are provided and, whenever possible, information on how to obtain the scale is given. In those cases in which the materials have not been copyrighted, the clinician is encouraged to reproduce these instruments and to use them in her own practice.

As described earlier, the clinician is encouraged to consult other, more traditional textbooks while reading this book. Some of the texts most useful for this purpose are listed below.

The reader is encouraged to read Sections Two and Three first. Then read the appropriate chapter in Section Four that applies to a specific patient with a particular psychiatric disturbance for whom pharmacotherapy may be indicated. In this manner, you will be able to integrate the information presented in this book with the reality of your own clinical material.

SUGGESTED READINGS

General References

Arana GW, Hyman SE. Handbook of Psychiatric Drug Therapy (2nd ed). Boston: Little Brown, 1991.

Bezchlibnyk-Butler KZ, Jeffries JJ, Martin BA. Clinical Handbook of Psychotropic Drugs (6th rev ed). Seattle: Hogrefe & Huber, 1996.

Ciraulo DA, Shader RI, Greenblatt DJ, Creelman W. Drug Interactions in Psychiatry. Baltimore: Williams and Wilkins, 1995.

De Vane CL. Fundamentals of Monitoring Psychoactive Drug Therapy. Baltimore: Williams and Wilkins, 1990.

Janicak PG, Davis JM, Preskorn SHP, Ayd FJ. Principles and Practice of Psychopharmacotherapy. Baltimore: Williams and Wilkins, 1993.

Kaplan HI, Sadock BJ. Pocket Handbook of Psychiatric Drug Treatment. Baltimore: Williams and Wilkins, 1996.

Schatzberg AF, Nemeroff CB (eds). Textbook of Psychopharmacology. Washington, DC: American Psychiatric Press, 1995.

Stahl SM. Essential Psychopharmacology. Cambridge: Cambridge University Press, 1996.

Child and Adolescent References

Green WH. Child and Adolescent Psychopharmacology (2nd ed). Baltimore: Williams and Wilkins, 1995.

Rosenberg DR, Holttum J, Gershon S. Textbook of Pharmacotherapy for Child and Adolescent Psychiatric Disorders. New York: Brunner/Mazel, 1994.

Werry JS, Aman MG (eds). Practitioner's Guide to Psychoactive Drugs for Children and Adolescents. New York: Plenum Medical, 1993.

Wiener JM (ed). Diagnosis and Psychopharmacology of Childhood and Adolescent Disorders (2nd ed). New York: John Wiley and Sons, Inc., 1996.

Periodicals

Child and Adolescent Psychopharmacology News. New York: Guilford Press.

Journal of Child and Adolescent Psychopharmacology. Larchmont, NY: Mary Ann Liebert, Inc.

Baseline Assessment for Psychopharmacologic Treatments

Introduction

The baseline assessment of a child or adolescent prior to initiating psychopharmacologic treatment is a complex process requiring careful evaluation of multiple psychological, physiological, and social parameters. Psychiatric illnesses are broad-based disorders involving disturbances in mood, cognition, and behavior that significantly affect many aspects of a child's or adolescent's functioning. Psychopharmacologic treatment is directed toward improving one or more of these disturbances. For this to occur, the various dimensions that psychiatric disorders present to the clinician must be not only identified and understood but also systematically evaluated and measured.

The importance of systematic assessment and objective measurement of the multiple domains of psychiatric disturbance cannot be overemphasized. Such assessment is necessary for a comprehensive understanding of any individual child or adolescent, and it provides the baseline for evaluating the outcome of treatment. After all, a demonstrated positive response to a particular type of treatment is the specific goal of psychopharmacologic intervention.

From this perspective, the clinician approaches the task of pharmacotherapeutic treatment with a critical attitude. The value of psychopharmacologic treatment in ameliorating or modifying specific psychiatric disturbances must be proved. Furthermore, it must be demonstrated that psychopharmacologic intervention is a necessary (it is unlikely to be sufficient) component of a comprehensive treatment program that is directed toward improving a patient's functioning across the multiple dimensions of his or her psychiatric disorder. Thus, psychopharmacologic intervention, while requiring specialized knowledge and a unique therapeutic model to administer, shares many characteristics of "good" treatment strategies in general.

The overall strategy for optimal psychiatric treatment in children and adolescents comprises the following features:

1. A clear psychiatric diagnosis

2. Identification and measurement of those features that are the target of treatment
3. A treatment "contract" with the patient (and when appropriate, the family)
4. Sophisticated knowledge about various treatment options and their relative risks and benefits
5. An understanding of the various interpersonal, psychological, family, social, and economic factors that can influence treatment
6. A useful methodology for determining efficacy and optimization of treatment
7. A constructively critical attitude about models of pathoetiology and how they relate to treatment
8. Knowledge of and proficiency in a model of therapeutics that can allow for the implementation and integration of various useful treatments

Effective psychopharmacologic intervention is based on the above-mentioned eight treatment principles, and it begins with an appropriate psychiatric diagnosis and assessment of those domains of disturbance that will become the focus of treatment.

The Baseline Assessment: General Issues

The baseline assessment provides the foundation on which psychopharmacologic treatment planning takes place. The baseline assessment is not unidimensional but comprises many aspects of an individual's functioning. Treatment can begin only after a comprehensive baseline assessment of these multiple domains has been completed.

Three separate but related areas comprise the baseline assessment:

- The patient and his or her symptoms
- The patient's family or living unit
- The patient's school or work and social environment

The baseline assessment of an individual patient must include a complete psychiatric history and mental status, the identification and measurement of specific symptoms that will be a focus of treatment (target symptoms), and a medical evaluation, with careful attention to baseline physical symptoms that may later be manifested as side effects of pharmacologic treatment. The assessment of other related areas (social, school, or family functioning) is also important because they may be of value in understanding either the specific pathoetiology of the illness or the more general nature of the patient's difficulties. These areas may also be identified as suitable treatment targets for pharmacotherapy or they may require separate interventions (apart from pharmacologic treatment) in order to improve the overall treatment outcome. For example, speech and language intervention may be required if the baseline assessment indicates that the patient has difficulties in this area.

Focused information about the patient's family is the second major component of the baseline assessment. This includes an understanding of the role of various family members in the patient's life (including those who do and those who do not live with the patient, such as a child in a reconstituted family), a complete psychiatric history of all family members, and identification of family experience with previous psychiatric or mental health treatments, either for the patient or for other family members. It is also essential to explore family value systems regarding psychiatric treatments in general and psychopharmacologic treatments in particular and to determine whether any specific cultural or religious beliefs may have an impact on psychopharmacologic interventions.

Third, the baseline assessment must examine the patient's school or work and social functioning. This includes consideration of academic performance, both current and past, work history (if applicable), current and past peer relationships, and current self-management ability, including independent living skills. This part of the baseline assessment often requires that information be obtained from sources outside the patient and family. For example, it will often be necessary to communicate with a child's or adolescent's schoolteacher or school counselor to obtain information on past and current academic and school performance.

In obtaining the information outlined earlier and described more fully in Chapters 3 to 5, the practitioner must evaluate the quality of the material obtained and the reliability of informants. For example, a severely depressed or anxious parent may overestimate the level of disturbance her child is presenting. In contrast, an adolescent concerned about social labeling or attending a psychiatric consultation under school, court, or parental duress may underplay symptom severity and even deny the existence of problems. If the practitioner is not cognizant of these potential confounds, significant diagnostic or measurement errors may occur.

Furthermore, studies of psychiatric symptom reporting in children and adolescents have shown that parents and children may differ in their perceptions of the identification or severity ratings of various psychiatric symptoms. In general, parents tend to be more reliable in the reporting of those symptoms that are externally observed, such as temper outbursts, conflicts with siblings and school, or peer difficulties. Children and teens, on the other hand, tend to be more reliable in the reporting of those symptoms that identify inner states, such as feelings of worthlessness, anxiety, and depression. If parent and child differ significantly in their reporting of either the presence or the severity of symptoms, a useful strategy is to discuss this disagreement nonjudgmentally with both parent and child together and to come to a consensus. There will be times when consensus is not possible, and it will be left to the professional judgment of the practitioner to evaluate and measure the symptoms in question.

At times it will not be possible for the clinician to obtain or clarify all the information needed to complete the entire baseline evaluation at one appointment. In many cases it will be possible to delay psychopharmacologic intervention until the necessary evaluations are completed. This should not, however, be put off too long (generally a maximum of 3 to 4 days), nor should pharmacologic intervention be delayed until every single "t" is crossed and every "i" is dotted. Instead, the clinician must decide when sufficient data are on hand to proceed with treatment. Interventions that jump in too quickly are as likely to be as unsuccessful as those that are unnecessarily delayed.

Of course, in some cases it may be necessary to begin pharmacologic treatment immediately (e.g., an agitated psychotic child or a suicidal depressed adolescent). In these cases the clinician will need to triage the value of information necessary, obtaining immediately what is of vital importance for beginning pharmacologic treatment and "filling in the blanks" as soon as possible.

Baseline Assessment: Interviewing Issues

One relatively common difficulty that some clinicians experience in conducting a baseline psychopharmacologic assessment is their reluctance to ask specific questions about symptoms and other pertinent issues. Often this reluctance may be understood as arising out of "insight"-oriented models of psychoanalytic assessment in which structured interviewing is seen as undesirable. Alternatively, some practitioners believe that direct questioning may damage patient rapport or "distort the transference." However, while respecting these traditional approaches to patient interviewing, it must be stressed that direct questioning is *essential* to the completion of a comprehensive and accurate baseline assessment for psychopharmacologic treatment.

An interview consisting predominantly of open-ended questions will not allow for the diagnostic evaluation and symptom measurement needed for psychopharmacologic intervention. While open-ended questions are a useful component of assessment interviews, the clinician must remember that direct but nonleading questions about symptoms and functioning are the most critical clinical tool of the baseline assessment. Often an open-ended question can be "twinned" with a specific, directed question for optimal information. For example, to elicit information about a child's or adolescent's mood, the clinician could begin with an open-ended inquiry, such as "How are you feeling inside?" and follow with a number of specific questions about various aspects of mood, such as "Have you been feeling down, low, or depressed?" The symptom-oriented descriptive interview is the "gold standard" for use in diagnosis and symptom ascertainment.

It should be noted that there is no evidence to suggest that direct questioning about symptoms damages patient-physician rapport. On the contrary, patients and parents frequently feel that the physician who uses direct questioning is keenly interested in them and takes their problems seriously by attempting to attain as much information as possible about them. Indeed, there is evidence that this direct questioning approach enhances the rapport between patient and family and the practitioner. The argument that direct questioning of a patient about his or her symptoms "distorts the transference" is perhaps best understood as an historical remnant that characterized the pre-psychopharmacologic treatment era.

The language of the interview must be appropriate to the developmental understanding of the child or adolescent. For example, a child may not clearly understand the meaning of the word *depressed* but may better identify the mood as "sad" or "crying inside." Similarly, a teenager may experience a depressed mood as a lack of normative affective range, sort of being "stuck in low gear," to

quote a 15-year-old girl with major depressive disorder. Thus the clinician may find that the adolescent will not describe his mood as "depressed" but will label it as "blah" or "flat." The skilled interviewer not only will use developmentally appropriate language but also will identify a range of useful descriptors for any one symptom.

Clearly, then, it is the role of the physician to identify and measure as objectively as possible the various components of the baseline assessment while taking into account the quality and reliability of the information obtained. Direct questioning regarding specific symptoms and associated features is imperative. These questions need to be developmentally appropriate and sensitive to the multiple descriptors that children and adolescents use to describe the same symptoms. In many cases it may also be necessary to use external sources to obtain information necessary for the completion of a baseline assessment. These may include mental health records, discussions with school or legal personnel, and interviews with family members not previously available. Informed consent to access these sources is, of course, essential, and in some jurisdictions it may also be necessary to use legally mandated methods (such as specific legal forms or documents) to obtain some or all of the baseline information needed.

In addition to conducting a supportive and directed interview, the clinician will need to identify and measure as accurately as possible the severity of various dimensions of psychiatric disturbance. This type of assessment is best accomplished using a variety of measurement tools, such as rating scales. These tools are applied in addition to and not instead of the diagnostic psychiatric interview. These measures are then used during treatment for baseline evaluation as well as to monitor outcome. Effective psychopharmacologic treatment begins with a proper assessment, the details of which are found in Chapters 3 to 5.

The Approach to Assessment for Psychopharmacologic Treatment— Practice Points

1. Psychopharmacologic baseline assessment must include evaluation of both symptoms and functioning across multiple domains.
2. The quality of information obtained during assessment must be evaluated, and if concerns regarding its validity are present, steps must be taken to provide the necessary clarity.

3. Direct questioning regarding symptoms and functioning is crucial to a proper psychopharmacologic assessment.
4. Developmentally sensitive questions must be used.
5. External sources of information are to be used whenever necessary.
6. A comprehensive baseline assessment includes a medical evaluation, a diagnostic psychiatric interview, and the application of various measurement tools to identify a diagnosis and to evaluate symptom severity.

SUGGESTED READINGS

Cantwell DP, Rutter M. Classification: Conceptual issues and substantive findings. In M Rutter, E Taylor, L Hersor (eds): Child and Adolescent Psychiatry: Modern Approaches. London: Blackwell Scientific, 1994, pp 3–21.

Costello A. Structured interviewing. In M Lewis (ed): Child and Adolescent Psychiatry: A Comprehensive Textbook. Baltimore: Williams and Wilkins, 1991, pp 463–472.

Cox A, Hopkinson KF, Rutter M. Psychiatric interview techniques (parts I and V). British Journal of Psychiatry, 139:29–37, 1981.

Klein RG. Parent-child agreement in clinical assessment of anxiety and other psychopathology: A review. Journal of Anxiety Disorders, 5:187–198, 1991.

Ollendick TH, Hersen M (eds). Handbook of Child and Adolescent Assessment. Needham Heights, MA: Allyn and Bacon, 1993.

Werry JS. Child psychiatric disorders: Are they classifiable? British Journal of Psychiatry, 161:472–480, 1992.

Wyatt RJ. Practical Psychiatric Practice: Terms and Protocols for Clinical Use. Washington, DC: American Psychiatric Press, 1994.

CHAPTER 3

Individual Baseline Psychiatric Assessment for Psychopharmacologic Treatment

The psychiatric component of psychopharmacologic treatment assessment begins with an interview of the individual patient, enriched by information supplied by his or her family whenever possible. In the absence of family, a legal guardian or health worker familiar with the patient should be included in the process. The purpose of the baseline interview is threefold:

1. To determine a psychiatric diagnosis or diagnoses for which pharmacologic treatment might be indicated (Table 3–1)
2. To identify and establish baseline measures for target symptoms suitable for pharmacologic treatment
3. To develop a therapeutic contract with the patient and family

The successful completion of these three components is necessary for establishment of a solid foundation for effective psychopharmacologic treatment.

During the initial interview, information from the patient and the family should be used, both to establish a psychiatric diagnosis and to assess the frequency, severity, and duration of symptoms. For example, in evaluating any symptom (i.e., sadness), information about its presence and severity should be obtained from both the patient and a parent or another individual who knows the child or adolescent well. This is necessary because in many cases a child and parent may present somewhat different evaluations of signs and symptoms of a psychiatric disorder, depending on their perspective or experience. In many cases the child or teenager may be more useful in characterizing internal phenomena, while a parent or other adult may be better able to describe external behaviors. For instance, a child or adolescent may be more able to inform the interviewer about the presence or absence of "sadness," including a description of its severity and duration, than the parent. Alternatively, a parent may be able to provide a better description of withdrawn behaviors and changes in social activities than a child or adolescent. Using both perspectives will allow the clinician to obtain a more comprehensive understanding of the signs and symptoms of the disorder and will provide a more thorough review of the diagnostic criteria necessary for diagnosis.

Although the potential for a seemingly never-ending assessment interview exists, with practice and the use of direct and systematic questioning, the entire baseline assessment (individual: psychiatric and medical; family; social-academic) should take no longer than a few hours. In some cases this may take substantially less time, as for example, when a child who is already in treatment for a well-defined psychiatric disorder is evaluated to determine whether pharmacologic intervention is reasonable. In such cases it may be possible to conduct the entire baseline psychiatric assessment in one session, particularly in the case of a second-opinion consultation or when a child's or adolescent's diagnosis and symptoms are well understood and the clinician is conducting a focused evaluation for a specific pharmacologic intervention (e.g., a schizophrenic adolescent in whom the initial response to antipsychotic treatment is suboptimal or a child with panic disorder [PD] in whom a pharmacologic intervention is being considered as an adjunct to ongoing psychological treatment).

The baseline individual psychiatric assessment

TABLE 3–1 **Child and Adolescent Psychiatric Disorders (DSM-IV) in Which Psychopharmacologic Treatment Should or May Be Indicated***

Major depression	Obsessive compulsive
Dysthymia	disorder
Generalized anxiety	Schizophrenia
disorder	Schizoaffective disorder
Social phobia	Schizophreniform disorder
Panic disorder with	Brief psychotic disorder
agoraphobia	Bipolar disorder
Panic disorder without	Attention-deficit hyper-
agoraphobia	activity disorder
Separation anxiety	Pervasive developmental
Tourette's disorder	disorders
Chronic motor or vocal tic	Selective mutism
disorder	Primary insomnia
Stereotypic movement	Enuresis
disorder	Narcolepsy
Sleep terror disorder	Intermittent explosive
Sleepwalking disorder	disorder
Trichotillomania	Bulimia
Borderline personality	
disorder	

*This list is not exclusionary, nor does it address symptoms that may be amenable to psychopharmacologic treatments that arise in the context of a disorder not identified. It is provided so that the clinician diagnosing or treating a child or adolescent with one of the above conditions will consider the potential role of one or more psychopharmacologic agents when developing a comprehensive treatment plan for a patient with that condition.

for pharmacologic treatment, described in detail later, must be tailored to the goals for which it is being made. It is not good clinical practice to provide the same baseline assessment for every child and adolescent regardless of the purpose of the assessment. Subjecting patients and their families to unnecessary evaluations on the basis of routine not only is unlikely to provide little new useful information but may be offputting to the patient, who may feel "assessed to death." Thus, prior to beginning the assessment for baseline psychopharmacologic treatment, the clinician must be clear about its purpose and should structure the evaluation accordingly. Some patients will require a full baseline assessment, as described later, while for others a more focused evaluation (using some but not all of the components to be described) will suffice.

This is not to say, however, that if a clinician has concerns about a previous diagnosis, or if new information is available that calls into question an earlier understanding of the case, these issues should be ignored. On the contrary, the clinician should undertake a full baseline assessment, as outlined later, when indicated. The physician may decide that this is necessary on the basis of information obtained either prior to seeing the patient

or during the course of a more focused evaluation. The point is that the clinician must tailor the baseline assessment to the needs of the patient and must be flexible enough to allow for whatever components of the baseline evaluation need to be performed.

Diagnostic Evaluation

A psychiatric diagnosis must be determined before psychopharmacologic treatment is begun. While in some communities the psychopharmacologist will also be the physician involved in the initial patient referral and mental health assessment, in others the psychopharmacologist will only be consulted regarding specific medication treatment issues. In either case the psychopharmacologist must personally establish or review the psychiatric diagnosis using rigorous assessment techniques. In communities where psychiatric care for children and adolescents is less readily available, the psychopharmacologic consultation may also be used as a method for increasing the awareness of other health practitioners regarding psychiatric diagnoses in children and teenagers. In those cases in which the psychopharmacologist acts as a consultant to another child psychiatrist or pediatrician, the consultation may also be of value for educating the practitioner about new developments in pediatric psychopharmacologic treatment.

Diagnostic evaluation should lead to a psychiatric diagnosis using currently accepted criteria-based categorical diagnostic classifications. Diagnoses should be determined using either the Diagnostic and Statistical Manual-IV (DSM-IV) or the International Classification of Diseases-10 (ICD-10) criteria. There is no place in psychopharmacologic practice for "diagnoses" such as emotional disturbance, behavior problem, adjustment difficulties, family problem, and difficulty in transition through the developmental tasks of adolescence, to name just a few. Often such labels are the product of sloppy history taking, lack of awareness of current diagnostic criteria, or etiologic biases using outdated, unvalidated models of child and adolescent psychiatric disorders.

CASE EXAMPLE

Avoiding the Diagnosis Does No One a Favor

T.F., a 16-year-old boy, had been an inpatient in an adolescent treatment center for 2 months. Consultation for psychopharmacologic intervention to assist in behavioral control was requested after his symptoms of irritability; mood swings; short-lived impulsive, aggressive outbursts; and unwillingness to participate in the center's group therapy program grew to such proportions that staff were considering discharging him from the institution. His problems had been diagnosed as "excessive adolescent narcissism" and "a failure to complete adolescent developmental tasks."

A detailed individual psychiatric diagnostic assessment revealed an ongoing hypomanic episode that had been preceded by a major depression. A family psychiatric history identified bipolar disorder in both the father and the paternal grandfather. Lithium treatment was instituted, although some members of the treatment center staff felt that this was likely to be therapeutically harmful because it would "medicalize T.F.'s problems" and he would no longer need to "take responsibility" for his behavior.

Seven weeks later T.F. was discharged to outpatient follow-up, showing good symptomatic control. A discharge conference revealed that a psychiatric interview using operational diagnostic criteria had not been carried out at the time of admission, and the family psychiatric history had not been obtained because the admitting mental health worker believed that such "intrusive questioning" would be inappropriate and he had not wanted to "use the medical model."

CASE COMMENTARY

In the case of T.F., failure to conduct an adequate diagnostic assessment at the time of admission to the inpatient treatment unit led to an inappropriate diagnosis that was based not on currently accepted criteria but on a specific theory of presumed underlying psychological conflicts. The treatment that this initial diagnosis led to was, not surprisingly, ineffective. In this case the patient's presenting symptoms and lack of response to a particular treatment program suggested that a diagnostic review, and not just an opinion about pharmacologic interventions for symptom control, was necessary. When a careful psychiatric evaluation using recognized diagnostic criteria was carried out, the resulting diagnosis led to more appropriate treatment, with subsequent positive results.

Given the current state of knowledge in psychiatric diagnoses of children and adolescents, it is important that the clinician make use of generally recognized diagnostic classifications (such as DSM-IV or ICD-10), while at the same time understanding their limitations. The use of such diagnostic systems does not negate the necessity of understanding the patient's difficulties using additional explanatory psychological or social models. The clinician who fails to use established diagnostic categories does so at the patient's peril.

In some cases the clinician may confuse the presenting problem with the diagnosis. Although these may often be similar or overlapping, they are not necessarily the same, and sometimes the presenting problem may only suggest the diagnosis. For example, a child presenting with "behavior problems at school" may turn out to have a diagnosis of one or more of the following: attention-deficit hyperactivity disorder (ADHD), conduct disorder, oppositional disorder, a specific learning disorder, or a specific communication disorder. A child whose behavioral problems arise from his or her attention-deficit disorder may experience a significant reduction in these difficulties with methylphenidate treatment. The same may not be the case when a phenomenologically similar problem behavior arises in the context of an oppositional disorder without a comorbid ADHD.

There are times when a clear-cut categorical psychiatric diagnosis is not possible or when the patient's symptoms fail to meet threshold criteria for a diagnosis. In these cases, the situation should be discussed with the patient, parent, or legal guardian and with the referring health professional. A provisional diagnosis may then be made and future diagnostic evaluations suggested. For example, a teenage male presenting with a nonorganic, nonaffective psychosis of 4 months' duration may fail to meet a diagnosis of schizophrenia by the criterion of duration of illness. In this case a provisional diagnosis of schizophrenia can be made in addition to the diagnosis of schizophreniform disorder. A decision to treat the patient psychopharmacologically in such a case is still valid as long as specific target symptoms for which pharmacologic treatment is indicated exist and the treatment plan calls for diagnostic re-evaluation at a specific time in the future.

Finally, it is important to remember that *a psychiatric diagnosis is a hypothesis*, albeit based on thorough assessment and rigorous application of operational diagnostic criteria. This hypothesis is used to suggest a prognosis for the patient's disorder and leads to a particular course of treatment. This hypothesis does not stand alone, is not immutable, and does not validate any pathoetiologic theory. *Because a diagnosis is a hypothesis, it must periodically be re-evaluated when new information becomes available or as treatment proceeds.* New information may lead to a change in diagnosis; thus, initial diagnoses should not be written in stone or presented to the patient and family as such. This understanding of what a diagnosis is and is not is essential, because it prevents the practitioner from locking in his or her thinking about a particular patient and encourages the use of periodic diagnostic reviews for all patients undergoing psychiatric treatment.

Periodic diagnostic re-evaluation is particularly important in treating children and adolescents whose first presentation of psychiatric disorders may often be atypical compared with the picture of the same disorder presenting in adults. For example, mania or hypomania onsetting in adolescents is generally characterized by irritability, mood cycling, and a mixed mood profile, often accompanied by psychotic features. In young children, manic symptoms may be predominantly those of aggressive outbursts, irritability, concentration difficulties, and impulsive-intrusive behaviors. The difficulties that even seasoned clinicians may have in cross-sectionally diagnosing these conditions in children and adolescents are well recognized. Because these and other disorders may become more clear-cut over time, and as a result may lead to the application of heretofore unused pharmacologic interventions, diagnostic re-evaluation becomes a necessary component of the ongoing psychiatric treatment of children and adolescents.

Another, often underappreciated, phenomenon underlines the importance of regular diagnostic re-evaluation in psychiatrically ill children and adolescents. Psychiatric symptoms are, by their very nature, highly variable. Their expression changes over time and is affected by multiple factors, including personality or coping style, life stressors and support networks, and peer or family influences. Thus, symptom variability is to be expected. In addition, psychiatric symptoms in children and adolescents are generally considered to be more variable than those found in adults with similar disorders. Too often, clinicians may unreasonably feel that psychiatric symptoms should be constant and unchanging. Such a perspective is not only incorrect but also unreasonable. Using a "medical" condition as an example, no physician would expect a patient with juvenile rheumatoid arthritis to demonstrate only the initial presenting symptoms (including the same affected joints) over the course of the illness, yet many clinicians working in the mental health field somehow expect that a major depression should always appear the same. Once these unrealistic expectations are confronted and the normative and

expected symptom variance is accepted, the clinician must then further realize that his initial diagnosis is not always the "last word" in classifying the patient's disorder.

Diagnostic re-evaluation is necessary not only for Axis I disorders; it is even more important for Axis II disorders because they are identified in children and adolescents. It is very important that the clinician not assign a primary Axis II disorder diagnosis without a very thorough consideration of possible Axis I disorders, including those in which the patient's symptoms may be subthreshold in number or in severity to satisfy current diagnostic classification. Furthermore, if a primary Axis II disorder diagnosis is made, the clinician should carefully review it within a few months, regardless of the patient's response to the treatment applied. Clinical experience suggests that this caution is especially important if the clinician is considering the Axis II diagnosis of borderline personality disorder, which in adolescents shows limited stability over time and may be very difficult to distinguish from the initial onset of an affective or psychotic illness.

Formal diagnostic interviewing is practiced by most child and adolescent psychiatrists and is now routinely taught in most training programs. Furthermore, many clinicians are becoming increasingly comfortable with using established diagnostic criteria (such as DSM-IV and ICD-10), even if they have not been formally trained in their use. However, diagnostic variability can be quite considerable, even amongst highly trained practitioners (Table 3–2). Although in some cases this variability may be explained by criterion variance (i.e., different diagnosticians use different criteria to make a specific diagnosis), more often this variability is caused by information variance (i.e., different diagnosticians use different questions or obtain different information in their attempts to identify operational diagnostic criteria). At times, observation or interpretation variance may also account for some degree of diagnostic variability. For example, different practitioners, particularly those using dissimilar models of etiology, may notice and remember different portions of similar pieces of information, or they may attach differing levels of significance to similar pieces of information.

While current diagnostic systems, such as the DSM-IV, offer clear operational criteria designed to decrease criterion variance, the potential for information, observation, and interpretation variance still exists. Thus, to decrease these other sources of diagnostic variance, in addition to the usual psycho-diagnostic interview used by most child and adolescent psychiatrists, the use of a

TABLE 3–2 **Areas of Potential Variance in Psychiatric Diagnosis**

Criterion variance	Different clinicians use different criteria for the same diagnosis. For example, one clinician may classify all teenagers who say they are feeling "depressed" and have occasional but fleeting suicidal thoughts as depressed, and another clinician will require that the teen meet full criteria for major depression as outlined in DSM-IV.
Information variance	Different clinicians use similar criteria for the same diagnosis but elicit different information, which is then applied to the same criteria. For example, one clinician may ask a child about depressed mood and obtain a negative reply, while another clinician may inquire about a "blah," "sad," "low," or "unhappy" mood and obtain a positive reply.
Observation or interpretation variance	Different clinicians identify or observe different features regarding similar diagnostic criteria. This may have a marked influence on the threshold for individual items, which will determine if the clinician then decides that the diagnostic item is present or absent. For example, one clinician may consider the all-black dress and unkempt, unwashed hair of an adolescent as evidence of a depressed mood, while another may see this as "teenage dress."

structured or semistructured diagnostic interview is desirable for child and adolescent psychopharmacologic treatment.

Structured Interview

A structured interview forces the interviewer (who often may not need to be a trained clinician) to ask specific symptom-oriented questions using a particular set format. Variation in how questions are asked is minimal, and thus structured interviews tend to be rather rigid in their application. In some cases further information may be obtained from more probing questions, but usually this is not allowed for in a structured interview. In complicated clinical cases, a sophisticated amount of interpretation may be necessary to understand a patient's or parent's responses to questions. This higher level of complexity may be lost when the interview is conducted by an interviewer who is well trained in the specific techniques of a particular structured interview but is not a seasoned clinician. Thus, a structured interview format, such as the Diagnostic Interview Schedule for Children (DISC), which is an excellent tool for use in epidemiologic research because it demonstrates good diagnostic reliability, may not be necessarily well suited to clinical psychopharmacologic practice.

Semistructured Interview

A number of semistructured diagnostic interviews for children and adolescents are available (see Suggested Readings). These must be administered by trained interviewers and are well suited for use by competent clinicians who have been taught how to conduct them properly. Some of the better known and clinically most valuable of these semistruc-

tured interviews are the Kiddie Schedule for Affective Disorders and Schizophrenia (K-SADS), the Diagnostic Interview for Children and Adolescents (DICA), the Child Assessment Schedule (CAS), and the Interview Schedule for Children (ISC). The K-SADS is available in present-state and epidemiologic versions and has recently been updated to allow for the determination of DSM-IV criteria and improved identification of anxiety and behavioral and substance use disorders. Computer algorithms for the DICA are available, but diagnoses developed by the exclusive use of these algorithms must be subjected to clinical verification.

It is the author's opinion, based on both clinical and research use involving a number of the above-mentioned semistructured interviews, that the K-SADS (using both present-state and epidemiologic versions concurrently) is perhaps the most clinically useful of the semistructured interviews available. Not only is it detailed and comprehensive, but it is relatively user friendly and also allows for individual symptom severity measurement as part of the diagnostic evaluation. The interview specifies that the child and parents be interviewed separately, which provides for a more complete evaluation of symptoms. Specific sections of the interview can also be conducted as a freestanding assessment for re-evaluation of a particular diagnosis following treatment. For example, the depression section can be administered by itself after a treatment course is completed to determine whether the patient still meets diagnostic criteria for a depressive disorder.

Whichever of the above-mentioned interviews is selected, however, the practitioner should obtain training in its application and use his or her clinical expertise to interpret the information obtained from the semistructured interview to determine psychiatric diagnoses.

Diagnostic Checklists

A busy clinical practice may not realistically lend itself to the use of either structured or semistructured diagnostic interviews, which can be unnecessarily time consuming, even for the most highly trained interviewer. In this case, it may be more useful to use a diagnostic checklist developed from current diagnostic criteria as an interview aid. Using this approach, the clinician conducts a detailed and comprehensive psychiatric interview and then identifies whether or not the patient fits into a recognized diagnostic category (e.g., learning disorders or anxiety disorders) and following that a specific disorder (e.g., reading disorder or PD without agoraphobia). It is important that the clinician first inquire about the various diagnostic groupings and then, if there is evidence suggesting a possible disorder within that grouping, proceed to a review of each of the potential disorders.

This type of review (Table 3–3) acts as a gateway to potential diagnoses of specific disorders. Once a diagnostic category is identified as possible, the clinician goes on to inquire about signs or symptoms of specific disorders within that category.

If the clinician using the general diagnostic checklist identifies that a patient may have a specific disorder within a particular category, she should then proceed to a more detailed review of all the disorders within that category. This is done using a disorder-specific checklist (see Table 3–4 for an example) for the most likely diagnosis within the general category. For example, if a clinician identifies that a patient may have a mood disorder and the patient's presenting symptoms are consistent with depression, the clinician then goes on to a detailed assessment of major depression using the specific diagnostic checklist for major depression. Using this disorder-specific checklist, the clinician identifies for *each diagnostic item* whether

TABLE 3–3   **General Diagnostic Checklist for Psychiatric Diagnosis in Children or Adolescents: Baseline for Psychopharmacologic Treatment***

Mark off degree of certainty regarding *each* of the following diagnostic categories using information obtained from the patient and parent or other appropriate informant.

Diagnostic Category	Likely	Not Likely	Unclear
Mental retardation			
Learning disorder			
Motor skills disorder			
Communication disorder			
Pervasive developmental disorder			
Attention-deficit/disruptive behavior			
Feeding and eating disorders			
Tic disorders			
Elimination disorders			
Separation anxiety			
Mutism/attachment/stereotypic movement disorder			
Organic induced disorder			
Substance-related disorder: Alcohol			
Substance-related disorder: Drugs			
Psychotic disorder			
Mood disorder			
Anxiety disorder			
Somatoform disorder			
Factitious disorder			
Dissociative disorder			
Sexual/gender disorder			
Eating disorder			
Sleep disorder: Primary			
Sleep disorder: Related or other			
Impulsive-control disorder			
Adjustment disorder			
Personality disorder			

If the score for any diagnostic category is *likely* or *unclear,* proceed to *each disorder-specific diagnostic checklist.*

*The successful use of this general diagnostic checklist is based on the clinician's knowledge of the specific disorders found in each of the categories, the utility of screening questions used to determine if a patient may fall into one or more of the above categories, and sufficient review of signs and symptoms to allow for a clinical judgment regarding *each* of the categories above.

TABLE 3–4 **Diagnostic Checklist for Child and Adolescent Depression**

Patient has two or more symptoms that suggest the presence of a depressive disorder *or* patient's parent or other responsible adult reports two or more symptoms that suggest the presence of a depressive disorder.

Symptom	Present	Present but Below Threshold	Absent	Unclear
Depressed or irritable				
Markedly decreased interest or pleasure				
Weight loss or insufficient weight gain				
Insomnia or hypersomnia				
Psychomotor agitation/retardation				
Fatigue or energy loss				
Feeling of worthlessness or guilt				
Concentration problems				
Death thoughts, suicidal				

Other criteria		
Change from "usual" state	Yes	No
Functional impairment	Yes	No
Other illness or drugs	Yes	No
Recent bereavement (≤2 mo.)	Yes	No
Lasted at least 2 weeks	Yes	No

Meets DSM-IV criteria for major depressive disorder: Yes   No   Unclear

that item is present, absent, or unclear. Following this, the clinician reviews other criteria (usual duration, functioning, etc.) for the disorder and then comes to a diagnostic decision about the presence or absence of that particular disorder.

In addition, if the clinician identifies that a patient may have a specific disorder within a general diagnostic category, she must carefully assess the presence or absence of all the related disorders within that category. For example, if a clinician determines that an adolescent may have a mood disorder, she must more carefully evaluate all the potential specific mood disorders: major depression, dysthymia, bipolar disorder, and cyclothymia. It is not sufficient to assess only the presence or absence of one of these disorders, and a negative finding for one specific disorder should not preclude the search for another disorder within that same category. For example, a finding that the patient does not meet criteria for a current major depressive disorder does not mean that the clinician should not then go on to determine the presence of a cyclothymic or dysthymic disorder. The identification of any one disorder within a general diagnostic category should likewise lead to careful review of all the other specific disorders within that category but also should lead the clinician to review those disorders known to be commonly found comorbidly with the identified specific disorder, even if they are found within other general categories that may have been scored as unlikely on the initial review. For example, a di-

agnosis of a major depression in an 11-year-old should lead the clinician to review the general category of anxiety disorders very carefully.

These types of diagnostic checklists (both general and specific) can be used during the interview as a type of memory prompt, or they may be completed immediately following the interview, prior to a final diagnostic determination. If the clinician finds that there is inadequate or unclear information on the basis of the diagnostic checklist, she should proceed to complete or clarify the information necessary for a proper diagnosis. In situations in which the clinician is still uncertain of the diagnosis following the use of a specific diagnostic checklist, the application of the appropriate section or sections (e.g., mania and schizophrenia for a youngster with a first-onset psychosis) of the K-SADS may be useful.

Use of a semistructured interview or a diagnostic checklist during baseline assessments for psychopharmacologic treatment will help decrease information variance and thus increase the validity of psychiatric diagnosis. The inclusion of such diagnostic aids in everyday practice is possible and clinically useful.

Developing a Problem List

In addition to establishing or confirming a baseline psychiatric diagnosis, the assessing clinician should develop a problem list. This should include not only the patient's diagnosis but additional areas that may be the focus of pharmacologic treatment or areas that are the focus of non-pharmacologic interventions. In some cases, such as the schizophrenic child already undergoing adequate social-psychological treatment, this may be a review of interventions already ongoing. In other cases, the clinician may identify other treatment targets for the first time.

The problem list should include the following:
1. Signs and symptoms that may be the focus of pharmacologic treatment (discussed later)
2. Medical issues of importance to the patient's care (discussed in Chapter 4)
3. Family, educational, social, and related issues (discussed in Chapter 5)

Diagnostic Evaluation—Practice Points

1. Determining a psychiatric diagnosis using a recognized classification system, such as DSM-IV or ICD-10, is necessary prior to beginning psychopharmacologic treatment.
2. Symptom-oriented descriptive interviewing is necessary to properly establish a psychiatric diagnosis.
3. Diagnoses are hypotheses leading to the treatment and prediction of outcome. They must be periodically re-evaluated and may be altered in light of new information.
4. The use of semistructured interviews or diagnostic checklists in establishing a diagnosis is preferred to unstructured methods of interviewing.
5. A problem list that identifies signs and symptoms—medical, social, family, and educational—and other targets of treatment should be developed.

Symptom Assessment and Measurement

Although psychiatric diagnoses must be determined prior to the initiation of treatment, the use of a psychopharmacologic agent in any specific case is dependent not only on the diagnosis but also on the specific symptoms that make up the patient's disorder. For instance, when a provisional diagnosis has been made, medication treatment for the illness may be indicated even if the diagnosis has not yet been clearly established. An example of this is prescribing a neuroleptic medication for a teenager with a psychotic illness that meets all the diagnostic criteria for schizophrenia except the 6-month time indicator. In other cases

pharmacologic treatment may be directed toward ameliorating specific symptoms arising in the context of a particular psychiatric disorder but not necessarily defining that disorder. Examples of this are the pharmacologic treatment of the self-mutilation that occurs in the context of an autistic disorder, the aggressive outbursts in a youngster with mental retardation, or severe agitation occurring during a manic psychosis.

Even when medications are prescribed to treat a specific disorder (such as major depression), the specific symptoms that make up the syndrome as it is expressed in the individual patient with the disorder must be identified as a focus of treatment. This is necessary because of the phenotypic heterogeneity of syndromal diagnosis. For example, although two adolescents may be given the diagnosis of major depressive disorder, each may have a number of specific diagnostic symptoms not shared by the other. Thus, in addition to a depressed mood, one may have early morning waking, suicidal thoughts, severe fatigue, anhedonia, decreased appetite, and weight loss. The other, in addition to a depressed mood, could present with difficulty falling asleep and prolonged daytime sleeping, reduced energy, concentration problems, decreased interest, increased appetite and weight gain, extreme rejection sensitivity, and no suicidal ideation. Although both depressed teens may be candidates for medication treatment, their symptom profiles differ and, accordingly, symptom outcome monitoring will differ. In addition, different medications might be selected on the basis of the different symptom presentation.

Thus, to direct medication selection, to improve outcome, and to permit comprehensive treatment monitoring, the clinician should use specific symptoms as the target of pharmacologic treatment. These target symptoms either (1) are part of the syndromal criteria of a psychiatric disorder (e.g., fatigue and lethargy arising with a major depression; auditory hallucinations in schizophrenia) or (2) arise as a result of, or are exacerbated by, a psychiatric illness (e.g., panic attacks that only arise during an episode of major depression; aggressive outbursts that are driven by paranoid delusions). Target symptoms should be:
1. Sufficiently distressing to either the patient or the patient's environment to warrant intervention (e.g., unhappiness and low mood for the depressed patient; frequent physical altercations occurring in the school classroom that are initiated by the conduct-disordered child)
2. Considered to impair "normal" functioning
3. Potentially amenable to pharmacologic treatment (e.g., panic attacks will often respond to

an appropriate medication, whereas lying will rarely, if ever, respond to any medication)

4. Able to be identified and measured (e.g., either the patient or other informant must be able to identify and quantify the mood, cognition, or behavior under evaluation)

Any target symptom will be made up of three components that may or may not exist independently of each other: intensity, frequency, and duration (Fig. 3–1). In evaluating the severity of each target symptom, the clinician must consider each of these three components. In many cases it is useful to think about these symptoms as mild, moderate, or severe. Each of these three components can be seen within this rating framework. For example, in rating the intensity of aggressive outbursts, the physician may consider them mild if they are only verbal in nature, moderate if they include minor degrees of property damage, and severe if they include major degrees of property damage or physical assault.

In assessing frequency of symptoms, a similar three-stage system can be used. Target symptoms may occur at different levels of frequency, ranging from occasional to constant. Different disorders may have recognized ranges over which such frequencies are known to occur, but in many cases the clinician may need to develop his own ratings from clinical experience. For example, verbal aggressive outbursts that occur once or twice daily can, in terms of frequency, be considered mild. Similar types of outbursts occurring two to four times daily can be considered moderate, and five or more times daily severe. At different levels of intensity, behaviors may exhibit different frequencies. For example, a child could exhibit severe frequency of mild aggressive symptoms and at the same time show a mild frequency of severe aggressive outbursts.

The duration of a symptom should also be in-cluded as a component of a target symptom. For example, an aggressive outburst may last a few seconds or it may last 10 minutes. The rating of duration in terms of mild, moderate, and severe should also be made within the context of the clinician's clinical experience because this parameter is often underreported in studies regarding the response of target symptoms to treatment.

Once these three components (intensity, frequency, and duration) have been identified and each has been evaluated as mild, moderate, or severe, the clinician should develop a list of target symptoms in which each symptom is summarized along each of these dimensions. Following this, a global rating for each symptom may be developed. An example of this applied to a child with aggressive symptoms, enuresis, and oppositional behavior is found in Table 3–5.

These components of target symptoms can vary over time and may be congruent with each other or independent of each other. Similarly, the overall summary evaluation of each target symptom itself can be expected to vary over time. It is important to appreciate the establishment and measurement of this symptom variability (discussed later) for the optimal assessment of both baseline and treatment outcome.

In some cases it will become apparent that target symptoms may also vary by place. For example, a child may show oppositional behaviors at home but not at school or in organized athletic or social activities. If such a pattern is identified within one or more target symptoms during the course of the baseline psychiatric assessment, this should suggest that a site-specific psychosocial intervention rather than psychopharmacologic treatment may be indicated.

Although it is useful to *conceptualize* target symptoms as described earlier, the optimal method by which to *measure* target symptoms is the use of rating scales. These scales, if they are available, often have the advantage of being reliable as well as symptom focused. They are generally easy to use and may provide an economical and efficient method for assessing and measuring target symptoms. They may be used to evaluate specific symptoms (such as aggression) or a number of related symptoms (such as scales for measuring the depressive or manic syndrome). They can be used by the patient (self-report scales), by the patient's parent or other informant (informant rating scales), or by a clinician during a patient interview (clinician rating scales). Scales that measure important aspects of a patient's functioning that may also be used to measure symptoms considered to be targets of treatment (such as social activities) are also available and provide an added dimension

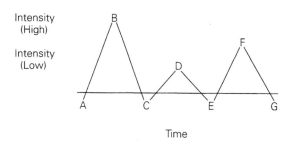

Symptom intensity, A-B, C-D, E-F
Symptom frequency, ABC, CDE, EFG
Symptom duration, A-C, C-E, E-G

FIGURE 3–1 Schematic Model of Psychiatric Symptom Description

TABLE 3–5   **Target Symptom Evaluation: Example of Clinical Rating**

Symptom Description	Intensity	Frequency	Duration	Summary
Aggressive outbursts	Moderate	Severe	Mild	Moderate
Enuresis	Moderate	Moderate	Moderate	Moderate
Oppositionality	Severe	Moderate	Moderate	Severe

to the assessment and treatment of a child's or adolescent's psychiatric disorder.

When adequate symptom rating scales do not exist or when a patient's unique presentation includes target symptoms not assessed by currently available rating scales, [the practitioner may wish to develop his own target symptom assessment tools for clinical use.] One useful method is to rate specific symptoms along the dimensions of intensity, frequency, and duration, as described earlier. This should be relatively easy to accomplish because these ratings would naturally follow from the clinician's conceptual understanding of target symptoms.

Another effective and clinically useful method for monitoring baseline symptom severity and potential symptom change with treatment is to adapt the 10 centimeter Visual Analogue Scale (VAS) line to any symptoms that are reported by a patient or a responsible informant. The patient, an independent informant (such as a parent), and the clinician can each then score the symptom-specific VAS line each time the symptom is evaluated (Table 3–6).

The clinical utility of using such a VAS-type methodology for rating target symptoms is that it can be customized to any patient and can be used to evaluate any symptom that either the patient, parent, or physician considers to be a needed focus for treatment. This method of measurement can also be used to complement other rating scales that could be used in a clinical situation but that do not identify target symptoms specific to a particular patient.

CASE EXAMPLE

Applying a VAS to Measure a Specific Target Symptom

N.G., a 14-year-old boy, was referred by his individual therapist for consideration of antidepressant treatment for "low mood." Although N.G. reported feeling "down," he demonstrated few of the expected cognitive and vegetative features of a major depression or dysthymic disorder. His family history was known to be negative for mood disorders but positive for PD and alcoholism in his mother and father, respectively. Diagnostic re-evaluation revealed a generalized anxiety disorder (GAD) with a secondary demoralization phenomenon. This diagnosis was discussed with N.G., his parents, and his individual therapist, and a joint decision was made to proceed to pharmacologic treatment directed at anxiety symptoms. Individual treatment was continued.

Following informed consent and patient education, treatment with buspirone was chosen by the patient in consultation with his mother. In addition to monitoring N.G.'s anxiety symptoms with the Hamilton Anxiety Rating Scale (HARS), the clinician selected a number of other target symptoms specific to N.G.'s situation and not adequately covered by the HARS to be monitored using a number of VASs. These VASs included the amount of anxiety felt overall at school and adequacy of peer functioning (playing with friends after school). In addition, a global assessment functioning question—"How do you think you (your son) has done overall this week?"—was added.

These specific target symptoms and global assessment were rated weekly by the clinician from information obtained at baseline assessment and during each reassessment visit independently by N.G. and his mother. This simple method (Figs. 3–2 and 3–3) proved to be a clinically useful measure of treatment outcome.

TABLE 3–6   **Visual Analogue Scale: Examples for Clinical Rating**

Getting along with parents:	0 _____ 10	
	(poor) (excellent)	
Getting to bed independently:	0 _____ 10	
	(poor) (excellent)	

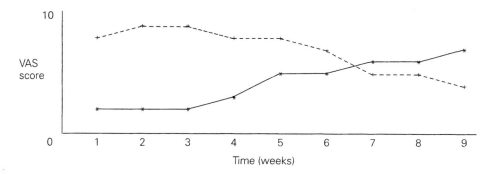

- - - - - Symptom: amount of anxiety felt at school, N.G. as informant. 10 = high anxiety; 0 = no anxiety.
——— Symptom: peer functioning (playing with friends after school), mother as informant. 0 = poor; 10 = good.

FIGURE 3–2 Use of a VAS to Measure Specific Symptoms in Buspirone Treatment of an Adolescent with Generalized Anxiety Disorder: An Example

CASE COMMENTARY

N.G.'s GAD was treated using busiprone. A reliable and standardized symptom assessment scale (the HARS; see later) was used to evaluate baseline symptom severity and treatment outcome. However, N.G. exhibited other symptoms that were felt to be reasonable targets for psychopharmacologic treatment. These were measured using a 10 centimeter VAS constructed for each specific symptom. Also, a VAS was used to obtain a measure of global functioning.

Both N.G. and his mother were used as informants to evaluate symptom severity. Their views were obtained independently of each other. This was necessary to decrease reporting bias in both the patient and parent. Regarding specific symptoms, N.G.'s evaluation of the level of anxiety that he felt at school (an internal symptom of his disorder) was used. N.G.'s mother's input was used to evaluate his peer

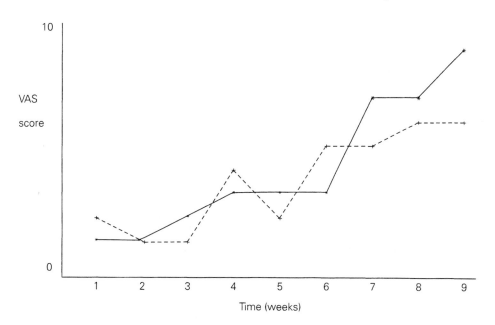

Global measure: "Overall, how do you think you (your son) has done over the past week?"
- - - - - N.G.'s ratings.
——— N.G.'s mother's ratings.
    0 = poor; 10 = good.

FIGURE 3–3 Use of a VAS to Measure Global Evaluation of Functioning in Buspirone Treatment of an Adolescent with Generalized Anxiety Disorder: An Example

functioning (an external sign of his disorder). This "tailoring"—asking the child or adolescent to evaluate internal symptoms of the disorder (such as anxiety, depression, worthlessness, etc.) and a parent or other responsible informant to evaluate external signs of the disorder (such as social activities, temper outbursts, school grades, etc.)—is often useful because it gives the clinician a broader appreciation of a patient's difficulties. In general, children and adolescents, if they are reliable informants, are more able to identify their own inner states than are observing adults. On the other hand, reliable parents may be more able to be objective regarding their child's or adolescent's external behaviors. In some cases, this approach may not work, as when a child does not understand, an adolescent denies internal symptoms, or a parent exaggerates external signs. In such cases both informants should be used to evaluate internal symptoms as well as external signs. Of interest is that in N.G.'s case both he and his mother reported similar trends in specific symptom evaluation and in their assessment of his global functioning.

Although VAS-type measures are clinically useful, they should not be used in place of well-known published symptom rating scales when these are available for the following reasons:

1. Many published rating scales have undergone extensive development and field testing and have been shown to be both reliable and valid instruments.
2. Some published rating scales have established norms; that is, they have been tested in nonclinical populations as well as clinical populations, and, in addition to measuring target symptoms, they offer some perspective as to how abnormal the symptoms under consideration are. This may be of importance in helping to determine whether a specific symptom is indeed significantly outside the normal range at baseline or if the change in a specific symptom following treatment has resulted in a normalization of that symptom (e.g., whether the amount of motor excess derived from the Revised Behavior Problem Checklist (RBPC) has been reduced following methylphenidate treatment).
3. Many published rating scales may have already demonstrated sensitivity to treatment effect.
4. If data are being kept for research purposes, it is helpful to collect them using instruments that are the industry standard to allow for comparisons across studies.

5. It is easier and less time consuming to use an already available scale with proven utility than to develop one's own and then test it to determine its clinical utility.

CASE EXAMPLE

Pitfalls of Doing It Yourself

Dr. P.J., a fourth-year resident in child psychiatry, was interested in using a scale to measure aggressive acts in a conduct-disordered adolescent referred to him for court-ordered psychiatric treatment. Dr. P.J. decided to develop his own aggression rating scale, keeping in mind the three components necessary to describe target symptoms: intensity, frequency, and duration. For clinical shorthand purposes, he chose to group these components together to determine an overall aggression severity rating scale. His scale consisted of the following:

Mild aggression: involves only verbal outbursts; occurs no more than two or three times per day and lasts a maximum of 5 minutes each time.

Moderate aggression: involves both verbal outbursts and property damage; verbal outbursts occur from three to six times daily and last up to 10 minutes at a time; property damage occurs at least once weekly.

Severe aggression: involves physical aggression such as hitting or scratching; occurs two or more times per week; verbal outbursts and property damage may also occur.

Dr. P.J. applied this scale using a self-report format in which his patient completed the scale while waiting for his weekly appointment. Five weeks after beginning cognitive approaches to anger control management combined with low-dose haloperidol (1 mg daily), the patient's aggression scale scores had changed from severe to mild. Dr. P.J. was proud of his success until he was contacted by the patient's probation officer, who informed Dr. P.J. of three recent incidents of physical assault perpetrated by his patient and another charge of breaking and entering that had stemmed from an incident at the patient's school. None of these incidents had been captured by the self-rating scale.

CASE COMMENTARY

This vignette illustrates that symptom rating scales are not without their difficulties and that their use involves clinical judgment. Dr. P.J.'s intentions were excellent, and he had realized the importance of assessing and evaluating target symptoms. Furthermore, he had thought a great deal about the measurement of aggressive symptoms and the unique characteristics expressed by his patient. Unfortunately, Dr. P.J. made two errors in measurement. The first error was that he "reinvented the wheel" by putting together his own scale when other clinically useful and better validated measures were available. Dr. P.J.'s second error was to fail to consider sufficiently the value of the information he was collecting. In this case the use of a self-report scale to determine aggressive acts in a conduct-disordered adolescent with a long history of illegal activities would be expected to provide less than optimally reliable information. In this case Dr. P.J. needed to use collaborative information obtained from a responsible adult.

Rating scales of any kind, be they reliable standardized measures or "shorthand" measures developed by the clinician to describe target symptoms, must be used with care and with full understanding of their strengths and limitations. Rating scales are not a panacea for the identification or measurement of target symptoms. Their use requires sophisticated clinical application.

Considerations regarding the use of rating scales to be kept in mind by the clinician include:

1. *Rater reliability.* In many cases different raters will rate a specific symptom or set of symptoms in a different way. A clinician may address this potential problem either by using one rater consistently or by training all raters who are using the instrument and then conducting periodic reviews of ratings to ensure that consistency is maintained over time. This is important in a clinical setting in which a number of different mental health workers may be involved in measuring target symptoms at different times or patient visits.
2. *Rater validity.* There are a number of issues regarding rater validity that are not specific to rating scales but also are not solved by rating scales.
   a. Self-ratings, especially by antisocial or conduct-disordered children and teens, are generally suspect because of underreporting. And many children or adolescents with attention-deficit disorder may have difficulty objectively evaluating their behaviors.
   b. Some raters will minimize their ratings of behaviors that they feel are "normal," regardless of what the scales specify. Others may use global impressions of the child

in their ratings of individual scale items and may disregard specific symptoms as having any stand-alone value. Scales completed by such raters will characteristically show a flat-line profile in which most symptoms receive the same score.
   c. Some raters may not be able to properly understand or use some rating scales. This is a potential problem in the use of self-report scales because children or adolescents with learning difficulties, low intelligence, or insufficient reading level may not be able to read or understand some scales. If such a situation occurs and self-report measures regarding target symptoms are felt to be necessary, the scale items can be read and explained to the child by a reliable adult, who then records the child's responses.
3. *Regression toward the mean.* Over repeated measurements, even in the absence of any significant subject change, many raters will tend to score behaviors as less severe. This problem is best addressed by obtaining multiple baseline measures (two or three ratings) prior to initiating any therapeutic intervention. The mean score of the two or three ratings should then be used as the baseline measure.

The strategy of making multiple baseline measures is a useful one, not only to avoid the regression toward the mean effect described earlier but also for other reasons, including the expected variability of symptoms over time. As discussed earlier, psychiatric symptoms are rarely static over time and can be affected by multiple factors, such as environmental stressors, interpersonal conflicts, and personality characteristics. Some symptom variation (intensity, frequency, or duration) is common over time. This symptom variability is often more pronounced in children and adolescents than in adult patients and must be accounted for during symptom assessment. The development of a valid baseline symptom measure must take this expected variability into account. Therefore, symptom ratings should be obtained at least twice during the baseline assessment, although three times, if clinically feasible, is preferable.

Target Symptom Assessment and Measurement—Practice Points

1. Target symptoms should be identified and measured as indicators for psychopharmacologic treatment and for monitoring outcome.

2. Target symptoms should be assessed either by using clinician-developed rating scales or by using the commonly recognized, clinically useful rating scales.
3. The use of symptom rating scales is based on a recognition of their benefits and potential problems.
4. Rating scales should be used to measure either individual symptoms or symptom clusters (syndromes).
5. Multiple time-separated assessments using symptom rating scales provide the optimal method for measuring baseline symptom severity.

While the various rating scales are generally used to measure symptom severity for purposes of baseline assessment and to assist in the monitoring of treatment, in some cases they may assist the clinician in the diagnostic decision-making process. These scales, however, are not meant to take the place of careful diagnostic interviewing. It is not acceptable practice to base diagnosis simply on scale application. Scales are tools that are meant to assist, not replace, clinical judgment.

Symptom Rating Scales Useful for Clinical Psychopharmacologic Practice

Many symptom rating scales are available for use in clinical psychopharmacologic practice. Those that are described here have been selected on the basis of the author's experience with their use, their sensitivity to medication effects, and the available research data on their validity and reliability. They comprise what can be considered a core group of symptom rating scales that would be of value to the child and adolescent psychopharmacologist involved in a busy clinical practice. Not all that are useful, however, are identified here, and the reader who wishes to explore other symptom scales should consult the references found at the end of this chapter for current reviews. In addition to the following discussion, a good general reference is the *Psychopharmacology Bulletin; Rating Scales and Assessment Instruments for Use in Pediatric Psychopharmacology Research* (National Institute of Mental Health, 21[4], 1985).

Scales Useful for Measuring Overall Symptomatology

There are two types of scales useful for measuring general symptoms. The first type simply gives a global impression of the severity of the patient's disorder by comparing the patient with other patients with similar problems in the clinician's practice. Obviously, the greater the clinician's experience, the wider the reference base for making this type of comparison.

The Clinical Global Impressions (CGI) scale provides this kind of comparison and also allows for measurement of change during treatment. The CGI also asks the rater to determine if, in his or her opinion, the observed change in symptoms over time is due primarily to a medication effect. The difficulty with this scale, apart from the lack of systematic study of its use in children and adolescents, is that attribution of clinical change to medication use may reflect to a great degree the bias of the observer, and in the author's opinion the section of the CGI that purports to determine medication effect (section 3, efficacy index) is of little or no value. Thus, the CGI should be scored only on sections 1 (severity of illness) and 2 (global improvement). Nevertheless, this scale does provide a simple and clinically useful measure of change, particularly when combined with one or more of the following general symptom assessment measures.

The second type of general symptom measures includes detailed questions about a variety of symptoms commonly described by patients with psychiatric difficulties. In addition to providing global scores, these measures can also be subdivided into categories that measure particular symptoms considered to reflect categories of dysfunction. Two clinically useful scales of this type are the Child Behavior Checklist (CBCL) and the Symptom Checklist 58 (SCL-58).

The CBCL and its related scales (the Teacher Report Form of the CBCL and the Youth Self-Report [YSR]) are among the most comprehensively studied of the child and adolescent rating scales available, and, while their sensitivity to medication effect remains uncertain, they have well-established psychometric properties. Designed to be completed by an independent rater (usually the parent) and developed for the age range 4 to 16 years, the CBCL provides information about a child's social functioning and behaviors. Eight subscales can be derived from the CBCL, and each provides a measure of a unique but not totally independent category (aggressive behavior, anxious-depressed, attention problems, delinquent problems, social problems, somatic complaints, thought problems, and withdrawal). The adolescent version (YSR) is a self-report instrument designed for use with adolescents ages 11 to 18 years; it may be of more value in providing valid information about internalizing rather than externalizing disorders.

The entire CBCL can be completed relatively quickly, and both the total score and specific subscale scores can be used to monitor treatment. In some cases the clinician may choose to limit patient monitoring to only those subscales that are a focus of pharmacologic intervention (such as aggressive behavior, attention problems, and social problems for a child with attention-deficit disorder).

The SCL-58 is a scale that lists 58 symptoms commonly described by patients with a psychiatric disorder. It is a self-report instrument in which the rater identifies the intensity of each listed symptom on a scale from 0 (none) to 4 (severe). The SCL-58 has shown sensitivity to medication treatment in pharmacologic studies of adolescents treated with antidepressants, neuroleptics, and thymoleptics. It can be further broken down into a number of categories (anxiety, depression, obsessive compulsive, somatic, and so on), each of which can also be used to monitor outcome.

The SCL-58 is routinely completed by most adolescents in 7 to 10 minutes, is directed more toward inner states than external behaviors, and can be completed by most patients with a grade 6 reading level. As such it is an ideal instrument to be completed by a patient while he or she is waiting to be seen by the clinician. It is not practical to use the SCL-58 with young children, who will have reading and comprehension difficulties with the instrument, but a parent or independent observer may complete it as an external rater of the child, although no data exist to substantiate the practice.

Scales Useful for Measuring Overall Symptomatology—Practice Points

> To monitor overall symptom change with pharmacologic treatment, use the CGI scale (parts 1 and 2) and either the total score or (if clinically indicated) the appropriate subcategories of the CBCL or the SCL-58.

Specific Rating Scales

Many rating scales for specific disorders (such as ADHD, mania, etc.) are available, and we have room here to discuss only some of them. In addition, new instruments are becoming increasingly available, and a vigorous market for the sale of these is flourishing. Accordingly, for each disorder found here, a select number of clinically useful rating scales are reviewed. For many of those recommended for general clinical psychopharmaco-

logic use, a copy of the scale is provided in the Appendix. When for copyright reasons the entire scale cannot be reproduced here, examples of sample items are provided, along with information about where the scale can be obtained. Wherever possible, I have attempted to include a clinically useful self-report, an informant report, and a clinician-scored scale for each disorder.

Depression: Major Depressive Disorder and Dysthymia

Although many depression rating scales are available for children and adolescents, no one scale can be unequivocally identified as optimal for purposes of monitoring treatment response to psychopharmacologic treatment. For children, the Children's Depression Inventory (CDI) has the advantages of good psychometric data and being relatively user friendly. Although not clearly a self-report scale (usually a clinician reads the scale items aloud to the child), it approximates the Beck Depression Inventory (BDI), a self-report scale, on which it was based. The Depressive Self-Rating Scale (DSRS) is an attractive alternative by virtue of the short time that it takes to complete it (only 18 items), but its clinical utility as a measure of treatment outcome is not known. Either one of these, however, is a reasonable choice for a depression self-report instrument for children.

For adolescents, the BDI has been the depression self-report scale most extensively studied (see Appendix). This scale has been shown to be sensitive to medication treatment in studies of antidepressants in this population. It is easy to administer, well tolerated by teenagers, takes 5 to 10 minutes to complete, and provides a useful self-report tool for evaluating clinical outcome in the pharmacologic treatment of depressed adolescents.

Informant rating scales are available for monitoring treatment outcome in child depression. The CDI has been modified for use as an informant rating scale and is a reasonable choice for clinical practice, particularly if the CDI is also being used to monitor the child's self-report of symptoms. The Bellevue Index for Depression (BID) can be used as an informant measure of a child's depressive symptoms. It is quite user friendly and takes about 10 minutes to complete. Both the CDI and BID have good clinical utility as informant measures for the assessment of pharmacologic treatment of depression in children, and either one is suitable for use in a child psychopharmacologic practice. No well-validated informant instruments are available for monitoring adolescents with this disorder.

Clinician rating scales for child and adolescent depression are based on direct clinical interview of the patient and should be used as part of the routine evaluation of treatment of every depressed patient. The School Age Depression Listed Inventory (SADLI) was designed specifically to assess depression in children but has seen limited use in treatment studies with this population. The section on depression from the semistructured diagnostic interview, K-SADS, provides perhaps the most comprehensive assessment of depressive symptoms and can be used to rate the severity of specific symptoms over time, as well as to establish the continued presence of the disorder itself. It takes 15 to 25 minutes to complete and has the additional advantage that it can be used for both children and adolescents.

No well-validated specific clinician rating scale has been developed for use in monitoring treatment outcome in depressed adolescents. The 17-item Hamilton Depression Rating Scale (HDRS), originally developed for adults, has shown sensitivity to medication effects in studies of adolescent depression. The HDRS takes about 10 minutes to complete, but many of the questions may be more suited to geriatric patients than to teen populations. However, this scale is available in various forms, including one that can identify some psychotic symptoms and one that has been modified to include symptoms of seasonal affective disorder.

Alternatively, the clinician may wish to use the Self-Rating Depression Scale which, although less reported on in studies of adolescent depression, nevertheless remains a useful rating scale for this population.

Mania (Bipolar Disorder)

The diagnosis of mania prepubertally is difficult and currently under active investigation. Mania more commonly onsets during the adolescent years, when it also may present with more atypical features, particularly with hostile and irritable mood swings and rapid mood cycling. If a diagnosis of mania is made, however, there are few if any validated instruments available for use in this population. Self-rating scales are of no value in this disorder, and no informant rating scales have been developed specifically for measuring manic symptoms in children or adolescents.

Clinician rating scales that have been used include the Manic-State Rating Scale (MSRS) and the Modified Mania Rating Scale (MMRS). Recent pharmacologic treatment studies of adolescent mania have used the MMRS as the major outcome measure, and it has been found to be user friend-

ly and reliable (see Appendix VI). The scale takes about 20 to 30 minutes to complete and is based on the clinician's interview with the patient as well as other information supplied by either a parent or a member of the nursing staff. The MMRS has also been found to be sensitive to treatment response in both inpatient and outpatient settings, and it is recommended as the rating scale of choice in manic adolescents. It is unclear whether the MMRS has similar utility in childhood mania, and the clinician faced with a patient presenting symptoms of mania may choose to develop a symptom rating scale based on the specific clinical characteristics of the child's disorder, using a VAS format, as described earlier. The depressive episodes of the bipolar disorder can best be monitored using the instruments previously described for depression.

Psychosis (Schizophrenia, Schizoaffective Disorder, Schizophreniform Disorder, and Organic Psychoses)

The schizophrenic disorders tend to arise during the adolescent and early adult years, but they do occur in children as well. Although there is a paucity of studies of the pharmacotherapy of schizophrenic disorders, neuroleptics remain the mainstay of treatment for adolescents and children alike. Of importance in monitoring treatment outcome in schizophrenia is the awareness that this disorder is composed of two types of symptom clusters: the positive symptoms, such as hallucinations and delusions, and the negative symptoms, such as apathy and anergy. Assessment and monitoring of the schizophrenic disorders must take into account both types of symptoms.

For children, perhaps the most useful available assessment and symptom evaluation scales are the Kiddie Formal Thought Disorder Scale and the Kiddie Positive and Negative Symptoms Scales. While formal psychometrics are generally lacking for these instruments and studies of their sensitivity to the effects of medication are few, if any, nevertheless they are the best of what are currently available and have the advantage of being adapted from adult scales with well-established clinical and research utility.

Symptoms of the schizophrenic disorders in adolescents can best be assessed using the scales developed for adult schizophrenic patients. The Positive and Negative Syndrome Scale (PANSS) provides an excellent symptom rating scale of both types of symptoms and produces a rating of general psychopathology as well. It is used in an interview setting, and in the hands of an experienced clinician it takes about 20 to 25 minutes to complete. Alternatively, the Scale for the Assessment of Negative Symptoms (SANS) and the Scale for the Assessment of Positive Symptoms (SAPS) could be used.

A more global scale, useful in the evaluation of any type of psychotic disorder (including manic or depressive psychosis), is the Brief Psychiatric Rating Scale (BPRS). This scale can be used in both inpatient and outpatient settings and is delivered by the clinician. Scores of individual items range from 0 to 6 and are completed following a clinical interview that is directed by the items on the scale. The BPRS (see Appendix VI) can also yield a number of subscales measuring thought disorder, behavioral disturbance, mood disorder, and anxiety. The scale is sensitive to medication treatment and provides a total score that can be used to monitor outcome and to determine the severity of a patient's disturbance by comparison with the numerous published studies in adults who have used the BPRS. Its routine use is highly recommended in the treatment of any psychotic adolescent.

For patients with organic psychosis, in addition to administering the BPRS the clinician must assess and carefully monitor the patient's level of consciousness and orientation. Some instruments developed for use in other populations are available for these purposes, but clinically the use of a simple checklist using a dichotomous measure (yes or no, present or absent) for each symptom category should suffice. As would be expected, this assessment is likely to be specific to inpatient services and should include orientation to person; orientation to place; orientation to day, month, year; alert; obtunded; comatose. This checklist should be completed by a health professional trained to make these assessments (a physician or nurse) and should be obtained at regular intervals; every 4 hours is suggested.

Anxiety Disorders (Generalized Anxiety Disorder, Panic Disorder, Obsessive Compulsive Disorder, Post-Traumatic Stress Disorder)

There are many anxiety disorders, and the choice of symptom rating scales will vary according to the type of disorder under consideration. Furthermore, there are relatively few, if any, disorder-specific (e.g., social phobia, PD, obsessive compulsive disorder [OCD], etc.) rating scales available that demonstrate clinical utility and medication sensitivity in this age group. In addition, many symptoms (both physiological and psychological) are found in a variety of anxiety

syndromes. With this group of disorders, the clinician may find himself or herself in the position of creating patient-specific symptom rating scales using a VAS format that can be applied as demonstrated earlier.

Although disorder-specific self-rating scales are generally unavailable, a number of more general rating scales—some of which measure both trait (long-standing and relatively stable components of a child's personal characteristics) and state (more short lived and possibly dependent on ongoing and relatively current external events) aspects of anxiety—are available and may be used to give an overall impression of the severity of anxiety experienced by a child suffering from any one particular anxiety disorder. However, the focus of some of these scales is such that the symptoms measured would be unlikely to be the target of pharmacologic treatments (e.g., specific fears or phobias, as measured by the Fear Survey Schedule for Children—Revised), and others have not been shown to be sensitive to monitoring medication effects. Given these caveats, nevertheless, the clinician should consider three rating scales for use in monitoring overall anxiety symptoms in children with a variety of anxiety disorders: the Child Anxiety Frequency Checklist (CAFC), the State-Trait Anxiety Inventory for Children (STAIC), and the Revised Children's Manifest Anxiety Scale (RCMAS).

The CAFC assesses a small number of physical symptoms of anxiety; it is relatively simple to administer in a clinical setting. The STAIC measures both state and trait aspects of anxiety and is suitable for self-reporting for children with a mid-elementary grade reading level. The CAFC takes about 5 minutes to complete, and the STAIC about 10 to 15 minutes. Used together these instruments provide a reasonable measure of general anxiety symptoms that will identify the severity but not the specificity of an anxiety disorder. They may also be of benefit in monitoring outcome in children with GAD or in children with separation anxiety disorder.

Self-report anxiety rating scales useful for teenage patients include the STAIC and the Beck Anxiety Inventory (BAI). Both scales are tolerated well by adolescents, but clinical experience suggests that older teens will generally prefer the BAI.

The RCMAS uses a self-report format comprised of 37 items to assess anxiety in both children and adolescents. It is not suitable for diagnostic purposes and should not be used as such. It is most useful as a general overall indicator of mixed anxiety symptoms that should be suitable for monitoring treatment outcome.

Although no age-specific clinician-administered scale that measures anxiety symptoms in adolescents is available, a scale commonly used to evaluate and measure anxiety symptoms in adults, the HARS, has demonstrated clinical utility in adolescent outpatient psychopharmacology clinics and has shown sensitivity to pharmacologic treatment. The HARS is a clinician-administered anxiety rating scale; it takes about 10 minutes to complete. It is comprised of two categories, somatic and psychological anxiety, which have been shown to have a differential response to medication treatment in at least one study of adolescents with PD. It is recommended for use with teenagers, both to monitor overall anxiety disturbance and specifically to evaluate treatment outcome in adolescents with GAD.

A potentially useful general measurement scale for anxiety is in preparation at this time, and early psychometrics seem promising. The Multidimensional Anxiety Scale for Children (MASC) is a self-report instrument that uses a 45-item scale to assess four factors of anxiety: physical anxiety, harm avoidance, social anxiety, and separation anxiety. Each of these factors can be monitored independently, and a total score provides a global evaluation of anxiety symptoms. (For more information on the MASC, see Stallings and March, under Suggested Readings at the end of this chapter.)

PD usually onsets in adolescence, although recent evidence suggests that it may occur in children as well, where separation anxiety may be the phenomenologic picture that is presented. No age-specific instruments for evaluating PD are available for children and adolescents. Clinicians treating patients with this disorder will need to develop their own instruments, or they may choose to use those that have been adapted for use with adolescents from instruments used in pharmacologic research studies of panic-disordered adults.

The three characteristics of PD that must be measured are:

1. The panic attacks themselves (intensity, frequency, duration)
2. Anticipatory anxiety (how worried someone is in anticipation of having an attack)
3. Phobic avoidance (what is avoided and how strongly because of fear of an attack)

Panic attacks are best monitored by a panic attack diary (see Chapter 9 and Appendix VI). The patient carries this diary at all times and marks down the intensity, frequency, and duration of every attack immediately after the attack has occurred. Changes in the number or severity of panic attacks can thus be measured when the panic attack diary is reviewed at regularly scheduled appointments.

Anticipatory anxiety is appropriately measured using a 10 centimeter VAS. The patient marks down how worried he or she has been over the past week that another panic attack may soon arise (0, no worry, to 10, extreme worry). Phobic avoidance is easily measured by asking the patient to identify the two things or places she most commonly avoids because of fears of having a panic attack while there. Some common responses are public transportation, movie theaters, restaurants, meetings at work, specific classes at school, and driving. For each item, the patient uses a 10 centimeter VAS to score the strength of her avoidance of that item over the past week.

Panic attacks and their associated disturbances (anticipatory anxiety and phobic avoidance) can thus be effectively and simply monitored. The experienced clinician should be able to evaluate the entire PD constellation in about 15 minutes.

The psychopharmacologic treatment of OCD has been the best studied of child and adolescent anxiety disorders, and the Leyton Obsessional Inventory—Child Version is the "gold standard" assessment and monitoring tool for children and adolescents with this disorder. The clinician treating adolescents with OCD, however, may consider using the Yale-Brown Obsessive Compulsive Scale (YBOCS), which evaluates the duration of symptoms (time spent on symptoms daily), symptom interference with functioning, degree of distress regarding symptoms, and the patient's ability and effort to resist or control symptoms. These ratings are provided for both obsessions and compulsions, and separate obsession and compulsion scores are provided, along with a total OCD score. The YBOCS takes about 10 minutes to complete and is the instrument of choice in assessing adults with OCD, for whom it has demonstrated good sensitivity to medication effects. It has shown excellent clinical utility during routine use in some adolescent psychiatry psychopharmacologic clinics. In addition, it provides a checklist of obsessions and compulsions that is useful for assessment purposes because teenagers with OCD are notorious for failing to mention certain obsessive or compulsive symptoms during the clinical interview, even if these symptoms are causing them serious distress and are significantly interfering with their daily functioning.

The Post Traumatic Stress Disorder (PTSD) Reaction Index and the Stress Reaction Index are symptom assessment tools for evaluating PTSD in children and adolescents. Their clinical utility as symptom rating scales is not known, however. And there is not sufficient information about their sensitivity to medication treatments. A 10 centimeter VAS scale on which each pertinent symptom is identified and scored remains perhaps the most clinically useful method for measuring treatment outcome in children and adolescents with this disorder.

No well-validated rating scales for measuring symptom severity or change with treatment are available for social phobia and separation anxiety disorder. The Social Phobia Anxiety Inventory for Children (SPAI-C) does show promise in ongoing evaluations and could be considered for the purposes of monitoring treatment outcome in social phobia. It is also available in a form for teenagers. Otherwise, for these disorders the HARS, combined with VAS ratings for each specific symptom, can be used to provide a useful measurement package that should be sensitive to treatment effect and can be quickly and easily completed.

Attention-Deficit Hyperactivity Disorder

ADHD is a syndrome comprised of symptoms of inattention, impulsivity, and hyperactivity. It is often found with disturbances of conduct, learning and language difficulties, problematic peer functioning, and (in a subgroup) symptoms of anxiety. The core symptoms for which pharmacologic treatment is usually sought, however, are those of inattention, impulsivity, and hyperactivity. Although most scales developed to assess and measure this core syndrome have been validated primarily on children, they have been used in studies of adolescents, and there is no reason to expect that these measures would not be sensitive to medication effects in teenagers.

A number of well-validated rating scales are available for use in monitoring treatment in ADHD. Two of the scales can be used both by clinicians and by informants (parents, teachers, childcare workers) alike and focus primarily on the core symptoms of inattention, impulsivity, and hyperactivity. The Childhood Attention Problems Scale (CAP) and the ADHD Rating Scale (ADHDRS) are user friendly and give total scores, as well as subscale scores for inattention and hyperactivity (CAP), and for inattention and impulsivity (ADHDRS). The use of either instrument to monitor symptom change in ADHD children and adolescents is recommended.

In children and adolescents with other difficulties associated with the ADHD syndrome, especially those with conduct, learning, or anxiety difficulties, the well-known Conners Abbreviated Symptom Questionnaire (CASQ) and its accompanying teacher (Conners Teacher Rating Scale, CTRS) and parent (Conners Parent Rating Scale, CPRS) rating scales are recommended. Parents will find the shorter of the two available CPRS

scales easier to tolerate. In addition to giving a total score (hyperactivity index), the Conners Scale will yield a number of useful subscales, including conduct problem, learning problem, psychosomatic, impulsive-hyperactive, and anxiety. An alternative strategy is to use one of the two core ADHD symptom rating scales (CAP or ADHDRS) and 10 centimeter VAS lines for specific related symptoms, such as anxiety or specific behavioral problems.

In contrast to many other child psychiatric disorders, a great number of rating instruments are specific to the various behavioral and cognitive features of ADHD. The following may be selected by the clinician for use with patients for whom these types of measurements are of value: Continuous Performance Task (CPT), Paired Associate Learning (PAL), actometer measures, and cancellation tasks. Also, the Gordon Diagnostic System and the Conners Diagnostic System are two readily available computerized assessment packages that provide some of the above-mentioned assessments in a user-friendly combination of scales.

CPTs are vigilance tasks, usually done on a computer, that are quite sensitive to medication effects of ADHD children and adolescents. They are best obtained from one of the companies that specialize in providing clinical measures to child and adolescent psychiatrists.

The PAL task is mostly a measure of short-term memory but seems to be sensitive to performance effort. PAL tasks are considered useful measures of medication effect on cognitive function. Actometers, on the other hand, can be used successfully to measure medication effect on motor activity. The wrist actometer is perhaps easiest to use in office psychopharmacologic practice, and it is relatively inexpensive. However, the clinician should be aware of some of the problems associated with the use of such a device including breakage and poor compliance by patients wearing the instrument.

Cancellation tasks, which are easy to administer and can be used in an office practice without the need for sophisticated equipment (a pencil, paper, and stopwatch the only tools needed), are sensitive to medication effect and have a history of use in the assessment and evaluation of treatment of children with ADHD. These time-limited tests ask the patient to identify and mark specific target letters or symbols on a page of many other letters or symbols that act as distractors (e.g., see the Talland Letter Cancellation Test in Appendix VI). Scoring is simple and can be done in a few minutes by the clinician, and the entire testing procedure takes only 5 to 10 minutes. In some cases the cancellation task can be administered and scored by a reliable informant (such as a teacher or parent), thus decreasing the time spent on instrument evaluation during the clinical interview.

As previously mentioned, the Gordon Diagnostic System and the Conners Diagnostic System consist of a number of tests, including a continuous performance test that may be of value in the assessment and evaluation of drug treatment for ADHD children and adolescents. Although relatively user friendly, these tests are comparatively costly to obtain and require an office practice in which computer assessments are easily available. They are relatively popular among some clinicians, but concerns have been raised about their overall sensitivity to medication effect, and it is unknown whether their routine use provides any significant treatment monitoring advantages for evaluating changes in attention over a properly administered cancellation task and an ADHDRS.

Autism and Mental Retardation

Rating scales for autism and mental retardation are discussed together because of the common occurrence of symptoms in these disorders that may be targeted for pharmacologic treatment. There is evidence that the Aberrant Behavior Checklist (ABC) is sensitive to medication effect in assessment of both autism and mental retardation, and it can be applied to both children and adolescents. It is available in both community and residential versions. Its 58 items can be broken down into useful subscales covering a wide variety of behavioral disturbances seen in these two disorders. These include irritability, lethargy, stereotypy, hyperactivity, and inappropriate speech. It is highly recommended for use in both children and adolescents with either autism or mental retardation.

The Childhood Autism Rating Scale (CARS) is a user-friendly 15-item behavior rating scale that can help in the diagnosis of autism and can be used to monitor outcome across a variety of treatment target symptoms. Its items measure the following: ability to relate to people; imitation; emotional response; body use; object use; adaptation to change; visual response; listening response; taste, smell, and touch response and use; fear or nervousness; verbal communication; nonverbal communication; activity level; level and consistency of intellectual response; and general impressions. The CARS takes about 10 to 15 minutes to complete by an experienced practitioner and is recommended for routine clinical use.

When used by trained observers, the Real Life Rating Scale for Autism provides an alternative rating scale for behavioral disturbances in autistic children and teenagers. It has been used in a number of pharmacologic studies of this disorder and,

while rather cumbersome to use, can provide a reasonable monitoring of a number of clinically useful subcategories, such as social relationships, language, sensory-motor responses, sensory responses, and affective responses.

Stereotypies can be monitored either by using the Timed Stereotypies Rating Scale or by simple counting. If a counting method is used, it is imperative that the particular stereotypic behaviors of interest are listed, with ample space provided on the scoring card to allow each event to be captured. Because stereotypies can come and go during the day, or can be accentuated by certain environmental factors, care must be taken not to inadvertently contaminate the results by inconsistent monitoring. A useful strategy is to score these behaviors at three or four set times daily using a 15 to 20 minute scoring "window."

Tourette's Syndrome

The physical and vocal tics of Tourette's syndrome can be monitored using a frequency count paradigm, as described in the section on the assessment of stereotypies in autism. The type of tic, its location, and its severity (0 = mild, almost not noticed, to 4 = severe, very obvious) should be noted. The patient's and parent's awareness of the tics should also be evaluated; a 10 centimeter VAS is sufficient for this purpose. Alternately, one of either the Hopkins Motor/Vocal Tic Scale, the Motor Tic, Obsession and Compulsion and Vocal Tic Evaluation Scale (MOVES) or the Tourette's Syndrome Symptom List can be usefully employed.

Bulimia

Bulimia is thought to onset in adolescence or young adulthood. Two rating scales may be of benefit in assessing and monitoring this disorder. The Eating Disorders Questionnaire (EDQ) is an extensive, detailed semistructured interview assessing a wide variety of eating disturbances. Section D, Binge Eating Behavior, can be used as a stand-alone measure of bulimic symptoms. As an alternative, the Bulimia Interview Form (BIF) provides a user-friendly daily binge-monitoring scheme that can be easily used by the motivated teen who is undergoing medication treatment for a bulimic disorder.

Aggression (Including Physical Violence, Theft, Lying, and Other Conduct Disturbances)

Although aggression is not a psychiatric diagnosis, it is often the focus of treatment for children and adolescents, particularly when it arises in the context of a psychiatric disorder. A number of scales are available for assessing and monitoring aggression. Self-report scales have not been well studied, and clinical experience suggests that in monitoring aggression or associated conditions, such as theft, lies, and other disturbances of conduct, ratings completed by informants are likely to be substantially more reliable than self-reports.

When aggression occurs as part of ADHD, it can be assessed using the CTRS and the CPRS, as described earlier. The RBPC can also be useful, particularly when a primary diagnosis of conduct disorder is the focus of treatment. For adolescents who are confined to residential or other such facilities in which medication treatment may be available, the Overt Aggression Scale (OAS), although developed and used mostly in studies of adults, is clinically useful. Care must be taken, however, to use the weighted scoring system of this scale. The Ward Scale of Impulsivity has been successfully used to measure a variety of aggressive and impulsive behaviors in adolescent pharmacotherapy. It is available in both inpatient and outpatient forms and can be used in self-report and informant formats. Finally, custom-made rating scales in which the most salient features of the individual's aggression profile can be identified and measured, preferably using continuous variables (e.g., hitting rate, from 0 = never to 4 = almost constantly) rather than dichotomous variables (yes or no) are often clinically useful.

The symptom scales reviewed in this chapter provide a core group of rating scales for clinical psychopharmacologic practice with children and adolescents. As further studies are conducted, new scales will be developed and some scales currently available will be further refined. The busy practitioner, however, should choose one or two rating scales per disorder and then, if indicated, custom design his or her evaluation package to suit the specific needs of any one patient. Only by trying a number of these suggested scales will the clinician find those that he or she feels are most useful in clinical practice. However, in all instances the following three considerations regarding the use of these scales must be kept in mind:

1. Rating scales are not diagnostic instruments but are used to develop baseline measures of symptom prevalence and severity, as well as to monitor outcomes from medication treatment.
2. Rating scales must be user friendly. It makes no sense to overload a patient or other informant with a plethora of rating scales, because this will usually not be tolerated or the

scales will be completed "just to get the darn things done," thereby decreasing their validity as tools for symptom monitoring.
3. Rating scales do not replace good personal clinical care; rather, they are incorporated into, and hence improve and enhance, good personal clinical care.

Specific Rating Scales—Practice Points

1. Choose one or more symptom rating scales as clinically indicated from those currently available that show reasonable clinical utility for the symptoms or disorder you are treating.
2. Custom design your own symptom evaluation package to suit the particular characteristics of your patient.
3. Be reasonable. Don't overload your patient with scales and don't expect rating scales to provide diagnoses or take the place of good personal clinical care.

SUGGESTED READINGS

Achenbach TM, Edelbrock CS. Manual for the Child Behavioral Checklist and Revised Child Behavior Profile. Burlington, VT: University of Vermont, 1983.

Angold A. Structured assessments of psychopathology in children and adolescents. In C Thompson (ed): The Instruments of Psychiatric Research. Chichester, UK: John Wiley, 1989, pp 271–304.

Cantwell DP, Rutter M. Classification: Conceptual issues and substantive findings. In M Rutter, E Taylor, L Hersov (eds): Child and Adolescent Psychiatry: Modern Approaches. London: Blackwell Scientific, 1994, pp 3–21.

Costello A. Structured interviewing. In M Lewis (ed): Child and Adolescent Psychiatry: A Comprehensive Textbook. Baltimore: Williams and Wilkins, 1991, pp 463–472.

Cox A, Hopkinson KF, Rutter M. Psychiatric interview techniques (parts II and V). British Journal of Psychiatry, 139:29–37, 1981.

Hodges K. Structured interviews for assessing children. Journal of Child Psychology and Psychiatry, 34:49–68, 1993.

Morgan S. Diagnostic assessment of autism: A review of objective scales. Journal of Psycho-educational Assessment, 6:139–151, 1988.

Orvaschel H, Ambrosin P, Rabinovich H. Diagnostic issues in child assessment. In TH Ollendick, M Hersen (eds): Handbook of Child and Adolescent Assessment. Needham Heights: Allyn and Bacon, 1993, pp 26–40.

Stallings P, March J. Assessment. In J March (ed): Anxiety Disorders in Children and Adolescents. New York: Guilford Press, 1995, pp 125–150.

Turner SM, Beidel DC, Dancu CV, Costello A. An empirically derived inventory to measure social fears and anxiety: The Social Phobia and Anxiety Inventory. Journal of Consulting and Clinical Psychology, 1:35–40, 1989.

Wells KC. Rating scales for assessement of conduct disorder in children and adolescents. In GP Sholevar (ed): Conduct Disorders in Children and Adolescents: Assessment and Intervention. Washington, DC: APPI Press, 1995.

Baseline Medical Assessment for Psychopharmacologic Treatment

A thorough medical evaluation of a child or adolescent is necessary prior to the initiation of psychotropic treatment. This is done for the following three reasons:

1. To identify any previously unrecognized medical condition that might be causing the patient's psychiatric symptoms (e.g., hypothyroidism causing depression, lassitude, and fatigue)

2. To provide a baseline for physiological parameters that may be affected by drug treatment (e.g., neutrophil counts with clozapine treatment, or height and weight measurement with long-term stimulant treatment)

3. To identify medical problems that may be exacerbated or complicated by pharmacologic treatment (e.g., cardiac conduction abnormalities that can be worsened by tricyclic antidepressants)

Physical assessments or repeated specific laboratory tests (e.g., electrocardiograms [ECGs], neurological evaluations, or serum thyroid hormone levels) may be necessary to monitor expected treatment-emergent side effects of pharmacologic agents. Such assessments might include, for example, monitoring the rate and rhythm of cardiac conduction in patients treated with tricyclics, evaluating hand tremor with neuroleptic treatment, or testing basal thyroid functioning in patients undergoing lithium treatment. The baseline medical assessment must be thorough enough to cover the three areas noted earlier but not so excessive as to subject the patient to unnecessary, and at times traumatic, investigations that are unlikely to provide any useful diagnostic or therapeutic information. While a comprehensive individual and family medical history and a physical examination are necessary at base-line, screening tests for the detection of occult medical conditions that might be causing psychiatric disorders provide a special problem for the practitioner. The issue of screening tests is discussed later in this chapter.

Baseline History and Physical Examination

The baseline medical history should cover the routine historical health information and general systems review that is consistent with standard clinical practice. An example of useful medical evaluation forms can be found in Figure 4–1 (medical history) and Figure 4–2 (physical examination). Routine completion of such forms and inclusion of this information in each patient's clinical record are good psychopharmacologic practices. In some cases the psychiatric practitioner may feel more comfortable asking pediatric or family medicine consultants to complete this portion of the assessment. However, care must be taken in the choice of consultant, as a rapid, incomplete, or cursory history and physical examination by a pediatrician or general practitioner is not acceptable for the purpose of baseline medical evaluation for psychopharmacologic treatment. If an external consultant is used for baseline medical assessment, the psychopharmacologist should, *at the very minimum*, review the medical history with the patient and the patient's family and perform those parts of the physical examination that will require consistent monitoring during the course of pharmacologic treatment (e.g., heart rate and blood pressure with antidepressants, and neurologic evaluation of extrapyramidal and motor functioning with neuroleptics).

Patient's Name: _____ Date: _____

Other Informant(s): _____

Spontaneously reported medical conditions: _____

Current: _____

Past (note date of onset and when resolved): _____

_____

_____

Probe for medical conditions not spontaneously reported:

CNS _____   Respiratory _____

Cardiac _____   GI _____

GU _____   Endocr _____

Musculoskel _____   Derm _____

ENT _____   Hearing _____

Vision _____   Other _____

Pubertal self-report: Female: Menses _____   Pubic hair _____

Male: Voice deepening _____   Pubic hair _____

Allergies: _____

Nonallergic reactions to medications: _____

Current medications and total daily dose (include side effects if any): _____

_____

Previous medications and total daily dose (include side effects if any): _____

_____

_____

Birth problems: _____

Childhood illnesses: _____

_____

Immunization record: _____

Hospitalizations (give dates and places): _____

_____

Specific issues: Trauma/Abuse: _____

Drug or alcohol use: _____

Sexual activity, contraception, other sexual concerns: _____

_____

Other issues: _____

_____

FIGURE 4–1   Medical History: Baseline Screening Assessment for Psychopharmacologic Treatment

Patient's Name: _____ Date: _____

Person(s) besides patient present during physical examination (give name and status, i.e., parent,

guardian, nurse): _____

General well-being and appearance: _____

Height: _____ Weight: _____ HR: _____

BP sit: _____ BP stand: _____

Head and neck (include goiter): _____

ENT: _____

Eyes (include disc and fundi): _____

Cranial nerves: _____

Respiratory: _____

Cardiac (auscultation): _____

Cardiac (pulses and other): _____

Abdominal: _____

Genitourinary (include breasts in girls): _____

Tanner stage: _____

Musculoskeletal: _____

Peripheral CNS: Reflexes: _____ Strength: _____

                  Coordination: _____ Motor: _____

                  Cerebellar: _____ Gait: _____

                  Cranial nerves: _____ Extrapyramidal: _____

Dermatologic (include acne): _____

Comments: _____

_____

_____

_____

FIGURE 4–2   Physical Examination: Baseline Screening Assessment for Psychopharmacologic Treatment

In taking a medical history, the physician should pay particular attention to the following:

1. Trauma, especially closed-head injury
2. Illicit drug and alcohol use, especially important for adolescents, who must be asked questions specific to *each* compound because they are often unlikely to volunteer this information spontaneously
3. Smoking, which may predict future substance use and may alter the metabolism of some medications
4. Past and current use of both prescription and nonprescription medications, including those compounds that many patients fail to consider as "real" medicine, such as oral contraceptives, analgesics, and antiallergy compounds
5. Sexual activity, especially for adolescents, to identify possible high risk for sexually transmitted diseases and to determine whether a female is likely to be or become pregnant during pharmacologic treatment

6. Sexual functioning, especially for adolescents, who may be quite hesitant to spontaneously express any concerns they may have in this area

In addition, important family medical history that must be recorded includes any genetic disorders with psychiatric manifestations (e.g., Huntington's chorea, Tourette's syndrome) and the presence of alcohol or drug use in other family members (including both prescription and nonprescription medications).

Baseline Laboratory Assessment

As discussed previously, baseline laboratory assessment is conducted for three purposes: (1) to screen for the possibility of an occult medical disorder presenting with psychiatric symptoms, (2) to confirm or validate a potential medical disorder identified by history or physical examination, and (3) to identify those physical parameters that may be affected by pharmacologic treatment.

Baseline Laboratory Screening Tests to Identify Occult Medical Illness

Screening may be defined as the examination by a single test or procedure of a population of apparently well people for the purpose of detecting those with a particular unrecognized disease or defect. The value of any screening test depends on its sensitivity in detecting a particular disorder and on the prevalence of the disorder it is expected to identify in the population in which it is administered. In conditions of very low prevalence, even tests with high sensitivity will often demonstrate a poor predictive value, and instead may even show a high proportion of false positive tests, in which individuals without the disorder are identified as having the disorder. For example, in a population in which the prevalence of a particular disorder is 1 percent, a test with the excellent sensitivity of 95 percent will show a positive predictive value of less than 9 percent.

Because the likelihood that any specific screening test will be useful in the diagnosis of an occult medical illness depends on the sensitivity of the test and the prevalence of the disorder that it is to identify in the population of interest, the value of a screening test in child and adolescent psychiatric disorders depends on the prevalence of occult medical illnesses that present with psychiatric manifestations as their only symptomatic feature.

In the child or adolescent patient with a negative medical history and physical examination, the prevalence of any specific medical disorder presenting with only psychiatric symptoms is likely to be exceedingly low. Thus, in the absence of signs or symptoms of a medical illness, the yield (positive predictive value) of any one specific screening test (even one with excellent sensitivity) is likely to be minimal.

Indeed, at the level of prevalence under discussion, the likelihood that any one screening test will provide a false positive result may be substantially higher than the likelihood that it will identify a true positive. The problem with false positive tests is well known. They often lead to more intensive, costly, and potentially traumatic investigations, all in the pursuit of an abnormal "laboratory value" or "roentgenographic shadow." This appreciation of the positive predictive value of screening tests and the potential negative consequences of false positive results must be kept in mind by the clinician as he or she determines what baseline laboratory tests will be ordered in any child or adolescent presenting with psychiatric symptoms.

For example, although it is well known that the onset of psychosis in adolescents may arise as a result of a space-occupying lesion of the central nervous system (CNS), the chance that a psychiatric practitioner will ever see such a case in his or her lifetime is small. Thus, while a silent brain tumor (a space-occupying lesion of the CNS that is not suspected following a thorough medical history and physical examination) *may be* causing the teenager's psychotic symptoms, it is exceedingly unlikely *to be* the cause of the psychosis. Therefore, the *routine* use of CNS imaging instruments such as computed tomography (CT), magnetic resonance imaging (MRI), positron emission tomography (PET), or single photon emission computed tomography (SPECT) as screening procedures for medical conditions that can lead to the presenting clinical picture of psychosis in a teenager should not be considered to be a necessary part of a baseline medical assessment.

If, however, a thorough medical assessment of the psychotic teenager raises historic or physical evidence that might suggest a CNS lesion (e.g., a history of recent onset headaches or long tract neurological signs discovered on physical examination), then, further follow-up investigations, involving some or all of the above-mentioned imaging tools, is indicated. In this case laboratory investigations are being used not as screening tests but as procedures to confirm or validate a diagnosis.

Given the caveats described earlier concerning the validity of baseline screening tests for medical illnesses presenting as psychiatric disorders in the absence of physical signs and symptoms, large numbers of "routine" laboratory or radiologic investigations are not necessary and indeed may lead to unneeded and clinically or economically unjustifiable consequences. The "shotgun" approach to baseline laboratory screening, in which multiple laboratory tests or prepackaged groups of laboratory tests are routinely ordered on every patient, is not only unnecessary but also not cost-effective. It provides no significant advantage to conducting fewer, but more specific, laboratory determinations based on a careful history and physical examination and on the physician's knowledge of psychotropic agents and their potential side effects.

Baseline Diagnosis-Confirming or -Validating Laboratory Investigations

Diagnosis-confirming or diagnosis-validating tests are, however, clearly indicated and should be used whenever clinically necessary. These can be considered necessary in two different instances. First, a positive medical history or physical finding suggestive of a previously unrecognized medical illness should be followed by the appropriate laboratory or radiologic investigations. Second, an ongoing medical disorder (such as diabetes mellitus) should be well characterized before psychopharmacologic treatment is started.

CASE EXAMPLE

"I feel depressed and I have no strength."

B.F., a 16-year-old boy, was referred for diagnostic reassessment and psychopharmacologic consultation for a treatment-resistant major depressive disorder. He had a history of 6 to 8 months of feeling tired, fatigued, and exhausted. He was described as unmotivated and as feeling hopeless and depressed. More recently he had been having fleeting thoughts about suicide. A family history of depression was present in a maternal aunt. B.F. had received individual psychotherapy and an adequate course of serotonin-specific reuptake inhibitor (SSRI) treatment without any symptom relief, and he appeared to be getting "worse."

A review of B.F.'s physical symptoms revealed that he was indeed feeling despondent and was tired and fatigued, but that he also had

physical weakness. He described how he had gradually lost the strength to shoot a basketball and was having difficulty climbing stairs at school. He had dropped out of his physical education classes because he did not have the strength to participate in them.

A short physical examination focused on his muscle strength clearly demonstrated muscle weakness in both the upper and lower limbs. Appropriate laboratory tests were obtained and the results showed severely low cortisol levels and mildly abnormal thyroid function tests. An endocrine consultation confirmed the diagnosis of Addison's disease, and necessary medical treatment was instituted, with an eventual good response, including amelioration of B.F.'s "depression."

CASE COMMENTARY

This case illustrates an appropriate use of diagnostic laboratory testing in a teenager thought to be suffering from a psychiatric disorder. The signs and symptoms suggestive of a significant medical illness were clearly present, and laboratory investigations were carried out not as screening but to provide specific diagnostic information.

Baseline Assessment for Concurrent Medical Disorders

The second indication for diagnostic baseline laboratory screening is in the patient with a psychiatric disorder who also has an ongoing medical illness. In this case baseline laboratory assessment provides necessary information for optimal patient management, regardless of whether the psychiatric disorder is thought to arise from the medical illness or to exist independently. In this instance the psychopharmacologist should work cooperatively with the appropriate medical specialist to ensure that proper combined medical and psychiatric care is delivered. In many cases in which medical illness complicates the psychiatric picture, ongoing conjoint management of the patient is indicated. If this is the case, face-to-face discussions with consultants is much preferred to the exchange of information through "consult letters" only.

Acute medical conditions may also onset during psychopharmacologic treatment, either as a result of the medication being taken (e.g., a fever and sore throat secondary to carbamazepine treatment) or independent of the medication used (e.g., leukemia). In these cases specific laboratory investigations (such as a complete blood count with suspected carbamazepine toxicity) are indicated and should be completed at the earliest signs of symptoms. A prudent course of action to follow if a serious medical side effect to pharmacologic treatment is suspected is to stop or quickly taper off the agent thought to be responsible for the condition. The medication can always be restarted if the medical condition is found not to be the result of the pharmacologic treatment.

Baseline Laboratory Assessment for Psychiatric Diagnosis

Special attention must also be paid to the desires of patients, parents, or some practitioners who seek a laboratory test to confirm that the patient has a "chemical imbalance" that explains the psychiatric disorder. This may particularly be an issue in those cases where previous psychosocial treatments have proved ineffective and patient and family are seeking a new treatment paradigm with high hopes of success. Alternatively, some patients or families are skeptical about a process that uses biologic interventions to treat what they consider to be a primarily psychological or socially based disturbance. In these and other cases, patient and family education about the diagnostic utility of laboratory or imaging testing is necessary. This issue is discussed more fully in Chapters 6 and 7. There is little to be gained and much to be lost in "diagnostic" laboratory testing in response to patient or parental pressures, or "just to see what the result will be."

CASE EXAMPLE

"This test will prove I have the disorder."

D.V., an 18-year-old boy with a 4-month history of major depressive disorder (MDD) was seen in consultation for diagnostic and treatment recommendations. His father was a family physician who himself had a similar disorder for which he was being treated. Mood disorders were found in both the father's and mother's biological families. D.V.'s father insisted that his son undergo a dexamethasone suppression test (DST) to "prove that the depression was a biological illness." D.V. initially resisted his father's demands, but when the consulting doctor agreed with his father, D.V. complied. When the DST showed normal cortisol suppression, both D.V. and his father became upset because they felt that this "proved" the depression was not a biological problem.

D.V. then decided not to use "pills" as part of his treatment because he reasoned that if there was no proof that his depression was biological (as established by the negative DST), there was no reason to use biological treatments. Some 10 weeks later he changed his mind and accepted medication treatment with fluoxetine with good results, but the time delay in instituting pharmacologic treatment led to his failing two of four school subjects, which he was obliged to make up at summer school.

CASE COMMENTARY

In this case example, a neuroendocrine procedure was inappropriately carried out as a diagnostic test for MDD in an adolescent. This investigation was not based on any substantive data suggesting that such a test was actually diagnostic for MDD in adolescents. On the contrary, all the available information suggests that the DST is not a diagnostic test for MDD in adolescents. The misapplication of this test may have played an important role in lengthening the course of the teenager's episode, compounding the patient's functional disturbance.

Specific Issues in Baseline Screening and Diagnostic Laboratory Evaluations

A number of special issues pertinent to the use of baseline screening and diagnostic laboratory investigations are important for child and adolescent psychopharmacologic treatment. These are neuroendocrine evaluation, neuroimaging, cardiac assessment, illicit drug identification, and the use of laboratory testing for psychiatric diagnosis.

Baseline Neuroendocrine Evaluation

At this time there is no evidence to support the use of basal neuroendocrine laboratory testing for either screening or diagnostic purposes in child or adolescent psychiatric disorders. Similarly, specific stimulation tests, such as the DST, the thyrotropin hormone releasing hormone (TRH) test, or the corticotropin releasing hormone (CRH) test have no demonstrated diagnostic validity for any child or adolescent psychiatric disorder. Finally, no neuroendocrine basal or stimulation test has been shown to clearly predict treatment outcome in any child or adolescent psychiatric disorder. Thus, good clinical psychopharmacologic practice does not include the use of either basal or stimulation (DST, TRH, and CRH) neuroendocrine testing for screening, diagnostic, or treatment outcome prediction purposes in this population.

Furthermore, although studies of cellular immunity, platelet imipramine and serotonin binding, and evaluation of various peripheral measures of catecholamine functioning have been reported in depressed, anxious, or behaviorally disordered children and adolescents, there is no diagnostic or predictive validity that supports the clinical use of these investigations in psychiatrically ill children and adolescents.

Baseline Neuroimaging

A number of assessments of CNS structure and function are currently available. These include CT, MRI, PET, electroencephalography (EEG), and SPECT. All require sophisticated technologies and considerable expense. Some are uncomfortable or even distressing to many patients. Young children, in particular, may be frightened by machines and the venipuncture necessary to perform various investigations. Some psychotic or manic adolescents may not be able to tolerate the movement restrictions necessary for optimal neuroimaging results. Thus, neuroimaging, although a potentially useful tool, is not without its difficulties.

At this time there is no evidence that routine neuroimaging screening in the absence of signs or symptoms of a neurologic disorder is of diagnostic or prognostic value in psychiatrically ill children or adolescents, and its use as part of the routine baseline medical assessment for psychopharmacologic treatment is not recommended. If, however, a neurologic problem is suspected on history or physical examination, the appropriate diagnosis-confirming neuroimaging investigations should be carried out.

Similarly, a screening EEG, which is often routinely ordered by many practitioners, has little if any value given the high prevalence of "abnormal" EEG findings in neurologically intact children and adolescents and the poor sensitivity of a single EEG recording in the diagnosis of seizure disorders (especially limbic seizures). If a seizure disorder is suspected from the patient's history, an EEG is indicated as a diagnosis-confirming investigation, and a neurologic consultation is necessary. Even if all investigations have proved inconclusive, a trial of an antiepileptic medication may be indicated depending on the clinical presentation. Other specialized EEG evaluations may at times be indicated, particularly if a condition such as narcolepsy, which often onsets in adolescence, is suspected. In this case referral to an appropriate sleep disorders clinic should also be made.

Baseline Electrocardiogram

The ECG is another potentially useful baseline assessment procedure, but like any other baseline medical investigation, its use should follow from a rational clinical indication, rather than from practitioner anxiety or a cookie-cutter approach to assessments. Thus, routine screening ECGs used to detect asymptomatic cardiac disease are not indicated and are unlikely to be of benefit. Similarly, ECGs are not necessary if the medications being considered are not known to have cardiac effects (such as valproic acid in the treatment of adolescent mania). However, if medications known to have demonstrated cardiac side effects are being used (such as tricyclics or lithium), then a baseline ECG is of value and repeat ECGs may be indicated during the course of treatment. It should be kept in mind, however, that occasional ECG monitoring will probably not identify those children who may suffer sudden cardiac death, as has recently been reported with the use of the tricyclic antidepressant desipramine. Rare events cannot be detected by routine monitoring, and a normal ECG does not mean that there is no underlying cardiac disease, nor that the patient will not experience a cardiac event. The practitioner, patient, and parents must be aware of this.

Baseline Drug Screening

Serum and urine monitoring for drugs of abuse may be of value, particularly in the following cases:

1. Adolescents for whom there is a high index of suspicion of drug use based on psychiatric or medical history
2. Patients with breakthrough mood or psychotic symptoms in the presence of adequate pharmacologic maintenance
3. Patients who are not responding to adequate trials of optimal pharmacologic or psychologic treatments

In addition, some drugs of abuse (particularly alcohol, cannabinoids, and over-the-counter antiemetic medications that contain diphenhydramine) may produce symptoms similar to the mood disorders of dysthymia or major depression, while other drugs of abuse (particularly amphetamines, cocaine and its derivatives, and hallucinogenics) may produce a psychotic picture with or without a mood component. Prudent psychopharmacologic practice includes awareness about and active pursuit of organic psychiatric disturbances that are chemically self-induced.

The clinician should be aware that the "footprints" of various drugs of abuse may be detected for different lengths of time following their use. As a rule of thumb, urine samples can be expected to show evidence of drug use longer than serum samples. Because different laboratories offer various methods of drug detection, the clinician should make sure that he or she is aware of the methods of analysis and collection and the limitations of various drug assays available in the particular laboratory being used.

Baseline Laboratory Monitoring Tests for Expected Physiological Changes

The third potential use of baseline laboratory tests is to establish initial reference points for those physiological parameters known or expected to be affected by *specific* psychopharmacologic treatments. For example, baseline laboratory evaluation of thyroid functioning is necessary if treatment with lithium is being considered, because the effect of lithium on thyroid functioning is well established, and thus thyroid functioning will have to be monitored during lithium treatment. Extensive thyroid function testing, however, is not indicated if treatment includes medications not known to affect the thyroid gland (such as neuroleptics). Similarly, hematologic monitoring (white blood count, platelets, hemoglobin) is indicated if carbamazepine treatment is considered but is not indicated for desipramine treatment.

Baseline Medical Evaluation—Practice Points

1. Conduct a comprehensive medical history and physical examination.
2. Use laboratory and other investigations rationally; avoid "shotgun screening."
3. Document clearly all medical information and use medical consultations when specifically warranted.

Side Effects: Identification and Measurement

Side effects occur commonly with pharmacologic treatment and must be carefully monitored. Because medication side effects are to be expected, patients and parents must be informed of the various expected side effects and the relative risk of their occurring. This information should be presented *prior to treatment* and in a clear educational format consistent with the cognitive level of the child or adolescent for whom it is intended. Details about the medications to be used, their potential benefits, and their possible side effects should be discussed fully with the patient and parent, and, whenever possible, written material should be provided. These educational issues are discussed more fully in Section Three.

Thinking About Side Effects

It may be helpful to categorize side effects as either nuisance or potentially physically/behaviorally problematic. Side effects occurring in either category often become rate-limiting factors in the use of pharmacotherapy, and it is important to identify and measure both types. A potential pitfall to be avoided is that of not taking seriously the so-called nuisance side effects associated with medication use. These include sweating, gastrointestinal upset, or headaches. While these may seem less "important" to the clinician when compared with side effects such as cardiac arrhythmia, orthostatic hypotension, or seizures, the nuisance side effects are very important to the patient and can in some cases significantly impact on his or her quality of life. In addition, nuisance side effects can become limiting factors in compliance with pharmacotherapy, thus potentially depriving the patient of a possibly useful treatment. Accordingly, it is essential that the pharmacotherapist not minimize or underplay the patient's experience of nuisance side effects just because they are less likely to cause significant physical or behavioral problems. They are experienced as distressing by the patient and must be taken seriously and dealt with as such.

Practitioners must be aware of the physical side effects, both acute and subacute, of the medications they prescribe. Acute side effects may be potentially life threatening and may require immediate intervention, including medical stabilization and rapid discontinuation of the offending compound. Acute effects include but are not limited to such effects as cardiac arrhythmia secondary to treatment with tricyclics, seizures occurring with clozapine treatment, and neuroleptic malignant syndrome and acute dystonia occurring with neuroleptics.

Subacute physical side effects are physiologic effects that may cause significant changes in body functioning but that are unlikely to lead to immediate negative consequences. These can usually be managed by modification of the pharmacologic treatment plan with strategies such as the following:

1. Dose adjustment, for example, to deal with a mild to moderate sinus tachycardia (100 to 120 beats per minute) onsetting with tricyclic treatment
2. Use of ancillary medications, such as procyclidine, to ameliorate neuroleptic-induced extrapyramidal symptoms
3. Changes in the timing of doses, such as taking clomipramine in the evening if sedation is a problem
4. Changing to another compound of the same class, such as changing from fluvoxamine to paroxetine (both are SSRIs) if nausea and vomiting occur with fluvoxamine

In most cases, one or more of these strategies usually improve or ameliorate the medication side effects. These strategies are also useful in addressing the nuisance side effects reported by patients.

Behavioral side effects may also occur secondary to treatment with medications, and these also can be categorized as acute or subacute. A high degree of suspicion is often needed to identify behavioral side effects because these are generally less well understood or appreciated by many practitioners. Acute behavioral side effects—such as increased self-mutilation or sexual disinhibition (occurring with benzodiazepine treatment) or aggression, severe irritability, suicidality, or inner tension (a part of the akathisia spectrum) following from neuroleptic use—require urgent intervention with either rapid discontinuation or significant reduction in the dose of the presumed offending compound and the application of acute psychiatric management as indicated (including short-term hospitalization to ensure patient safety).

It is important to consider the possibility of behavioral side effects during pharmacotherapy. If these side effects do occur but are not identified, the possibility exists that the practitioner may incorrectly increase the medication dose, thinking that the observed symptoms are a result of the initial disorder. For example, a manic adolescent who becomes increasingly disinhibited when treated with a benzodiazepine might not be recognized to be exhibiting a benzodiazepine-induced behavioral adverse event, and the benzodiazepine dose may be raised to treat his or her "agitation." Similarly, a psychotic child treated with neuroleptics may experience akathisia, which might be misinterpreted as agitation or increased psychotically driven behaviors and inappropriately treated with higher doses of the neuroleptic. This obviously will only make the situation worse,

and this type of circular pattern—with the cause being used to treat its effect—is to be avoided at all costs.

If the clinician is uncertain as to whether a particular symptom or set of symptoms is a behavioral side effect of psychopharmacologic treatment, the prudent course is to assume that it might be and to institute appropriate interventions, such as dose reduction, immediately. By using this strategy, it should become readily apparent within a relatively short time if this was indeed the case.

The emergence of subacute behavioral side effects may arise directly from the medication itself or may complicate the physical side effects induced by the medication because of the particular psychological characteristics of the patient. For instance, the mild sexual disinhibition that can accompany benzodiazepine treatment is an example of a subacute behavioral side effect arising directly from the medication itself. An example of psychological distress that is dependent on the personal characteristics of the patient and arises from that person's unique experience of a physical medication side effect is the worry and distress that some (but not all) adolescents experience secondary to the emergence of mild to moderate forms of lithium-induced acne.

CASE EXAMPLE

"I was worried but now I'm sexy."

P.S., a 16-year-old girl with a long history of anxiety symptoms, had undergone a variety of nonpharmacologic treatments with limited effect and was referred to her therapist to determine whether the addition of a medication might be of value in ameliorating her symptoms. Diagnostic evaluation confirmed a diagnosis of generalized anxiety disorder (GAD), and occasional panic attacks were noted, though not at the frequency to qualify for panic disorder (PD). These attacks, however, were very distressing to P.S. and were beginning to complicate her social and vocational functioning.

After a discussion of the various pharmacologic treatment options, P.S. and her parents elected to try the benzodiazepine clonazepam. Treatment was started with a dose of 0.25 mg daily and was increased systematically over 2 weeks to a dose of 2.5 mg daily. On this dose, P.S. reported feeling "the best I have ever felt." Her parents, however, reported that she had become intrusive, more talkative, and more obviously sexually preoccupied. Quite out of character, she was flirting with boys in the shopping mall to the point that her girlfriends were apparently becoming embarrassed by her behavior.

When seen, P.S. showed no core symptoms of mania but was mildly disinhibited. She reported much less baseline anxiety and fewer worries. She heard her parents' concerns but felt that it was "the real me that is now coming out." The possibility of behavioral disinhibition with benzodiazepine treatment had been raised with P.S. and her parents prior to the initiation of pharmacotherapy. At that time, they had been advised that should such a phenomenon occur, the best approach would be to decrease the dose of the medication and to observe the effect. Although P.S. was certain that her behavior was not due to a side effect of the medication, she agreed to follow the management strategy previously identified.

P.S.'s clonazepam was gradually reduced to 1.75 mg daily. After a week at this dose she was no longer as intrusive, talkative, and flirtatious as previously. Her anxiety symptoms, while not as subjectively improved as at the higher clonazepam dose, were significantly better than at baseline. She now felt that perhaps the medicine had "made me a bit too loose" and accepted treatment at the lowered dose.

CASE COMMENTARY

The case of P.S. illustrates the induction of mild disinhibition as a behavioral side effect of benzodiazepine treatment. In this case the clinician had increased the medication too rapidly to a relatively high total daily dose without evaluating the effect of the medication on target symptoms at lower doses. The patient understood her behavior purely in psychological terms, and—while it may (or may not) have been true that there was "a real me" that needed "coming out"—the appearance of these behaviors coincident with treatment, followed by a decrease in these behaviors following a decrease in the dose, suggests that they were a side effect of pharmacotherapy.

The importance of this case is twofold. First, the prescribing clinician was too hasty in his introduction of the medication and did not conduct proper symptom evaluations at lower doses. Second, it would have been too easy to accept P.S.'s psychological explanation of her behavior as being "true" and to have not tested the "truth" of this assertion, particularly if the clinician had

not been aware of the potential for behavioral side effects from the medication. This may have led to inappropriate and ineffective psychological intervention. Fortunately, the physician was aware of this possibility and had informed the patient and parents about this prior to beginning treatment. This, and a critical attitude toward simple models of understanding behavior (be they psychological or biological), led to the proper course of action: testing the hypothesis of a behavioral adverse effect by decreasing the dosage of the medication.

Both kinds of subacute behavioral side effects (those introduced by a direct pharmacodynamic effect and those that are psychological consequences of medication treatment) often require changes in the pharmacologic treatment plan or the addition of other modes of intervention. A number of the following strategies may be useful:

1. Changing to another medication with similar effects, such as changing from lithium to valproic acid for the adolescent who is extremely distressed by the appearance of lithium-induced acne
2. Addition of specific nonmedication interventions, such as nutrition counseling for the adolescent concerned about weight gain secondary to the use of tricyclics
3. Intermittent use of medications as needed to deal with situation-specific issues, such as adding propranolol to decrease lithium-induced tremor because of self-image concerns that arise only when the adolescent will be in a stressful social situation (such as reading onstage at a school assembly)

Education About Medication

Education about medication or "meducation," as it could be called, is an essential component of proper psychopharmacologic treatment (see Appendix II). Although patient education is discussed in detail in Section Three, a number of points bear identification here.

First, all consumers (child, teen, and parent or other responsible adult) should be informed about his or her medical care. With regard to the use of medications, they need to know the following:

1. What are the medications being used for?
2. What are the medications expected to do and when?
3. What (common) side effects can reasonably be expected?
4. What (uncommon) side effects may happen occasionally or rarely?

5. What activities, foods, drinks, etc., should I avoid or be careful about?
6. What other medicines should I avoid or be careful about?
7. What do I do if I (or my child) experience difficulties that may be medication related?

Second, it is unreasonable to tell a patient or parent about a particular medication and expect him or her to understand all about it, to remember all the important details, and to voice all the reasonable concerns in one sitting. More useful and more helpful is the provision of specific "meducation" programs for patients and their families. If this is not possible or feasible, then increased time should be spent discussing medication issues. Often concerns about medication use may take up two or three meetings and can be expected to arise occasionally during treatment as well. These concerns should be carefully and immediately acknowledged, and every effort should be made to deal with them appropriately.

Third, an important adjunct to verbal instructions regarding specific medications is the use of printed material, often in the form of handouts, which provide information about the medicine that the patient is taking. Such handouts will help in the educational process, and the patient can keep them and refer to them during the duration of treatment. Various examples of such handouts can be found in the pertinent chapters of this book in which the uses of specific medicines or classes of medicines are described. Handouts are available from pharmacists, pharmaceutical companies, and health care institutions. It is useful for the clinician to make such printed material readily available to patients and families alike.

It is also necessary for the practitioner to be aware of a number of developmentally specific issues regarding the identification and measurement of side effects in children and adolescents. These are as follows:

- Questioning about side effects must be direct, detailed, and systematic because many children and teenagers may fail to report on their own treatment-emergent physical or behavioral symptoms.
- The use of medication-specific side effect questionnaires is to be encouraged in the identification and monitoring of treatment-emergent adverse events. These are discussed further later in this chapter.
- A parental report about side effects (again elicited in a direct, detailed, and systematic manner) should be obtained whenever feasible, especially in younger children.
- Children and adolescents are in a stage of rapid physical development, and the effect of

most psychotropic medications on these processes is often not clearly known. Thus, particular attention must be paid to monitoring the essential aspects of normal growth, such as height and weight, especially in those patients for whom long-term pharmacologic treatment is indicated.

- Side effects are often most pronounced during periods of dose escalation, dose change, or medication withdrawal, and side effect monitoring should be increased during these phases of pharmacologic treatment.
- Some children and adolescents or their parents may be hypervigilant regarding medication side effects and may either attribute common or usual physical sensations to a medication effect or may report substantially higher than usual levels of distress for any one treatment-emergent side effect. Thus, the use of specific placebo techniques (*n* of 1 studies) and systematic side effect monitoring should be routinely considered in this population.
- All medication treatment must take place within the context of sufficient patient and parent education about the medicine to make them informed consumers and to instruct them in its proper use.

Side Effects: Identification and Management—Practice Points

1. Side effects are common, so expect them and systematically look for them.
2. Side effects can be both physical and behavioral.
3. Educate the patient and family about potential side effects.
4. Both acute and subacute side effects require active management.
5. Improperly managed side effects lead to treatment noncompliance.

Monitoring Side Effects: The Use of Symptom Rating Scales

Not all physical or behavioral disturbances that arise during the course of pharmacologic treatment are side effects of the medication. True treatment-emergent side effects (those physical and behavioral disturbances that arise from a specific pharmacologic treatment) must be distinguished from the following:

1. Symptoms arising from an unrelated medical condition, for example, nausea and vomiting secondary to a viral gastroenteritis

2. Symptoms arising from a concurrent social or environmental disturbance, for example, aggressive or self-harm incidents that occur secondary to severe family dysfunction
3. Symptoms that are part of the psychiatric disorder under treatment, for example, difficulty falling asleep in the depressed child
4. Symptoms that arise from the pharmacologic treatment of an unrelated condition, such as diarrhea secondary to erythromycin treatment of a chest infection
5. Symptoms that were present prior to initiating pharmacologic treatment but that are later ascribed to a medication effect by either the patient or parent

CASE EXAMPLE

"If you've got side effects, it has to be the antidepressant."

M.B., a 13-year-old girl, presented with a 7-month history of major depression that had been refractory to treatment provided by her primary care physician. Following a detailed baseline assessment that confirmed the initial diagnosis and a thorough review of past interventions, the patient and family agreed to a trial of fluoxetine for M.B.'s depressive symptoms, although M.B.'s father expressed serious doubts about the value of using medicines to treat a "psychological problem" and felt that she should "just get a handle on herself."

Some 2 weeks following the initiation of medication treatment, which to that point had been free of side effects, M.B. developed a low-grade fever and a frequent cough. A clinical diagnosis of *Mycoplasma* pneumonia was made by her family physician, and a course of erythromycin was begun. About 3 days following the onset of antibiotic treatment, M.B. developed nausea and diarrhea. Her father attributed her physical symptoms to the fluoxetine, and, in spite of discussions with the psychopharmacologist and family doctor, who identified the erythromycin as the medication most likely to induce these symptoms, M.B. discontinued her fluoxetine treatment.

CASE COMMENTARY

Prediction of, education about, and careful identification of treatment-emergent side effects are especially important in the psychopharmacologic management of children and adolescents. Pharmacotherapy for psychiatric disorders is still relatively new in this population and is yet insufficiently validated for many potential indications. There are, however, many instances in which pharmacotherapy can be quite helpful, and compliance with medication treatment is necessary. Treatment-emergent side effects, particularly if they are unexpected or severely distressing, may lead to treatment noncompliance.

In M.B.'s case, the presence of a parent who "did not believe" in medications complicated the picture, yet this is a reality often faced by clinicians. Strongly held opinions about both the dangers of medications and the presumed supremacy of purely social or psychological treatments of child and teenage psychiatric disturbance may be held by patients, family, friends, other physicians, and mental health professionals alike. There is often a reluctance on the part of some patients, families, or mental health professionals to attempt psychotropic treatments, even when their use is clearly indicated. Perhaps as a result of such attitudinal bias, it may too often be assumed that any physical or behavioral symptoms arising after the initiation of psychopharmacologic treatment are caused by the medication. Improving the patient's and family's knowledge and understanding of the appropriate use and anticipated adverse events of psychopharmacologic treatments is thus a necessary component of good clinical care.

Thinking About Treatment-Emergent Side Effects

Treatment-emergent side effects may be of two types. First, a symptom previously not present may arise for the first time following the initiation of pharmacologic treatment, such as inhibited orgasm or tremors onsetting some 2 to 3 weeks after treatment with an SSRI was begun. Second, a symptom previously present at baseline (prior to the initiation of the medication) may undergo significant exacerbation, such as mild and infrequent headaches becoming severe and frequent following the onset of treatment with a monoamine oxidase inhibitor.

Thus, proper side effect monitoring must determine the following:

1. Is the symptom treatment emergent, or was it present before treatment began?
2. What is the severity of the symptom and has this changed from baseline?
3. What is the frequency of the symptom and has this changed from baseline?
4. What is the likelihood that the symptom is caused by the psychotropic agent?

In order to properly address these issues, the physician *must* monitor side effects using consistent and detailed assessment techniques. In clinical psychopharmacologic practice the best way to achieve this is to use medication-specific side effect scales (MSSES), which combine physical and behavioral symptoms with information obtained from medical evaluation of the patient (such as specific neurologic examination, heart rate, blood pressure, etc). Although a number of excellent side effect monitoring instruments are available for research purposes, they tend to be overinclusive and offer no real advantages for routine clinical use over side effect scales that are designed for specific medications. Such MSSES also have the advantage of being able to more easily identify side effects that are unique to a particular medication (e.g., hair loss with valproic acid treatment) and are less time consuming to complete. In addition, they can be easily further customized to any one particular patient's experience by adding categories such as "other effects" for measurement. Examples of clinically useful MSSES are described in the relevant chapters of this book and can be found in Appendix IV.

The MSSES include scales for use with various antidepressants, lithium, various anticonvulsants, benzodiazepines, buspirone, stimulants, typical antipsychotics (e.g., chlorpromazine, haloperidol, perphenazine, etc.), and the atypical antipsychotics (clozapine and risperidone). These scales are designed to be used by trained raters, either physicians or nurses, and should ideally be completed by the same rater at every patient visit. Younger patients, or those the rater feels may be unreliable in their responses, should be interviewed with a responsible adult, such as a parent or group home staff. Questions that can be potentially embarrassing to the patient, such as sexual side effects, may be left to be completed during a more private time of the interview. If the patient is being treated with more than one medication at a time, each medication should be evaluated using its own specific side effects scale.

Every MSSES *must* be completed at least once *prior* to beginning treatment with a psychotropic agent. This is *essential* because without this information, obtained at baseline while the patient is medication free, it will be next to impossible to determine whether or not a particular symptom or other complaint is likely to be treatment emergent. When using an MSSES, the patient is instructed to give an overall impression of how he or she has been feeling with regard to each listed side effect since the last visit. Following this, direct questions regarding the presence or absence of each listed side effect should be asked. If a symptom is identified as present, further direct questions of clarification designed to rate the severity of the symptom should be asked. These questions should be phrased in such a way as to allow the rater to determine the intensity, frequency, and duration of the symptom in question.

For example, regarding the side effect of headaches, the initial question would be something such as, "Have you experienced any headaches since I saw you last?" If the answer is in the affirmative, the rater should probe using the following types of questions:

Could you describe them to me?

When did they start?

How often do they occur?

How long do they last?

How much do they hurt?

Do you get any other sick feelings with them, such as an upset stomach?

Do they stop you from doing anything that you would otherwise like to do, such as playing with your friends or watching television?

Do you do anything to try to help them go away?

Do you take any medicine for your headaches?

What kind of medicine, and how often do you take it?

Why do you think you are having these headaches?

It is always important to try to determine the patient's or parent's understanding of possible side effect symptoms. This may help the practitioner evaluate whether or not the reported symptom is indeed a treatment-emergent side effect and may occasionally lead to a therapeutic intervention that, without knowledge of the patient's view of his or her symptom, may not be obvious to the practitioner.

CASE EXAMPLE

"This medicine may be the death of me."

K.C., an 11-year-old boy, was being treated for Tourette's syndrome. His treatment plan included a special education placement, individual and family counseling, and low-dose pimozide. He had been observed to be uncharacteristically morose for a couple of weeks, but a review of his case had not identified any understandable reason for this. During a side effects assessment as part of the routine monitoring of his pimozide treatment, he reported the occurrence of occasional headaches that had been more prominent during the last month. He was worried that he might have a brain tumor and had begun to think about this possibility daily, particularly because he remembered that an aunt of his had died of a brain tumor a few years earlier. He knew that Tourette's syndrome was familial and thought that brain tumors were also. Reassurance from the physician and discussion of this issue by K.C.'s family and counselor led to both a decrease in headaches and a return of his more lively self.

CASE COMMENTARY

As this vignette illustrates, there is much more to proper pharmacologic treatment of children and adolescents than simply prescribing and monitoring medications. The clinician must also always strive to understand what the child or adolescent is feeling or thinking and why. Although MSSES can assist in the identification of treatment-emergent symptoms, they do not explain them. That is the task of the clinician.

In using the MSSES found in Appendix IV, the clinician rates each symptom on a 5-point scale, from 0, indicating no symptom present, to 4, indicating the symptom is severe. The intensity, frequency, and duration of the symptom are evaluated to determine degree of severity. Each scale point is an overall severity rating, the clinician's best estimate of the combination of symptom intensity, frequency, and duration.

Scoring of the MSSES can be conducted in two ways. First, the total of all individual side effect scores can be tabulated to give an overall side effect score. Second, individual side effect scores or groups of side effect scores (e.g., gastrointestinal side effect made up of the combined scores of nausea, vomiting, abdominal distress, diarrhea, and constipation) can be determined. Thus, the practitioner can follow both total and specific symptom ratings over time.

Whatever the MSSES chosen for use, it must be completed prior to the initiation of pharmacologic treatment and routinely at each patient visit thereafter. If the MSSES is not completed prior to beginning medication treatment, the practitioner will not be able to properly judge whether or not any particular physical or behavioral complaint or symptom is a treatment-emergent side effect. Furthermore, in monitoring side effects the clinician must review both the total and specific item scores over time. Simply reviewing total scores may hide specific treatment-emergent side effects that can show increasing severity over time, even while total side effect scores decrease or remain relatively static. For example, an increase of 2 points on a 5-point scale for any individual side effect should be cause for careful evaluation of that symptom and possible changes in medication management, as outlined earlier (Fig. 4–3).

Figure 4–3 shows two distinct patterns. First, the

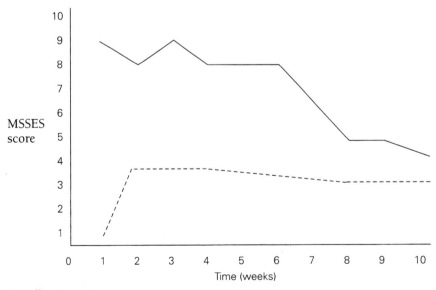

—— Total side effects score
- - - Gastrointestinal side effects score

FIGURE 4–3   Using an MSSES for Monitoring Antidepressant Treatment in an Adolescent with Major Depression: An Illustration

total MSSES shows a high level at baseline (week 1), which has decreased substantially by week 10. This decrease in total MSSES is often found, and it tends to parallel clinical improvement in the psychiatric syndrome. Second, the gastrointestinal subscale clearly shows the development of treatment-emergent side effects that plateau and then gradually disappear. In this case, the patient and physician decide to not make an intervention for the gastrointestinal side effects, hypothesizing that the patient would develop tolerance to this adverse effect. In this case at least, such an approach worked, in large part because the patient was prepared for this potential side effect and was able to tolerate it without discontinuing treatment.

The clinician should not be surprised to find MSSES scores decreasing with successful medication treatment. Indeed, studies of depressed teenagers treated with desipramine and manic teenagers treated with divalproex sodium show that successful medication treatment is correlated with decreased total MSSES scores at treatment endpoint compared with baseline. This occurs because physical symptoms are often part of the psychiatric syndrome and improve as the disorder is ameliorated with pharmacologic intervention.

For the practitioner choosing to use one of the available non–MSSES, the following scales are currently available:

1. Dosage Record and Treatment Emergent Symptom Scale (DOTES)
2. Treatment Emergent Symptom Scale (TESS)
3. Subjective Treatment Emergent Symptom Scale (STESS)

These scales are all published by the U.S. Department of Health and Human Services. Other useful assessment and side effect rating scales can be found in the 1985 National Institute of Mental Health–sponsored special issue of the *Psychopharmacology Bulletin* (DHHS publication ADM 86–173), which can be obtained from the Superintendent of Documents, Government Printing Office, Washington, DC 20402.

Monitoring Side Effects: The Use of Symptom Rating Scales—Practice Points

> 1. Differentiate treatment-emergent side effects from other causes of physical or behavioral symptoms.
> 2. Remember that antimedication or antitreatment biases may lead to incorrect labeling of physical or behavioral symptoms as medication side effects.

> 3. Complete a specific side effect scale for each medication used prior to initiating pharmacologic treatment.
> 4. Always use MSSES to measure and monitor treatment-emergent side effects at regular intervals during treatment.
> 5. Evaluate both total and specific side effect scores over time.
> 6. Always obtain the patient's and family's understanding of specific treatment-emergent side effects.

Special Issues in Side Effects Monitoring

Three special issues arise in side effects monitoring: (1) the use of specific scales designed to evaluate neurologic symptoms, (2) the frequency of side effect monitoring, and (3) therapeutic drug monitoring.

Neurologic Side Effects

A number of scales are available for measuring and monitoring specific neurologic signs and symptoms that may arise as a result of treatment with neuroleptics. These scales all require careful physical evaluation of the patient by a trained clinician. Although modified versions of some of these scales are included in the specific antipsychotic MSSES found in Appendix IV, the physician should be familiar with those instruments that are often used in the research literature to measure and monitor extrapyramidal and tardive dyskinesia symptoms. In addition, one or more of the following neuroleptic specific side effect scales may be used in addition to the MSSES found in Appendix IV. This can be completed less frequently than the MSSES, such as for annual or biannual case reviews of children and adolescents treated with antipsychotic medications (Appendix III).

Although not specifically developed for use with children and adolescents, two useful extrapyramidal side effect rating scales are the Simpson–Angus Scale for Extrapyramidal Symptoms and the Chouinard Extrapyramidal Symptom Rating Scale. The Chouinard Scale also provides for the assessment of involuntary movements. The Abnormal Involuntary Movement Scale (AIMS) is the standard rating scale for assessing tardive dyskinesia and has been successfully applied in evaluating neuroleptic-induced movement disorders in children and adolescents.

As with all side effect rating scales, the clinician choosing to use one or more of these listed must complete them prior to initiating antipsychotic drug treatment and at specific regular intervals during the course of neuroleptic treatment. These scales are particularly useful during the treatment of acute psychosis in which significant side effects are expected to occur and when these side effects may onset rapidly and require rapid intervention. In such cases these scales may be more reasonably applied on a daily basis.

The Physical and Neurological Examination for Subtle Signs (PANESS)—Revised is a detailed semistructured interview that must be conducted by a trained examiner. While its use provides a detailed neurologic evaluation, including "soft signs," this scale is not recommended for routine clinical use because it is time consuming to administer and unlikely to provide any further useful information than can be obtained from the physical examinations included in the MSSES found in Appendixes III and IV.

Frequency of Side Effect Monitoring

The frequency of side effect monitoring is described in upcoming chapters as part of the approach to using specific psychotropic agents, but it is important for the clinician to be aware of the conceptual framework used to guide side effect monitoring. This framework consists of the following three major components:

1. Educate the patient and family about treatment-emergent adverse events.
2. Obtain adequate baseline assessments, both medical (symptom measures using the appropriate MSSES and physical examination) and laboratory (those physiological measures that will probably be affected by medications).
3. Determine the optimal monitoring strategy for each patient and each medication.

Items 1 and 2 have already been discussed in this chapter and will be further elaborated for specific disorders and medications in later chapters. Regarding item 3, the critical issue here is the importance of the clinician's understanding of both patient and medication variables and how they interact. Many side effects are often subjective evaluations (or in the case of a parent's observing a child, a subjective-objective evaluation) of various signs and symptoms. Some of these signs and symptoms may be entirely or mostly explained by the pharmacodynamic effect of medication. In other cases only a portion or even none of the identified effects will be explained by pharmacodynamic effects of the drug. In most cases, however, there will be a dynamic interplay between pharmacodynamic and personal-social factors.

The astute clinician must recognize the complexity of this interplay and be careful not to jump to conclusions about the "psychological" or "pharmacodynamic" pathoetiology of subjectively reported side effects.

As a general rule of thumb, side effect monitoring should consist of both face-to-face (appointment-based) contact and available telephone contact. Appointment contact should be set up in anticipation of the expected onset of side effects. Thus when medications are introduced or when doses are raised it is reasonable to see the patient 2 to 4 days later (depending on the medication) as the dose modification kicks in. These visits should be focused on side effect monitoring only and do not need to be overly long; usually 15 to 20 minutes should suffice. Each visit should consist of a general review of the patient's experience of the medication and then an application of the relevant MSSES. Physical examination—neurologic, heart rate, blood pressure, etc.—should also be performed at this time. If ancillary investigations are necessary (such as an ECG), these can also be completed.

Available telephone contact is a useful and indeed necessary component of good psychopharmacologic practice. Many patients or their parents are quite concerned about potential side effects of medications. Some are hypervigilant about them. If a patient or parent does not feel that he can access the clinician or someone on the clinical staff with questions or problems relating to side effects, he may often discontinue potentially effective treatments because of needless worry. On the other hand, some patients or parents may proceed in the opposite direction and continue using a medication that may be harmful.

Such availability of the clinician will not only provide a "safety net" for the patient and parents but also will create a therapeutic framework in which the importance of respectful medication monitoring can be taught to both patient and family. The "art" of this from the physician's perspective is to provide enough structure to assist the patient and parents to develop the necessary skills and confidence that will allow them to take over reasonable medication monitoring. Because this is a learning process, the clinician can expect to find (in some cases more than others—remember the dynamic interplay of subjective experience of side effects) that telephone contact may be more frequent at the onset of treatment and will gradually subside as the patient and family become more comfortable with the process.

Directions regarding telephone availability should be made clearly to the patient and the family. An information sheet regarding the medication should be given to the patient and parents, and a telephone number where the physician can be reached should be provided. Who the patient or parent should contact when the clinician is not available should also be identified. In some clinics a competent health professional, such as a registered nurse, may be identified as the initial contact person. Patients and parents should be asked to call if they have any *medication-specific concerns.* Other therapeutic issues (besides concerns about the safety of the patient or others) should be left to regularly scheduled appointments. Patients and parents should be helped to identify those medication-related issues that might be urgent (such as sudden onset of a rash, fainting, etc.) and those that might not be (such as dry mouth, trouble sleeping). Urgent matters should be dealt with immediately, and less urgent matters can be dealt with at the end of the clinician's day.

In some cases, such availability may be seen as an open invitation to engage the clinician in a variety of nonmedication monitoring issues. In other cases this telephone availability may become an objective measure of the general distress experienced by the patient or parent, expressed as concern about medications and side effects. The clinician must be aware of these possibilities, and if she or he is concerned that these are driving the telephone contact must deal with them therapeutically in the context of a face-to-face appointment. Clinical experience using this method, however, suggests that it is the exception rather than the rule that issues other than learning how to adequately evaluate and monitor medication treatment drive telephone contact.

Therapeutic Drug Monitoring

Therapeutic drug monitoring (TDM) is an issue that has relevance to the evaluation of treatment-emergent side effects and one that is often poorly understood. TDM is the measurement of drug levels in body fluids (predominantly blood) and the use of those levels to adjust drug dosage based on a well-referenced "therapeutic range" for any one specific drug. Thus TDM may be used clinically for the following purposes:

1. To titrate pharmacologic treatment to produce an optimal effect
2. To avoid toxicity
3. To monitor compliance

This use of TDM is based on clearly determined efficacy and toxicity ranges for any specific compound. Efficacy and toxicity ranges, however, may not be identical, and the therapeutic level is defined as that range of drug

serum concentration above which the probability of adverse effects increases and below which the probability of a satisfactory clinical response decreases. Thus, a drug level outside the established therapeutic range in any specific patient may or may not signal either an ineffective or potentially toxic amount.

TDM is most useful if putative therapeutic levels have been established for particular compounds across the life cycle, because age and pubertal status are known to affect both the pharmacokinetic effects (the physiological factors that determine the delivery of a particular medication to its target tissue) and the pharmacodynamic effects (what a particular medication does when it reaches its target tissue) of many drugs. Regarding pharmacokinetics, most psychotropic medications exhibit first-order kinetics, which means that the amount of drug that is eliminated from the body is directly proportional to the amount in the blood. For these drugs, knowledge of their serum or plasma half-life (the amount of time it takes to clear a specific drug to half of its initial concentration) will help the clinician determine their steady-state concentrations. Usually, if dosing is constant, the steady-state concentration can be said to have been reached at the time of 4 to 6 half-lives. Any alterations in this process (e.g., liver disease that affects drug metabolism or erratic compliance) will be pharmacokinetically reflected in serum or plasma drug concentrations that differ from those predicted.

Regarding pharmacodynamics, although the amount of drug reaching target tissues is important for its effects (hence the importance of pharmacokinetics), what a drug actually does when it reaches the target tissue is fundamental to both its therapeutic and its adverse effects. This relationship between a drug's concentration and its effects is fundamental to the issue of TDM. Therapeutic ranges are concerned with the pharmacodynamic effects of medications. Specific serum or plasma concentrations of any drug are related to, but do not necessarily predict, a drug's therapeutic and adverse effects profiles.

Furthermore, because the parent drug and its metabolites may not exhibit similar therapeutic or toxic effects, the TDM of only the parent compound may provide a false sense of security for the clinician with regard to potential drug toxicity. For example, the desipramine metabolite, 2-hydroxy-desipramine, while not known to exhibit an antidepressant effect, is generally considered to be significantly more cardiotoxic than its parent, desipramine. Similarly, a major metabolite of carbamazepine shows significant neurotoxic activity in the absence of any well-documented antimanic effect. Some of these metabolites (such as 2-hydroxy-desipramine) are relatively easily measured and are available for clinical use; others are not. Thus, if only parent drug levels are measured, some patients may be found to show significant toxic effects, even when the serum levels are in the "therapeutic" range.

In addition, clinical endpoints of defined efficacy for any particular therapeutic range may differ. In pediatric medicine, for example, the serum range of theophylline needed to improve pulmonary function and exercise tolerance in asthmatic children is well known. Less well established are the effects of theophylline on such parameters as school performance and social development. In child and adolescent psychopharmacology, while some study of therapeutic ranges for symptom improvement has been undertaken in a number of disorders (e.g., the relationship between serum imipramine levels and symptomatic improvement in depressed children), much less is known about, and almost no study has ascertained, the relationship between functional outcome (such as school performance or peer relationships) and serum levels of any specific medication.

Developmental psychopharmacology is still a recent innovation in studies of pharmacokinetic and pharmacodynamic effects of psychotropics. Much of the recent interest in this field has taken place in geriatric psychopharmacology, and few large-scale studies directed at eliciting this information in children and adolescents are available, for almost any compound. In child and adolescent psychopharmacology, sufficient information for a few compounds may exist to estimate a serum range above which adverse effects are found to occur more commonly. However, there are few if any sufficiently studied compounds for which serum drug ranges for therapeutic efficacy have been clearly demonstrated. It is essential that the child and adolescent psychopharmacologist not make the assumption that therapeutic ranges developed from studies of adults will also apply to children and adolescents as well. The issue for the psychopharmacologist treating children and adolescents is how to rationally use TDM in the context of the issues just raised. Guidelines for TDM are found in Table 4–1.

When using TDM, care must be taken to ensure that the proper time has elapsed between the last oral dose and blood sampling. The proper time for lithium, the tricyclics, and the anticonvulsants valproic acid and carbamazepine is about 12 hours between the last oral dose and blood sampling. Usually this is accomplished by drawing blood in the morning if the medication is taken

TABLE 4–1 Guidelines for Therapeutic Drug Monitoring in Children and Adolescents

1. Therapeutic ranges are guidelines that supplement but do not replace careful clinical monitoring of side effects and symptom improvement.
2. TDM should be used to target medication dosage for those compounds in which therapeutic ranges have been suggested in children and adolescents. These include lithium, the tricyclics imipramine and nortriptyline, and the antiepileptic medications used for mood stabilization—valproic acid and carbamazepine.
3. TDM should be used in those situations where the therapeutic range of a specific compound may be relatively narrow and extremely wide fluctuations in serum levels for any one single oral dose are known to commonly occur, for example, a 6- to 10-fold variance in combined imipramine/desipramine levels in children or adolescents treated with imipramine.
4. They should be used in those clinical situations in which
   a. Concentration-dependent toxicity can occur with conventional dosages in patients who slowly metabolize specific drugs.
   b. The therapeutic index is narrow, such as lithium.
   c. Combinations of drugs are used such that one compound may significantly affect the metabolism of another compound (e.g., fluoxetine can raise the serum levels of desipramine and barbiturates can lower the levels of carbamazepine).
5. TDM should be used with those compounds that autoinduce their own metabolism (such as carbamazepine).
6. TDM should be used when clinical response to optimal oral dosing is significantly below what is expected following an adequate trial of treatment or when unexpected or severe side effects occur.

during the evening of the previous day. Obviously, some changes to this schedule may be necessary given the realities of patient and parent schedules. If an outpatient laboratory near the patient's home is used instead of the practitioner's usual laboratory facility, it is important for the laboratory to document the actual time that the blood sample was drawn so that the clinician will be able to properly evaluate the drug level reported. Furthermore, as many patients may use laboratory facilities that are unfamiliar to the clinician, it is important for the physician to understand the type of assay used to determine drug levels and to know the therapeutic ranges established by each laboratory for that particular assay used by a particular patient.

In using TDM, overmonitoring is to be discouraged and undermonitoring provides no useful information. Serum levels of a medication must be obtained in such a manner as to reflect the steady-state level of the drug being measured. Knowledge of a specific medication's pharmacokinetic properties is thus essential for proper

TDM. For example, when monitoring lithium levels, it is of little value to obtain a serum lithium level sooner than 3 to 4 days following the last dose adjustment because the new steady-state level will not yet have been reached. Indeed, in this case overmonitoring may lead to a dosing strategy that will result in the elevation of serum lithium levels to outside the therapeutic range. Once a therapeutic level of a drug in a specific patient has been established (two serum levels within the therapeutic range separated by at least the same time as the drug half-life), TDM can be ordered less frequently, every 2 to 4 months unless clinically indicated earlier (e.g., lithium levels must be evaluated if severe vomiting or diarrhea occurs, and the onset of new treatment-emergent side effects may suggest a need to monitor serum levels). The value of TDM for monitoring compliance in children and adolescents has not been established and cannot at this time be recommended as a routine procedure, although it may be useful in those cases in which the physician suspects that the patient might be a rapid metabolizer. Discussion of TDM for specific medications is found in the appropriate chapters that illustrate their use.

Special Issues in Side Effects Monitoring—Practice Points

1. Specific neurologic side effect scales for neuroleptic treatment can be a useful adjunct to clinical monitoring scales.
2. Establish an optimal and flexible schedule for monitoring side effects using a combination of face-to-face (appointment) and telephone availability structures.
3. TDM is indicated for certain medications and in specific clinical situations, but overuse of TDM is to be avoided.

SUGGESTED READINGS

Adams M, Kutcher S, Bird D, Antoniw E. The diagnostic utility of endocrine and neuroimaging screening tests in first onset adolescent psychosis. Journal of the American Association of Child and Adolescent Psychiatry, 35:67–72, 1996.

Bailey A. Physical examination and medical investigations. In M Rutter, E Taylor, L Hersov (eds): Child and Adolescent Psychiatry: Modern Approaches. London: Blackwell Scientific, 1994, pp 79–93.

Clein PD, Riddle MA. Pharmacokinetics in children and adolescents. Child and Adolescent Psychiatric Clinics of North America, 4:59–75, 1995.

Gabel S, Hsu LKG. Routine laboratory tests in adolescent psychiatric inpatients: Their value in making psychiatric diagnoses and in detecting medical disorders. Journal of the American Academy of Child Psychiatry, 25:113–119, 1986.

Geller B. Psychopharmacology of children and adolescents: Pharmacokinetics and relationships of plasma/serum levels to response. Psychopharmacology Bulletin, 27:401–409, 1991.

Greenblatt DJ. Basic pharmacokinetic principles and their application to psychotropic drugs. Journal of Clinical Psychiatry, 54(Suppl):8–13, 1993.

Hughes C, Preskorn S. Pharmacokinetics in child/adolescent psychiatric disorders. Psychiatric Annals, 24:76–82, 1994.

McLeod HL, Evans WE. Pediatric pharmacokinetics and therapeutic drug monitoring. Pediatric Review, 13:413–421, 1992.

Paxton JW, Dragunow M. Pharmacology. In JS Werry (ed): Practitioner's Guide to Psychoactive Drugs in Children and Adolescents. New York: Plenum Publishing, 1993, pp 23–55.

Popper C (ed). Psychiatric Pharmacosciences of Children and Adolescents. Washington, DC: American Psychiatric Press, 1987.

Preskorn SH, Burke MJ, Fast GA. Therapeutic drug monitoring. Psychiatric Clinics of North America, 16:611–645, 1993.

Wallach J. Interpretation of Diagnostic Tests: A Synopsis of Laboratory Medicine (5th ed). Boston: Little, Brown and Company, 1992.

Other Useful Baseline Assessments for Psychopharmacologic Treatment

A more comprehensive determination of the efficacy of psychopharmacologic treatment in children and adolescents can be made if a variety of other issues are considered. Thus, psychopharmacologic treatment may include the baseline evaluation of one or more of the following selected areas: family functioning, overall functioning, academic functioning, speech and language ability, and institutional assessment. Detailed knowledge about many of these areas is also useful for understanding the context—both family and institutional—in which psychopharmacologic treatment will occur. Other parameters, such as social and academic functioning, may themselves be a focus or target of pharmacologic treatment. Speech and language assessment is of value in selected cases in which problems in these areas are suspected because unidentified speech and language difficulties may contribute to the development or maintenance of psychiatric disturbance.

Family Assessment

For the purposes of psychopharmacologic treatment, the family unit is viewed as a powerful environmental influence on the child or adolescent presenting with a psychiatric disorder. This influence is understood as having the potential to modulate or influence the course of the illness and the outcome of treatment. Hence identifying certain aspects of family functioning and understanding how the family comprehends and deals with psychiatric disturbance in its members are

very important for psychopharmacologic treatment.

The family of a child or adolescent with a psychiatric disturbance is not a priori seen as "sick" or "dysfunctional," and the psychopharmacologist appreciates that interpersonal or systemic difficulties that may be found within any particular family are most likely to be multifactorial in nature and often may reflect the effect of a particular psychiatric illness on the child or adolescent. Similarly, in most cases no reasonable purpose is served in attempting to explain the entire pathoetiology of the patient's disorder as a specific or necessary outcome of family functioning. In addition, the psychopharmacologist must appreciate the burden that a severe psychiatric illness of one or more of its members can have on even a very well functioning family and should not be quick to label all problems in family functioning as resulting from some type of long-standing family pathology. On the other hand, the psychopharmacologist must keep in mind that some families do have problematic styles of interpersonal interaction that may have an impact on a child's psychiatric illness either to increase morbidity or to decrease treatment response. Even if the family is contributing to the patient's problems, however, blaming the family is unlikely to be productive and may actually be harmful.

Families often come for pharmacologic intervention after psychotherapeutic modalities of treatment have not provided the hoped-for outcome. Furthermore, parents of psychiatrically ill children or teenagers may often blame themselves for their child's problems. Sometimes other health professionals have directly or indirectly given the parents the message that their child's difficulties are primarily or even solely the result of family conflicts or poor parenting styles. The psychopharmacologist should approach the family without preconceived etiologic hypotheses about family dysfunction being the cause of psychiatric disorders, and must provide the family with understanding, support, education about the specific psychiatric illness, and help with those areas of family functioning that are problematic. The clinician must remember that, just as family functioning may affect symptom expression in a child or adolescent, the child's psychiatric illness may create problems in the family. Thus family assessment of a number of key areas should be part of the baseline evaluation completed prior to psychopharmacologic treatment. These areas include:

1. History of family psychiatric illness and family psychiatric treatment
2. Family attitudes toward psychiatric treatment in general and pharmacologic treatment in particular
3. Specific areas of functional disturbance (such as communication or role definition) and their impact on the manifestation of the child's disorder or treatment outcome
4. Cultural issues that may help in understanding the patient and family better or that may impact on the pharmacologic treatment of the child's illness

Family Psychiatric Illness and Psychiatric Treatment

An important area of investigation in family assessment is the determination of possible psychiatric illness in one or more family members other than the identified patient. Psychiatric disorders often cluster in families. For example, depressed children and teenagers may have a mood-disordered parent or one with an anxiety or substance use disorder. Children with obsessive compulsive disorder (OCD) may have a parent or sibling with an anxiety disorder or Tourette's syndrome. Psychotic adolescents may have a family member with schizophrenia. In some cases these psychiatric disorders have not previously been identified in another family member. In other cases, they may have been suspected or even diagnosed, but for one reason or another not effectively treated. The presence of an ongoing psychiatric illness in another family member may significantly affect either the child's or adolescent's clinical presentation or response to treatment.

CASE EXAMPLE

"I can't go to school even though I feel better."

S.P., a 10-year-old girl, has generalized anxiety disorder and occasional mild panic attacks (once or twice a month). Combined psychological and buspirone treatment at a dose of 5 mg given three times daily was successful in decreasing the severity of her anxiety symptoms and improving her school attendance. Even with good symptom control, however, she still missed about one quarter of her school days. A review of her difficulties regarding attendance raised the possibility that S.P. was missing school to comfort and care for her mother. Discussion of this problem with the mother and child identified that the mother suffered from an untreated panic disorder (PD) and that she felt more comfortable having her daughter at home with her when she was having a "bad day." Referral to another psychiatrist led to effective treatment of the mother's PD, with subsequent marked improvement in S.P.'s school attendance.

CASE COMMENTARY

In S.P.'s case the presence of a psychiatric disorder in another family member negatively affected her social and academic functioning, even when her own symptoms had improved significantly. Providing effective treatment for a family member whose own psychiatric illness has an impact on that of the identified patient is a necessary part of optimizing treatment outcome for a child or adolescent.

A potential problem regarding the issue of a family member with substance abuse can be avoided if this problem is identified and appropriate proactive procedures are put into place prior to treating the child or adolescent. Clinical experience suggests that some parents or other family members may use a child's medication for their own purposes, although the prevalence of this problem is not known. This may be a problem in particular with benzodiazepines when a family member is a drug or alcohol abuser. In such a scenario it is necessary to identify this situation as a possibility and to devise a system for monitoring medication abuse quickly should it occur.

In other cases the presence of a psychiatric disorder in a family member may be a clue to a psychiatric diagnosis in a child or adolescent presenting with atypical symptoms. In addition, successful response to a particular medication in a parent may be used to guide the selection of a particular pharmacologic treatment in the child with a similar disorder.

CASE EXAMPLE

Mood Problems or Normal Adolescence

V.J. was a 12-year-old girl with a 3-month history of "difficult behavior," including temper outbursts, mood swings, irritability, "hyper-epi-sodes" (where she would go for days at a time with minimal sleep), grandiosity, and the emergence of new oppositional behaviors both at home and at school. Six weeks prior to being seen, V.J. began to smoke and to drink alcohol, and her parents were concerned that she was experimenting with marijuana. A consultation with the family physician had led to the diagnosis of "normal adolescent rebellion," with the advice that "she will grow out of it." The problems continued, however, and began to escalate. V.J. stopped attending school because she was convinced she did not need to graduate to be successful and also because she hated the "rules."

Although V.J. did not meet formal diagnostic criteria for a mood disorder, her family history was positive for bipolar disorder on her father's side (uncle and grandfather) and for depression (mother) and alcohol abuse (grandfather) on the mother's side. Because her behavior was out of character, a provisional diagnosis of possible bipolar disorder was considered. And because V.J.'s uncle had had a well-documented positive response to lithium, pharmacologic treatment using lithium at a daily dose of 1050 mg, with steady-state serum levels achieved between 1.0 and 1.1 mEq/L was begun with V.J. Seven weeks following initiation of lithium, V.J. experienced almost complete symptom resolution, was once again attending school, and had stopped smoking and using alcohol.

CASE COMMENTARY

In the case of V.J., the presence of a clear family history of mood disorders (including bipolar disorder) suggested that she might be experiencing an atypical and early onset of mania-hypomania. This information led to a psychopharmacologic intervention that would not have necessarily been considered otherwise. Her response to treatment, although it did not prove that she indeed had a bipolar disorder, nevertheless suggested that she might and provided a well-documented intervention for the future.

Family Attitudes Toward Psychiatric and Psychopharmacologic Treatment

Family attitudes toward psychiatric treatment, particularly pharmacologic treatment, can have a major impact on patient compliance. For example, if a parent or other family member conveys the message—either direct or implicit—that taking medications for a psychiatric disorder is a "bad thing," it may be quite difficult for the child or adolescent to continue pharmacotherapy. This is particularly true if the patient is a child who is totally dependent on a parent for medication administration. This problem may be further compounded when parents have differing views on whether or not their child should take medication. These issues must be clarified early on in treatment because they can significantly contribute to the success or failure of pharmacotherapy by affecting compliance.

CASE EXAMPLE

Is It Father or Mother Who Knows Best?

M.E. was a 7-year-old boy with a diagnosis of attention-deficit hyperactivity disorder (ADHD). He was somewhat oppositional but did not meet diagnostic criteria for oppositional defiant disorder (ODD). He was not conduct disordered, nor was he anxious. He was underachieving at school and had begun to develop problems in the classroom as a result of his impulsive and motoric behaviors. Treatment with methylphenidate was suggested and heartily endorsed by the father but only tentatively agreed to by the mother, who felt that dietary manipulation and clearing of "environmental toxins" would be more appropriate. Nevertheless, the clinician prescribed methylphenidate beginning at a dose of 5 mg to be taken twice daily. At a follow-up visit 3 days later, M.E.'s parents quarreled about the value of his taking medications, and the mother admitted that she had not been giving M.E. any "pills" because, although she had agreed to a methylphenidate trial, she had heard from friends that this medicine was highly addictive and turned children into "zombies." She restated her belief in dietary manipulation and toxin removal as the more appropriate treatment and refused to return for pharmacotherapy.

CASE COMMENTARY

This case illustrates problems with compliance in psychopharmacologic treatment when parental issues regarding the use of medications are not adequately dealt with. In a case such as M.E.'s, a more appropriate approach than that taken by his clinician would have been to introduce a trial of dietary manipulation and "toxin" removal (within reason) for a specified length of time (2 to 3 weeks), with the use of methylphenidate beginning only if these approaches failed. Alternatively, a double-blind placebo trial of methylphenidate using an ABAB design may have been suggested. This is discussed more fully in Chapter 7. Either of these two interventions might have been more palatable to M.E.'s mother and might have prevented her from terminating her son's treatment. In this case the clinician's use of one of the alternative strategies described earlier might or might not have been helpful, and the clinician would have had to address the individual and marital issues of the parents. At the very least, the identification of this issue early on in pharmacologic treatment would have been appropriate, and proactive intervention should have been applied.

Occasionally, this family-patient interaction may take on an unusual flavor, as described in the next case.

CASE EXAMPLE

Sneaking Drugs
Behind the Family's Back

C.S. was a 17-year-old girl who had been recently discharged from the hospital following her second admission in a manic state. During her first manic episode she had responded well to treatment with carbamazepine, and she was maintained at a prophylactic dose similar to her treatment dose. Four months after her first hospital discharge, at the urging of her mother (who also suffered from bipolar disorder and who was well known for her treatment noncompliance) and her uncle (a trained but not medically practicing psychiatrist living in another country, who followed the teaching of R. D. Laing and who did not "believe" in "drugs"), she discontinued her medications and promptly relapsed.

Following her second hospital discharge, C.S. was continued on her carbamazepine. Once again she was advised by her family to discontinue medication, although heroic attempts had been made by the hospital treatment staff to elicit the support of her mother for continued pharmacotherapy. This time, however, C.S. refused to follow the directives of her family and told her doctor that she was taking her medicines in secret because, although her mother felt medicines were bad for her, she herself realized that they were necessary to help stabilize her mood.

CASE COMMENTARY

This case is no doubt unusual, but it does illustrate well the importance of knowing parental and family attitudes toward psychopharmacologic treatment of a child or adolescent. In this case, because the patient was older than the legal age of consent, the clinical treatment team worked directly with the adolescent, while at the same time trying to help her mother understand the importance of pharmacologic treatment. Had the patient been younger than the legal age of consent in the jurisdiction in which the case occurred, the physician would have had to consider using legal means to assist the patient in obtaining appropriate treatment. These issues of consent are discussed in Chapters 6 and 7.

Family Functional Difficulties and Psychopharmacologic Treatment

At times the pattern of family functioning may significantly affect psychopharmacologic treatment of a child or adolescent. Although this situation may occur within the context of a family that showed significant dysfunction prior to the onset of the child's or adolescent's disorder, even developmentally normative family perturbations may have an impact on treatment compliance. Medication treatment can also become the focus of parent-child conflicts, and in adolescents may become one of the battlegrounds on which the war of independence is waged.

CASE EXAMPLE

Just Who Is in Charge Here?

D.G. was a 14-year-old male with a long history of ADHD that had been successfully treated with methylphenidate and educational assistance. Difficulties arose when he decided that he would stop his medications because he was now a teenager, was no longer a child, and was the one who "made those decisions now." His parents responded by refusing to allow him to discontinue his medications. The situation escalated into a major conflict, with no ground given by either side. D.G.'s parents felt that their appeals to "reason" were met with "irrational responses." D.G. argued that he knew what was best for him because "this is my body and my brain." The impasse was solved by asking D.G. to share responsibility for taking his medications with his doctor and not with his parents. In addition, a medication holiday was instituted, with symptom rating scales done prior to medication discontinuation and later, 2 weeks following medication discontinuation. The outcome of these strategies was that D.G. began to once more take his medications but using a different strategy. He took methylphenidate on those school days when he had a heavy "thinking class load" and not on those days when he had "mostly spares, gym, and lunch." His parents were helped to see this process as part of D.G.'s growing up and willingness to assume responsibility for himself. Although this was probably not optimal pharmacotherapy, D.G. was satisfied with the results and, although his grades did go down slightly, his parents eventually became satisfied as well.

CASE COMMENTARY

Not all parent-adolescent conflicts in which medication use is an issue have such a positive outcome as in D.G.'s case, but this vignette illustrates that this issue, when it arises, must be addressed psychotherapeutically and educationally in order to provide the best possible pharmacologic management, although this may not always be the optimal pharmacologic management. The principle that "half a loaf is better than none" is often evoked during the psychopharmacologic treatment of the adolescent.

Family Cultural Beliefs and Psychopharmacologic Treatment

Cultural issues often arise in the family context and in some cases may have an impact on pharmacologic treatment. These issues are quite varied and range from specific religious beliefs to "home remedies" to other culturally specific models of intervention. In many cases, awareness and understanding of these issues may help present the pharmacologic intervention in a framework that makes it more understandable to the family. In other cases these issues can significantly negatively affect the course of pharmacologic treatment.

CASE EXAMPLE

Eye of Newt and Horn of Toad Are Bound to Help

R.C. was a 16-year-old boy who was hospitalized following treatment of a manic episode. His psychiatric history revealed that he had experienced a previous depressive episode of 5 months' duration at age 15, and that he had not received any treatment for this episode. R.C.'s family had recently emigrated from China, and the paternal grandparents who had come as part of the family lived with R.C. and his parents and played an important role in family decision making. These grandparents were very skeptical of Western methods of medical treatment.

A few months after his discharge from the hospital and after a period of relative mood stability, R.C.'s mood control became problematic. Serum lithium levels were within the therapeutic range of 1.0 to 1.2 mEq/L, and R.C. denied taking any illicit drugs. A drug screen, however, was positive for an "unidentified substance." A review of these findings with R.C. and his family revealed that R.C.'s grandmother had been augmenting his lithium treatment with "Chinese home medicines," which she made up from various roots and over-the-counter compounds. All attempts to involve the grandmother in discussions about R.C.'s treatment were unsuccessful. R.C.'s father consented to supply examples of some of the over-the-counter substances used in the preparation of the home remedies. Examination of these substances revealed the presence of sympathomimetic compounds. The family was educated about the potential for drug interactions and the possible effect of unknown substances in the home remedies on R.C.'s mood control. In spite of ongoing clinic staff efforts in this area, however, R.C. continued to use home remedies.

CASE COMMENTARY

In the case of R.C., the influence of non-Western methods of treatment had the effect of producing unhelpful complications because of drug-drug interactions with his psychopharmacotherapy. In some cases, as illustrated here, in spite of a clinician's best attempts, such mixing and adding continue. Faced with such a situation, it is useful for the clinician to meet with the family members who are insisting on "doing it their way." The purpose of this meeting is not to blame family members or dismiss their knowledge. Rather, it should be seen as an opportunity for the clinician to determine how the family thinks about and understands psychiatric illness, who the decision makers in the family are, and whether there is any common ground regarding therapeutics.

For example, it may be possible to combine nontoxic home remedies with rational psychotropic therapy. If such is the case, the clinician should have the intended home remedy chemically analyzed in order to determine whether such a combination is indeed safe. In many cases a variety of different home remedies may be available, and one of them may cause no known harm.

As demonstrated in these cases, the clinician must be aware of multiple family issues that can have an impact on the psychopharmacologic treatment of the child or adolescent. At the very least, the clinician must conduct a family assessment as part of the baseline interview process that takes into account the issues identified earlier. The family history protocol found in Figure 5–1 can be used to ensure that the necessary areas have been covered in the family assessment.

The establishment of a positive collaborative relationship between the physician and family is essential, and for this reason it is not appropriate for the initial family assessment to be completed by a mental health practitioner other than the psychopharmacologist. Should particular problems in family functioning be identified from this initial assessment, further specialist evaluation may be indicated. In some cases, long-standing family difficulties or severe family problems arising as a result of the child's illness may need particular interventions for optimal outcome, which can then be arranged as necessary.

Use of Scales in Family Assessment for Psychopharmacologic Treatment

Some relatively useful and user-friendly family evaluation instruments suitable for psychopharmacologic assessment are available, and the clinician may decide to incorporate one of the following into his or her baseline assessment package. The rationale for using any of these measures, however, has to be clear. Will the results obtained be useful in developing a treatment plan? Will the "cost" of completing yet another and potentially time-consuming form be negatively experienced by the patient and family? What is the value of the family assessment scale for diagnosis or monitoring of treatment?

In many cases the results obtained by using a family assessment schedule will not justify the time spent or the rationale for doing so. Using the screening form found in Figure 5–1, a skillful clinician should be able to identify those family issues that may be expected to have an impact on psychopharmacologic treatment. While there is nothing to be gained by using any of the following instruments as screening tools for family dysfunction, judicious use of one of the following measures may help clarify particular difficulties in families that the clinician has identified as exhibiting functional problems.

The general scale of the Family Assessment Measure (FAM) is a series of 50 statements about family functioning. Each statement is scored on a letter scale from "a," indicating "strongly agree," to "d," indicating "strongly disagree." Useful information can be obtained from scores submitted independently by the patient and one parent, but the input of both parents (when possible) is preferred. A scoring sheet showing normative ranges and assessing a variety of family functions (including such items as communication, social desirability, role performance, etc.) is produced from the score sheets. This scale takes about 20 to 30 minutes to complete and must be filled out independently by each family member. Clinically, it is useful for identifying areas of problematic family functioning, and sharing the results of the FAM with the patient and parents may be a useful part of the illness education process (see Chapters 6 and 7), in which the relationship between family functioning and illness outcome is discussed.

The FAM is copyrighted and much too long to reproduce in this volume; thus, it is not available in the appendixes. The scale, scoring key, and psychometric information are available from Multi-Health Systems, Inc., 908 Niagara Falls Boulevard, North Tonawanda, NY 14120–2060, USA. Clinicians practicing in Canada can write to Multi-Health Systems, Inc., 65 Overlea Boulevard, Suite 210, Toronto, Ontario, M4H 1P1.

The Family Adaptability and Cohesion Scales (FACES) II is a 30-statement questionnaire that is completed by the child or adolescent. It requires a grade 6 reading level and takes about 10 to 15

Patient's Name: _____ Date of Assessment: _____

Family Members Living at Home and Relationship to Patient (establish birth or adopted status): _____

_____

_____

_____

_____

Family Members Living Outside the Home and Relationship to Patient: _____

_____

_____

_____

_____

Family Psychiatric Illness (for each family member: diagnosis, treatment, outcome): _____

_____

_____

_____

_____

_____

_____

Family Attitudes Toward Psychopharmacologic Treatment (positive and negative): _____

_____

_____

_____

_____

Family Cultural or Religious Factors (describe and evaluate): _____

_____

_____

_____

Other Issues Arising from Family Assessment That May Impact on Pharmacotherapy:_____

_____

_____

_____

FIGURE 5–1   Family History Protocol for Psychopharmacologic Treatment

minutes to complete. FACES II (available from D. Olsen, PhD, Family Social Science, University of Minnesota, St. Paul, MN 55108) is based on the circumplex model of family functioning and measures three dimensions of family behavior: cohesion, adaptability, and communication. Results can be compared with normative data, and the scale has been successfully used to evaluate family functioning in studies of adolescent bipolar disorder.

A related instrument, the Parent-Adolescent Communication Scale, can also provide useful baseline information. The Parent-Adolescent Communication Scale is comprised of 20 items, each of which is scored from 1, "strongly disagree," to 5, "strongly agree." The teenager completes the scale twice—once for the mother and once for the father (as appropriate). Population norms are available for comparative purposes, and the results of this assessment may provide some appreciation of the adolescent-parent potential for conflict regarding pharmacologic treatment.

One area in which the use of one or more of the above-mentioned family assessment instruments is necessary is when family functioning is a target of psychopharmacologic treatment. For example, it is now well appreciated that the behavior of a child with significant ADHD may be clearly related to disturbed family function or to difficulties in dyadic relationships between the child and a parent. Treatment of the ADHD child with methylphenidate alone (in the absence of family counseling) may, in some cases, significantly affect improvement in family or dyadic relationships. In such a case family functioning may well become a focus or target of psychopharmacologic treatment, and the appropriate baseline and follow-up evaluations of family functioning should be made using one of the instruments designed for this purpose.

Family Assessment—Practice Points

1. Evaluations of specific areas of family functioning are useful for optimal psychopharmacologic treatment.
2. The following family issues should be included in baseline family assessment: history of psychiatric treatment, attitudes toward psychopharmacologic treatment, specific difficulties in functioning, and cultural or religious attitudes toward psychopharmacologic treatment.
3. The use of specific family assessment scales should be for focused diagnostic, and not for screening, purposes.

4. If family functioning in general or a segment of family functioning in particular is a focus of psychopharmacologic treatment, then it is necessary to use the appropriate scale to determine baseline levels of disturbance and to evaluate outcome.

Social and Interpersonal Functioning

Psychiatric illnesses affect multiple areas of a child's or adolescent's functioning. At times the social and interpersonal morbidity arising from the disorder may persist even after the symptoms of the illness have come under relatively good control. This morbidity may then give rise to a variety of other problems that could affect the child's or adolescent's quality of life. Continuing functional impairment as a result of a psychiatric disorder might also become a risk factor leading to relapse or might result in the development of another related psychiatric illness. For example, a severe and prolonged depressive illness may bring on the loss of past positive friendships and school failure, which may then lead the patient toward substance or alcohol abuse. At this time it is not known whether these functional impairments require additional specific treatments, such as vocational counseling or individual psychotherapy, beyond the basic support and counseling that occur as part of psychopharmacologic treatment (see Chapters 6 and 7). Thus, social and interpersonal functioning may legitimately be targeted as a focus of psychopharmacologic treatment.

A number of scales have been developed that are of value in the identification and outcome evaluation of a child's or adolescent's functioning. A few such scales found to be of clinical utility in general office-based psychopharmacologic treatment are described here. The clinician should select one scale that will best meet the needs of the patient and not subject the patient and family to a battery of functional assessment scales that may all measure more or less the same area of interest. Although some of the scales are available in self-report form only (e.g., the Sickness Impact Profile—Adolescent Version [SIP-AV]), they can be easily amended for informant scoring as well.

Unlike symptom rating scales (see Chapter 3), scales that measure social or academic functioning are unlikely to show rapid responses to treatment. Accordingly, when developing a treatment monitoring strategy (see Chapters 6 and 7), the clinician should plan to use only these scales at baseline and two or three times thereafter. More frequent use is unlikely to demonstrate any clinically significant information and will simply give the patient and family more things to do while they wait for their appointment.

The SIP-AV is a self-report instrument developed for use with psychiatrically ill teenagers by modification of the SIP adult version. Although psychometrics for the SIP-AV are lacking, it has been used in psychopharmacologic and outcome studies of mood-disordered adolescents and in clinical work with a variety of psychiatric disorders found in older children and adolescents (see Appendix VII). It consists of 53 statements about various aspects of a teen's life and provides a total functioning score as well as subscores measuring sleep and rest, daily work around the house, contact with family and friends, concentration and problem solving, and social activities. Used at baseline and at reasonable intervals during treatment, it provides an overview of how teenagers and older children perceive themselves to be functioning. The suggested schedule of use is at baseline, at the expected treatment midpoint, at the expected treatment endpoint, and at the follow-up treatment review.

The Autonomous Functioning Checklist (AFC) is a user-friendly informant (usually parent) scored instrument that provides a good measure of multiple areas of a teenager's current functioning (see Appendix VII). An individual's score on the AFC can be compared with population norms, and the scale has demonstrated clinical utility in adolescent psychopharmacology clinics. This scale takes 10 minutes to complete and should be used following the same schedule as outlined earlier for the SIP-AV.

A less comprehensive self-report instrument that predominantly measures social support is the Social Health Battery developed by the Rand Corporation in 1978. Although the scale was not designed for use with psychiatric patients, it has reasonable psychometric properties and an age of application beginning at 14 years. The scale takes 5 to 7 minutes to complete and provides a total score that measures overall social support as well as two subscales: social contacts and group participation. It is unclear whether this scale is sensitive to treatment change, and it is included in this section for consideration by the clinician faced with a teenage patient (such as an 18-year-old with schizophrenia) in whom the development of useful social supports is part of the overall treatment plan.

Another potentially useful instrument for measuring adolescent functional health is the Duke Health Profile (DUKE). This is a 17-item self-rating scale that takes 5 to 7 minutes to complete and provides an overall health score plus five health subscores: physical health, mental health, social health, perceived health, and self-esteem (see Appendix VII). It may be particularly useful in assessing and monitoring the generic health status of adolescents suffering from conditions such as mood and psychotic disorders that have well-established negative effects on physical well-being. Although only recently available and untested in psychiatric populations as such, the DUKE nevertheless should be considered for use if the psychopharmacologist has a relatively large population of adolescents with mood or psychotic disorders in his or her clinic population.

An adequate scale for baseline and treatment follow-up in terms of assessing overall functioning is the Global Assessment of Functioning Scale (GAFS). This is available in both child and adult versions, and the clinician can reasonably choose to use the adult version for older teenagers. The GAFS (see the DSM-IV) is scored by the clinician following a comprehensive assessment of the patient. Psychological, social, and occupational/school functioning is collapsed to create a general overall functioning score ranging from 90 (excellent) to 1 (exceedingly poor). The GAFS provides a reasonable shorthand overview of the clinician's perception of the patient's functioning. Optimal use of this scale should avoid overapplication, and completion of the GAFS at baseline and at the time of expected acute treatment termination is sufficient. For children or teenagers undergoing long-term psychopharmacologic treatment for chronic conditions, GAFS evaluations completed at intervals of 4 months provide a reasonable monitoring of overall functioning.

Three additional scales that may be of value in assessing and monitoring social and interpersonal functioning in children are the social competence section of the CBCL, the Vineland Adaptive Behavior Scales, and the School and Social Disability Scale (SSDS).

The Vineland Adaptive Behavior Scales are available in two forms: the Survey Form and the Classroom Revision. Useful in assessing a variety of social and functional domains, they can be completed by interviewing a parent, other caregiver, or a child's classroom teacher.

The SSDS (see Appendix VII) is a clinician-scored 7-point scale that is designed to measure functional improvement in school and social functioning during treatment. The baseline score on this instrument for each child or adolescent is always 0, and the patient is rated as improved (mildly, moderately, greatly) or worse (mildly, moderately, greatly) at specific evaluation points, usually at 3- to 4-week intervals. In regular clinical practice, the SSDS is time efficient and simple to complete, and provides a sensitive indicator of change over time. Information obtained from the patient, parent, and school official (teacher or guidance counselor) is used to make the ratings.

A number of fairly popular assessment tools, used in particular by clinicians whose therapeutic training has been predominantly in psychodynamic models of intervention, have no role to play in the baseline evaluation necessary for psychopharmacologic treatment. Neither the Rorschach Inkblot Test (even when scoring using Exner's Comprehensive System Workbook) nor the Thematic Apperception Test (TAT) is of any value in diagnosis or outcome measurement. The administration of these tests provides no useful information and simply increases assessment time and cost. Accordingly, neither of these should be used.

Social and Interpersonal Functioning—Practice Points

1. Social and interpersonal functioning is useful to assess both for baseline evaluation and as a target for treatment.
2. Functional assessment scales are less likely than symptom rating scales to show rapid changes in response to treatment, and thus should be used less frequently than symptom rating scales to monitor outcome.

Academic Functioning

Knowing a child's or adolescent's current and past school performance is essential for a comprehensive understanding of his functioning. Psychiatric disorders by themselves may have a significant negative impact on a child's ability to do well in school. For example, the difficulties in concentrating and loss of interest that are part of a depressive syndrome often lead to a drop in grades. In addition, long-standing school problems may provide a clue as to the nature of the patient's current problem or may be important in understanding comorbid or associated difficulties that present along with the primary psychiatric disorder. In some cases the school may not have been aware that the child or adolescent suffered from a psychiatric disorder and may have inadvertently contributed to his difficulties by identifying a "behavior" or "emotional" disturbance and instituting unnecessary and ineffective interventions. Also, side effects of many psychotropics may impede learning and decrease academic success. A teacher should thus be aware of medication-induced

problems, such as difficulties with concentration, memory, and drowsiness, in the pupil taking particular psychotropics. Appropriate modifications to the school curriculum might need to be made to optimize academic outcome. Thus, a school assessment is an important part of a baseline evaluation for psychopharmacologic treatment.

CASE EXAMPLE

He Is Either Mad, Sad, or Bad

M.F., a 13-year-old boy living in a small rural community, was referred for psychiatric evaluation at the insistence of his parents. He had just been expelled from the local school for disruptive behavior but his parents felt he was depressed. Psychiatric assessment determined a diagnosis of ADHD, oppositional disorder, and a possible speech and language problem. A review of school records indicated that M.F. had been "hyperactive" and "difficult to keep focused on his school work" since he had started school. He had shown serious difficulties in spelling and reading, and by the time he was in sixth grade he was significantly below grade level in both areas. His teachers consistently reported that he was "always acting silly," "he is the class clown," "he can't settle down to do any work," and "he is not interested in school." His family physician, who had been consulted regarding M.F.'s problems, felt that M.F. was "probably just a bad kid."

Following the diagnostic evaluation, M.F.'s treatment consisted of pharmacologic management of his ADHD, further evaluation of his speech and language difficulties, meetings with his parents and representatives of the school to develop school-based behavioral and remedial teaching interventions, and a discussion with his family doctor about symptoms and associated problems of children with ADHD.

CASE COMMENTARY

In this case, M.F.'s ADHD had been noticed but not diagnosed. The school's attempts at intervention not only had been unsuccessful but had most likely contributed to his deteriorating academic and social functioning. In a case such as this, the results of a thorough assessment and diagnosis should be made available to the appropriate school authorities, and their assistance should be enlisted in developing and implementing a treatment plan for the child. This is most usefully done in a meeting with teachers and school administrators in a nonjudgmental, supportive, and educational manner. If this meeting and the subsequent intervention are successfully accomplished, the clinician should not be surprised at the high number of school-initiated referrals of all sorts of "problem children" that will be directed her way.

Thinking About the Academic Assessment

A comprehensive academic assessment should include the following:

1. Review of school grades from elementary school to the present
2. Review of teachers' written comments regarding behavior at school from early elementary school to the present
3. Review of an attendance profile, noting tardiness, absences, and the reason given to explain them
4. Review of any educational diagnostic testing or standardized grade level tests (if available)
5. Review of past and current extracurricular activities
6. Note of any specific academic or social strengths or weaknesses (including parental concerns, if available)

The clinician should also have a general idea of what skills and processes a child usually develops at a specific time in his or her academic career (Table 5–1).

An academic assessment form that is useful for clinical psychopharmacologic practice is shown in Figure 5–2. This form can be completed by interviewing either the patient (if a responsible adoles-

cent) or a parent. Whenever possible, information should be corroborated by examination of school records and discussion with the classroom teacher or other school officials (guidance counselor, vice-principal). Many clinicians feel that no evaluation of a child or adolescent can be considered complete without a discussion with the patient's classroom teacher. This practice is strongly recommended, but the legal and consent issues that may apply in different jurisdictions must be considered. A good guideline is to obtain and document in the clinical record the patient's consent or assent as well as the parent's consent prior to contacting any school official.

If specific educational concerns, such as a potential learning disorder, are identified from the baseline academic assessment, then further detailed educational diagnostic investigations are indicated. These are best conducted by a teacher or educational psychologist who is expert in their administration and scoring. Similarly, if the initial educational assessment identifies speech, language, or communication difficulties, referral for further specialized evaluation is in order.

Although the preferences of educational evaluators will vary, the following standardized tests are likely to be of benefit in delineating academic and learning problems possibly experienced by the patient:

1. Wide Range Achievement Test—Revised (WRAT-R)
2. Peabody Individual Achievement Test—Revised (PIAT-R)
3. Woodcock-Johnson Psycho-Educational Battery—Revised
4. Wechsler Intelligence Scale for Children III (WISC-III)
5. Test of Non-Verbal Intelligence (TONI)
6. Slosson Intelligence Test—Revised (SIT-R)

The clinician interested in further information about these tests should consult the references cited at the end of this chapter.

It should be kept in mind that these tests are not considered suitable for monitoring treatment outcome because they are relatively insensitive to pharmacologic interventions, so they should be used for baseline assessment only. A further caution in interpreting the results of these tests is indicated. Most educational diagnostic tests can be influenced greatly by the mental state of the patient at the time of testing. Thus, the results obtained from any educational testing conducted while the subject is suffering from an acute psychiatric illness (such as a major depression) may not be a valid reflection of that individual's academic capabilities. For these reasons, comments from the tester as to the subject's motivation, application to

TABLE 5–1 **Proposed Developmental Timetable for the Acquisition of Academic Skills and Processes in Children and Adolescents**

Grade	Skill and Process
Kindergarten	Acquisition of motor, language, learning, and socialization skills
Grades 1–3	Development of acquired motor, language, literacy, mathematics, and social skills
Grades 4–8	Application of these skills in learning new knowledge and further development of literacy, mathematics, and social skills
Secondary school	Development of specialized knowledge or skills in multiple domains and refinement of social skills

Name: _____ Age: _____ Date: _____

Current School: _____ Telephone: _____

School Contact: _____ Teacher's Name: _____

Current Grade: _____ Expected Grade: _____

  or   or

Current Credits Earned: _____ Expected Credits Earned: _____

Current Courses and Last Grade Obtained in Each: _____

_____

_____

Past Academic Performance:

Elementary School (give grade average obtained; list learning problems identified, if any; note grade failures, if any):

First: _____ Fifth: _____

Second: _____ Sixth: _____

Third: _____ Seventh: _____

Fourth: _____ Eighth: _____

Secondary School (give grade average obtained; list learning problems identified, if any; list all subjects in which grades fall below a C; note grade failures):

Ninth: _____

Tenth: _____

Eleventh: _____

Twelfth: _____

Thirteenth (if applicable): _____

Results of Previous Academic Testing, If Any (give dates and grade level at time of testing):

_____

_____

_____

Previously Identified or Suspected Speech, Language, or Communication Problem (e.g., "learning exceptionality" and type of special program recommended):

_____

_____

FIGURE 5–2 Academic Baseline Evaluation for Psychopharmacologic Treatment

Results of Previous IQ Testing, If Any (give dates and full scale; verbal and performance scores if available):

_____

_____

_____

_____

Current Participation in Extracurricular School Activities (identify interscholastic activities with an *):

Sports: _____   Clubs: _____

Music/Drama: _____   Student Associations: _____

Other: _____ .

Past Participation in Extracurricular School Activities (give dates; identify interscholastic activities with an *):

Sports: _____

Clubs: _____

Music/Drama: _____

Student Politics: _____

Other: _____

Identified Academic or Social Strengths: _____

_____

_____

Identified Academic or Social Weaknesses: _____

_____

_____

Parental Concerns (if any): _____

_____

_____

School Concerns (if any): _____

_____

_____

(This form was developed with the assistance of Mr. Peter Chaban, Metropolitan Toronto Separate School Board, and Mr. Doug Quackenbush, North York Board of Education, Toronto, Ontario, Canada. It may be easily modified to fit local differences in descriptive educational terms or academic structures.)

FIGURE 5–2 *Continued*

task, and general functioning in the testing situation are extremely useful in interpreting the results. If there are concerns that the child's or adolescent's mental state is such that the results of academic tests may be significantly distorted, repeat testing conducted when the patient has been relatively symptom free for 3 to 4 months is advisable.

In addition to baseline academic evaluation and psychoeducational testing, if indicated, ongoing liaison with the school is an important part of psychopharmacologic treatment. This has been described best in the treatment of children with ADHD, but it applies equally well to children and adolescents with psychiatric illnesses such as major depression, bipolar affective disorder, schizophrenia, and OCD who are attending regular community or private schools. If the patient is in a specialized treatment setting, this type of ongoing school-physician liaison is usually built into the overall treatment plan. Outside of specialized settings, such as hospital clinics or therapeutic day programs, school-physician communication is more difficult to establish, but it is vitally important that every reasonable attempt be made to facilitate such interaction because it will be of tremendous benefit to the patient.

Communication between the school and physician may include educating the classroom teacher or school health personnel about the child's disorder and the possible side effects of medications. Particularly with younger children, the school may be willing to take on the responsibility of dispensing a lunchtime dose of medication, if indicated. Such cooperative planning will require written consent from the patient and family, and the logistics of this will have to be considered prior to the initiation of pharmacotherapy.

Medication side effects such as drowsiness, direct cognitive difficulties arising as a result of the illness (such as concentration problems with depression), and psychological and social adaptations to the illness may all have an impact on school success. The physician who is actively involved in liaison with the school can suggest program modifications such as reducing course loads, tailoring courses to the child's strengths, allowing increased time for project completion, and using oral examination procedures. These kinds of interventions may be the key to the successful integration of pharmacotherapy and school performance.

Although many clinicians are sensitive to the practitioner-school interaction when treating young children, some may neglect this particular aspect of care when dealing with adolescents. However, the physician-school interface is equally important in this age group, and the clinician should take an active role in advocating for his patient with the responsible school personnel. Particularly important is the delicate balance between respecting the teenager's autonomy while at the same time providing the needed educational support to optimize treatment outcome without casting the adolescent into a sick role.

Academic Functioning—Practice Points

> 1. An evaluation of a child's or adolescent's academic functioning is a necessary component of the baseline assessment for psychopharmacologic treatment.
> 2. Depending on the results of the baseline assessment, specific educational diagnostic testing may be indicated.
> 3. Ongoing liaison with the child's or adolescent's school is needed to optimize treatment outcome.

Speech and Language Assessment

Speech and language problems are frequently found in child and adolescent psychiatric populations. In some cases they may occur as part of the pathoetiology of the disorder; in other cases they may reflect central nervous system maturation or development problems; and in still others they may occur independently of the psychiatric illness. When severe, as in autism, speech and language problems are not difficult to identify. In most disorders, however, the speech and language problems are more subtle, and their identification requires attention on the part of the assessing clinician. Because the presence of a speech or language problem may require specialist evaluation and intervention, the clinician should perform a screening assessment of speech and language function at the time of diagnostic evaluation.

Clarification of the age at which the child first began to speak in two- to three-word phrases (usually beginning at about 18 months) is a useful starting point. Children who fail to acquire phrase speech by 2.5 years should be considered as demonstrating speech delay and require further evaluation. During the clinical interviews, particular attention should be paid to the child's level of comprehension. If there are concerns about this (the child seems "spacey" or "in a fog," makes comments out of context, or seems to be forgetting instructions or simple information), then further evaluation of auditory comprehension, auditory memory, and attention is warranted.

Speech articulation problems are generally less likely to indicate a central nervous system language processing problem, and the normal variability in the developmental gradient of pronouncing specific letters must be considered. Nevertheless, articulation problems may lead to psychosocial or academic difficulties and should be treated when they cause functional impairment.

More recently, a child's pragmatic skills are being subjected to closer scrutiny. If difficulties such as waiting one's turn in a conversation, maintaining appropriate distance between self and other, and being unable to appreciate what further information the listener needs to understand what is being said are apparent, further evaluation of this part of language function is indicated. In some cases a problem in pragmatic function in the presence of normal comprehension and auditory memory may suggest a clinical picture of Asperger's syndrome.

Speech and Language Screening—Practice Points

1. The clinician should be aware of speech and language problems that may arise in the context of a psychiatric disorder.
2. Baseline screening for speech and language problems should include a history of language development as well as assessment of verbal comprehension, verbal memory and attention, articulation, and the pragmatic aspects of language.

Institutional Assessment

Although the term *assessment* is perhaps inappropriate for the evaluation that the psychopharmacologist should make about the institutional context of his patient, an awareness of particular institutional issues is necessary for conducting optimal psychopharmacologic treatment.

Children and adolescents spend much of their time in institutions. For most this institution is a community or private school. For some, it is a therapeutic environment, such as a day hospital, group home, or other residential facility. For others, it is a correctional setting. Staff attitudes and institutional cultures can be very important in providing for successful pharmacologic interventions. The active participation of institution staff, such as teachers or childcare workers, may be required for informant input regarding treatment outcome. Indeed, sometimes the request for psychiatric intervention has come from the institution because of staff concerns about the child's mood or behavior.

CASE EXAMPLE

When Supports Do Not Support

J.I. and E.N. were 18-year-old boys with schizophrenia living in two different mental health group homes. Both were outpatients in the same hospital medication clinic and participated in the same day treatment program, where they had become friends. Both J.I. and E.N. were being treated with injectable neuroleptic medications and had experienced good symptomatic control of their illness with minimal side effects. Both had been in remission for about a year. At one clinic visit E.N. announced quite unexpectedly that he had decided to stop taking his medications. His stated reason was that he needed to be in control of his treatment. He was adamant that the medicines were not helping him but were keeping him in a "chemical straitjacket." His opposition to continued treatment was intense and out of keeping with his usual attitudes to medications. At one point in the conversation he threatened to sue the doctor if any more medicine was given to him, stating, "You can't assault me like that." There was no evidence of any psychotic symptoms.

A meeting held with staff in E.N.'s group home to discuss this issue revealed that a new "house director" had been appointed some 5 weeks earlier. This director held very strong negative opinions about the use of medication to treat psychotic illness and confronted the physician about using "chemical straitjackets" to "control people who were different." She had advised E.N. and a number of other residents to stop taking their medicines and had suggested that they consider charging the doctor who was prescribing the medications with assault.

Discussion of this issue proved fruitless, and even the intervention of E.N.'s parents and the advice of his friend J.I. were not sufficient to change E.N.'s mind. Eight months following this episode, E.N. stopped attending his day program. Soon thereafter he was admitted to another hospital in an acute psychotic state.

CASE COMMENTARY

Although not all institutional opposition to medication treatment is as dramatic or obvious as described in this case, nevertheless, it does occur. Furthermore, unlike this example, such opposition may be more difficult to identify when the negative views about pharmacotherapy are more subtle. For example, a member of the staff might "forget" to dispense the medication or "forget" to complete routine evaluations of mood or behaviors. Should such issues arise with some frequency, an urgent meeting between the physician and institutional staff is necessary.

In many cases, the participation of institutional staff in structuring or monitoring psychopharmacologic treatment occurs in a reasonable and positive manner. Successful cooperation between clinician and an institutional setting is often possible and is usually based on the following foundations:

1. Face-to-face meetings at the onset of treatment
2. Education about the disorder, the medications, and the medication treatment goals
3. Staff training for specific monitoring tasks (such as use of rating scales)
4. Ongoing communication between clinician and institution

Face-to-Face Meetings at Treatment Onset

Although a meeting between the physician and institutional staff can be time consuming, it is nevertheless essential for building a positive cooperative climate. Such a meeting serves a number of useful functions. First, it allows for the development of a personal relationship between the clinician and staff of the institution. Second, it identifies who the child or adolescent's primary caregivers will be. Third, it identifies a liaison person from the institution (in some cases this may be the child's primary caregiver). Fourth, it identifies a structure for communication between institution and clinician. This should include both routine, regularly scheduled feedback sessions and procedures for contacting the clinician or institutional representative when an urgent problem arises. Fifth, such a meeting provides a forum for sharing the results of the child's or adolescent's assessment and providing education to the institution staff about the nature of the illness, target symptoms of pharmacologic treatment, optimal combinations of other treatment strategies with medications, expected outcome with psychopharmacologic treatment, nature and type of evaluation of treatment, and information about medication delivery (doses, time of day) and anticipated adverse events.

Education About the Disorder, the Medications, and Medication Treatment Goals

Reviewing the details of the baseline assessment with institutional representatives is essential. This review not only will provide them with a good thumbnail sketch of the child's functioning across a variety of dimensions, but will be of value as they work to develop institution-based interventions that will complement psychotropic treatment. Useful discussion about how to proceed with a variety of psychological, social, and educational interventions should arise from such a review.

It is useful for the clinician to review the diagnosis and to provide education about the child's or adolescent's disorder. It is not enough to state that a young teenager suffers from schizophrenia. A discussion of what the disease is, its phenomenology, how it is expressed in this particular adolescent, its optimal treatment, and its prognosis is a necessary part of this education. In addition, suggestions of further readings or the provision of educational materials about the illness is usually welcomed by most institutional staff, who by and large are interested in learning more about the illnesses that afflict the children and teenagers with whom they are working.

Education about the medications a client is taking is essential. In some cases the staff will already be somewhat familiar with a specific medication, if, for instance, other children or teenagers they have been involved with have taken the same or a similar drug. Still, a review of the medication, including its anticipated therapeutic effect, potential adverse effects, and limitations is necessary. Clinical experience suggests that in many cases information about medications is not known by the staff, often because it has never before been provided. In some cases incorrect or "off-base" information about a specific medication may have been acquired by some staff members. In this case the medication education review will serve to clarify and correct such misconceptions.

As part of this "meducation" discussion, the clinician should make available to the institution staff medication information material that is similar to that provided to the patient. These handouts or readings will be of great value to the treatment staff, particularly with regard to discussions of potential adverse effects. Not only should these effects be identified and described, but the staff needs to review how they should be dealt with if they arise. For example, it is not usually helpful for the clinician to tell a day treatment mental health worker to "watch out for dystonia." Instead, the clinician should describe what a dystonia is, how it manifests itself, and what the staff member should do if she suspects this is occurring. It is useful for the institutional staff to have immediate telephone access to the clinician should an urgent problem arise.

The clinician should also remember to discuss with the institution staff what the targets of medication treatment are, what the expected time line for improvement is, and how improvement will be determined. Equally as important, the clinician must clarify the limits of the effects of medication. In many cases teachers and other institutional staff have unrealistic expectations about what medication treatment can actually achieve. In some cases these expectations will be too high or will be directed toward problems that are not amenable to modification by psychotropics. In such cases treatment staff may become disillusioned with what they perceive to be minimal gains. On the other hand, some staff members may have unrealistically low expectations of medication treatment. These may range from such ideas as "medicines will not help" to an acceptance of suboptimal symptom response to psychopharmacologic treatment because they do not appreciate what the maximal potential response can be. In this case treatment staff may avoid using the medications entirely or may fail to optimize pharmacologic therapy. A frank and detailed discussion of these issues will help the institutional staff better understand the parameters of psychopharmacologic treatment.

If staff of an institution will be dispensing medication (such as a noon-hour dose of methylphenidate), it is important that the physician review with them the dose and dose timing. Staff members will also need to know what to do if medication doses are inadvertently missed. And they will need advice on how to proceed if they are concerned that the presence of side effects may make an additional medication dose at a prescribed time inadvisable. These and other issues arising from staff involvement in dispensing medications should be addressed and discussed by the prescribing clinician.

Staff Training for Specific Monitoring Tasks

Whenever informant rating scales are used in an institutional setting to assess treatment outcome, it is the responsibility of the physician to elicit the cooperation of the individuals who are performing this function. In some settings this may already be in place, while in others it may need to be part of the education about the disorder and its treatment. If institutional staff input is necessary

for monitoring outcome, it is essential that the clinician ensure that staff members who will be doing the evaluative tasks (such as completing symptom rating scales) are properly trained in the use of the instruments. If this training has not previously taken place, or if the clinician is uncertain as to the reliability of the information that will be obtained, the clinician must provide the necessary training.

While the need for proper training applies to all institutional settings, it is of particular importance in a community or private school setting, where the clinician is working with teachers who may not have had the training necessary to participate properly in such a venture. The time and effort spent by the physician in meetings, discussion, and training at the onset of monitoring will prove invaluable later. Regular communication throughout the monitoring period is also necessary, and feedback of the results to the staff member (teacher or childcare worker) at the conclusion of every treatment trial is vital.

Ongoing Communication Between Clinician and Institution

Ongoing communication with a school or treatment center is of value, particularly when pharmacotherapy is long term and the medications or the illness may have an impact on a child's or adolescent's ability to perform adequately in the classroom or other social setting. In this context, it is important that the clinician share information about the patient's status with institution personnel. In a school setting, modifications to the school curriculum or academic expectations may need to be made to optimize a child's or adolescent's school success. In this case, cooperative planning involving the clinician, patient/family, and school is necessary. In other institutional settings, such as day treatment or residential programs, changes in the child's or adolescent's clinical status may require modification of pharmacologic or nonpharmacologic treatments. Such modifications will require discussion and joint planning between institution staff and the prescribing clinician.

Two clinically useful strategies for optimizing ongoing communication between the clinician and an institution are the identification and use of a preset structure of clinician-institution meetings and the clarification of responsibilities for therapeutic decision making.

A child's or adolescent's ongoing psychopharmacologic treatment will be enhanced if regular meetings are held between the clinician and institution staff to review the child's progress and to chart future interventions. Such meetings should be scheduled on the basis of the clinical situation of the child or adolescent. In some cases, for example, soon after admission to an institution or during periods of symptom exacerbation — when the child's clinical situation is somewhat unstable — these meetings may need to be held more frequently, as often as once every week or two. At other times, if a child's or adolescent's clinical condition is relatively stable, such meetings can be held less frequently. Even in the presence of a stable clinical condition, however, these meetings should be held. Once every 3 to 4 months is a useful guideline. Not only will this structure ensure the maintenance of the important personal connection between the clinician and the institution staff, but such meetings can be used for educational purposes or for developing strategies regarding maximization of the patient's treatment outcome.

In addition, the clinician should ensure his availability if an emergency situation regarding the use of psychotropics (such as an acute dystonia or an overdose) occurs. The clinician's telephone number should be kept by the institution, and contingency plans should be made, including use of an appropriate emergency facility, in the event that the clinician or his delegate cannot be reached or a life-threatening situation requiring immediate medical intervention occurs.

Clarification of the roles of various caregivers is necessary for optimal clinician-institution cooperation. Ideally, this should be done at the time of the first meeting between the clinician and institution staff. Otherwise, clinical experience clearly indicates that confusion and conflict among the various caregivers often arise. For the clinician, it is important that she clarify who will be responsible for making the decisions about overall treatment planning. In some cases the clinician will be solely charged with this responsibility. In other cases the clinician will have little or no say in overall treatment strategy, and her role will be limited to that of a consultant on medical or psychopharmacologic issues alone. In still other cases this responsibility will be shared by the various caregivers. In this situation the clinician must be certain that decision-making guidelines are clear and that an appropriate structure exists for dealing with potential conflicts about treatment decisions.

Furthermore, a physician prescribing psychotropic medications for a child or adolescent must ensure that institution staff not inadvertently "double doctor." And the clinician prescribing psychotropic medications must insist on being informed if the patient is seen by another physician and is prescribed medication, regardless of the type of medication. At the very least, this will serve as a check on potential drug-drug interactions that some physicians who are less experienced in the use of psychopharmacologic compounds in children and adolescents may not anticipate. In all cases in which ongoing cooperative care is carried out, however, the clinician must ensure that he is aware of and understands the legal ramifications of those responsibilities involved in the ongoing joint care of a patient. These are discussed further in Section Three.

Institutional Assessment—Practice Points

1. Understanding the institutional context in which the child or adolescent operates is important for providing optimal psychopharmacotherapy.
2. Institutional factors such as staff biases may affect treatment outcome and need to be identified and discussed.
3. Ongoing cooperative liaison with schools, correctional facilities, and other treatment centers will be necessary to properly evaluate treatment outcome and to provide long-term psychopharmacologic care.

SUGGESTED READINGS

Berger M. Psychological tests and assessment. In M Rutter, E Taylor, L Hersov (eds): Child and Adolescent Psychiatry: Modern Approaches. London: Blackwell Scientific Publications, 1994, pp 94–109.

Doll EA. Vineland Social Maturity Scale: Manual of Directions (revised). Circle Pines, MN: American Guidance Service, 1965.

Howell KE, Morehead MK. Curriculum-Based Evaluation for Special and Remedial Education. Columbus, OH: Merrill, 1987.

Jansky JJ. Assessment of learning disabilities. In C Kestenbaum, DT Williams (eds): Handbook of Clinical Assessment of Children and Adolescents, Vol. 1. New York: New York University Press, 1988, pp 296–311.

Quackenbush D, Kutcher S, Robertson H, Boulos C, Chaban P. Premorbid and postmorbid school functioning in bipolar adolescents: Description and suggested academic interventions. Canadian Journal of Psychiatry, 41:1–7, 1996.

Racusin GR, Moss NE. Psychological assessment of children and adolescents. In M Lewis (ed): Child and Adolescent Psychiatry: A Comprehensive Textbook. Baltimore: Williams and Wilkins, 1991, pp 472–485.

Reynolds C, Kamphaus R (eds). Handbook of Psychological and Educational Assessment of Children. New York: Guilford Press, 1988.

Shinn MR (ed). Curriculum-Based Measurement: Assessing Special Children. New York: Guilford Press, 1989.

Towbin KE. Evaluation, establishing the treatment alliance, and informed consent. Child and Adolescent Psychiatric Clinics of North America, 4:1–14, 1995.

Planning, Initiating, and Providing Psychopharmacologic Treatment

The following practical issues that impact on the success of pharmacologic interventions for child and adolescent psychiatric disorders need to be considered and dealt with in the planning and initiation of psychopharmacologic treatment:

1. Patient and parent education about the child's or adolescent's illness
2. Patient and parent education about psychopharmacologic treatment
3. Patient and parent education about specific medications
4. Clinical setting
5. Common practical issues in psychopharmacologic treatment
6. Design of psychopharmacologic treatment trials
7. Consent to psychopharmacologic treatment

This section includes two chapters that deal with these issues. Chapter 6 deals with the importance and practical aspects of providing education to patients and their families regarding the specific psychiatric disorders and how they should be treated. In addition, this chapter provides useful clinical guidelines as to how to deal with information about psychopharmacologic treatment in general and specific medication education strategies. Chapter 7 provides information on how to structure an outpatient clinical service to provide for optimal psychopharmacologic treatment for children and adolescents. Common problems encountered by clinicians when initiating and continuing psychotropic interventions are discussed. Finally, the important issue of consent to treatment and some useful strategies for designing treatment trials with psychotropic medications are reviewed.

Educational Issues in Child and Adolescent Psychopharmacology

An educational approach to understanding the child's or adolescent's psychiatric disorder and its treatment is a fundamental principle that underlies the provision of psychopharmacologic care. This approach to treatment involves a therapeutic relationship among the clinician, patient, and parent that is based on a joint understanding of the problem and an informed joint decision on how it should be treated. The patient and his family are encouraged, and indeed actively helped, to be informed consumers about their psychopharmacologic care. Responsibility for treatment is shared among the clinician, the patient, and the family (if applicable). This is a very different approach to treatment than that advocated by many psychodynamic or family therapy practices. In this pharmacologic treatment paradigm, the clinician takes on the role of a good medical practitioner whose job it is to understand the patient and to work with the patient and, when appropriate, the patient's family to ameliorate the signs, symptoms, and functional disturbances that, when taken together, define a psychiatric disorder.

Patient and Parent Education About the Child's or Adolescent's Illness

Children, adolescents, and their families often come to psychiatric attention already carrying a stigma. Many feel, often with some justification, that their friends, acquaintances, teachers, or employers will look down on them, think less of them, or demonstrate prejudicial feelings toward them because they or their child has a mental illness. In some cases concern about this stigma has led them to avoid or delay treatment until the problems have become so severe that available support and coping mechanisms have broken down. In some cases these children, teens, or their families are further burdened by self-blame and self-doubt. Often such views have been encouraged by commonly held ideas that people who develop a mental illness are somehow "deviant" or "constitutionally weak" or "less than a whole human being." In many cases parents blame themselves, feeling that they have "somehow failed my child" or "caused this to happen to him." Again, such views are often encouraged by popular albeit incorrect understandings of the pathoetiology of psychiatric disorders.

One of the first tasks of the clinician is to be sensitive to how the child or adolescent and his parents (and other family members) feel about the illness. In many cases supportive listening followed by a discussion of the psychiatric illness as another type of medical disorder will be very helpful to both patient and family. In this discussion it is useful to use well-known and popularly understood analogies in which psychiatric disorders can be compared with medical illnesses. For example, many patients and their families know about someone or even know someone who has a seizure disorder. In most cases people will understand that although the seizures themselves may seem unusual or frightening, they are merely manifestations of a body part (in this case the brain) that is not functioning optimally. Some patients or their parents may also know that it was not that long ago that people who had seizure disorders were shunned, thought to be possessed, or ostracized. As improved understanding about the causes of seizures and better treatments for them developed, this negative but popular view gradually changed. Now most people with a seizure disorder are treated no differently from anyone else with a chronic medical disorder such as diabetes or rheumatoid arthritis.

The use of such educational analogies will in many cases help patients and their families begin to deal with the social stigma surrounding psychiatric illnesses, which, although changing, is still unfortunately too common. Furthermore, a patient and his parents should be told what the psychiatric diagnosis is and what this diagnosis means. It is altogether too common in a consultative clinical practice to see children and adolescents who have a clear psychiatric diagnosis (such as schizophrenia, bipolar disorder, generalized anxiety disorder [GAD], etc.) who say that they have never been told what their diagnosis is. Often this lack of information is not caused by poor diagnostic ascertainment on the part of a previous clinical assessment. The diagnosis may be even documented in the patient's clinical record, yet the patient or parent does not seem to know what it is.

Sometimes this lack of information may be caused by denial on the part of the patient or parents. At other times patients or parents may profess not to know in order to check or validate what they have already been told against another clinician's opinion. However, clinical experience suggests that although such cases do occur, in many instances the patient or parent has never been told what the psychiatric diagnosis is.

There is no reason to withhold a psychiatric diagnosis from a patient or parent. Patients need to know what they are dealing with in order to engage in the necessary psychological processes that should accompany such knowledge. On a pragmatic level, they will need to know a diagnosis in order to have some idea about the expected outcome and to be able to work effectively with mental health professionals to plan appropriate treatments.

Some clinicians may feel that providing a patient with a psychiatric diagnosis is a form of social disgrace, a type of negative labeling that in and of itself will predict a negative outcome. Such viewpoints have had their day and have been found wanting. There is simply no reasonable evidence to support this type of argument. Others may feel that the use of nonspecific identifiers will be better accepted by the patient or family. As one practitioner explained, "It won't be so hard for them to deal with the idea that their child has an emotional problem as it will be for them to deal with the idea that their child has schizophrenia." This type of diagnostic euphemism and the thinking that accompanies it have no role in the psychopharmacologic treatment of children and adoles-

cents. Not only does this perspective demonstrate a poor understanding of the psychological coping processes that patients and their families need to deal with in the face of a psychiatric illness, but it assumes that the patient and family are incapable of understanding or dealing with reality. This is clearly not a good foundation on which to build a treatment alliance.

Given the importance of informing the patient and parents of the psychiatric diagnosis, the purpose and limits of the diagnosis must be also explained to them. As discussed previously, a psychiatric diagnosis is a hypothesis that suggests a particular prognosis and directs treatment. It needs to be critically evaluated over time, as the response to treatment becomes clear and new information is obtained. This caveat about the child's or adolescent's diagnosis should not, however, be presented in such a way as to raise false hopes in either patient or parent. In all cases the clinician must be clear about the limitations of his understanding, yet comfortable in the presentation of the psychiatric diagnosis.

The clinician must also explain what is meant by a particular psychiatric diagnosis. In many cases the patient or parent will have a popular yet incorrect appreciation of what a particular psychiatric diagnosis is actually describing. For example, many people still think that *schizophrenia* means the same thing as "split personality." In other cases patients and their parents will need to know the difference between the use of a particular term in describing a common and nonpathological state and its use as a psychiatric diagnosis. One such often confused term is *depression,* which to many people means an expected, ubiquitous, and self-limiting mood of relatively short duration, while to the clinician it means a pathological state characterized by specific persistent and significant affective, cognitive, behavioral, and vegetative disturbances accompanied by serious functional difficulties. It is important that the clinician and patient are speaking the same language.

In some cases a clear-cut psychiatric diagnosis may not be possible. In this case the physician must identify one or more tentative diagnoses and decide on one provisionally. This decision and the reasoning behind it should be shared with the patient and family as appropriate. In many cases presenting a number of alternatives when the clinician is himself unsure has the effect of enlisting the patient or parents in the process of further diagnostic clarification.

Once a psychiatric diagnosis has been established and shared with the patient and family, a frank and informative discussion abut the illness can begin. In most cases the patient and family are relieved to discover that the difficulties can be understood, that a fair amount is known about the problem, and that there is something that can be done to help.

Education about the child's or adolescent's psychiatric disorder should ideally take place within three different but related contexts. These are (1) discussions with the clinician about the illness, (2) reading about the illness, and (3) organized community or institutional resources.

Discussions with the Clinician

The clinician must be certain to provide sufficient time to discuss the illness with the patient and the family. Discussion should include an outline of how the disorder is characterized, some idea of the current understanding about its pathoetiology, and what its expected outcome—treated and untreated—might be. This information must be presented in a developmentally appropriate manner so as to facilitate understanding. In many cases, and always when young children are involved, the clinician must explain the illness in language that the child as well as the parent can understand. Often this necessitates two levels of explanation, with one being easily interchanged with the other as the clinician alternates between addressing the child and the parent.

"Doctorspeak" should be avoided. Patients and parents will not usually understand what is meant by the phrase "you have a formal thought disorder complicated by systematized delusional material and auditory hallucinatory experiences." They are much more likely to appreciate the information that is conveyed in everyday language, such as, "Your mind is often playing tricks on you, making you think things are happening that are not really happening, and making you hear and see things that are not really there." Medical or psychiatric terms that the patient or family will need to know should be introduced and defined. For example, if the patient is psychotic, the patient and family will need to know what is meant by the word "delusion."

The discussion should be structured so as to allow the child or adolescent and parents to ask questions about the diagnosis and all aspects of the illness itself. It is usually best to deal with these questions as they arise and not to save them until the end of a long and tedious monologue. Every attempt should be made to ensure that, as much as possible, a two-way flow of communication occurs. And it is unrealistic to expect the patient or parents to absorb all the information provided or to raise all the questions that they have in one sitting. In most cases additional meetings scheduled soon after the first will be necessary.

Finally, it must be emphasized that this information-sharing and educational discussion is not a lecture to a classroom of eager but emotionally uninvolved students. On the contrary, effective illness education is a therapeutic encounter in which the fears, worries, and emotional distress of the patient and family must be anticipated, explored, and sensitively dealt with.

Reading About the Illness

The clinician should encourage the patient and parents to read about the illness. If possible, at the initial discussion the practitioner should provide some written information about the diagnosis and the disorder. Useful handouts suitable for clinic use are available through a variety of sources. In general, professional organizations such as the American Academy of Child and Adolescent Psychiatry provide user-friendly information packages that can be purchased by the clinician at a nominal cost. This type of information should be made freely available to patients and family.

The physician should also have available a printed list of books and magazine articles that address specific psychiatric illnesses of children and adolescents. Such a list will be useful to the patient and parents as they seek appropriate information.

Finally, the clinician should be as flexible as possible in supporting the patient's or parent's search for information about the illness. In some cases this search may lead to information that is not only incorrect but potentially harmful. In other cases this will lead to information that is out-of-date and based on an understanding of psychiatric illness that has not stood the test of time or empirical research. This type of broad net approach is not to be avoided. On the contrary, it is to be encouraged because it will allow the patient or family to raise conflicting issues with the clinician and to engage in a frank and critical review of the value of this information. It is much better that these issues arise openly and are addressed at the onset of treatment than that they remain hidden and make themselves known at a later date.

Organized Community or Institutional Resources

Many patients or their families find that illness-specific support groups (such as the National Depressive, Manic-Depressive Association, The Schizophrenia Society, and the Attention-Deficit Hyperactivity Support Group) provide helpful and at times therapeutic resources. Such groups are also able to suggest useful reading material about specific psychiatric disorders and may be able to provide books, articles, videos, or other educational materials, often at minimal cost. The clinician should refer the patient and parents to the closest appropriate community support group.

Many clinicians find it helpful to give patients and their parents a single-page handout that identifies the diagnosis, lists suggested treatments, and identifies sources for further self-directed education about the illness. A prototype of such a useful form (Diagnosis and Treatment Suggestions) can be found in Table 6–1.

Patient and Parent Education About Psychiatric Illness—Practice Points

1. Be sensitive to what having a psychiatric illness means for a patient and his family.
2. Clearly inform the patient and family of the psychiatric diagnosis and explain in understandable terms what it means.
3. Encourage and assist the patient and family to pursue self-education about the illness.

TABLE 6–1 Diagnosis and Treatment Suggestions for Child and Adolescent Psychopharmacology

This single-page outline is being provided for you as a summary of your (your child's) psychiatric diagnosis and potentially useful treatments. Sources that your doctor feels are useful for you to consult for further information about the diagnosis and its treatment are also listed. Please review some or all of these prior to your next meeting with the doctor so that you will have an opportunity to find out more about the diagnosis and its treatments. If you wish to consult sources of information not listed below, please feel free to do so. Bring any questions that you have regarding your (your child's) diagnosis to the next meeting and discuss them with your doctor.

Provisional Diagnosis:

Other Related Diagnoses:

Other Possible Diagnoses:

Treatment Options:

	Pharmacologic	Psychological	Family	Other
1.				
2.				
3.				
4.				
5.				

Treatments that your doctor feels may be most useful to begin with are identified with a check mark.

Suggested Sources of Further Information:

1.

2.

3.

4.

5.

Patient and Parent Education About Psychopharmacologic Treatment

The success of psychopharmacologic treatment depends a great deal not only on the proper choice of the specific medication for a particular disorder or symptom but also on the compliance of the patient with the prescribed treatment. *Compliance* may be defined as patient adherence to a specific treatment plan developed conjointly by patient and physician. In the psychopharmacologic treatment of children and adolescents, the issue of compliance is much more complicated than with adults because not only the patient but also the parents, other family members, and often institutions or legal authorities may be involved. Thus, with the addition of various layers of interested parties, all with their own perspectives and viewpoints, a greater likelihood of problems leading to treatment noncompliance arises. Many factors contribute to patient compliance, but the following factors are the most common reasons patients prematurely discontinue a potentially effective treatment:

1. Side effects of treatment
2. Initial clinical improvement
3. Denial of illness
4. Family, peer, or social pressure
5. Confusion about the illness or its optimal treatment
6. Idiosyncratic personal reasons ("meaning" of medication use)
7. Effects of the illness itself (e.g., hopeless, delusions about poisoning)
8. Previous negative experience with medical treatments
9. Previous negative experience with psychotropic medications
10. Cost of treatment
11. Misinformation about psychotropics (e.g., drugs are addictive)
12. Unreliability of responsible adult (e.g., medication dispensing)

Although it may not be possible to fully address all the reasons for noncompliance for any single patient, and no one of these issues is known to predominate in determining noncompliance, many of these issues may be effectively dealt with in the context of a supportive and respectful therapeutic relationship in which the patient and family understand the various essential aspects of pharmacologic treatment.

The importance of this therapeutic relationship cannot be overemphasized. Psychopharmacologic treatment is not simply the act of prescribing a medication. It is a comprehensive approach to the physician-patient relationship that is based on these specific principles:

1. Competency
2. Collaboration
3. Evaluative-based care
4. Flexibility
5. Effective communication

These five issues must be identified and practically addressed to improve the probability of success with pharmacotherapy. Although in actual practice they overlap, they are discussed here separately to highlight the complexities and importance of each.

Competency

The physician must demonstrate competency in a variety of areas, including psychiatric diagnosis; course and natural history of psychiatric illnesses; detailed knowledge about a variety of potential treatments (including biological and nonbiological) for specific disorders or symptoms; knowledge about specific medications, including their pharmacokinetics and pharmacodynamics; and potential side effects and drug interactions. Psychopharmacologic treatment is directed toward ameliorating either specific psychiatric syndromes or particular behavioral, mood, or cognitive symptoms. A particular psychopharmacologic treatment is indicated by the type of disorder, the nature of the symptoms, or both. Choosing the correct medication requires the ability to determine exactly what medicine is needed, what medicine is not to be used, what condition or symptom the medicine is being prescribed for, how much of the medication is needed, and how long it is needed.

In most cases in child and adolescent psychiatry, medications are part of a comprehensive treatment program that may contain a variety of behavioral or other psychosocial interventions. In many cases medications not only will improve a child's or adolescent's symptoms and functioning but will also enhance the efficacy of psychosocial interventions. Optimal psychopharmacologic treatment is thus realized when applied concurrently with interventions specifically designed to ameliorate a number of aspects of the child's or adolescent's difficulties. The physician, therefore, must know which other types of treatment are likely to be helpful, not only to decide if or when to prescribe a medication (perhaps nonmedical rather than pharmacologic treatments are indicated, such as exposure therapy for phobias) but also to determine whether adding a medication to an ongoing psychosocial treatment is likely to be worthwhile. For example, adding an antidepressant medication to primal scream therapy as a treatment for adolescent depression is less likely to be therapeutically useful than adding an antidepressant to cognitive-behavioral treatment.

Physicians need to know when a medication is indicated for treatment and what type of medication is indicated, as well as when a medication is not indicated for treatment. Compared with adult psychiatry, in child and adolescent psychopharmacology clinical decision making regarding optimal use of psychotropics is more difficult because research in this area is not comprehensive and enough may not have been completed to allow for the establishment of clear guidelines. In such cases the physician must not only recognize the limits of his own knowledge but must also be able to deduce from the information that is available potentially helpful medication interventions. In addition, the physician must show the ability to properly use an objective methodology to assess and evaluate treatment. This is discussed further in Chapter 7.

A host of medications are currently available for treating mental illnesses in children and adolescents. For many disturbances more than one potentially useful drug is available. At times different classes of medications may provide useful results, such as lithium or valproate in the treatment of acute mania. The physician must be able to evaluate critically the various outcome probabilities of any one medication compared with a medication from an alternative class. Often this will occur in a situation of less than optimal information, in which the necessary head-to-head scientific comparisons will either not have been reported or indeed not have been conducted. In other cases, studies will indicate that different medications from the same general class of drugs (such as various antipsychotics) will have similar therapeutic effects. In this situation the choice of a specific agent may well be dictated by comparative side effect profiles or patient preference. The physician must be aware of these issues and can best prepare himself for dealing with them by acquiring in-depth knowledge about a number of compounds from each of the medication classes and by using these medications consistently.

For example, exhaustive knowledge about two or three tricyclic medicines should suffice for the optimal and rational use of this class of medications. These medicines, of course, should be selected on the basis of available knowledge about indications and side effects for each compound in the class, with the choice of the final few taking into account the need to properly characterize the class as a whole. To extend the tricyclic example further, the physician could choose from the following: imipramine—a primary amine with predominantly noradrenergic activity and demonstrated use in enuresis and attention-deficit hyperactivity disorder (ADHD); desipramine—a secondary amine with primarily noradrenergic activity with demonstrated use in attention-deficit hyperactivity disorder; and clomipramine—a mixed noradrenergic/serotonergic compound with demonstrated efficacy in obsessive compulsive disorder (OCD). Having chosen these three (or other reasonable selections), the clinician should then develop sufficient experience in their use. This experience is obtained by preferentially using the chosen tricyclic compounds consistently instead of choosing from the entire range of tricyclic possibilities. Using a small number of class-representative medications will over time lead to the development of expertise with each of these specific medications, an expertise that may take much longer to develop if the clinician tries to use all members of the tricyclic family that are currently available.

Finally, the physician must be able to recognize and acknowledge the limits of her knowledge. The phrases "I don't know" or "I am not sure" need to be part of every physician's language, but particularly so in a fledgling field such as child and adolescent psychopharmacology. Of course, these phrases need to be matched with, "But I know of a way to find out." Therapeutics in child and adolescent psychiatry in general are poorly studied, and clinicians' therapeutic choices may often rely more on physician preference and training than on demonstrated efficacy. While psychopharmacologic treatments generally derive from scientific and rigorous evidence, in many cases this knowledge is still fragmentary or deductive in nature. To pretend otherwise is to deceive the patient or the family. To acknowledge this while maintaining hope about the outcome of treatment and at the same time to apply what is known in a manner that allows for optimal evaluation of outcome are to initiate and manage potentially effective treatment. This is the task of the clinician.

CASE EXAMPLE

A Psychosis Is a Psychosis

P.H., a 17-year-old boy, was referred by his family physician for a second opinion because the physician was concerned that in spite of ongoing treatment P.H. was not improving. A diagnostic assessment revealed a withdrawn adolescent who would sit in a corner of the room and laugh quietly to himself. Although he avoided eye contact and showed no common social behaviors such as greeting the clinician, he would answer questions when directly asked.

A history of progressively withdrawn behavior over 1 to 2 years was elicited. At the time of referral he was not attending school, and while he had never had many friends, those few who he usually spent time with no longer contacted him. His personal hygiene had deteriorated, and he tended to sleep most days and watch television or video movies at night. He had covered the windows in his room with blankets and told his mother that he needed to do so to block out radiation.

On direct questioning, P.H. was found to be delusional. He described auditory hallucinations of two male voices, which often spoke to each other and made rude or humorous comments about people who were present in the room with him. He was convinced that radiation from space was being beamed at the earth, and thus he avoided the daylight and would go outside only after dark. He described messages on the television station that were being sent to him in code, although he could not identify exactly why that was occurring. He had told his friends about his concerns and, according to him, they teased him about these ideas so he had gradually begun to avoid them. He was concerned that they might be involved in a program of space radiation against the earth.

The family history was remarkable for "odd" and "eccentric" people on P.H.'s father's side. An aunt had been treated in a psychiatric hospital in another country. No diagnosis was known. Another aunt had lived the life of a recluse. Further information about the extended family was not available.

P.H.'s father was described by P.H.'s mother as "cool and distant." He had few friends and preferred to spend most of his nonworking time (he was employed as a computer programmer) working in his woodshop building "sets" for his extensive model train collection. P.H.'s mother worked as a salesclerk in a clothing store and enjoyed the company of many friends. P.H.'s parents noted that their marriage had been "on the rocks" for many years and that they had contemplated a divorce about 1 year ago. At that time P.H.'s behavior had become more noticeably problematic, and they sought assistance from their family physician, who referred them to a community mental health treatment program that specialized in family counseling. P.H.'s problems were identified as behavior designed to "keep his parents

together," and family therapy was offered. Seven months of weekly family therapy had been unsuccessful both in solving the parental relationship difficulties and in addressing P.H.'s behavior, which continued to deteriorate. The family stopped treatment, and P.H.'s parents decided to "wait until he grew out of the phase he was in." When a number of months passed with no improvement, they once again contacted their family physician, who referred P.H. for psychiatric evaluation.

CASE COMMENTARY

The case illustration of P.H.'s gradual development of a schizophrenic illness describes an unfortunate scenario in which a clear psychotic process with a classical presentation continued for a prolonged period of time without proper treatment. In P.H.'s case, a proper psychiatric diagnostic assessment was not completed, and his behavior was explained by the uncritical application of an inappropriate pathoetiologic model. Family difficulties were assumed to be "causing" the patient's problem, and insufficient attention was paid to P.H.'s obvious individual psychopathology. While his parents may well have benefited from psychotherapeutic help, that intervention alone was not sufficient or proper treatment in this case. Furthermore, when the chosen intervention showed little or no positive effect, no attempt was made to critically review the case to try to understand why the expected improvement had not occurred.

This case describes an all too common occurrence in the psychiatric treatment of children and adolescents, that is, the application of a single etiologic model as both the explanatory and treatment framework for behavioral disturbances in this population. In most cases, simple unidimensional or one-book models do not apply either in identification of psychoetiologies or in the application of single therapeutic approaches.

Physician competency is not enhanced by single-model constructs applied to a wide variety of patients, be those models hypotheses about pathoetiology or applications of specific treatment methods. It does not matter whether these constructs are psychological, social, or biologic, the competent clinician must use a variety of models to fully understand and effectively treat patients with psychiatric disorders. Furthermore, the competent clinician understands that she is using models and knows the limits of their applicability. Finally, the competent clinician realizes that models of understanding behavior may or may not pass the test of critical evaluation, that is, the demonstration that treatment based on particular pathoetiologic constructs actually works. Not only must the competent clinician know and be able to critically assess various theories of pathoetiologies and treatments, but she must be able to apply the most appropriate model for each individual patient and be prepared to change her understanding and type of treatment if initially optimally applied interventions are unsuccessful. In brief, if the model doesn't fit, the problem is probably more likely with the model than with the patient.

Collaboration (Patient, Parent, Physician)

The most useful framework of clinical care for modern-day psychopharmacologic treatment is that of collaboration between the physician and the patient and family—shared decision making—regarding treatment. Although the physician retains the role of "expert," this is not expressed through a dictatorial or paternalistic approach. Rather, the physician works together with the patient and family to provide information and to give advice. All aspects of decision making, including type of treatment, duration of treatment, methods of evaluation, and course of action if treatment is unsuccessful, are shared with the patient and family. Responsibility for compliance with the treatment plan is also shared. As one clinician so bluntly synthesized this perspective, "The physician's job is to give the best possible advice. The patient's [family's] is to make reasoned decisions about accepting the advice."

At times this process may prove to be challenging and in many cases will involve greater time spent with patient and family than would otherwise be allocated in a nonshared decision-making model. In some cases, the physician may have to intervene with a pharmacologic treatment, even if the patient or family is uncomfortable with it or opposed to it. Such cases are rare, however, and tend to arise only occasionally in emergency circumstances, such as neuroleptic treatment of acute psychosis in which the patient, family, or treatment staff are at risk or when a patient is incompetent to give consent. In these rare cases (discussed in more detail in Chapter 7 under issues of consent), the physician may revert to a model of care, in which emergency intervention occurs "in the child's best interests." Even in these situations, however, a therapeutic framework that approaches the collaborative model should be a goal, and a frank discussion of the physician's understanding of the clinical situation, an explanation of his responsibilities, and the acknowledgment of patient or parent disagreements are helpful in the maintenance of this therapeutic approach.

CASE EXAMPLE

Sharing the Decision Making About Treatment

B.C. was a 16-year-old girl with a nonpsychotic major depressive disorder of 7 weeks' duration. Her family history was positive for unipolar depression in both her mother's and father's relatives. Following a diagnostic evaluation and education about the illness, the physician met with the patient and her family to discuss treatment. Various psychotherapy options were outlined, including cognitive-behavioral treatment, interpersonal therapy, and social skills training. In addition, the use of various medications, such as serotonin-specific reuptake inhibitors (SSRIs), buspirone, and buproprion was discussed. Although the physician's advice was to combine an SSRI with cognitive psychotherapy, B.C. decided that she wished to pursue interpersonal therapy instead. Her family was willing to support her in this decision, and the therapy was arranged, with the proviso that if significant improvement had not occurred within 10 weeks, the issue of medication use would be reviewed.

Ten weeks later, B.C. and her family were seen once again. Her baseline Beck Depression Inventory (BDI) had dropped from 21 to 9, and her 17-item Hamilton Depression Rating Scale (HDRS) had decreased from 19 to 10. Although she still exhibited a number of depressive symptoms, many of these had substantially improved from the time of her previous assessment. Her parents reported that she was less moody and irritable and was more socially active, and they felt that she was "getting better." A decision was made for B.C. to continue in her interpersonal therapy for another 8 weeks and then to re-evaluate once again.

When next seen, B.C. was continuing to do well. Her BDI was now 6 and her HDRS score was 9. She no longer met diagnostic criteria for a major depressive disorder, and although she still exhibited some depressive symptoms (particularly difficulty in concentrating and sleep problems), they were mild. Her parents reported that she was "pretty well back to normal" and voiced no specific concerns about her. Both B.C. and her parents felt that her therapy was going well, and plans for discontinuation of weekly sessions and a setting up of monthly "psychotherapy boosters" had been made with B.C.'s therapist. Further discussion resulted in an exploration of the probability of future depressive episodes, the possibility of developing a bipolar disorder, the development of a signs and symptoms checklist (for relapse identification, see Appendix II) to be used if patient or parental concerns about B.C.'s mood arose, and the importance of early intervention in a future developing depressive or hypomanic episode. B.C. and her parents agreed to contact the physician again at any time in the future should her mood begin to change again.

CASE COMMENTARY

In this case, although the patient chose a treatment alternative other than that suggested by the physician, the collaborative model of shared decision making provided a framework for the physician to support the patient's choice (given that her decision was not unreasonable) and at the same time to offer a structure for objective evaluation of the therapeutic efficacy of that decision.

Application of this collaborative model does not mean that the physician abrogates his responsibility for patient care. Shared decision making does not mean that the clinician agrees to support any and all treatment decisions made by the patient or family. Should the patient choose an intervention that the physician knows is unlikely to be effective or potentially harmful, the physician does not "go along with it." In that scenario, the clinician is obliged to inform the patient (family) that he does not support the decision, and this should be written into the clinical record. However, even when this does occur, the physician does not "bar the door" should the patient and family wish to try a more reasonable alternative at a later time.

The decision-making process regarding clinician support of a treatment decision made by a patient or family is not always easy. At times it may be difficult to determine if the selected treatment is or is not reasonable. It may be even more difficult if the patient (or family) chose a treatment with which the clinician is less familiar. The questions in Table 6–2 should be asked by the clinician when a patient or family decides to choose a treatment that he has not recommended. If these questions can all be answered in the affirmative, the patient's/family's choice is much more likely to be reasonable than if one or more questions are answered in the negative. In uncertain cases the clinician may find that filling out this questionnaire with the patient and family is a useful therapeutic exercise.

The collaborative model of shared decision making is defined by the following nine essential components:

1. The physician respects the rights, abilities, and limitations of each patient and his or her family.
2. The physician provides clear and understandable information about the rationale,

TABLE 6–2 **Guideline Questions for Evaluating Patient and Family Decisions Regarding Nonrecommended Treatments***

Patient's Name: _____ Date: _____

Questions	Answers	
Has the treatment been properly shown to be effective in this condition?	Yes	No
Are the expected adverse effects of this treatment known to the patient, family?	Yes	No
Are the expected adverse effects of this treatment within reasonable limits?	Yes	No
Are there no contraindications for this treatment in this patient?	Yes	No
By choosing this treatment does the patient allow him/herself access to other clearly effective and less dangerous interventions?	Yes	No

*If one or more answers are scored "No," the clinician should carefully assess his support of the patient's/family's treatment decision.

efficacy, and availability of a number of treatment alternatives.

3. The physician provides advice as to potentially optimal treatment choices based on his knowledge of the expected outcome of various treatments, not on his "school" or "orientation."

4. The patient and/or family decides what type of treatment will be given.

5. As long as this decision is reasonable (i.e., the selected treatment appears to be effective, side effects of the selected treatment are within acceptable limits, the patient does not exhibit any contraindications to the selected treatment, and the patient does not deny himself access to a clearly more effective and less dangerous other form of treatment), the physician supports the patient and family decision.

6. The physician and patient/family identify the method by which, and time frame within which, treatment efficacy will be determined.

7. In case the selected treatment is not shown to be effective, alternative methods of treatment are discussed and provisionally agreed to before the outcome of the chosen method of treatment is evaluated.

8. Responsibility for the proper maintenance of the chosen treatment is shared by the patient/family and the physician.

9. Changes in the chosen treatment are to be made only following the agreement of all participating parties—physician, patient, and family.

The use of this collaborative model allows for a supportive, flexible approach to psychopharmacologic intervention, while at the same time firmly grounding psychiatric treatment within an evaluation-based paradigm.

Evaluative-Based Care

Therapies, whatever their nature, rationale, or theoretical orientation, must stand the scrutiny of objective evaluation. For all treatments it must be demonstrated using appropriate scientific methods that they:

1. Do what they are said to do
2. Do so within a reasonable time
3. Do not cause more harm than good
4. Do not deny the patient accessibility to other proven helpful treatments
5. Are cost effective

Although these characteristics are usually determined by methodologically rigorous large-scale studies in a variety of populations, they are demonstrated in everyday clinical care through the use of knowledge acquired from properly conducted treatment outcome studies and through the use of systematically applied and continuously measured criteria of outcome. Even in situations in which definitive information regarding a chosen intervention is available from multiple rigorously conducted treatment outcome studies, the use of within-treatment evaluative rigor is still necessary because data obtained from the analysis of population "means" may not be applicable in the case of any individual patient. In the absence of clear treatment guidelines derived from multiple scientifically valid investigations, this internal or within-treatment evaluative rigor is even more necessary.

For proper evaluation of treatment outcome, the following considerations must be met:

1. Treatment targets are clearly identified prior to treatment initiation.

2. Treatment targets are properly measured.

3. Optimal treatment strategies are followed.

4. Treatment targets are again properly measured following the application of optimal treatment strategies.

5. The measures of treatment targets at the completion of treatment are properly compared with those same treatment target measures that were conducted prior to treatment initiation.

CASE EXAMPLE

"Well, I think she's better, maybe?"

L.S. was an 8-year-old girl who had been diagnosed by her pediatrician as having Tourette's syndrome. She was referred for a psychopharmacologic assessment and treatment recommendations. A diagnosis of Tourette's syndrome was confirmed, and child and parents agreed to a medication trial of haloperidol. Treatment was initiated with a daily dose of 0.5 mg daily and was increased to 1.0 mg daily within 1 week.

After 4 weeks of continuous haloperidol treatment, a reassessment was completed. L.S. did not feel that the medications were helping. She stated that she was not having any more fun than previously, even though she had been taking the medicine, and stated that children at school were still teasing her. Furthermore, L.S. complained that she was getting headaches, which she attributed to the medicine.

L.S.'s parents felt that her tics had decreased in frequency but complained that her behavior at home had not improved. Specifically, they noted that she continued to argue with her brother and still would not take responsibility for keeping her room tidy. They also stated that L.S. was occasionally complaining of headaches. The physician noted a few mild facial tics during the office visit. There were no vocal utterances. He consulted his initial assessment note and found that he had written down, "a few mild to moderate facial tics" and "no vocalizations noted." L.S. wanted to stop the medications. Her parents wanted the dose increased.

CASE COMMENTARY

This case illustrates an all too common scenario in clinical treatment. The quandary regarding decisions about what next to do with L.S.'s medications arose out of a failure to apply the collaborative model of care within an evaluative-based context.

First, the physician had neglected to identify specific target symptoms for medication treatment with the child and her parents. Second, the physician had not completed any objective and valid baseline ratings of target symptoms or of potential side effects. Thus, when the time came to determine whether treatment had been effective, partially effective, or ineffective, the clinician had no objective measure of outcome by which to make this determination. The only criteria that were available to guide further treatment decisions were his own anecdotal typed notes and subjective opinions of the patient and her parents.

Furthermore, although the patient was complaining of headaches, the physician could not determine whether these were indeed treatment-emergent side effects or had been present prior to initiation of medications. Thus, the physician could not determine whether the headaches were a side effect of the medication. To further complicate matters, the expectations of the physician, child, and parents for the medication treatment were different. The physician expected the medication to decrease tic frequency. The patient expected the medication to make her have more fun and to stop the other children at school from teasing her. The parents expected the medication to improve their daughter's behavior at home. Conflict about how to proceed with further treatment arose because each participant in this process had different expectations (e.g., targets) of medication effect. Unfortunately, not all these targets were reasonable, and all were quite different one

from another. All these problems may have been avoided had a proper baseline assessment, education about medication treatment, and objective evaluation of treatment outcome using a collaborative care model been completed.

There is no place in psychopharmacologic practice for initiating interventions that do not include as part of their evaluation strategy adequate measures of treatment outcome across a variety of dimensions.

Flexibility

Psychopharmacologic treatment demands practitioner flexibility in the provision of care. This flexibility is of two sorts. First, the practitioner must be able to "go with the flow" and at times support reasonable patient decisions about treatment that in her opinion may not be the first choice, as in the case of B.C.

The second dimension of flexibility is that of the practical structure of the kind of clinical care that is delivered by the physician. Patient need and not practitioner preference or traditional practice is the model used in the delivery of psychopharmacologic care.

CASE EXAMPLE

How Often and for How Long Do I Need to See You?

Y.N. was an 18-year-old girl who presented with a 3-month history of panic attacks. Although she had experienced a few episodes of panic attacks 3 years earlier, they had been mild and infrequent. At that time she had been assessed and had been taught cognitive approaches, which had been successful in dealing with these attacks. Because this psychotherapeutic strategy was effective, it was felt that pharmacologic treatment was not indicated. She agreed to return to the physician if the problem became too much for her.

At the time of her second assessment she was experiencing between 6 and 10 full-symptom panic attacks per week. Her cognitive techniques, which she was continuing to apply, were no longer helpful in controlling her symptoms. Although most of her panic attacks were described as mild or moderate, one or two each week were quite severe. She described anticipatory anxiety and identified phobic avoidance, particularly of grocery stores, because a particularly severe attack had occurred while she had been waiting in line at the supermarket 2 weeks earlier.

After appropriate baseline evaluation, Y.N. chose pharmacologic treatment with clonazepam to augment her cognitive interventions. This was initiated with a test dose of 0.25 mg given at noon on the day after her official visit. Because Y.N. was anxious about taking the medication, she asked to speak to the physician at the time she took her first tablet. This was accommodated by having her telephone the doctor at the time she was taking the first tablet and about 1 hour later, although she was told that if she needed to, she could call before the hour had passed.

When Y.N. called postmedication ingestion, she was happy to report that she was not experiencing any side effects, something she had been worried would occur immediately following the first medication dose. She was instructed to take clonazepam at a dose of 0.25 mg daily 1 hour before bedtime, was given an appointment in 3 days, and was instructed to call the physician if any problems with her medications occurred.

Y.N. was seen as scheduled for about one-half hour, during which time her symptoms and side effects were reviewed. The dose was raised to 0.25 mg, given twice daily, and she was scheduled to be seen again in 3 days. Two days following the last appointment, she called to say that she was experiencing a "terrible panic attack" and accepted reassurance and support over the telephone. At her next visit her medication was increased to 1 mg daily in divided doses, and she was scheduled to be seen in 3 days. Two days later she called to say that she was feeling "really good" and that she just wanted to let her doctor know that she was experiencing no side effects. She kept her next appointment and reported a significant decrease in her panic attacks. She was reminded that a period longer than 2 days (the length of time that she had been feeling "great") was needed to properly evaluate the potential therapeutic effect of the medicine.

Her dose was maintained at 1 mg daily, and she decided that her next visit could wait until a week had passed. About 5 days later, she telephoned to say that she had experienced two mild panic attacks but had been able to apply her cognitive techniques, which she felt had helped. When seen at her next appointment, her panic attacks diary showed only two mild partial symptom attacks, each lasting for less than 5 minutes, over the past week. She still reported anticipatory anxiety, but this had decreased greatly and, although she still felt "queasy" about going into grocery stores, she was not avoiding them as before. She was experiencing no side effects and felt that she should be able to "go for 2 weeks" before her next appointment. She did want to make sure, however, that she could call if any problems arose.

CASE COMMENTARY

This case illustrates the type of physician flexibility needed for good psychopharmacologic treatment. The patient's clinical condition and the exigencies of treatment dictate the frequency and duration of patient visits. In addition, telephone contact with the physician is available for the patient should any questions or concerns arise during treatment. In the early phases of treatment, contact with the patient is more frequent as the medication dose is adjusted and side effects are carefully monitored. As symptomatic improvement occurs in the presence of minimal treatment-emergent side effects, patient monitoring decreases in frequency, again dictated by patient need.

The importance of this flexibility cannot be overemphasized. Careful patient monitoring during the early stages of treatment can identify and ameliorate problems as they emerge. The patient's concerns about medication use and symptoms are clearly and effectively dealt with in a supportive and rational manner. The knowledge that the physician is a telephone call away provides reassurance for patients or their families that, should any problems arise, help is readily available.

This model of care is very different than the traditional psychotherapeutic hour provided routinely one, two, or three times a week. Some practitioners will need to change the patterns of their practice to accommodate this different model of care. The traditional single-office, single-practitioner practice using a psychiatric care delivery structure developed in the mists of history and uncritically continued into the present will need to be modified to more effectively deal with the proper application of modern psychopharmacologic treatment strategies. How this type of clinical structure can be established is described in Chapter 7.

Effective Communication

Medical licensing authorities in Canada report that about 80 percent of patient or parent complaints about physicians can be traced back to

CHAPTER 6 / Educational Issues in Child and Adolescent Psychopharmacology **89**

problems in communication between the physician and the patient. This finding underscores the recognized clinical necessity for good communication between the clinician and the patient or family. Clear, direct, and supportive communication is necessary for effective psychopharmacologic treatment. Patients and their families must understand the following:

1. The diagnosis and what it means (acute and chronic issues)
2. The treatment proposed, its anticipated outcome, and expected side effects
3. Alternative treatments available, their reported efficacy, and their side effects
4. Estimated length of treatment and mode of outcome evaluation

These issues are more complicated in the psychopharmacologic treatment of children and adolescents than in the treatment of adults. Information must be presented to patients in a form and at a level that take into account their developmental ability to reason and understand. As discussed earlier, "doctorspeak" must be avoided, and the meaning of commonly used terms must be defined. Furthermore, family and other issues may have an impact on the effective communication of all of the above. In many cases, family, individual, or social dynamics will need to be identified, understood, taken into consideration, and therapeutically addressed for effective communication to occur.

CASE EXAMPLE

"What do you mean depressed? He's just lazy. Why, when I was young. . ."

S.A., a 13-year-old boy with a 2-year history of dysthymia, was referred for psychopharmacologic treatment by his pediatrician. A detailed assessment revealed a comorbid diagnosis of generalized anxiety disorder (GAD) that predated the onset of the dysthymia, and one clearcut episode of major depression accompanied by problematic social and academic functioning, which had come on about 1 year into the dysthymia, had lasted for 7 to 8 months, and had subsequently spontaneously remitted, leaving a continued dysthymic profile.

The family history was positive for panic disorder (PD) and substance abuse on the father's side, but no clear identification of a psychiatric illness was apparent on the mother's side. S.A.'s father was a "self-made hard-nosed businessman" by his own description. He saw his role in the family as that of setting goals and achieving them. S.A.'s mother was a primary school teacher whose self-appointed task was that of providing affective support in the family. Two other children, one aged 19 and one aged 11, were doing well.

At the time of diagnostic assessment, S.A.'s baseline BDI score was 19 and his baseline HDRS score was 13. The diagnosis was discussed with the family and patient together. Although S.A. and his mother were comfortable with the assessment and diagnosis, S.A.'s father was not. He felt that S.A. was "bone lazy" and needed to "get a grip on himself and get to work." At that point during the session, the clinician elected to approach the problem using an information- and education-based approach. Although the father was more willing to consider a psychiatric disorder after a detailed discussion about depression, its diagnosis, and its effects on teens, it was not until the clinician presented the father with a copy of the DSM-III-R—in which he could read and identify the description of the syndrome and its specific symptoms—that the father felt more comfortable with the diagnosis. Following this, a decision to attempt pharmacologic treatment with paroxetine was agreed to, and concurrent cognitive psychotherapy was begun.

CASE COMMENTARY

This case illustrates both clinician flexibility and effective communication within the specific dynamics of a family unit with a psychiatrically ill youngster. It also shows how written material may be very useful in providing the necessary diagnostic and pharmacologic information for a patient and family. Indeed, it is suggested that, whenever possible, the clinician provide written information about the disorder, its treatment options, and the specific pharmacologic agents recommended. If this information is summarized on a single sheet of paper that is given to the patient and family, they can pursue their educational process regarding pharmacotherapy in a more reasonable and useful way. A prototypic Diagnosis and Treatment form is found in Table 6–1. This can be used as is, with the clinician filling in the specific information. Or the clinician may choose to make up a variety of such forms, all using a similar outline, in which the appropriate information about specific diagnoses and treatment is already outlined.

A useful approach in the nonemergency case is to provide the patient and family with a diagnosis and information about the disorder and its possible treatments, followed by an opportunity for them to ask questions and voice their concerns. This can then be followed by a period of about a day or so during which they can obtain further information about the illness and its treatments. In addition to reading materials provided by the physician, the patient and family should be encouraged to obtain further information on their own, both through reading (a list of suitable references can be provided on the form in Table 6–2) and discussion with others. The patient and family can then be seen again, at which time questions arising from their self-directed research about the disorder and its treatments are answered. In this way, a collaborative treatment approach can be developed.

Such a process, used at the time of diagnosis and prior to the onset of treatment, is very valuable. First, it provides the patient and family with the information they need to make a reasonable decision about treatment. Second, it does not force them to accept a single-model approach to understanding the problem and encourages them to educate themselves about the disorder and its various treatments. Third, it provides the patient and family with greater autonomy and control of the treatment, thus eliciting ownership and enhancing compliance. Fourth, it can help identify interpersonal and family dynamics that may interfere with effective treatment and allow for these issues to be dealt with "up front." Finally, it underscores the following previously identified basic principles of the therapeutic relationship:

1. Physician competency: The physician is knowledgeable about diagnosis and treatment, provides useful scientifically valid information about the disorder and its treatments to the patient and family, and assists and encourages the education of the patient and family about the illness and its treatments.
2. Collaboration: Realizing that shared decision making needs active, informed participation of all parties involved, the physician encourages and facilitates this process.
3. Evaluation-based care: The physician presents a model of objective, measure-based outcome evaluation as the method for directing treatment rather than an intervention-based approach selected through practitioner preference or hypothesized pathoetiology.
4. Flexibility: The physician is willing to consider reasonable treatment alternatives brought forward by the patient or family and provides a structure in which this is possible.
5. Effective communication: Both verbal and written materials are presented, with enough time allowed for the patient and the family to digest the information and to develop an understanding of the disorder and its possible treatments.

Patient and Parent Education About Psychopharmacologic Treatment— Practice Points

1. Be aware of and monitor the factors that affect compliance with psychopharmacologic treatment in children and adolescents.
2. Understand and practice the five basic principles that underlie the therapeutic relationship necessary for psychopharmacologic care.

Patient and Parent Education About Specific Medications

Educating the patient and parent about the use of specific medications in the treatment of the patient's disorder begins with their understanding that one or more medicines may be potentially useful and that medication should be seriously considered as a treatment option. In some cases such a suggestion will be welcome news to a patient or parent. In other cases this suggestion will be met with skepticism, worry, or concern. At times, negative reactions to such a suggestion may be caused by previous personal experience with drug treatments (both psychiatric and nonpsychiatric); child or parent belief about the value or advisability of treating behavioral, mood, or cognitive disturbances with "drugs"; or misinformation or disinformation obtained from the popular media or other sources about the proper use of medications in psychiatric disorders. The physician must be aware of such potential negative reactions and anticipate the patient's and family's responses to the suggestion that medications may be necessary or at least indicated in treatment.

In discussing the use of medications with the patient and his family, the following issues need to be addressed.

1. What evidence is there that medications will be either necessary or helpful?
2. How can medicines help this problem? How do the medicines work?
3. Will using medicines make me (or my child) a different person?
4. Will I (or my child) become addicted to the medicine?

These issues may not be mentioned by the patient or parent(s), even if they are concerned about them, but the clinician should bring them up. Once they have been identified and discussed, more focused reviews of medications that are likely to be helpful in the particular case can be conducted.

What Evidence Is There That Medications Are Either Necessary or Helpful?

This excellent question should be asked more often by both clinicians and their patients about all forms of psychiatric treatment. Regarding medications specifically, the physician should briefly discuss how evidence for efficacy of treatment is determined (case studies; open trials; double-blind, placebo-controlled trials) and what specific evidence from each of these progressively more valid methodologies is available to support the use of a medication in the treatment of the patient's (or child's) psychiatric disorder.

How Can Medicines Help This Problem? How Do the Medicines Work?

To answer these important questions, the clinician should provide a brief overview of current models of understanding regarding the possible biological pathoetiology of the patient's (or child's) disorder and how the medication is thought to work in this context. Descriptions that are too superficial are not useful, and descriptions that are too detailed will only be confusing. A happy medium should be the goal of this discussion. Visual aids or drawings may be useful for illustrative purposes.

Will Using Medicines Make Me (or My Child) a Different Person?

This question raises an important distinction between the use of pharmacologic treatment to address a pathologic condition as distinct from such usage affecting a normative state. This is an essential but often difficult distinction for the patient and parents to grasp. Most children and some adolescents may not appreciate the fundamental complexities of this issue. The physician can best address this question by stating that the medicine is used to treat an illness, not to change who or what a person is. For patients and parents who are able to understand the complexities involved, the physician may decide to use the following guideline to discuss the relationship between a disorder (such as depression) and a person with the disorder: When the symptoms of the disorder are under control (e.g., the person no longer feels unhappy or sad most of the time), the person may

think that he or she has changed. While this feeling is true, it is not the person who has changed but the disorder that has now gone. The person is no longer being affected by a disorder that was itself actually changing that person.

Will I (My Child) Become Addicted to the Medicine?

This extremely common concern is almost always present, even though it is not usually raised by patients or their families. Perhaps fueled by irresponsible and uninformed popular reports, or by professionals who themselves do not understand the issues related to addiction, many patients or families are worried that using psychotropic medications properly will invariably make them addicted. Nothing could be further from the truth, and the clinician must take time to discuss with a patient and parents the difference between addiction and the use of medications to treat a pathological condition.

Many patients and families think that if they take a medication, even once, they will be "hooked forever." Others think that if they take a medication for any length of time, this means they are addicted to the medicine. Others confuse the concept of physiologic dependence with addiction. Still others are certain (in the face of any solid evidence) that "psychological addiction" (itself an unuseful and generally unsubstantiated concept) characterizes all psychotropic medication use. In discussing these issues with patients and their families, the physician must identify and clarify these misconceptions and describe what the risk of addiction actually is. In most cases the use of a medical analogy, such as insulin treatment for diabetes or antiinflammatory medications for arthritis, will help facilitate understanding.

A full, frank, and informed discussion of these general issues will assist the patient and his or her family in their decision making regarding the use of psychotropic medications in general. However, moving to the more specific, the clinician should help the patient and parents understand that any treatment involves a careful consideration of the risks and benefits of using that treatment and, of equal importance, of not using that treatment. Thus, on the basis of her knowledge of the scientific literature and clinical experience, the clinician should provide the patient and parents with her reasonable estimate of treatment success, both with and without the use of medications. Simply stated,

1. What are the risks and benefits of using these medicines?

2. What are the risks and benefits of not using these medicines?

Proceeding further from the general to the specific, the clinician will need to provide sufficient information to the patient and family to help them decide whether or not to select a particular compound for their treatment—in other words, to help them determine their own view of the risk/benefit ratio of treatment.

In many cases more than one medication may be suggested as a viable treatment choice. In such a case it is important that the clinician review with the patient and family the various pros and cons of each potentially useful compound. This review should ideally include a discussion of all of the following issues:

1. What are the medication choices for this condition?
2. What is the anticipated therapeutic effect of each medication?
3. What are the side effects of each medication?
4. What are the anticipated costs of each medication?

These issues should be addressed not only by themselves but also in comparison with other alternative treatments. Obviously, if only one medication is indicated, such comparisons are not necessary. Similarly, if multiple medications (five or more) are potential choices, it is not unreasonable for the clinician to inform the patient or family of this but to suggest three or four choices for review.

If urgent pharmacologic intervention is not needed, the clinician should encourage the patient and family to discuss their various options further if they wish. In many cases the patient and family may want to learn more about the medications before making a final decision; they can use the Diagnosis and Treatment Suggestions handout (Table 6–1) obtained from the clinician to assist them in the process. In other cases, the patient and family will want to begin medication treatment immediately and will choose to pursue the collection of further information and its subsequent discussion concurrently. Either course of action is reasonable. If urgent pharmacologic intervention is necessary (such as for severe panic attacks or psychosis), the clinician should advise the choice of the second option.

Once a specific medication is selected, more detailed information about the use of that medication needs to be made available to the patient and family. This helps provide a review of the purpose of treatment, the potential side effects, and the anticipated time of onset of expected therapeutic efficacy and to ensure that issues unique to the use of that medication are known.

CASE EXAMPLE

"I know my lithium."

G.D. was a 15-year-old boy who experienced an acute manic episode. He responded well to lithium treatment. In the hospital he underwent extensive education about his illness and his medication. At the time of his discharge, he and his parents were given a lithium information sheet that outlined important issues related to his taking of the medication.

Five months later, G.D. presented to the hospital emergency room. He had become ill with the flu and had experienced about 1 day of vomiting and diarrhea. He had stopped taking his lithium because he understood that his body would save lithium in situations when he lost body fluids, specifically sodium-containing fluids. His parents had suggested that because of the prolonged duration of his symptoms he should have a lithium level taken, and when G.D. agreed they brought him to the emergency room.

When G.D. was seen he had no physical signs of lithium toxicity. A serum lithium level taken in the emergency room was 1.1 mEq/L. His outpatient psychiatrist was notified, and G.D. was advised to continue to refrain from taking his medications for the rest of the day. A follow-up visit with his outpatient psychiatrist was arranged for the following day.

CASE COMMENTARY

This case illustrates an appropriate patient and family response to lithium monitoring that can be generalized to psychotropic medications as a whole. Providing written material about specific medicines, knowing what to do in particular situations, and knowing the optimal dosage for a medication will all improve the conduct of psychopharmacologic treatment and help safeguard patients who may be taking compounds that have toxic effects if not used properly. A useful medication information outline that can be adapted for use with a variety of psychotropic medications is provided in Figure 6–1 and reproduced in Appendix II. Routine clinical use of such an outline, which is provided to both patient and family, is to be encouraged.

A number of other educational issues need to be identified whenever psychotropic medications are prescribed. For adolescents in particular it is essential to provide appropriate advice about the ef-

Patient's Name: _____   Date: _____

The information you find on this page is designed to help you take your medication properly. If you have any questions about your medicine, call _____ during office hours. If there is any urgent question or you are experiencing side effects at any time, call _____ or come to the hospital emergency room and bring this paper with you.

Name of medicine(s):

Time medication is taken and amount of medicine taken at each time (dose):

Side effects to be aware of:

What to do if you get side effects:

Drugs (prescription and nonprescription), foods, and other things to avoid:

Other important things:

FIGURE 6–1   Medication Information Form

fect of the medicine on driving. Many medications may decrease a driver's reaction time, and teens should be advised not to drive if taking one of these substances. In addition, teens should be advised not to use any illicit drugs or alcohol because of potential drug-drug interactions and the negative effect of some of these substances on the natural course of the disorder. Adolescents will appreciate the clinician who has a clear, reasonable, and informed perspective on these issues. Being a "nice guy" or turning a blind eye to substance use is of no therapeutic help to teenage patients.

Other issues that should be addressed with teenage patients include pregnancy and birth control. Because some medications may have teratogenic effects, these should be outlined at the onset of treatment. Some drug-drug interactions decrease the efficacy of oral contraceptives, and

teens should be informed of this and encouraged to use other birth control techniques if they are sexually active. These issues are usually best discussed with the teen privately.

Education about medications should begin as soon as they are suggested for treatment and should include both verbal and written material. If the patient is hospitalized, a medicine education or "meducation" group is useful. In this forum, patients learn about medication issues in general and their own medication specifically. Individualized "homework" sessions can be prescribed to be completed by individual patients or small groups of patients between group sessions. In addition, patients benefit from the support of others with similar problems and can share their concerns, frustrations, and successes. Nursing, medical, and pharmacy staff may all play an active role in group and individual teaching/learning sessions.

The use of a group educational format also helps the child or adolescent deal with some of the psychological issues that arise from the use of medications. Peer expectations can be predicted and dealt with in the relative safety and support of a therapeutic structure. The classroom feeling that a well-functioning meducation group can create is a familiar learning environment for most children and adolescents, and this is useful in decreasing anxiety and encouraging active learning about their medications and illnesses. A useful set of instruments for such a group is found in Appendix II.

Patient and Parent Education About Specific Medications—Practice Points

1. Understand, identify, and therapeutically deal with the commonly held concerns that patients and families have regarding the use of psychotropic medications.
2. Provide sufficient verbal and written information so that the patient and family are well-educated consumers with regard to their medications.
3. Provide medication-monitoring handouts to assist patients in managing their medications.
4. Identify and monitor lifestyle issues that will affect medication treatment.

SUGGESTED READINGS

Bastiens L. Knowledge, expectations and attitudes of hospitalized children and adolescents in psychopharmacological treatment. Journal of Child and Adolescent Psychopharmacology, 2:157–171, 1992.

Bastiens L, Bastiens D. A manual for psychiatric medications in teenagers. Journal of Child and Adolescent Psychopharmacology, 3:M–1 to M–24, 1993.

Facts for Families. American Academy of Child and Adolescent Psychiatry, P.O. Box 96106, Washington, DC 20090.

Mattar M, Markello J, Yaffe S. Pharmaceutic factors affecting pediatric compliance. Pediatrics, 55:101–108, 1975.

Seltzer A, Roncari I, Garfinkel P. Effect of patient education on medication compliance. Canadian Journal of Psychiatry, 25:638–645, 1980.

Singer M, Shear N. The SAFFR MD informed patient decision making check-list for the use of prescription medications: a foundation for responsible risk management. Canadian Journal of Psychiatry, 3:172–174, 1996.

CHAPTER 7

Pragmatics of Psychopharmacologic Treatment in Children and Adolescents

A number of issues of practical importance in child and adolescent psychopharmacologic care need to be considered by the clinician. These include:

1. Setting up and operating a clinical outpatient service designed to provide the type of service delivery demanded by modern models of psychopharmacologic care
2. Common practical issues in psychopharmacologic treatment
3. Informed consent
4. Design of pharmacologic treatment trials

Each of these issues is discussed in detail in this chapter.

Outpatient Clinical Service Delivery

The realities of modern outpatient child and adolescent psychiatric care have developed from the inclusion of psychopharmacologic treatments in what have traditionally been primarily individual or family psychotherapy practices. Accordingly, it is not reasonable to expect that structures of delivering this care should remain unaltered. Furthermore, the availability of relatively new and time-saving technologies, the need to provide an educational focus to treatment, and the increasing realization that reliable and repeated measurements of treatment targets and side effects are necessary all ensure that the traditional single-person practice using 1 therapeutic hour (or a significant part thereof) is no longer adequate to meet new care demands.

A model of outpatient practice more suited to the new exigencies of modern caregiving is that of the child and adolescent psychopharmacologic clinic, in which both pharmacologic and psychosocial treatments can be provided. Such a clinic should be set up so as to facilitate and optimize care. Such a clinic will require particular types of personnel, equipment, and office space.

Personnel

It is impractical and unnecessary for the single physician to attempt to provide good outpatient care that includes sophisticated psychopharmacologic treatment. The use of other well-trained medically and psychosocially competent staff members who work with a physician is much more appropriate. A team approach to care optimizes service delivery. In some cases it may be difficult to find staff members who are already trained in this type of work, and the physician may need to spend the time and energy ensuring that team members learn the appropriate skills. In addition, regular review of these skills (at least once a year), including the use of rating scales, will be necessary to ensure that all members of the treatment team are working in a reliable fashion.

The members of such a treatment team will be identified by the tasks that the new model of care demands be performed. These tasks include the following:

1. Patient intake and scheduling
2. Diagnostics and treatment planning
3. Measurement and monitoring
4. Delivery of identified interventions
5. Financial record keeping and accounting

The staff needed to assist in the smooth operation of a busy outpatient child and adolescent psychopharmacologic clinical practice is identified from an appreciation of the above-mentioned care-related tasks. In many cases competent individuals who have good skills in one area can be trained to take on other related tasks. For example, a registered nurse will be needed to deal with the medically related issues arising from the delivery of psychopharmacologic treatment. There is no reason, however, that this same individual cannot be trained in the application of specific rating scales that are used to assist in the monitoring of adverse events and treatment outcome. Some clinicians find that competent nurses, particularly those with previous experience in psychiatry, may often appreciate the opportunity to obtain further specific psychotherapeutic training. A registered nurse who combines the skills necessary for medical monitoring with expertise in a specific psychotherapy (such as cognitive-behavior therapy) will be a valuable member of the clinic team.

Administrative functions, including bookkeeping and office management, can often be performed by one individual. This person must have the skills necessary to perform specific office tasks (such as intake and reception), but also needs skills in interpersonal relations. The value of such skills cannot be overemphasized. An intake worker or receptionist who is curt, hasty, or inattentive will not only put off patients, parents, and referral sources, but may cause considerable chaos if appointment scheduling and record keeping are not properly handled. Perhaps more importantly, this individual will often be the first telephone contact for a patient or parent in distress and will need to know how to respond appropriately. Training sessions in which such potential scenarios are practiced are often helpful.

Appointments will not generally follow the 1-hour rule. Instead they should be scheduled to provide sufficient time to carry out the necessary therapeutic task. To some practitioners it may seem like a novel approach to alter the care delivery schedule to meet the needs of the patient.

Appointments will generally be of four different types: diagnostic, decision making or educational, therapeutic, and evaluative. Diagnostic appointments may be expected to last from a minimum of 1 to a maximum of 2 hours, depending on the complexities of the case. For example, a patient seen for a specific consultation regarding recommendations for psychopharmacologic treatment can usually be carefully and systematically evaluated and given feedback in 50 to 70 minutes. It will take substantially longer to appropriately assess a patient referred for initial diagnosis and treatment. Dictating a short consultation note or completing a Psychopharmacology Consultation Summary Form (see Appendix II) to be sent out to the referral source should take another 10 to 15 minutes. There is no evidence that marathon assessments lasting 4 to 6 hours (or even days) that are popular in some outpatient settings provide any better or more useful diagnostic information than can be obtained within the time frame just described.

The overall assessment time for a consultation request can be shortened by the routine use of a Psychopharmacology Consultation Request Form. The intake person completes this form using information obtained from the referral source at the time the referral is made. Thus the information is always available when the patient and family are seen. Clinical experience suggests that if such forms are mailed out to referral sources with instructions to be completed and returned before the patient's scheduled appointment, chances are very good that the consulting clinician will never see the referral form. A copy of this form can be found in Appendix II.

Decision-making or educational appointments will usually be with patients and families who have already completed the diagnosis or initial psychopharmacologic consultation. The clinician will be familiar with the case and the issues that need to be addressed. A decision-making session will be directed toward coming to a joint decision (patient, family, and physician) about treatment using the collaborative model described in Chapter 6. For this type of meeting the patient and family have already had a preliminary discussion about the disorder and its treatment and are returning following further study and self-education about available options. They are meeting with the clinician to make a decision about interventions. This type of session should be clearly goal oriented, that is, a decision about treatment must be made. After this the treatment monitoring and evaluation framework will have to be put into place. This type of appointment should take only 30 to 40 minutes, with 5 to 10 minutes required for appropriate documentation. This type of session is like a gas; it will expand to fill the container in which it is kept.

An educational appointment is one in which a patient (or family) requests additional time to discuss issues related to his (or their child's) illness and its treatment. While this often has a therapeutic purpose and effect beyond the transmission of information, it is necessary to try to clearly define the goals of this meeting. This meeting should not be used for personal or family therapy treatment. Rather, it should be well focused, although it should be conducted in a sensitive and supportive manner. Such a session could be expected to last

20 to 30 minutes, followed by a few minutes for appropriate documentation. In many cases the physician does not need to conduct this session. A well-trained and competent nurse or other mental health worker who is familiar with the patient and family should be able to take on this task and complete it successfully. In some cases the physician's presence for a short time during such a session can be useful in clarifying issues that may have arisen earlier or during the meeting.

Therapeutic appointments are of two kinds. One type is the psychological (cognitive, behavioral, interpersonal) or family therapy treatment that can be carried out by either a physician or other clinic staff (nurse, social worker, educator) trained in its implementation. The other is the medication-monitoring appointment, in which the therapeutic and adverse effects of medication treatment are assessed.

For the first type of therapeutic appointment, it is not necessary, or indeed desirable, for the physician to personally provide specific individual psychotherapies or family therapy to every patient. In many cases such therapies are not indicated and do not need to be part of a comprehensive treatment plan. In other cases practitioners with more specialized training and skills in a particular treatment modality (such as cognitive-behavior therapy for children with obsessive compulsive disorder [OCD]) are available. In this case it is reasonable for the specialist to work closely with the clinician, although the responsibility for monitoring and evaluating treatment efficacy should remain with the specialist. This type of therapy appointment has traditionally been approximately 1 hour in length. However, therapy goals, not tradition, should dictate timing. One might find that a variety of therapy appointment time slots of various lengths provide optimal flexibility.

The purpose of the medication-monitoring appointment is to evaluate the efficacy and adverse events related to medication treatment. Such evaluation requires the determination and documentation of necessary laboratory and physical parameters (such as heart rate, blood pressure, and neurologic examination). In most cases Medication-Specific Side Effect Scales (MSSES) and other rating scales will be used. Again, it is not necessary for the physician to take on this entire task. This can be reasonably shared with a nurse who is competent in both physiologic and psychological measurement. Such an individual can also provide injections (e.g., for long-acting antipsychotic medications) and telephone counseling regarding medications for issues that do not require the physician's immediate attention.

Generally, the time required for a medication-monitoring visit will range from 20 to 30 minutes, depending on the complexities of the case. In many cases, the physiologic monitoring and some of the psychological monitoring can be conducted by the clinic nurse. When the physician sees the patient, she should review the information obtained by the nurse, complete those evaluations that remain to be done, and ensure that the appropriate documentation has been completed.

Treatment evaluation meetings take place after a particular course of treatment has been completed and a formal assessment of its efficacy is to be carried out. This requires a detailed review of all of the data compiled in the patient's clinical record and a determination, using the appropriate techniques, of any change in the target symptoms. In many cases, external information (such as that obtained from teachers, counselors, therapists, and others) will have to be synthesized and interpreted. This review is conducted in conjunction with the patient and parents, and decisions about further treatment are made at this time. It will usually take about 45 to 60 minutes to properly conduct this type of session, followed by about 10 minutes for proper documentation. If all the information has been collated and analyzed beforehand (this can often be done by a clinic nurse or well-trained intake worker/receptionist), this block of time can be shortened somewhat, but not as much as might be expected.

Given the different types of sessions and the estimated time requirements of each, it will quickly become apparent that scheduling may become very complicated. The use of a computerized appointment program that can be custom designed by an experienced programmer, if necessary, and a competent receptionist/intake worker/secretary to manage it is needed. Although it will take some time to set up such a system and "debug" it, such scheduling flexibility is necessary to allow the individualized needs of various patients receiving psychopharmacologic treatment to be met.

Equipment

The modern psychopharmacologic outpatient practice will require more equipment than standard office items familiar to most practitioners. These items are identified by the functions of the clinic. For example, the medical management of patients will require a small examination room where appropriate baseline physical examinations or medical monitoring can be conducted. If a nurse is to draw blood for laboratory analysis, a small centrifuge and a refrigeration unit will be needed. Since most rating scales and other diagnostic and monitoring instruments are available on computer, the clinician may find that placing computer terminals in easily accessible locations will reduce paperwork and save time previously spent on manually scoring rating scale results.

Office Space

This clinic model will require careful consideration about space needs. In some cases one or more clinicians may decide to form a group practice to be able to share function-specific space (e.g., waiting area or sample preparation room). In other cases a child and adolescent psychiatrist may join up with a larger medical group made up of pediatricians or family physicians. Whatever the structure chosen, there should be space for a small but well-stocked education and reading materials library that can be used by patients and their families. Ideally, this library should be next to the waiting or reception area, where more than one patient and family can be expected to congregate. Such a waiting area should also have facilities to assist patients and families in the completion of various rating scales that they will often be filling out while waiting to be seen. In addition, such a waiting area or small reading space could be the repository for the various handouts and information booklets that the clinician is using as patient education materials.

Model of Outpatient Clinical Care for Integrated Child and Adolescent Psychopharmacologic Practice— Practice Points

1. New models of care require new structures for service delivery.
2. The use of a clinic model that provides for both medical and psychosocial care is more appropriate than a single-practitioner, one-office practice.
3. The practical necessities of providing integrated psychopharmacologic care rather than traditional practices will dictate staffing, equipment, and space requirements.

Common Practical Issues in Psychopharmacologic Treatment

Issues commonly arising when psychopharmacologic intervention for children and adolescents begins are the following:

1. Developing and identifying the integrated treatment plan
2. Initiating medication
3. Choosing the initial or first-choice medication

4. Establishing the optimal frequency of patient contact
5. Optimizing initial pharmacotherapy
6. Dealing with treatment resistance
7. Communicating with patients and parents about psychopharmacologic treatment
8. Continuing and discontinuing medication treatment

Developing and Identifying the Integrated Treatment Plan

Before initiating psychopharmacologic treatment, the clinician must consider how the psychotropic intervention will fit into the overall treatment plan. If this process is systematically conducted, the optimal integration of multiple interventions can be planned best by considering the following items:

1. Diagnosis
2. Type of treatments selected (pharmacologic and nonpharmacologic)
3. Expected duration of each treatment
4. Measures for evaluating outcome (efficacy and adverse events)
5. Options for further interventions
6. Responsibility for provision of treatments
7. Responsibility for overall treatment management
8. Structures for ensuring optimal monitoring and decision making

In some cases the clinician can operationalize this treatment planning in a way that is useful for the patient and family, as well as meeting his or her own record-keeping needs. Many clinicians find it useful to outline the overall treatment plan in a written form that can be kept in the clinical record and given to the patient and family. This practice will help minimize misconceptions about the treatment plan. If the clinician has concerns about the reliability of a patient or family member in adhering to a collaborative constructed treatment plan, the patient and family may be asked to sign the written form, which outlines the treatment plan. This form can then be considered a treatment contract. Figure 7–1 is an example of such a treatment contract.

In every treatment plan, the goals of pharmacologic intervention are the same, namely:

1. Amelioration of the symptoms of the disorder
2. Improvement of patient functioning and quality of life
3. Prophylaxis against relapse

Initiating Medication

A number of issues that are specific to the use of medication must be considered by the clinician at

Patient's Name: _____ Date: _____

This form is provided as a review of the reasons for your treatment, the type of treatment you and your physician have agreed to, the anticipated length of this treatment, and the method of determining if your treatment is effective.

Diagnosis (name of the problem):

Target symptoms (what we expect to improve with treatment):

Type of treatment selected (what we have chosen to do to help):

Talking therapies (include name and frequency):

Social therapies (include name and frequency):

Medications (include name, dose, and frequency):

Other treatments (include name and frequency):

Onset of therapeutic effect (how long before we expect to see improvements):

Duration of treatment (when we will evaluate if the treatment has been helpful):

Outcome measures (what we will use to determine if treatment has helped):

Further options (what we will do if treatment has not been fully successful or what we will do to continue helpful treatment):

FIGURE 7–1   Patient/Parent Information Regarding Treatment Plan: A Treatment Contract

the time pharmacotherapy is begun. The clinician's approach to initiating the specific psychopharmacologic components of the overall treatment plan includes the following:

1. Identifying and measuring the target symptom
2. Identifying and measuring treatment-emergent adverse events
3. Making a reasonable choice of medication
4. Educating patient and family about the medication
5. Initiating treatment with a test dose strategy
6. Starting with an appropriate dose
7. Identifying a reasonable target dose range
8. Identifying an expected length of treatment
9. Titrating the medication to target dose range
10. Maintaining the target dose and evaluating efficacy

Identifying and Measuring the Target Symptoms

Do not rely on clinician or patient/parent impressions alone. For each treatment target, always use at least one or more structured evaluation instruments. Whenever possible, combine a self-report with an observer report measure. For each target treatment, complete the appropriate symptom rating scales before beginning treatment and at appropriate intervals thereafter.

Identifying and Measuring Treatment-Emergent Adverse Events

Do not rely on clinician or patient/parent impressions alone. For each medication used, complete the appropriate MSSES (see Appendix IV) before beginning treatment and at appropriate intervals thereafter.

Making a Reasonable Choice of Medication

The choice of medication should be based on the physician's knowledge of the various potentially useful compounds available and the unique characteristics of the patient. Selection of medication follows discussion of the symptom and treatment with the patient and family.

Educating Patient and Family About the Medication

Ensure that the patient and family are aware of the potential risks and benefits of treatment and assist them in developing the knowledge and skills necessary for them to understand and monitor treatment.

Initiating Treatment with a Test Dose Strategy

While most patients will not demonstrate an allergic or otherwise severely untoward acute reaction to a medication, it is prudent to have the patient take the first dose of any medication at a time when access to necessary medical assistance is available if problems do arise. For example, do not advise a patient to take a medication for the first time when he is traveling far from home. Other, perhaps less obvious suggestions are: Do not advise the patient to take the first dose of a new medication at night, and do not begin a patient on a new medication (unless it is an urgent matter) just before a holiday weekend.

Starting with an Appropriate Dose

In most cases there is nothing to be gained by prescribing "loading" doses of medications. On the contrary, much is to be lost, because this type of approach may induce significant side effects without providing any additional beneficial treatment effect. Furthermore, in many children and adoles-

cents, therapeutic doses of medication (e.g., clonazepam in panic disorder (PD); see Chapter 9) are substantially *lower* than for adults with a similar diagnosis. Beginning at a high dose can lead to unnecessary and potential problematic overmedicating.

Identifying a Reasonable Target Dose Range

On the basis of knowledge of the literature and clinical experience, set an initial total daily dose target for the medication that you expect will provide a reasonable therapeutic effect for the patient. Keep in mind the unique pharmacokinetic and pharmacodynamic effects of the medication and the individual variability in these features. Most medications have a target dose range, and it is reasonable to set your first target dose somewhere in the middle of that range.

Identifying an Expected Length of Treatment

Most patients and their families will not know how long pharmacologic treatment will need to proceed before they can expect significant symptom improvement. This length of time can vary considerably across different disorders (e.g., enuresis should respond within a week of attaining the proper treatment dose, while depression will take 6 to 8 weeks or even longer) or across different medications used to treat the same disorder (e.g., anxiety symptoms will usually respond within a few days to adequate benzodiazepine treatment but will require 2 weeks or so if buspirone is used). Be sure to inform the patient and family of the expected length of pharmacologic treatment before they will observe symptom improvement. If this is not done, the patient may prematurely discontinue a potentially effective treatment before it has had a chance to demonstrate its efficacy.

In determining the expected duration of treatment before clinical improvement is achieved, it is essential that the clinician understand the relationship between the attainment of steady-state pharmacokinetics and the therapeutic components of the pharmacodynamic response. In most cases it will be necessary for a patient to attain and maintain the steady-state serum or plasma level of the medication with which he is being treated for the necessary length of time. Thus compounds with different serum or plasma half-lives will take different lengths of time to achieve therapeutically associated steady-state levels. This factor must be considered when estimating expected treatment duration. The adverse-event components of most compounds' pharmacodynamic effects, however, usually do not follow a similar pattern, and many are associated with maximal serum levels or the rate at which the maximal serum drug concentration occurs.

Titrating the Medication to Target Dose Range

Using treatment-emergent side effects and therapeutic outcome as a guide, titrate the medication to target dose range. In many cases early dose increments will not be associated with treatment efficacy, and knowledge of the compound's pharmacokinetics (half-life, metabolism) and the systematic evaluation of treatment-emergent adverse events (using the appropriate MSSES; see Section Two and Appendix IV) will guide initial dose increments. Increasing the dose too quickly will usually increase adverse effects, while increasing the dose too slowly will delay the onset of the therapeutic effect.

Maintaining the Target Dose and Evaluating Efficacy

Once the target dose has been reached, maintain the medication dose at this level for a reasonable length of time, provided side effects are tolerable. This length of time is the period previously identified as necessary for the reasonable determination of therapeutic efficacy. For example, allow 8 weeks for paroxetine treatment of major depression, a few days for clonazepam treatment of PD, and 12 weeks for fluvoxamine treatment of OCD. Avoid the temptation to increase the dose of a medication if the patient shows an initial response followed by a plateau period, as long as this phenomenon occurs during the dose maintenance phase. Appropriate evaluation of the effect of the initial target dose can only be made after adequate time has passed.

Choosing the Initial or First-Choice Medication

In many cases more than one medication may be a reasonable choice with which to initiate treatment. In this case the clinician should be able to develop a rational reason for the choice of one compound rather than another. Reasons such as "I've always done it this way" are not acceptable. Familiarity with a particular medication must be tempered by rational evaluation of alternatives.

Other, perhaps newer compounds may be therapeutically just as good or even better and may have fewer side effects. Reasons such as "It looks good in the advertising" are totally unacceptable as the basis for any rational decision making about pharmacotherapy.

Because the choices of medicines are numerous and the possible indications for their use are varied, no simple formula can be devised to determine the optimal first choice. Instead, you should ask yourself the following questions about the candidate first-choice compounds:

1. Which of the compounds available has demonstrated treatment efficacy in children and adolescents with the same disorder or symptoms as the patient I am about to treat?
2. If more than one medication shows some degree of therapeutic efficacy, which evidence is stronger, and have any comparisons among these various possibilities been carried out?
3. Which medications are the least likely to cause serious or life-threatening adverse events?
4. Which medications require additional laboratory or other physiologic monitoring (e.g., venipuncture or electrocardiogram [ECG]) to ensure their safety or therapeutic efficacy?
5. Which medications are the least likely to cause annoying or distressing subjective adverse events?
6. Does my patient have any physical or psychiatric contraindications to the use of one or more of the potential first-choice medications?
7. Is there a family history (preferably in a first-degree relative) of a good therapeutic response to a particular medication among those that are potentially useful for my patient?

After answering these questions, you should be able to determine a short list of potential medications that can then be discussed with the patient and family so that a joint decision about a first-choice treatment can be made.

Establishing the Optimal Frequency of Patient Contact

Frequency of patient contact is another issue that must be addressed during the initiation of treatment. In many cases practitioners are accustomed to using a 1-hour, once-a-week patient visit to deliver psychiatric care, even though there is no reasonable evidence that this type of visit is the most effective model available. In addition, this model of service delivery is usually based on tradition or practitioner preference rather than on a rational evaluation of patient need.

Patient contact during psychopharmacologic treatment cannot be based on such a model. The use of medications forces the clinician to schedule appointments on the basis of two factors: (1) monitoring side effects and (2) evaluating treatment outcome. In most cases patient contact will have to be more frequent during the initiation phase of pharmacologic intervention and will decrease over time as treatment becomes more established. In many cases telephone contact should be integrated into a face-to-face meeting schedule. Telephone contact will suffice to deal with minor issues as they arise, and face-to-face evaluations can be reserved for more formal assessment points. Be prepared to deal with urgent medical problems that can occur outside of regularly scheduled visits. Most successful child and adolescent psychopharmacologists are routinely "on call" for their patients in case of an emergency. They find that patients and their parents rarely take advantage of this, but both patient and parent appreciate the chance to "touch base" if problems occur.

You will also need to consider unique patient and medication variables in developing an optimal frequency of monitoring for each patient. In terms of patient or family variables, if a patient or her family is exceedingly anxious about medication treatment, for example, slightly more frequent contact than usual may be indicated. In some cases, as in a suicidal adolescent, more frequent monitoring may serve additional therapeutic purposes. In other cases ongoing medical concerns (such as liver disease) may require more frequent medication monitoring.

In terms of medication variables, issues of efficacy and adverse events are important. Some medications, such as a benzodiazepine, will be expected to demonstrate therapeutic efficacy quite rapidly (within 2 to 3 days), while others, such as buspirone, will be unlikely to show efficacy until later on in treatment (within 2 to 3 weeks). Most medications, however, will demonstrate their adverse effects shortly after the initiation of treatment or when changes in dosage are instituted. Thus treatment-monitoring strategies will differ, depending on whether therapeutic efficacy or tolerability is the focus of attention.

A reasonable guideline regarding the necessary frequency of medication monitoring is to schedule face-to-face monitoring sessions for those times at which medication variables (side effects, therapeutic effects) and patient variables (anxiety about treatment, specific illness-related concerns)

are most likely to need evaluation. Telephone contact or urgent visits can be used on an as-necessary basis for other times that concerns arise. In general, monitoring visits will need to be more frequent at the initiation of pharmacotherapy and will usually focus on tolerability during this time. Once the initial target dose is reached and the initial maintenance phase begins, monitoring visits will usually become less frequent and will focus equally on efficacy and tolerability.

The amount of time needed for each monitoring visit will also vary depending on patient need. In most cases more time is needed at the onset of pharmacologic treatment because the patient and family will have many questions or concerns about the medications that need to be addressed. Furthermore, one of the goals of good pharmacologic treatment is to help the patient and family become well-educated consumers who know how to monitor medication use properly. This is a skill that does not arise "de novo" in most cases. On the contrary, it must be learned, and this learning takes some time. Thus, monitoring sessions occurring later in the course of a patient's ongoing care can in general be expected to be shorter in length as the patient and family become more comfortable with the medication.

However, a minimum time expectation for each monitoring visit should be defined given the measurement goals that need to be accomplished at each patient visit. In most cases, one or two MSSESs (see Appendix IV) will be completed, as well as one or two other rating scales designed to evaluate treatment outcome. In many cases, a brief and focused physical examination, including heart rate, blood pressure, or neurologic evaluation, may be necessary. Appropriate documentation of this must also take place. In addition, each medication-monitoring visit occurs in the context of a supportive therapeutic relationship, and the time necessary for this must also be considered. Taking all these issues into consideration, and depending on the complexities of the problems that the patient is experiencing, most medication-monitoring visits will last 20 to 30 minutes.

Because the frequency and duration of patient contact are individualized using the two-factor model outlined earlier, it is not possible to create a rigid framework that can be applied for all patients. Instead, the variables described earlier should be considered in developing an individualized optimal monitoring schedule for each patient. The monitoring schedule profiles that follow provide examples of how such individualized schedules might be structured at the initiation of psychopharmacologic treatment.

EXAMPLE 1

Initiating Pharmacologic Treatment with a Serotonin-Specific Reuptake Inhibitor in a Depressed 12-Year-Old Girl

Medication Issues Under Consideration

1. When side effects are most likely to occur—1 to 3 days
2. When medication dose should next be raised—5 to 6 days

Patient Issues Under Consideration

1. Patient and parent anxiety about medication treatment—low
2. Parent knowledge about treatment—good
3. Specific illness-related concerns, such as suicidality—none
4. Specific medical concerns—none

Diagram of Anticipated Medication Monitoring Sessions at Treatment Onset

```
      B  T     F        F* T     T      F*
Day 1  2  3  4  5  6  7  8  9  10  11  12
```

B = Begin medication treatment—starting daily dose of 5 mg, fluoxetine
F = Face-to-face office visit to assess side effects
F* = Same as F, but dose was increased
T = Telephone contact to monitor patient progress, especially side effects

EXAMPLE 2

Initiating Treatment with Buspirone in a Young Adolescent Boy with Generalized Anxiety Disorder

Medication Issues Under Consideration

1. When side effects are most likely to occur—1 to 3 days
2. When medication dose should next be raised—3 to 4 days

Patient Issues Under Consideration

1. Patient anxiety about medication treatment—high

2. Patient knowledge about treatment—average
3. Specific illness-related concerns, such as suicidality—none
4. Specific medical concerns—none

Diagram of Anticipated Medication Monitoring Sessions at Treatment Onset

```
      B  F     F* T     F* T     F      F+
Day 1  2  3  4  5  6  7  8  9  10  11  12
```

B = Beginning medication treatment—starting daily dose of 10 mg
F = Face-to-face office visit to assess side effects
F* = Same as F, but dose was increased
F+ = Same as F, but therapeutic effect was measured
T = Telephone contact to monitor patient progress, especially side effects

EXAMPLE 3

Initiating Clonazepam Treatment of Panic Disorder in a 10-Year-Old Girl

Medication Issues Under Consideration

1. When side effects are most likely to occur—1 to 2 days
2. When medication dose should next be raised—2 to 3 days

Patient Issues Under Consideration

1. Patient and parent anxiety about medication treatment—high
2. Parent knowledge about treatment—poor
3. Specific illness-related concerns, such as suicidality—none
4. Specific medical concerns—none

Diagram of Anticipated Medication Monitoring Sessions at Treatment Onset

```
      B  F  T  F*  T  F*+   T      F+       T
Day 1  2  3  4  5  6  7  8  9  10  11  12
```

B = Beginning medication treatment—starting daily dose of 0.25 mg
F = Face-to-face office visit to assess side effects

F* = Same as F, but dose was increased

F⁺ = Same as F, but therapeutic effect was measured

F*⁺ = Same as F*, but therapeutic effect was measured

T = Telephone contact to monitor patient progress, especially side effects

EXAMPLE 4

Patient Monitoring over the Long Term: Clomipramine Treatment of an Adolescent with Obsessive Compulsive Disorder

Medication Issues Under Consideration

1. When side effects are most likely to occur—1 to 3 days after dose initiation and changes
2. When medication dose should next be raised—5 to 7 days following previous levels to steady-state target level
3. Late-onsetting side effects—yes, cardiac

Patient Issues Under Consideration

1. Patient anxiety about medication treatment—low
2. Patient knowledge about treatment—average
3. Specific illness-related concerns, such as suicidality—moderate
4. Specific medical concerns—none

Diagram of Anticipated Medication Monitoring Sessions

B F F* T F* T F* T F* F* F F⁺ F⁺

Week 1 2   3   4   5 6 7 8 9

B = Begin treatment with medication—25 mg total daily dose

F = Face-to-face office visit to assess side effects or therapeutic effect

F* = Same as F, but with a dose adjustment

F⁺ = Same as F, but with therapeutic outcome assessed

T = Telephone contact

The patient contact pattern illustrated here shows that the type and frequency of each patient contact change over time. This change is driven by patient need not practitioner preference.

Optimizing Initial Pharmacotherapy

Medication treatments should be delivered in such a manner as to optimize their therapeutic effects. Initial daily target doses may or may not lead to optimal pharmacotherapy, and it may be necessary to change medication doses in order to optimize the effect. Once the appropriate initial treatment maintenance phase has passed, the first question that the clinician must ask with regard to optimization of pharmacotherapy is: Is the patient continuing to show signs and symptoms or does the patient continue to show significant functional impairment arising from the disorder?

If the answer to this question is yes, then the initial pharmacotherapy may not have been optimized. This now needs to be determined. Some questions useful in helping the clinician determine if the initial pharmacotherapy has been optimized are as follows.

1. What is the known and expected maximal effect of medication treatment in this condition?

   In some disorders, symptom reduction of 30–50 percent from baseline is generally considered the best that can be expected. Accordingly, if the patient shows a response less than this, it might be reasonably considered that treatment has not been maximized. However, the opposite is not necessarily true. The patient who shows a 50 percent symptom reduction may not have achieved the best that can be obtained in his or her *particular case.*

2. Was the predicted total daily dose target correct?

   The amount of medication initially chosen could have been incorrect. It may have been too low, or it may have been too high. The clinician should review her expectations of the target dose range, paying considerable attention to both possibilities.

3. Has the patient been taking a reasonable amount of the medication (within the expected total daily dose target range)?

   The operative word here is *taking*. Obviously if compliance is poor, then this important factor in determining response has not been optimized. The use of therapeutic drug monitoring may, in some cases, be helpful in this determination.

4. Has the patient been taking the medication

properly over a sufficiently long period of time?

As described previously, if maximal symptom improvement may take 8 weeks and the patient has been taking the medication for 4 weeks, this criteria has not been fulfilled. Time must take its proper course.

5. Are there any particular medication or patient characteristics that may relate to this matter?

The most important issue to consider here is that of the rapid hepatic metabolizer who may need larger than predicted doses to experience a therapeutic effect. Therapeutic drug monitoring may be helpful in this determination.

6. Is the patient exhibiting treatment-emergent side effects that limit increasing the total daily dose of the medication or that mask the therapeutic outcome?

Here the answer is yes, no, or maybe. At times the side effects experienced may be less distressing to the patient than the symptoms of the disorder. In such cases the patient may choose to tolerate the medication or even increase the dose if no other treatment alternatives are available. In other cases the side effects of the medications may be confused with the symptoms of the illness. This must be carefully considered, and if the clinician is not certain, a dose-lowering strategy may help clarify the issue.

If after considering these questions the clinician is concerned that pharmacotherapy with the initial medication has not been optimized, the plan of action should be as follows:

1. Identify a new (higher or lower) target dose for the medication.
2. Gradually increase or decrease the medication to that dose.
3. Use treatment-emergent side effects to guide dose increments.
4. Maintain the new target dose for a sufficient length of time.
5. Evaluate the outcome of this strategy.

This same five-point plan can be initiated at any time during treatment to determine optimization of pharmacotherapy. This plan does not need to be limited to evaluation of the initial pharmacologic effect because clinical conditions can change over the duration of treatment, and these may require alterations in the ongoing pharmacotherapy.

Two practical points arise from this approach:

1. The process of determining optimization to initial pharmacotherapy may take a considerable length of time.

This is true. For example, in OCD, this could take 4 months or longer.

2. The optimized total daily medication dose that is obtained may lie outside the predicted therapeutic dose range.

As long as the treatment-emergent adverse events do not harm, endanger, or significantly distress the patient, and the pharmacotherapy is properly and adequately monitored, doses that show efficacy may fall outside the expected range. All therapeutic ranges are exactly that—ranges. While most patients will fall within the expected range, some will fall outside it, both above and below. The clinician is treating the patient, not a drug level.

If, however, after considering these issues the clinician is quite certain that the patient is compliant and that optimization of pharmacotherapy has been attained but therapeutic response is not optimal, the clinician should proceed to the following:

1. Review the diagnosis.

Perhaps the patient is not responding because she has a disorder other than the one for which treatment was being prescribed— for example, a psychosis instead of OCD or mania instead of attention-deficit hyperactivity disorder (ADHD). In this case, the correct diagnosis will suggest another treatment.

2. Review the choice of medication.

Perhaps the wrong medication was chosen and applied; for example, buspirone was given to a child with PD. In this case, use the correct treatment.

3. Review concurrent psychosocial interventions.

Perhaps the patient is not receiving appropriate and effective psychotherapeutic interventions. If this is the case, add these to the medicine.

4. Review other factors.

Perhaps the patient is experiencing environmental or family factors that are mitigating against a positive therapeutic outcome. If this is the case, develop strategies to deal with these factors.

5. Consider the possibility that the patient is abusing drugs or alcohol.

This is especially important with adolescents. Always ask direct questions regarding drug and alcohol use, and follow up with the appropriate blood and urine tests. Know what tests to order and don't forget to screen for over-the-counter compounds.

6. Consider the possibility that your patient may be treatment resistant.

Dealing with Treatment Resistance

In some cases, patients will not show a therapeutic response to optimized initial pharmacotherapy. They may show no response or, more usually, they may show a partial response. These patients are referred to as *treatment resistant* or *treatment refractory*. In many cases, however, patients who are thought to be treatment resistant in reality have either been incorrectly treated (usually because the initial diagnosis was wrong) or have not had their initial pharmacotherapy optimized. Thus, the first step in dealing with treatment resistance is to review the diagnosis and then to optimize the initial pharmacotherapy, as described earlier.

Some patients, however, will actually be treatment resistant to initial pharmacotherapy. This may happen most commonly for one of the following two reasons:

1. The patient cannot tolerate a medication at a dose necessary for a therapeutic effect.
2. The patient experiences none or only partial symptom relief after initial optimization strategies have been put into place.

Treatment resistance can be addressed using a number of different strategies, namely:

1. *Substitution.* This is achieved by stopping the initial pharmacotherapy and using a medication different from that used initially. This medicine may be chosen from the same class (e.g., paroxetine instead of fluoxetine for depression) or from a different class (e.g., desipramine instead of methylphenidate for ADHD).
2. *Augmentation.* This is achieved by continuing with the initial pharmacotherapy and adding another medication to the first in order to enhance the therapeutic response. For example, clonazepam can be added to fluoxetine in OCD or lithium to paroxetine in major depressive disorder (MDD). The added compound is known or expected to lead to a combined effect that is greater than the sum of the individual compounds.
3. *Combination.* This is achieved by simultaneously administering two or more psychoactive agents that are known to be independently effective in a particular disorder. Compounds that are known to demonstrate unique and different mechanisms of action should be used. An example of this strategy is the use of a serotonin-specific reuptake inhibitor (SSRI) combined with a tricyclic antidepressant (TCA) in major depression.

The clinician trying to determine which of these three pharmacologic strategies to choose when faced with a treatment-refractory case should consider the following questions:

1. What information is available about the use of one or more of these strategies?

   Have any studies been reported in the literature regarding the various options? If none have been reported, what is the probability of success if one is chosen over the other? Is one option known to be associated with more serious adverse effects than the other? Will one take longer than the other? Have head-to-head comparisons of the various options been conducted?

2. What are the unique characteristics of the patient?

   Is there a medical or psychiatric feature of the patient that would suggest the advantage of one strategy over the other? What would the patient or parents prefer to do?

Reviewing these issues carefully should assist the physician in choosing among the available strategies.

Once the physician and patient embark on one of the three choices, there are the following three potential outcomes:

1. A maximal therapeutic response is obtained.

   The clinician should now proceed to maintain and monitor treatment.

2. A partial therapeutic response is obtained.

   The clinician should now proceed to optimize treatment.

3. Very little or no therapeutic response is obtained.

   The clinician should now consider additional substitution, augmentation, or combination strategies.

An important clinical point that arises when an augmentation or combination strategy proves successful is determining exactly what led to the success. Two explanations are probable:

1. The combined treatment (initial plus augmenting or combining strategy) was necessary.

   In this case both treatments will need to be maintained.

2. The augmenting or combined treatment would have led to the same result if it had been applied on its own.

   In this case one treatment (the initial one) is not necessary and thus should probably not be maintained.

The only way the clinician can determine which of these two probable explanations is more likely is to discontinue the initial pharmacotherapy at some later point in time and evaluate the effect of this change. If the augmenting or combining agent had been previously used successfully as a monotherapy in the patient, however, the clinician can be reasonably certain that a discontinuation strategy will lead to loss of therapeutic efficacy. In this case there is little to be gained and much to be lost in attempts to switch the patient to monotherapy.

Communicating with Patients and Parents About Psychopharmacologic Treatment

A number of important issues regarding communication with patients and parents about psychopharmacologic treatment often arise in clinical practice. These include the following:

1. Unrealistic anticipation regarding the time of onset for therapeutic effect
2. Confusing and possibly contradictory information about treatment
3. Unplanned and nontherapeutic discontinuation of successful treatment

These issues are described and discussed in the following sections.

Unrealistic Anticipation Regarding Onset of Therapeutic Effects

CASE EXAMPLE

> **"It was not working so I stopped taking the medicine."**
>
> W.E. was a 17-year-old girl who had been "anxious her entire life." She was referred for pharmacologic treatment after intensive insight-oriented individual psychotherapy had not provided effective symptom reduction or improved social functioning, although W.E. felt that it had helped her "understand myself better." Diagnostic assessment confirmed a diagnosis of generalized anxiety disorder (GAD). No comorbid disorders were identified. A Hamilton Anxiety Rating Scale (HARS) scored at baseline was 24, and functional difficulties were identified in social, school, and workplace situations. These were further specified and rated as to severity using various visual analogue scales.
>
> A family history was consistent with anxiety disorders on the mother's side of the family, where the maternal grandmother had severe difficulties compatible with a DSM-IV diagnosis of social phobia and a maternal sister had been treated for panic attacks. The father's family history showed depression in the paternal grandmother, which had been successfully

treated with tricyclic medications, and excessive alcohol use in a paternal uncle. W.E.'s father was a successful financial consultant who was "prone to depression," for which he had received "counseling" in the past, and W.E.'s mother was an editor, working out of the family home, who described significant anxiety symptoms and a history of alcohol use that was currently "under control." W.E.'s mother had recently sought psychiatric help, had been diagnosed with GAD, and had started psychotherapy and imipramine.

Following informed discussions with W.E. and her parents, it was decided that W.E. should continue with her psychotherapy and try buspirone for amelioration of anxiety symptoms. Outcome measures were identified, and the treatment was discussed with her psychotherapist, who agreed with the medication trial and offered to provide an independent evaluation of W.E.'s progress. Treatment was initiated with 5 mg given twice daily and, in the absence of side effects, this was increased after 3 days to 5 mg given three times daily.

When seen 4 days following the last dose increase, W.E. stated that she was no longer taking the medication. Although she had not experienced any adverse effects, she had discontinued the buspirone because "it was not working." Further discussion revealed that although the expected time for the onset of buspirone's anxiolytic activity had been discussed, W.E. had expected to feel better immediately. When this had not occurred, she concluded that the medication was not effective and thus should not be continued. After further education and support, W.E. returned to taking buspirone and experienced significant symptomatic and functional improvement that began 2 to 3 weeks following stabilization on 20 mg daily.

CASE COMMENTARY

This case illustrates a very common clinical issue arising with the use of most psychopharmacologic compounds. Indeed, it occurs so often that it could be called the *aspirin anticipation syndrome*. Many patients or the parents expect all medications to work the same way, and the most common model that they have experienced regarding medication effect is that of analgesics or antipyretics. In this model, the therapeutic effect of the medication is almost immediate, within hours or sooner. Thus, even though the physician may clearly inform the patient and family that therapeutic onset will be delayed and may provide the time line for the expected onset of action, patient and family experience derived from the aspirin model, coupled with expectations of a positive result, may lead to disheartenment when no clinical effect is readily apparent.

In discussing the expected onset of the medication effect, in addition to providing information about when the therapeutic effect might be expected, the clinician should clearly identify this common, unrealistic anticipation of immediate effect. Calling it the *aspirin anticipation syndrome* provides a useful label that the patient can remember later during the initial treatment-monitoring visits.

Confusing and Possibly Contradictory Information About Treatment

CASE EXAMPLE

"What should I do? I'm getting different information from my doctors."

S.C. was a 14-year-old girl with a diagnosis of PD. She had been referred by her primary care physician for pharmacologic intervention because counseling and buspirone at a dose of 30 mg daily had not provided adequate control of her symptoms. Psychiatric assessment confirmed a diagnosis of PD with a past history of a major depressive episode that had spontaneously remitted. Family history was positive for dysthymia, GAD, and PD on the mother's side and for alcoholism on the father's side.

As part of the discussion about the disorder and its treatment, the clinician mentioned that buspirone was not indicated for treatment of PD and reviewed the medications that might be of benefit. After further reading and discussion of the medication options, S.C. and her parents decided to try low-dose fluoxetine. Accordingly, 5 mg of fluoxetine, to be taken in the morning, was prescribed and a letter to that effect was dictated to the referring physician.

Two days later, S.C.'s mother telephoned and told the doctor that she had withheld S.C.'s medications on the advice of the referring physician. As she had understood the conversation, the primary care physician had told her that fluoxetine treatment might lead to suicide, confirming what she had read in the newspapers. Although this had been discussed with S.C. and her family prior to treatment, S.C.'s mother wondered why she was getting contradictory advice from two doctors. Furthermore, she stated that the primary care physician was certain that buspirone was a very safe medicine used to treat anxiety problems. She could not understand why two doctors differed on the use and value of a medication.

CASE COMMENTARY

This case illustrates an unfortunate and hopefully preventable problem, that of different and contradictory messages being given to patients by mental health professionals. In some cases, this may be caused by differing philosophical perspectives. In other situations, such as the case described here, this may be caused by different competencies. To prevent this problem from occurring, the psychopharmacologist should, whenever possible, know the referring professional and feel comfortable in working together with him or her. This is especially important if two professionals are working together to provide different aspects of a patient's care, such as psychotherapy and pharmacology. If this is the model of care chosen, written acknowledgment of each practitioner's role and an a priori decision on how to deal with therapeutic disagreements should be made. The patient and the patient's family need to know the parameters of this agreement and to agree to it as well.

In some situations, as illustrated here, professional differences of opinion may arise. In the case just described, the primary care physician was providing information at odds with that provided by the consultant, and the consultant's information and treatment plan were more appropriate. However, regardless of the merits of the particular case, patient and family confusion can easily arise if two professionals provide different information. In most cases clear and open communication between professionals should ensure that such problems do not arise. If communication problems that cannot be resolved do occur, the psychopharmacologist should not agree to participate in the care of any patient for whom he feels improper treatment is being provided by a conjoint clinician. By prescribing medication for a patient the clinician takes responsibility for that patient's care and therefore must agree to the value and validity of interventions prescribed by others involved in the case.

A perhaps more common variation of this scenario is the case in which a patient or parent receives contradictory and often incorrect information about medications from friends, relatives, the media, or other sources. Sometimes, medication myths or horror stories are prominently featured in print or electronically. In many cases these stories are told out of context, embellished, misunderstood, or otherwise distorted. Yet they negatively affect patients' and parents' perspectives on medications, often in inverse proportion to their validity. The clinician should be aware of these factors and discuss at the outset such issues as what to do with conflicting advice and how to handle differing viewpoints of involved physicians.

Unplanned and Nontherapeutic Discontinuation of Successful Treatment

CASE EXAMPLE

"I was all better so I stopped the medication."

E.S. was a 17-year-old girl with a 7-month history of major depressive disorder. She was treated with a combination of interpersonal therapy and the SSRI medication paroxetine at a dose of 20 mg daily. Eight weeks of this treatment resulted in significant symptom reduction, and her baseline Beck Depression Inventory (BDI) score of 19 dropped to 7, with her Hamilton Depression Rating Scale (HDRS) baseline score of 17 dropping to 8.

Five weeks following this improvement, E.S. returned to the clinic complaining of a return of all her symptoms. Her BDI had increased to 21 and her HDRS was now 17 again. In discussing the situation she revealed that she had terminated all treatment because she had been doing so well and felt that she was "cured." She had not realized that it was necessary to continue treatment beyond symptomatic improvement. These issues are discussed in the next part of this chapter and are addressed in all chapters in Section Four under the long-term pharmacologic treatment of specific disorders.

CASE COMMENTARY

This case illustrates an important issue in psychopharmacologic treatment. Many disorders for which pharmacologic interventions are indicated are chronic illnesses and can be expected to last well into the adult years, or even over the entire lifespan. In addition, their appearance in the child or adolescent years may

predict a more severe course than if they first began in adulthood. Relapse rates in many of these disorders are significant but may often be reduced with appropriate maintenance pharmacotherapy. Thus, effective medication treatment should be extended beyond the acute phase of the illness.

Continuing and Discontinuing Medication Treatment

Patients need to be educated about the expected course of their particular disorder and the pharmacologic interventions that may improve the length of their remission or provide prophylaxis against future exacerbations. Treatment, both pharmacologic and psychological, should continue past the time during which acute symptom resolution occurs. Unfortunately, there is little specific child or adolescent literature on optimal pharmacologic treatment types, dosages, or lengths of time necessary to prevent relapse or to increase the duration of remission. Guidelines extrapolated from studies in adults may be used in the treatment of specific disorders to guide pharmacologic treatment past the acute phase.

For example, it is well known that depressive disorders onsetting in youth recur in adulthood. Each episode is associated with marked symptomatic distress and functional impairment. Furthermore, multiple episodes may also induce long-standing physiologic, interpersonal, or functional disturbances that not only contribute to poorer long-term outcome but may increase the individual's vulnerability to future episodes of the illness (more depressions) or lead to other related disorders (such as dysthymia or substance abuse).

Long-term treatment of children and adolescents can be conceptualized as consisting of two phases. The first is consolidation, and the second is continuation. Consolidation treatment identifies that time from the resolution of the acute episode until the time the highest risk of relapse has passed (about 6 to 8 months for most disorders and 1 year for schizophrenia). Continuation treatment covers the time from the end of the consolidation phase until the end of the time when all possible recurrences of the disorder have passed. In many illnesses, the continuation phase may last many years, or indeed may be lifelong. Pharmacologic treatment in both these phases shares the following goals:

1. Maintain symptom remission.
2. Ensure compliance with pharmacotherapy.
3. Identify relapse or recurrence early.
4. Intervene immediately at the earliest signs of relapse or recurrence.

Information obtained from studies in adults and data available from clinical experience and ongoing investigations into maintenance treatment of children and adolescents suggest that continuing effective pharmacotherapy beyond the acute phase of the illness will significantly decrease the probability of relapse and will improve long-term outcome. Just how long such pharmacologic treatment should be continued and at what dose for what specific disorder are not well established. In most cases, however, the following guidelines can be applied:

1. Continue pharmacotherapy at the same dose required for initial improvement for at least 6 to 8 months following full symptom resolution.
2. Continue to monitor the patient over this time. If full functional resolution has not occurred, consider increasing the length of time of continued pharmacotherapy.
3. If an adequate therapeutic response to treatment has occurred and has been maintained as described earlier, consider gradually discontinuing medications so as not to induce a treatment withdrawal syndrome or precipitate a relapse.
4. Do not rush to withdraw medications if the patient is entering a part of her life cycle in which a relapse, if it occurred, would have serious and severe consequences for the future (e.g., prior to university entrance examinations).
5. If breakthrough symptoms occur during medication withdrawal, return the patient to the full maintenance dose of the medication as quickly as clinically possible.
6. Once pharmacotherapy has been discontinued, continue to monitor the patient at reasonable intervals to ensure that symptoms of the disorder have not recurred.
7. Provide the patient and parents with the information they need to adequately self-monitor symptoms of relapse. A relapse identification handout that can be used for this purpose is found in Appendix II.
8. If symptoms recur, treat them immediately with the same medication at the same target dose as was previously found to be effective in promoting remission. Do this even if the symptoms are mild.
9. If the patient has experienced two or more episodes of the disorder, consider maintenance therapy for a minimum of 1 to 2 years prior to reviewing the possibility of attempting medication withdrawal again.
10. In addition to providing optimal maintenance pharmacotherapy, assist the patient in obtaining other psychosocial interventions to improve interpersonal, social, and academic/vocational functioning as necessary.

Patient monitoring during long-term pharmacologic treatment should follow the guidelines described earlier. As already discussed, no single, rigid schedule can be developed to fit all potential scenarios. Each patient's long-term medication-monitoring schedule will need to be individualized using the previously identified variables to determine the frequency and duration of contact.

Diagnostic Re-evaluation

In many cases, the long-term maintenance pharmacotherapy of a patient will provide opportunities for the treating physician to review the patient's diagnosis as well as the treatment course to date. As previously discussed, a diagnosis is a hypothesis that must be re-evaluated when new information about the patient, course of the illness, or response to treatment is obtained. Ideally, this re-evaluation should be conducted routinely once a year and should include the following:

1. Review of the initial presentation, including the diagnostic instruments used (semistructured interview, DSM checklist)
2. Review of the course of illness up to the date of evaluation, including the onset of new symptoms and the offset of previous symptoms
3. Review of response to treatment, including symptoms, social or academic functioning, etc.
4. Evaluation of new information not available at the time of the initial diagnosis, such as a more detailed extended family history
5. Patient reassessment using a semistructured interview (such as the K-SADS; see Section Two)

Ideally, this type of diagnostic re-evaluation will include not only the physician but other members of the treatment team as well. The patient and family should be active participants in this process.

Diagnostic reassessment can have one of two results, and either outcome is reasonable. Either the initial or working diagnosis will be confirmed, or serious doubt will be raised about the validity of the first diagnosis. Should the diagnosis be confirmed, the treatment plan (suitably modified to achieve identified goals) can be carried out as usual. Should the initial diagnosis be questioned, changes in the treatment plan may need to be made.

Other, less obvious results from this type of

diagnostic reassessment may also occur, including:

1. Providing a forum for the patient and family to voice their opinions and concerns regarding the initial or working diagnosis
2. Providing the patient and family with a better understanding of the strengths and limits of psychiatric diagnosis and demonstrating that the physician is not closed minded but is willing and actually eager to challenge his own perspectives
3. Providing a supportive forum for the patient, family, and members of the treatment team to further their education about the illness and its treatment. This may be of particular importance if new therapies are available that were either not considered or not available earlier

Design of Psychopharmacologic Treatment Trials in Clinical Practice

Although many psychopharmacologic treatments follow the tried-and-true method of comprehensive baseline assessment, prescription, and careful outcome evaluation, the effectiveness of any particular pharmacologic treatment may occasionally not be readily apparent. At times other non-medication effects may account, at least in part, for outcomes attributed to the medicine. It is very important that the clinician have a reasonable certainty that the medication that she is prescribing is providing the desired therapeutic effect. This is particularly important when recognizing that the therapeutic effects of placebo treatments in children and adolescents can be considerable. In the estimation of some experts in this field, depending on the disorder under consideration, placebo effects may be expected in 30 to 40 percent of cases or even more.

CASE EXAMPLE

"How do I know if it's the medicine that is making the difference?"

F.V. was a 7-year-old boy who was referred by his family doctor for assessment and treatment of "hyperactivity." A detailed diagnostic assessment confirmed a diagnosis of ADHD, and appropriate baseline measures were completed. After discussions with F.V. and his parents, a decision was made to begin treatment with methylphenidate.

An "n of 1" single-case design trial was initiated using an ABAB design. Using parent, child, teacher, and physician ratings, the physician found clinically significant change in both the ADHD Rating Scale and Connors Scale scores (see Section Two) for a description of these instruments) at the times that F.V. was being treated with methylphenidate. During periods of placebo treatment, his scores returned to baseline (Fig. 7–2).

As a result of this single-case trial, F.V. was treated with methylphenidate at a dose of 10 mg, given in the morning, at noon, and in late afternoon. With this treatment and a number of concurrent behavioral interactions, his behavior, academic performance, and family functioning showed improvement. He was not experiencing any significant side effects. Six months later, his parents wondered if F.V. still required the medication or if the behavioral interventions alone would now be sufficient. In order to answer this question, another "n of 1"

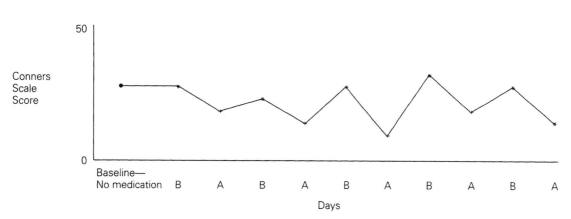

A = active drug; B = placebo.

FIGURE 7–2   Methylphenidate Treatment of a 7-Year-Old Boy with ADHD: Outcome Measures, ABAB Design

ABAB single-case design trial was undertaken. The results clearly showed a clinically significant effect of medication compared with placebo (Fig. 7–3).

CASE COMMENTARY

This case illustrates a useful approach to the common clinical problem of distinguishing the effect of medication from placebo in determining both the utility of beginning treatment and the necessity of continuing treatment.

The placebo effect can be defined as the expectancy of a positive outcome that occurs within the interpersonal interaction between physician and patient. This produces a therapeutic effect in the patient that is independent of the effect of the prescribed intervention. The placebo effect is a powerful force found in all of medicine, including psychiatric medicine. This effect operates regardless of the type of therapeutic encounter and is found in psychological, social, and physical treatments alike. Proof of the efficacy of any specific treatment must therefore account for the expected placebo effect, which may account for a significant percentage of responses.

Obviously, if a sustained placebo response to medication occurs, then the possibility arises that such a response might persist in the absence of continued medication use. Thus, it is worthwhile to differentiate those patients whose clinical symptoms remit because of placebo factors from those whose symptoms remit because of an active medication effect. Some of the former may be expected (with careful ongoing monitoring) to maintain their improvement free from the side effects associated with medication use. Those from the latter group will need to take medication, and their side effects, although remaining a risk of treatment, are tolerated because of the positive effect of the medicine. Considerable evidence now exists that many children and adolescents who demonstrate a placebo response may relapse fairly rapidly. Thus continued monitoring of response is necessary.

In studies of psychopharmacologic treatment in large numbers of subjects, the placebo effect is controlled for by the inclusion of a *placebo group*. In clinical work, however, placebo effects are difficult to distinguish from an active medication effect in any one individual. Some types of psychopharmacologic treatment can be clarified using a special controlled intervention design called the *single-case design* or the *"n of 1" study*. Methylphenidate treatment for ADHD, for example, uses this design; this is discussed more fully in a subsequent chapter.

The single-case design has a number of features that make its use in clinical practice invaluable in those situations in which it can be applied effectively. First, the single-case design can often answer a question that a large-scale treatment trial of any medication cannot: Will the treatment in question work for this specific patient? In any report of a medication trial, a variety of responses will be obtained in the population studied. Some patients will show a very positive response, others will demonstrate minimal or even worsening effects, and still others will be somewhere in between. Because of this diversity of response, even in studies with clearly demonstrated positive results, no large clinical treatment study can be unequivocally generalized to any individual patient. Thus, the questions that clinical treatment studies answer about the value of a particular treatment in a specific patient are as follows:

1. Which treatment is likely to work (and at what dose)?

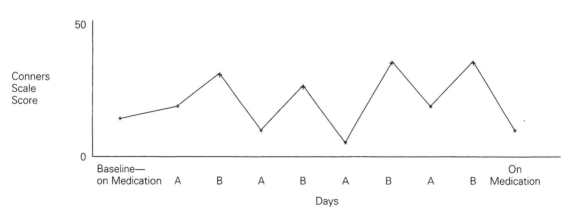

A = active drug; B = placebo.

FIGURE 7–3 ABAB Treatment Withdrawal Design for Methylphenidate Treatment

2. Which treatment is unlikely to work?
3. What side effects might reasonably be expected from a particular treatment?

In addition, single-case designs offer an empiric approach to evaluating treatment outcome and can help control for extraneous factors that occur during an intervention. This includes but is not limited to the placebo effect. Additional intervening variables may include such things as environmental effects, social supports, and nonspecific psychological events. These extraneous factors are continuously operating and may explain patient changes that the clinician wishes to attribute to his treatment, whether that treatment is psychological, social, or physiological. The design of the "n of 1" study is such that it allows for more valid inferences to be drawn about the impact of any specific intervention.

An "n of 1" study is useful in those cases where the following factors are found:

1. The disorder is diagnosable.
2. The target symptoms can be clearly identified and reliably measured.
3. The onset and cessation of the medication effect are relatively rapid.
4. The medication has previously demonstrated a positive treatment effect for the symptoms under evaluation in similar patients.
5. Continuous assessment of symptoms is possible.

When these conditions are met, an "n of 1" approach not only is useful but is the preferred method of initiating treatment because it can quickly and reasonably provide information about the clinical efficacy of the intervention under consideration.

Although a variety of single-case designs are available and can be modified to fit most clinical situations, two such "n of 1" methods are commonly used in everyday clinical practice. These are the ABAB design and the multiple-baseline design. These are briefly described here, but for further reading about these and other single-case designs the interested reader should consult the Suggested Readings list at the end of the chapter.

The ABAB design is essentially an on-off-on-off treatment paradigm in which the active treatment (the medicine) is switched to an inactive or inert substance (the placebo) and then this process is repeated. If the "on" mode shows a positive treatment effect as determined by the use of reliable evaluative methods over the baseline condition, and this effect returns to baseline once the active condition is replaced by the inactive condition (the "off" mode), this suggests that the active or "on" condition led to the observed change. If this same effect can be replicated, this provides further

confirmation that the observed change was most likely caused by the active treatment. For absolute certainty, of course, this ABAB design must be continued to infinity. However, real life intervenes, and the replication of treatment effect using continuous observations with reliable methods across two active and two inactive intervention modes provides sufficient evidence of treatment efficacy for usual clinical practice.

One important aspect of a successful single-case design trial is the careful assessment of baseline symptomatology. Psychiatric symptoms, like any medical symptoms, vary over time. Also, there may be situational effects in which symptoms vary with the patient's activities or location. For example, excessive motor activity might be most noted in a classroom or home setting compared with a playground, or attention problems may be more evident in a classroom in which many pupils are engaged in active learning as opposed to a small, quiet space where one-to-one instruction is available. Thus baseline symptom evaluation must be of adequate length and must be performed across sufficient situations to provide a proper measure of both time and site issues in symptom expression.

Following from this, the various intervention modes (A, B, A, B) must be of sufficient duration to allow for symptom measurement and must be performed across all indicated sites. A useful guideline is to try to make each intervention block the same length of time as the baseline assessment. This will provide a better evaluation of treatment response than using block times that are significantly shorter or longer than the baseline period.

Another useful type of the single-case design is the multiple-baseline design. In this design, two or more symptom baselines are determined and then each is assessed for treatment effect. Alternatively, a particular problem is identified and then evaluated specifically for different settings. For example, if different doses of a medication are to be evaluated for their effect on a number of possibly independent symptoms of ADHD (methylphenidate for motor hyperactivity or for attention), baseline assessment of each symptom should be obtained and then different doses of medication can be evaluated in turn for each of the symptoms independently. In this manner, determination of the optimal medication dose to improve motor hyperactivity, the optimal dose to improve attention, and the dose that provides the best effect on both symptoms together can be made.

When properly used, single-case designs can improve clinical practice by helping to evaluate the effect of a particular treatment in any individual case. Treatment can then be continued as is, augmented, modified, or discarded. Single-case designs can be readily improvised for a variety of clinical problems, as long as the criteria for their use (as outlined earlier) are met. They can also be used over the course of an intervention to determine whether a particular treatment is still effective over time or if it needs modification. Although some concerns about the use of such "n of 1" studies have been raised, including the issue of substituting a placebo for a treatment already known to be effective, if proper consent is obtained and if the answers to be provided outweigh the risks, the use of single-case designs in everyday clinical practice is to be supported.

Designs of Pharmacologic Treatment Trials—Practice Points

> 1. Single-case treatment designs provide a useful means for evaluating treatment response to medications.
> 2. In those cases in which single-case designs are applicable, they should be used at the onset of pharmacologic treatment to determine response.
> 3. Single-case designs are useful in determining whether ongoing pharmacologic interventions are of continuing therapeutic benefit.

Issues of Consent to Treatment

Consent to treatment is a fundamental part of the therapeutic relationship that in effect constitutes a contract between the provider and consumer of treatment. Valid consent is necessary for treatment and implies both willingness and capacity on the part of the consumer to allow the treatment process to occur. It is important to consider consent not as a one-time occurrence but as an ongoing basis for treatment.

The concept of consent to treatment is based on both legal and ethical perspectives. Legal guidelines may vary among jurisdictions; hence the practitioner must know the legal guidelines regarding issues of consent as they apply to the jurisdiction within which the practice is located. Ethical considerations also have an impact on consent to treatment, and the practitioner must understand that these are not unidimensional but may reflect differing cultural, religious, and personal values that are brought to the therapeutic relationship. Thus, the conceptual framework of consent to treatment is exceedingly complex, and while the complexity of this concept must be recognized, it must not lead to either therapeutic inertia or excessive or inappropriate standards of practice that are based primarily on fears of possible litigation.

Consent to treatment implies competency to give consent. This is perhaps best understood as a person's ability to make informed decisions on his own behalf. Competency, to be demonstrated in the consumer, as outlined by Janicak, Davis, Preskorn, and Ayd (see the Suggested Readings list), includes the following:

1. Ability to communicate
2. Presence of intact immediate-recent memory
3. Intact orientation
4. Adequate intellectual functioning (both abstract and logical processing)
5. Intact reality testing
6. Age (elderly and the young)

Once these have been established, other factors related to a person's understanding should be established. These include:

1. The consumer shows evidence of making a treatment choice.
2. The treatment choice made shows a reasonable outcome of success.
3. The treatment choice is made on the basis of rational reasons.
4. The consumer making the treatment choice demonstrates an ability to understand the risks, benefits, and alternatives to the choice she has made.
5. The consumer understands the potential harmful consequences that may occur if treatment is not accepted.

Competent patients have the right to refuse treatment. As previously stated, the legal guidelines and procedures for determining an individual's competency for decisions regarding medical treatment vary across jurisdictions, and the physician must be aware of those that apply in her setting and follow them.

In order to assist the consumer in the process of giving consent to treatment, the practitioner is obliged to provide the patient with information that can be used in his or her deliberations. This information is characterized by the following criteria:

1. It must be accurate. Information should be based on available scientific knowledge and not merely on the theoretical orientation or clinical experience of the practitioner.
2. It must be comprehensive. Details of the treatment must be outlined. In pharmacotherapy this includes the risks, expected benefits, and unique features of the medications under discussion. In addition, an estimation of the likelihood of success and the expected time for symptom resolution should be provided.

3. It must be sensitive to the consumer's concerns. The patient must be given an opportunity to ask questions and demand clarification of any issues regarding treatment.
4. Alternatives to the proposed treatment must be identified. The patient must be made aware of other treatment options, if they exist, along with the known evidence of their efficacy and their risks and benefits.
5. Consequences of inappropriate choice must be made clear. The physician must inform the patient of the potential consequences of not accepting treatment of demonstrated efficacy or of choosing a treatment without demonstrated efficacy.

In dealing with information regarding psychopharmacologic treatments for children and adolescents, many of the above-mentioned information-based parameters for informed consent are not adequately characterized. Often this is because insufficient data regarding the use of any specific medication in any particular disorder of children or adolescents are available. In many other cases the information about the efficacy or potential adverse effects of nonpharmacologic treatments is either insufficient or lacking. Thus the clinician is forced to provide advice regarding treatment on the basis of less than adequate information. It is important that the patient and parent understand that their decisions will be based at times on less than perfect knowledge.

Some physicians will use labeling guidelines confirmed by the Food and Drug Administration (in the United States) or the Health Protection Branch (in Canada) as rigid criteria for decision making and consent regarding the use of psychotropics in children and adolescents. This is inappropriate because approval of use for medications is not limited to the labeling guidelines that accompany them. Furthermore, in many cases, especially in children or younger adolescents, the labeling guidelines are based on little if any empirical information regarding the use of the drug in that age group because the necessary investigations have not been carried out.

The issues of consent to treatment become more complicated when children under the age of majority are involved. In addition to the complexities of competency to give consent found in adult psychiatric patients, there are other legal and developmental considerations. In many jurisdictions, children have an indirect legal relationship with the clinician, and difficulties stemming from this (as discussed later) may arise. Furthermore, developmental issues regarding the level of cognitive understanding are at play for children and some adolescents. Many younger patients may not be able to consider and evaluate the various parameters of treatment options available to them or may not be able to properly assess the impact of a choice of one treatment over another or of treatment over no treatment. Thus, responsible adults, usually the parents or legal guardians, are given the responsibility for providing consent to treatment. This legal imperative, however, should not limit the physician's involvement in providing the necessary information about proposed medication treatment and support to the child, albeit at the appropriate developmental level. In this situation, which is respectful of the dignity of the child as well as within the legal framework of consent, the child's *assent* to treatment is obtained, as well as parental or legal guardian consent to treatment.

Parents or legal guardians are expected to act in the best interests of the child and to provide the legal requirement for the giving of consent to the treatment of minors. Thus, the clinician must also evaluate the competency of the responsible adult in providing consent for pharmacologic treatment of a legally defined minor. Furthermore, the involvement of many individuals, all having some say in the potential treatment of a child, may lead to even further complexities. Family issues may come into play, such as when two parents disagree on what constitutes appropriate treatment. In these situations, the physician not only must exercise wisdom and therapeutic skill but may be placed in the difficult situation of overriding parental or legal guardian decisions in response to what he considers the best interests of the child. In these cases legal interventions, including judicial orders to treat, may be necessary, and the therapeutic relationship among child, parent, and physician will obviously be strained. Often effective, open communication may prevent such a situation from occurring, but the possibility of potential conflict should not prevent the physician from following through with her obligation to the child.

CASE EXAMPLE

Overriding the Parental Decision in Treatment of Child Psychosis

K.B. was a 6-year-old boy who was brought by his mother to the emergency room of a children's hospital. She gave a history of K.B. showing increasingly unusual behaviors, including staring off into space, mumbling and laughing to himself, eating sporadically, urinating in his bedroom, and talking in a language that she did not understand. She denied any significant premorbid difficulties but dated K.B.'s problems to about 1 month previously.

On examination K.B. did not make eye contact and huddled in a corner of the room, refusing to play with toys or look at picture books. He occasionally produced gutteral sounds, and although he seemed to understand what was being said, he would not or could not speak, even to answer direct questions. At times he would approach his mother and sit with her; then he would get up and walk away. At one point he sat facing the wall and began to babble and sway but stopped immediately when he was asked about his behavior.

The attending physician was concerned that K.B. was showing possible psychotic symptoms and wanted to admit the youngster to the hospital for observation and further assessment. K.B.'s mother became upset when this was suggested to her. In further discussions she told the physician that she felt that K.B. was possessed by the spirit of a popular singer who had died about the time that K.B. was reported to have begun his unusual behavior. She felt that exorcism of this spirit was needed and stated that she would take K.B. home and arrange for this to occur. She told the examining physician that she had only wanted to have a doctor see K.B. to make sure that he did not have cancer.

Attempts made to obtain corroborative information to her story were unsuccessful. According to K.B.'s mother, there was no other responsible adult living in the family home, and she refused to divulge the name of K.B.'s primary care physician. She refused to listen to any suggestions that K.B. be admitted and turned down an offer to be able to stay in the hospital with him. She was fully informed about the diagnostic possibilities and the necessity to perform a proper assessment. She remained adamant that demon possession was the cause of K.B.'s problems and then refused to let the physician continue his attempts to speak to her son.

When she was informed that the physician was obligated to act in what she perceived to be the best interests of the child and that in the physician's opinion K.B. needed a proper psychiatric assessment and hospitalization, she demanded that the doctor and the hospital release her son immediately. Furthermore, she threatened to bring legal action against the physician for her actions. The appropriate child protection authorities were contacted, and temporary guardianship of the child was arranged. K.B. was admitted to the hospital for a psychiatric assessment. His mother was subsequently admitted to an adult mental health unit in a nearby institution.

CASE COMMENTARY

This case illustrates an extreme situation in which the child's parent was judged not to be acting in the best interests of the child. In such cases, the treating physician is obliged to invoke appropriate legal measures when in his best judgment these are necessary to ensure that a legal minor has access to necessary reasonable medical interventions.

At times, the child's or adolescent's developmental stage or family dynamics may lead to difficult issues regarding consent to treatment. In situations where the biological parents are divorced yet share joint custody and disagree as to the appropriate medical intervention, the physician should meet with each parent individually and then with them jointly. Occasionally a further consultation with another physician may be useful. If treatment is indicated and the impasse cannot be overcome, the physician may need to explore the pertinent legal issues that impact on the child's right to appropriate medical treatment.

Adolescents may pose a special problem in terms of consent to treatment. Psychological issues of independence or conflict with parents or other authority figures may lead to a teenager's refusal of treatment. In these situations clear, direct, but nonthreatening discussions with the adolescent are helpful. In addition, depending on the severity of the clinical situation, the physician may need to allow the teen a period of time of refusal before treatment is accepted. Adolescents may sometimes benefit from a short period of reflection time and usually a few days are sufficient. If this goes on too long, the patient may simply be refusing treatment. Another useful intervention is to identify the course of treatment as an experiment in which the teen and physician are joint participants. And it is not uncommon for teens to change their minds about treatment, sometimes more than once, in response to peer and other environmental influences. The physician providing pharmacologic treatment for adolescents must be prepared to "hang in there" because the personal relationship between clinician and teen is essentially the ground in which pharmacologic treatment grows. The following case example illustrates these points.

CASE EXAMPLE

Hanging In There with the Anxious Teen

A.F. was an 18-year-old girl who was referred for pharmacologic treatment of OCD of 6 years' duration. Following a detailed assessment and baseline evaluation, a course of treatment consisting of behavior therapy and clomipramine was suggested. A.F.'s parents were in favor of this, but A.F. was opposed. She stated that she did not believe in treatment with "drugs" and did not see how behavior therapy could possibly help her because it did not make any sense to her. She was, however, willing to "drop by and see the doctor in a week or so to just talk a bit." She refused to read anything about OCD compulsive disorder because she felt it was "all propaganda anyway."

When A.F. was seen again, she talked about her friends and school. Although she remained very symptomatic, she continued to refuse treatment and still would not accept any written material about the disorder. She did agree to "drop by again." At the conclusion of A.F.'s third visit, she asked if there was anything to read about OCD that "wasn't propaganda," meaning that it was available outside the doctor's office. She was told about the book, *The Boy Who Couldn't Stop Washing*.

Four days later A.F. telephoned to say that she wanted to discuss treatment because she had read the book. When next seen she stated that she had decided to take the medications but not the behavior therapy because she still felt that behavior therapy did not make sense to her. She was given information about clomipramine and asked to discuss this with her parents and anyone else that she wanted to. She was also encouraged to find out more about behavior therapy because of its demonstrated efficacy. She was very surprised to find out that her doctor also did not know exactly how behavior therapy worked and took on the challenge of finding out more about this type of treatment. Her physician suggested that A.F. could think about her OCD as a scientific puzzle and its treatment as an experiment to be carefully conducted and assessed. She was intrigued by this idea.

At her next visit A.F. stated that she had decided to try a combination of behavior therapy and medication treatment. She became an active participant in the treatment experiment.

CASE COMMENTARY

This case illustrates the relatively common dynamic processes at play in the pharmacologic treatment of teenagers. Neither autocratic nor laissez-faire approaches are useful. Treating the teen with respect while holding gently but firmly to clinical expertise and allowing the time

necessary for the development of a trusting relationship are all essential components of the therapeutic process of adolescent treatment.

Another common issue arising in pharmacologic treatment of adolescents is that of confidentiality. Teenagers are often concerned that information shared with their physician remains confidential, especially with regard to their parents. It is important that this issue be openly addressed at the beginning of treatment so that all parties—patient, family, and physician—know what the boundaries will be. It is suggested that all information arising from therapeutic interaction between teen and physician remain confidential, except for information that may lead to significant harm to the teen or to others. Information in this category includes such issues as suicidality, drug abuse, and serious criminal activity. Teens should be assured that if the physician feels that issues arise that in his opinion require parental awareness, these will be discussed with the teen before the parents are involved, except in an emergency situation in which this is not possible. The vast majority of adolescents have no difficulty with these guidelines, and making them explicit at the onset of treatment will be helpful to the teen, parents, and practitioner alike.

The issue of pregnancy arising during pharmacologic treatment is a difficult one that has complicated legal and ethical components. Legal directives regarding pregnancy issues with respect to minors vary across jurisdictions, and the physician must be aware of these. In many cases, however, this issue may arise for an adolescent who has reached the age of majority. In this situation, medical imperatives (such as potential teratogenic effects of medications), as well as ethical and legal factors, must be considered as the physician attempts to work with the patient to identify and choose an appropriate course of action.

In some cases, or even as a general rule, the physician may wish to append a documentation of consent to the patient's clinical record. Although in most cases a note summarizing the pertinent issues is sufficient, the form in Figure 7–4 is offered as a checklist and consent documentation. Many clinicians find it useful to have the patient and parent sign this document and then to append it to the clinical chart.

Issues of Consent to Treatment— Practice Points

1. Fully informed consent to treatment following the above-mentioned guidelines

Patient's Name: _____ Date: _____

Parties present: _____

The following have been discussed with the above individuals on the above date:

_____ Psychiatric diagnosis   _____ Expected efficacy of suggested treatment(s)

_____ Purpose of treatment   _____ Expected side effects of suggested treatment(s)

_____ Types of available treatments   _____ Confidentiality

_____ Known efficacy of available treatments   _____ Emergency procedures

_____ Known side effects of available treatments   _____ Expected medical procedures

_____ Expected outcome with no treatment

_____ Suggested treatment(s) (describe): _____

The following were issues or questions regarding the treatment raised by the individuals identified above:

_____

_____

_____

_____

_____

_____

In my opinion the patient (name: _____) and/or parent(s)/legal guardian(s)

(name: _____) understand the diagnosis, prognosis, treatment options, the

evolving nature of knowledge about medical diagnoses and treatment, and the expected risks and benefit

of the proposed treatment. In my opinion (name: _____) is competent to give

informed consent for the following pharmacologic treatment(s):

_____

_____

_____

_____

_____

_____

Physician signature: _____ Date: _____

Patient signature (where appropriate): _____ Date: _____

Parent signature (where appropriate): _____ Date: _____

Legal guardian signature (where appropriate): _____ Date: _____

FIGURE 7–4   Psychopharmacologic Treatment Review Form

must be obtained from the patient and family (as appropriate) before beginning pharmacologic intervention.

2. The child's legal and developmental status may require modifications in obtaining consent to treatment. In these cases assent to treatment should be obtained.

3. Information about treatment must be presented in a manner that is suitable for the child's level of cognitive development.

4. The use of a consent to treatment document signed by patient and parent(s) or legal guardian, as appropriate, is encouraged.

SUGGESTED READINGS

Cheng TL, Savageau TA, Sattler AL, DeWitt TG. Confidentiality in health care: A survey of knowledge, perceptions and attitudes among high school students. Journal of the American Medical Association, 269:1404–1407, 1993.

Guyatt G, Sackett D, Adachi J, et al. A clinician's guide for conducting randomized trials in individual patients. Canadian Medical Association Journal, 139:497–503, 1988.

Janicak PG, Davis JM, Preskorn SHP, Ayd FJ. Principles and Practices of Psychopharmacology. Baltimore: Williams and Wilkins, 1993.

Mardr J, Mulle K, Stallings P, Erhardt D, Connors CK. Organizing an anxiety disorder clinic. In JS March (ed): Anxiety Disorders in Children and Adolescents. New York: Guilford Press, 1995, pp 420–435.

Nurcombe B, Partlett DF. Child Mental Health and the Law. New York: Tree Press, 1994.

Popper C. Medical unknowns and ethical consent: Prescribing psychotropic medication to children in the face of medical unknowns. In C Popper (ed): Psychiatric Pharmacosciences of Children and Adolescents. Washington, DC: American Psychiatric Association Press, 1990, pp 125–161.

Towbin K. Evaluation, establishing the treatment alliance, and informed consent. Child and Adolescent Psychiatric Clinics of North America, 4:1–14, 1995.

Wallace AE, Kofoed LL. Statistical analysis of single case studies in the clinical setting: The example of methylphenidate trials in children with attention-deficit hyperactivity disorder. Journal of Child and Adolescent Psychopharmacology, 4:141–150, 1994.

White L, Tursky B, Schwartz GE (eds). Placebo: Theory, Research and Mechanisms. New York: Guilford Press, 1995.

Clinical Practice of Child and Adolescent Psychopharmacology

The clinical use of psychotropic medications with children and adolescents depends on the therapeutic value of these compounds. Therapeutic value is determined by establishing clearly the efficacy and treatment-emergent side effects of a medication used in treating the symptoms and functional impairments of psychiatric illness in children and adolescents. In many instances in child and adolescent psychopharmacology, therapeutic value as described here has not yet been scientifically determined. However, reasonable evidence for therapeutic value exists, although such evidence is based on fewer clearly validated criteria than are often available for psychopharmacologic treatment in adults.

Given the current state of knowledge regarding psychopharmacologic treatment in children and adolescents, the clinician should apply the following criteria to evaluate the strength of valid support for the use of medications in this population:

1. Evidence of therapeutic value arising from properly designed double-blind clinical research conducted in children and adolescents.
2. Evidence of potential therapeutic value arising from properly designed open clinical research conducted in children and adolescents.
3. Evidence of potential therapeutic value arising from properly designed double-blind clinical research conducted in adults.
4. Evidence of possible therapeutic value arising from extensive clinical experience in using psychotropic agents to treat children and adolescents.

Certainly, there is a hierarchy of evidence in this list. Psychotropic treatment based on the first criterion is on much firmer ground than treatment based on the fourth criterion alone. In reality, therapeutic evidence for treating children and adoles-

cents with psychotropics is usually based on more than one of the above-mentioned criteria. However, in many cases information obtained from double-blind, placebo-controlled studies of various compounds is still lacking. Given this situation, the clinician must ensure that he knows what information is available and passes this on to the patient and parent. The issues arising from this state of current knowledge have been discussed in detail in previous chapters.

Even in the optimal knowledge scenario, however, the practitioner still faces uncertainty in the application of scientifically derived knowledge to the patient who presents to his care. Psychopharmacologic information is often not easily transferable from the research laboratory or the double-blind clinical trial to the physician's office. In all cases, general information available about treatment with psychotropics must be applied to the unique characteristics of each individual patient.

For example, clinical trials of antidepressants usually randomly assign all participants to either the study drug or the placebo (and in some cases a reference drug as well). Inclusion and exclusion criteria apply to all patients equally, creating, as much as possible, a relatively homogeneous study group. This does not occur in the clinician's office or hospital ward. Important patient-specific factors such as comorbidity, past history of treatment (pharmacologic and psychosocial), family history, social milieu, and economics will all influence decisions regarding psychopharmacologic treatment.

Furthermore, in clinical trials treatment is protocol driven and deviations from the protocol are not permitted. The subject is "slotted" into the treatment. In real-life clinical psychopharmacologic practice, the model used attempts to adapt the psychotropic treatment to the patient. This may necessitate many deviations from standard protocol, as long as these deviations make clinical sense and are subject to careful objective scrutiny. Hence, clinical practice can never be as cut and dry as research studies are.

Currently, most psychiatric texts and psychopharmacologic review articles present information about psychotropic medications in the format of the studies that have been undertaken to determine their therapeutic value. While valuable for transmitting information about medications and their potential clinical utility, this format is not sufficiently helpful to the clinician attempting to treat a psychiatrically ill patient. In most texts the vital questions of clinical care usually remain unidentified or unanswered. These vital issues are as follows:

1. How do I decide whether or not to treat?
2. Given a particular clinical presentation, how do I choose which medication is best or is at least more appropriate?
3. How do I begin treatment, and how do I titrate the dose?
4. How long does treatment last, and how should I decide when and how to stop?
5. What are the common side effects (not lists of every possible symptom ever reported in the use of a particular drug), and how do I deal with them?
6. What do I need to tell the patient and parents about the medicine and the treatment?
7. What problems commonly arise in treating patients with this medication?
8. Are there any "clinical pearls" that I can't find in research reports that would help me treat my patients better?

The purpose of Section Four of this book (Chapters 8 to 17) is to provide clinically relevant information that answers these questions and others that commonly arise in everyday psychopharmacologic care. As a result, the chapters are organized not by class of drug but by type of psychiatric disorder or psychiatric symptoms. This, after all, is how patients present. They will not arrive in one's office with the sign "needs antipsychotics" nicely stamped on their shirts. In the real world, they have depressions, psychoses, anxiety, symptoms of aggression, and so on. They have families, friends, and unique personal characteristics. Treatment with psychotropics must begin from the realization that medications are used to treat people. People are not defined by the medications that are being used to treat them.

In each chapter in this section the various medications of therapeutic value are identified and the process of clinical decision making is described. Then, chosen medicines (and the reasons for this choice) are described in clinically relevant detail,

and appropriate acute and chronic models of treatment are elucidated. Where reasonable alternatives to treatment (apart from those chosen) occur, these are identified and the reader is directed to that chapter of the book in which that particular compound or group of compounds is discussed.

Commonly occurring problems are identified and solutions are suggested. When available, "clinical pearls" are dropped. What to do and what not to do in specific instances are discussed. How to deal with treatment resistance is described. Whenever possible, methods of evaluating outcome are presented.

Each chapter uses one or more case histories to identify and illustrate the issues. This is done to bring life to scientific data and to make the information relevant and understandable to practitioners and trainees alike. The cases are all taken from clinical experience. They represent both successes and failures of pharmacotherapy. They are the human frame on which to hang the clothing of clinical psychopharmacologic practice.

Because many medications can be used in a variety of disorders, detailed information about every potential medicine is not necessarily found in every chapter. For example, fluoxetine, a serotonin-specific reuptake inhibitor, can be used to treat obsessive compulsive disorder or major depression. This medicine will be discussed in detail in one chapter, and references to this detailed discussion are provided in the other chapters in which its use might be considered. In some cases a medication may be the first choice in more than one disorder. In that case it is described fully in one chapter, and in other chapters a different medication is discussed in its place. When this occurs, the reader will be advised that such is the case and will be directed to the appropriate part of the book in which the first-choice compound is described.

Every attempt has been made to make the chapters readable and clinically relevant. As in other parts of this book, no references break the flow of the text. Selected further readings that are felt to be useful for clinicians are suggested at the conclusion of each chapter.

SUGGESTED READINGS

Adams S. Prescribing of psychotropic drugs to children and adolescents. British Medical Journal, 302:217–218, 1991.
Kaplan S, Simms R, Busner J. Prescribing practices of outpatient child psychiatrists. Journal of the American Academy of Child and Adolescent Psychiatry, 33:35–44, 1994.
Klein R, Abikoff H, Barkley R, Campbell M, Leckman J, Ryan N, Solanto M, Whalen C. Clinical trials in children and adolescents. In R Prien, D Robinson (eds): Clinical Evaluation of Psychotropic Drugs: Principles and Guidelines. New York: Raven Press, 1994, pp 457–508.

CHAPTER 8

General Issues in the Psychopharmacologic Treatment of Anxiety Disorders

A number of anxiety disorders may first manifest themselves in childhood or adolescence. These are panic disorder (PD) (with or without agoraphobia), generalized anxiety disorder, specific phobia, social phobia, obsessive compulsive disorder (OCD), post-traumatic stress disorder, and acute stress disorder. Other anxiety-type syndromes more specific to childhood, such as separation anxiety disorder, may be a unique behavioral manifestation of attachment difficulties. Alternatively, particularly for separation anxiety disorder, they may be a *forme fruste* of an anxiety disorder, such as PD, in which the observed behavioral disturbances either are a developmentally appropriate response to symptoms of panic or encompass a cluster of activities reflecting the anticipatory anxiety or phobic avoidance of the PD constellation. In addition, anxiety secondary to acute medical conditions may occur.

Pharmacologic interventions for anxiety disorders in children and adolescents are still in the early stages of development but, apart from the behavioral treatment of phobic states, they represent the largest body of currently available scientifically valid information regarding any treatments of these disorders, psychological, biologic, or social. Thus, while it may seem prudent to delay pharmacologic interventions to determine whether a nonpharmacologic treatment will be effective, no scientific evidence exists to support this perspective. On the other hand, in the absence of sufficent valid study, the rationale for early and aggressive pharmacologic interventions for conditions that may be adequately addressed nonpharmacologically, such as OCD, are also lacking.

In this situation thoughtful clinical considerations must guide treatment, and the physician should neither press nor withhold pharmacologic interventions simply on the basis of her beliefs about what is best. Available treatment literature in studies of affectively ill or psychotic adults suggests that early pharmacologic interventions improve both acute and long-term outcomes. Whether this information pertains to the treatment of anxiety-disordered children and adolescents is not clear, but it should not be ignored in favor of the dictum that the least intensive intervention should be performed first—a practice that is often followed in spite of the lack of evidence to support it.

One potential conceptual issue that may have an impact on the treatment of child and adolescent anxiety disorders is the view that these syndromes are relatively benign or "mild." Unfortunately, this is not the case, and the extensive morbidity and high economic cost of the anxiety disorders, at least in adults, have recently been identified. The relationship between specific anxiety disorders such as PD and suicide is also relatively well established. Given this evidence, the clinician considering competing treatment options for the various child and adolescent anxiety disorders must carefully weigh not only the potential short-term risks and benefits of any one particular treatment but also the potential long-term effects of providing suboptimal interventions.

Another important issue to consider in the treatment of child and adolescent anxiety disorders is the natural course of the various illnesses. This is important in at least two different respects. First, the natural course of the particular illness itself is important. For example, although confirming scientifically valid studies are generally unavailable, the natural course of PD seems to be one of intermittent waxing and waning. Often occasional panic attacks will be followed by months or years of a relatively panic symptom–free state, only to be shattered by the onset of frequent and at times severe panic attacks. In other cases, panic attacks may reappear and disappear quickly, perhaps to manifest themselves again years later. Treatment of a disorder with such a variable natural course is very different from treatment of a disorder with a pattern of continued and relatively constant severity.

Many of the anxiety disorders exhibit this pattern of changes in symptom intensity over time. Some disorders, such as OCD, may even show variations in specific symptoms, as when one particular obsession or compulsion decreases in severity or disappears altogether, only to be replaced by another. In some cases this may be associated with changes in the individual's environment. In other cases these fluctuations seem to occur with a rhythm independent of external influences.

This type of fluctuating course may make it difficult to determine treatment success. A clinician who happens to prescribe a particular treatment at a time that the patient's disorder is in the process of a spontaneous improvement may incorrectly attribute the change in symptoms to the treatment. In this case it appears that the treatment is effective, even if it actually has no effect on the natural course of the disorder. Alternatively, a clinician who applies a partially effective treatment at the time that the patient's disorder is in the process of a spontaneous relapse may incorrectly conclude that the treatment is completely ineffective or indeed contraindicated.

When the above-mentioned issue regarding the natural course of anxiety disorders is considered together with the high estimated placebo effect of intervention in many of these disorders (other than from OCD), the clinician must be careful when choosing, applying, and evaluating any treatment, including pharmacotherapy, in anxiety disorders. At the very least, the severely limited applicability of single-case reports in suggesting useful interventions must be kept in mind.

Second, a particular anxiety disorder may lead to or precede the development of another psychiatric illness. For example, studies of adolescent-onset depression have identified a significant number of patients in whom a clear-cut anxiety disorder predated the onset of the depressive illness. It is not yet known if early and effective intervention in the first illness would have prevented the development or diminished the severity of the second. Neither is it known if the treatment of the second disorder (in this case depression) is optimally identical to the treatment for the same syndrome occurring "de novo," that is, without a preceding anxiety disorder. Studies in adults suggest that the comorbidity of an anxiety disorder such as PD with another psychiatric illness such as depression is associated with a poorer treatment response and a more malignant long-term course. It is important to acknowledge these issues in the treatment of child and adolescent anxiety disorders.

Given the current state of knowledge about the clinical course and efficacies of various treatments for child and adolescent anxiety disorders, the high economic costs of such treatments, and the well-established morbidity associated with them, it is suggested that, contrary to much current clinical practice, relatively aggressive early interventions that include the consideration of appropriate pharmacotherapy may be indicated to improve current symptoms and to maximize long-term outcomes. The nature of these early interventions should be guided by the severity of symptoms and the degree of functional disability that they create. In cases in which symptom severity and functional disability are moderate to severe, combined pharmacologic and psychological interventions are suggested from the onset of treatment. In cases in which symptoms and disability are mild, more time may be taken to determine whether psychological treatments may by themselves be of value. In any case, good clinical practice demands that the clinician consider these issues and discuss them with the patient and family to come to a joint decision about the treatment plan that will be followed.

Although it is recognized that anxiety disorders are frequently found to be comorbid with other anxiety disorders, mood disorders, or attention-deficit disorder, their psychopharmacologic treatments are discussed separately because they are diagnosed as separate entities. Given the different clinical approaches to the psychopharmacologic treatment of PD compared with the other anxiety disorders, PD is discussed in a chapter of its own. Pharmacologic treatment of comorbid states is reviewed as appropriate.

Issues in the Treatment of Anxiety Disorders—Practice Points

1. Anxiety disorders are serious psychiatric disorders with significant short- and long-term morbidity requiring effective treatments.
2. Consider maximal initial interventions (combined pharmacotherapy and psychotherapy) for anxiety disorders with moderate to severe symptomatology and functional impairment.

SUGGESTED READINGS

Kendler KS, Neal MC, Kessler RC, et al. Major depression and generalised anxiety disorder: Same genes, (partly) different environments? Archives of General Psychiatry, 49:716–722, 1992.

Leon AC, Portera L, Weissman MM. The social costs of anxiety disorders. British Journal of Psychiatry, 166 (Suppl 27):19–22, 1995.

Leonard HL (ed). Anxiety disorders. Child and Adolescent Psychiatric Clinics of North America, 2:563–838, 1993.

March J (ed). Anxiety Disorders in Children and Adolescents. New York: Guilford Press, 1995.

Salvador-Carulla L, Segui J, Fernandez-Cano P, Canet J. Costs and offset effect in panic disorders. British Journal of Psychiatry, 166 (Suppl 27):23–28, 1995.

Psychopharmacologic Treatment of Panic Disorder

Panic disorder (PD) is an anxiety disorder characterized by severe, often spontaneous panic attacks complicated by anticipatory anxiety (worry of having another panic attack) and phobic avoidance (avoiding those situations in which panic attacks have occurred or may be precipitated). For clinical treatment purposes, panic attacks are conveniently classified as:

- Induced or spontaneous
- Mild, moderate, or severe
- Full (four or more symptoms) or partial

In addition, the duration of panic attacks is timed, and the rapid crescendo and decrescendo pattern of the typical panic attack may be followed by a period of variable length in which the child or adolescent feels shaky and distressed. Many children may not be able to verbalize the psychological or physiologic symptoms they are experiencing, or they may interpret their symptoms in developmentally appropriate ways that may make it difficult for the clinician to identify the state as a panic attack. Of particular interest is the possibility that hyperventilation syndrome, well described in the pediatric literature, may be a presentation of a panic-type disorder.

Given these features, the diagnosis of PD in children and young adolescents may not always be clear-cut. A high degree of clinical suspicion and detailed direct questioning is necessary to identify a potential PD. In many cases, especially in young children, a panic-like syndrome (consisting of periodically occurring poorly characterized fears accompanied by symptoms of autonomic arousal) may indicate an underlying PD. The possibility of PD must be considered in any child or adolescent presenting with a recent onset of anxiety symptoms or avoidance behaviors, including refusal to attend school.

CASE EXAMPLE

"I can't sleep because . . ."

R.A. was a 6-year-old boy who was referred for assessment of problems in getting to sleep. Four months prior to assessment, he had suddenly started fretting about going to bed and occasionally came into his parents' bed at night. When asked what his concerns about going to bed were, he stated that he had bad dreams about terrible ghosts and dying. These "dreams" occurred infrequently and were not consistent with night terrors. Over time he began to avoid going to bed because of these dreams and began to demand that his mother sit with him until he fell asleep. If he awoke during the night he would seek out his parents' bed, even if he had not had a bad dream, because he was afraid he might have one. Even when he fell asleep in his parents' bed, he would occasionally wake up feeling very "scared." Interventions attempted prior to R.A.'s assessment had been reassurance and a bedtime hygiene program. These had not been effective, and his anxiety about going to bed increased. He also complained about breathing problems and "stomachaches."

On assessment R.A. voiced the fears described earlier. On direct questioning he endorsed seven or more physical symptoms of panic, which he described as "scary fast." Also, he was able to describe rapid-onset feelings of dread and doom, which he interpreted as meaning that his parents would die "because that would be the worst thing in the world." He described waking up from sleep with these feelings, thoughts, and physical symptoms and stated that he had been having similar feelings during the day as well. He was worried that he would have these feelings at school because he had felt "scared" for no reason in his class a number of times. A few weeks prior to his appointment, he had begun to try to avoid going to school.

A family history was positive for depression in his mother and, although a clear diagnosis could not be made from the information available, "anxiety problems" were described by his maternal grandmother as well. R.A.'s father denied any psychiatric disorder, and his family history was not known because he was an only child whose parents had died while he was a senior in high school.

A tentative diagnosis of PD was made. It was determined that in R.A.'s case, nocturnal panic attacks were occurring more commonly than daytime panic attacks by a ratio of four to one. Because of the severity of the symptoms and R.A.'s increasing functional impairment, appropriate baseline assessment was followed by a successful treatment program, including education about PD, "thinking the scary thoughts away" (cognitive therapy), and medication.

CASE COMMENTARY

In R.A.'s case the diagnosis of PD was not considered, possibly because of the atypical clinical presentation. Indeed, at first glance and in the absence of a careful history, he might have been diagnosed as suffering from separation anxiety disorder. It is not known, however, if this atypical presentation is actually atypical or simply considered so because the developmentally appropriate questions needed to elucidate the diagnosis were not asked. The simple take-home message in assessing anxiety-like symptoms in children is to probe carefully for signs and symptoms of a PD using developmentally appropriate language.

In adolescents PD is generally easier to diagnose but still is often not considered as a diagnosis until many unnecessary medical investigations have been performed. In a recently completed placebo-controlled, double-blind treatment study of adolescents with PD, the investigators noted that, on average, the teens with PD had seen physicians four times for physical complaints arising from panic attacks prior to the identification of their problems as PD. In many of the cases the diagnosis had first been considered by either the teen or a parent and not by their primary care physician. Many clinicians treating large numbers of adolescents with PD have found that a number of these teens have been treated with inhalant bronchodilators following a presumptive diagnosis of "asthma." Proper respiratory flow studies and assessments by pulmonary specialists have not confirmed the initial "asthma" diagnosis. In these cases a proper medical diagnosis is necessary and if asthma is not confirmed, discontinuation of the use of inhalant bronchodilators is indicated because some of these compounds can actually induce or increase the symptoms found in panic attacks.

CASE EXAMPLE

"I think it's a panic problem, not just growing up."

H.I. was a 14-year-old girl who presented with a 7-month history of panic attacks and "difficulty coping." Her problems had become much worse over the last month and a half prior to assessment. Her primary care physician had considered a possible diagnosis of PD because her mother was under his treatment for the same problem.

H.I. had been well until she experienced her first panic attack. The episode was of mild severity and occurred while she prepared for an overnight school trip. H.I. had never before experienced any difficulty with separation or overnight stays away from home, and she had spent two summers away at camp. This first episode was followed shortly thereafter by two more attacks, both of a mild nature. At that time H.I. was seen by a counselor at her school, who told her she was anxious about growing up and being away from her mother. H.I.'s mother was unhappy with this explanation and sought medical advice from her own physician, who felt that H.I. might be experiencing panic attacks but not PD and advised cognitive therapy to deal with the episodes.

Although H.I. did not choose to be treated at that time, she felt relieved to know that her symptoms were not part of normal growing up and that she might be able to exert some control over them. In addition, both H.I. and her mother decided that they would "keep an eye on things," and if the panic attacks became more frequent or severe, H.I. would seek further interventions.

Over the next 4 months, H.I. experienced a few spontaneous limited-symptom panic attacks but was able to manage quite well. Five weeks prior to her referral, she developed severe spontaneous full-symptom attacks, about five to six per week. She also reported a number of milder attacks, about two or three per week.

H.I.'s symptoms were so severe that she began to worry about having another attack. Because one of her attacks had occurred in a restaurant, she resolved never to eat out again and refused to accompany her friends even to the local "hamburger joint." As the attacks continued, she became increasingly frightened about having an attack while traveling on public transit because she felt she would be trapped there. Soon she was having difficulty leaving the house alone, even to walk to the corner store. She would go out accompanied by a parent but not with her friends. Although she forced herself to attend school, her peer relationships suffered, and she felt that she might stop going to school altogether. She described having suicidal ideas during one of the episodes, and she felt these ideas were secondary to the intense fears and resulting hopelessness she was feeling.

A family history revealed PD in H.I.'s mother and a variety of anxiety problems in her aunts and uncles (of which there were seven). One uncle was described as "having a real drinking problem." H.I.'s father denied any psychiatric disorder but admitted that he had had difficulties with alcohol as a young man; these had been successfully treated by his joining Alcoholics Anonymous. H.I.'s paternal grandfather (deceased) was described as a "cleaning nut," and by description was thought by the physician to have suffered from obsessive compulsive disorder (OCD).

A diagnosis of panic disorder was made. No other psychiatric syndromes were identified. H.I. was described as "tending toward stubborn" and "having a mind of her own," and this attitude was identified as a problem in her relations with other members of the family. H.I. and her parents were given feedback about the diagnosis and education about PD and its treatment. H.I.'s mother had been successfully treated with imipramine and was currently taking 150 mg daily with relatively good symptom control. She also used cognitive techniques to help her with occasional mild breakthrough panic symptoms. She wanted H.I. to be treated with similar interventions, but H.I. had her own ideas about what she wanted to do.

CASE COMMENTARY

This is a classic presentation of an adolescent-onset PD. In its initial stages it is mild and the attacks occur infrequently. The distress experienced by the teenager is often interpreted as a response to an environmental stressor. As time goes on, the disorder may suddenly declare itself with frequent, severe attacks, followed rapidly by the development of anticipatory anxiety and phobic avoidance. When this occurs the diagnosis should no longer be in doubt, although in many cases it continues to be missed. In other cases the disorder may continue with a pattern of occasional partial-symptom panic attacks accompanied by mild to moderate functional impairments, which make diagnosis more difficult.

Initiating Pharmacologic Treatment for Panic Disorder

Three treatment options are available for PD in children and adolescents: serotonin-specific reuptake inhibitors (SSRIs), tricyclic antidepressants (TCAs), and benzodiazepines (see Table 9–1). As in all child and adolescent psychiatric disorders, the psychotropic medication chosen should be used within the context of a supportive psychotherapeutic relationship and should be part of a comprehensive treatment program, which may include cognitive-behavioral or family interventions. Because results of ongoing studies of the antipanic effects of the monoamine oxidase A inhibitor moclobomide are not yet conclusive, traditional monoamine oxidase inhibitors (MAOIs) (phenelzine and tranylcypramine) are not advised for use in children and adolescents because of problems with dietary compliance and the frequent side effect of orthostatic hypotension seen with these compounds in this population. Although at least one child psychopharmacology text advises that antidepressants are the treatment of choice in child and adolescent PD, there is no valid evidence to support this assertion.

In the face of insufficient evidence for the demonstrated efficacy of certain compounds in treating child and adolescent PD, the clinician will need to be guided by the literature that is available, information obtained in studies of adults with this disorder, and the risks and benefits of certain candidate compounds in children and adolescents. Applying this strategy, Table 9–1 can be constructed.

Using the information in Table 9–1, the clinician can tailor the choice of medication to the patient's profile. For example, the adolescent with a past history of depression who now presents with mild to moderately severe panic attacks and minimal functional impairment may be a good candidate for SSRI treatment. On the other hand, the child or adoles-

TABLE 9–1 **Comparative Pros and Cons of Psychotropic Agents in Treating Panic Disorder in Children and Adolescents**

Compound	Pros	Cons
Serotonin-specific reuptake inhibitors	Evidence for effect in adults Relatively well tolerated Relatively safe in overdose Some evidence for antidepressant effect in children or teens	? Evidence in children/teens Relatively slow onset of action High cost May induce mania Potential drug-drug interactions
Tricyclic antidepressants	Evidence for effect in adults Low cost	? Evidence in children/teens Many side effects Relatively slow onset of action Can be fatal in overdose No evidence for antidepressant effect in children/teens May induce mania Many drug-drug interactions Can show withdrawal effect
Benzodiazepines	Evidence for effect in adults Some evidence in children/teens Generally well tolerated Very safe in overdose Rapid onset of action Low cost	Can show withdrawal effect May show dependence effect May be abused by high-risk group Potential drug-drug interactions

cent with no prior history of depression who presents with moderate to severe symptomatology and noticeable functional impairment may be a candidate for treatment with a benzodiazepine. Other patient information of note is the presence or absence of prior or current substance abuse or a family history of alcoholism, particularly in the male offspring of adult male alcoholics. In the latter case, for example, the clinician may advise the patient that the potential risk for abuse of benzodiazepines may be increased and suggest a nonbenzodiazepine pharmacologic intervention. The initial psychopharmacologic choices for the treatment of PD are an SSRI medication or a benzodiazepine medication. If an SSRI is chosen, use fluoxetine or sertraline. If a benzodiazepine is chosen, use clonazepam. Some clinicians prefer to use a lower dose (75 to 100 mg of imipramine) as a first-choice medication. If this is to be considered, a careful risk/benefit discussion of this alternative needs to be undertaken with the parents and patient.

Baseline Evaluations

Medical Considerations

Medical considerations are outlined in Section Two. Of particular importance is the evaluation of those physical parameters that may be affected by pharmacologic treatment. Because the expected treatment will include SSRIs or benzodiazepines, the Medication-Specific Side Effects Scale (see Ap-

pendix IV for the MSSES for antidepressants and benzodiazepines) is suggested as a baseline physical assessment.

The onset of treatment-emergent side effects is expected to occur during the initiation of treatment and on dosage escalation. If benzodiazepines are used, withdrawal effects may be noticed when the dosage is decreased. At these times more frequent physician monitoring is required.

Laboratory Considerations

Laboratory investigations should assess those physiologic parameters that pharmacologic treatment may affect, both in the short term and, because chronic treatment may be indicated, in the long term as well. Expected treatment will include either an SSRI, such as fluoxetine, or a benzodiazepine, such as clonazepam. No routine baseline laboratory investigations or diagnostic screening tests are necessary with benzodiazepines. A pregnancy test is suggested for potentially fertile females if an SSRI is to be used.

Psychiatric Considerations

The constellation of PD is comprised of three related features: panic attacks, anticipatory anxiety, and phobic avoidance. Pharmacologic treatment is directed toward each of these features. Baseline evaluation should include those symptoms that are the target of pharmacologic treatment. The following baseline measures are suggested.

Panic Attack Evaluation

A panic attack diary (see Appendix VI), provides a clinically useful measure of many variables associated with panic attacks. A detailed panic attack diary is provided in Kutcher, Reiter, and Gardner (1995). Alternatively, the clinician may wish to use a less comprehensive but still clinically useful short version, as shown in Figure 9–1.

The panic attack diary is taken home by the patient, and panic attacks are logged as they occur. Younger children may need the assistance of their parents and should be instructed to tell their mother or father whenever one of the episodes has occurred, even if it has been mild. The physician then reviews the panic attack diary with the patient (and, if appropriate, the parents as well) at the premedication visit to obtain a better understanding of the qualitative aspects of the panic attacks and to satisfy himself that the patient has identified symptoms that are indeed panic attacks.

Anticipatory Anxiety Evaluation

Anticipatory anxiety is defined as the anxiety or worry experienced by an individual in anticipation of having a panic attack. Perhaps the most clinically useful method of monitoring anticipatory anxiety is to use the 10 cm Visual Analogue Scale (VAS), shown in Figure 9–2.

The VAS is best completed by the patient during office visits. For younger children, the clinician can ask them questions about their anticipatory worries and use their answers to mark a severity score. Parents should also be asked their opinion about their child's anticipatory anxiety and should independently complete a VAS. Both child and parent scores, especially when combined, provide valid measures of treatment outcome. Most adolescents are able to self-rate on the VAS, but the clinician should review their ratings with them to ensure that they have understood the instructions and that they are not underreporting the severity of their anticipatory symptoms.

Name: _____   Recording Date: _____

For each panic attack, please note the time it occurred, the length of the attack, and the severity of the attack (1 = mild, 2 = moderate, 3 = severe).

Please use a different page for each day of recording.

Number	Time of Onset	Length of Attack in Minutes	Severity
_____	_____	_____	_____
_____	_____	_____	_____
_____	_____	_____	_____
_____	_____	_____	_____
_____	_____	_____	_____
_____	_____	_____	_____
_____	_____	_____	_____
_____	_____	_____	_____

Please go on to the next page for the next day's recording. Thanks.

If you have more attacks today than there is room on this page to record, please use another page but put today's date on the top and clearly label that page as page 2. Thanks.

Remember to bring all the pages of your diary to your next appointment with your doctor.

FIGURE 9–1   Panic Attack Diary: Short Version

Name: _____ Date: _____

Overall, how worried or anxious are you about having another panic attack? Please indicate the severity of this worry or anxiety by making a mark through the line below, where the strength of the worry or anxiety corresponds to the following scale:

0 = not at all worried or anxious about having another panic attack
to
10 = very worried or anxious about having another panic attack

0 _____ 10

FIGURE 9–2 Visual Analogue Scale for Monitoring Anticipatory Anxiety

Phobic Avoidance Evaluation

Phobic avoidance, defined as the child's or adolescent's conscious decision to avoid situations or places because of fear that another panic attack may occur there, is an important feature of PD. In many cases this phobic avoidance may lead to severe functional impairment. Thus, it must be a target of medication treatment.

The measurement of phobic avoidance has two components, (1) the actual situation or location avoided and (2) the strength of the avoidance. Both of these components of phobic avoidance must be evaluated when treating PD.

A variety of situations or locations may be avoided by the patient because of fear of having a panic attack while there. Perhaps the most useful clinical approach to this issue is to explain to the patient (and parents, where indicated) what phobic avoidance is and then to ask the patient to generate his own list of avoided situations and locations. Then a standard list of situations and locations commonly avoided by patients with PD can be completed. It is always useful to review with the patient (and parents, where indicated) the entire list of situations and locations found in Figure 9–3, even if the patient has already spontaneously reported one or more items not on the list. A simple check mark is

Name: _____ Date: _____

Situations

_____

_____

_____

_____

_____ Going to school

_____ Going out of the house

_____ Speaking in public

_____ Standing in line

_____ Traveling alone

_____ Driving alone

_____ Being in crowds

Locations

_____

_____

_____

_____

_____ School

_____ Theaters

_____ Restaurants

_____ Cars

_____ Stores or malls

_____ Bridges

_____ Buses or subways

FIGURE 9–3 Phobic Avoidance Checklist

sufficient to indicate the presence of phobic avoidance.

In completing the list in Figure 9–3, the clinician must be careful to identify whether the patient can tolerate the situation or location on his own. For example, if a patient can go out of the house but only if accompanied by a parent, sibling, or friend, he meets the criteria for having phobic avoidance of "going out of the house." Developmental issues also come into play here. Many children and young adolescents do not usually travel alone on buses or subways or go to malls. In this case the clinician must judge the level of avoidance expressed by the child when accompanied by a parent, sibling, or friend. If a child has usually enjoyed going to the mall and now refuses to go, complains about going, or uncharacteristically fusses, the clinician must consider the presence of phobic avoidance. Similarly, if a patient can enter a theater only when accompanied by a parent and that patient previously was able to attend with friends, then phobic avoidance must be considered.

The strength of phobic avoidance is best measured by having the patient select the two most severely avoided situations and locations as identified from the Phobic Avoidance Checklist (see Fig. 9–3) and completing a VAS for each. If the patient cannot identify two situations, then at least one is useful (Fig. 9–4).

As with the anticipatory anxiety VAS described earlier, children and some young adolescents may need the clinician to score the Phobic Avoidance VAS from information derived from direct questioning. Some older children and most adolescents will be able to score the scales themselves. In these cases the clinician should review the scales to ensure that the patient has understood the instructions and has not under represented the severity of avoidant symptoms. With younger children and some teenagers, independent parental completion of these scales is of value, and both child and parent scores should be considered in evaluating the outcome of treatment.

Initiating Pharmacologic Treatment of Panic Disorder

CASE EXAMPLE

"I can make my own choices."

H.I. did not want to be treated with the same medication that her mother was receiving. After discussion with her parents and the consulting physician, she chose fluoxetine as the pharmacotherapy and agreed to cognitive ther-apy to help her "use her mind to deal with the panic attacks." H.I. was given a short-version panic attack diary (see Fig. 9–1) and was asked to complete it over a 5-day period. This length of time was chosen because her panic attacks were severe and had already demonstrated a relatively constant frequency over the 2 to 3 weeks prior to assessment. It was felt that this length of baseline assessment would provide a reasonable evaluation of the panic attacks and at the same time not prolong the wait for active pharmacologic treatment. At the same time, H.I. and her parents were given further information about panic attacks and their treatments and about fluoxetine. They were encouraged to read about the subject on their own and to contact the physician if any concerns or increasing difficulties arose prior to the next visit.

Treatment of Panic Disorder: Use of the SSRI Fluoxetine

The efficacy of various SSRI compounds in treating PD has not been clearly demonstrated for children or adolescents, but studies of adult patients suggest that many of these compounds may be useful. Although controlled studies support the use of clomipramine in adult PD, the nature, frequency, and severity of side effects of this compound in children and adolescents suggest that other, better tolerated medicines (such as the more SSRI fluoxetine) should be a first-line choice.

As a group, the SSRIs (fluoxetine, sertraline, paroxetine, and fluvoxamine) are thought to demonstrate their effects primarily through blockade of serotonin reuptake in the central nervous system (CNS). They have little or no effect on noradrenergic or dopaminergic neurotransmission. They are currently indicated for treatment of depression in adults, and fluoxetine in some jurisdictions is approved for the treatment of bulimia and OCD. SSRIs tend to be better tolerated than TCAs and are relatively free of cardiovascular complications compared with TCAs. They are also demonstrably less lethal in overdose, and initial suggestions about their effects in attempted suicide have not been confirmed. On the contrary, all evidence available to date clearly indicates that not only does treatment with SSRIs in depressed patients not increase suicide rates but rather it decreases suicide rates. (For further information regarding SSRI medications see Chapter 11.)

SSRIs have been implicated in the onset of mania and hypomania in adults and adolescents and

Name: _____ Date: _____

People who have panic attacks often are afraid or worried about getting an attack in a particular place or while doing a specific activity. This fear or worry is part of panic disorder and sometimes stops people from doing things that they might usually do or from going places that they might usually go. This is called phobic avoidance.

You and your doctor have identified the following most severe situations that you have begun to avoid because of fears or worries about having a panic attack:

1. _____

2. _____

For each of these situations, please mark the strength of your avoidance (how strongly you resist doing these things) with a mark that cuts across the following line at the level of your avoidance:

0 = I do not avoid doing this by myself.
        to
10 = There is no way that I will do this by myself.

For situation number 1:

_____
0   10

For situation number 2:

_____
0   10

You and your doctor have also identified the following most severe locations or places that you have begun to avoid:

1. _____

2. _____

For each of these locations, please mark the strength of your avoidance (how strongly you resist going to these places) with a mark that cuts across the following line at the strength of your avoidance:

0 = I have no problems going there by myself.
        to
10 = I will not go there by myself.

For location number 1:

_____
0   10

For location number 2:

_____
0   10

FIGURE 9–4 Visual Analogue Scale for Rating Phobic Avoidance

have a number of potentially significant drug-drug interactions that may be problematic. The serotonin syndrome is perhaps the most common concern when SSRIs are taken together with other compounds that affect CNS serotonin functioning, such as lithium, tricyclics, MAOIs, and other SSRIs. If this occurs, the patient may be expected to complain of nausea, diarrhea, chills, headache, palpitations, or muscle twitching. Severe cases can progress to excitation, delirium, and possibly seizures. Thus, care must be taken not only to avoid concomitant administration of these compounds but also to ensure that any serotonin-type medications taken before the onset of SSRI treatment have been fully eliminated prior to the prescription of SSRIs.

Fluoxetine is perhaps the most studied of the SSRIs in the psychopharmacotherapy of children and adolescents, and it has been used to treat major depression, PD, bulimia, attention-deficit disorder (ADHD), aggressive outbursts, Prader-Willi syndrome, and various anxiety disorders (see Chapter 10) and compulsive-type behaviors such as trichitillomania. Although it is not officially approved for use in child or adolescent PD, clinical experience and a growing body of literature on adults suggest that it may be a useful and relatively well-tolerated pharmacologic treatment in this population.

Fluoxetine is a compound that facilitates serotonergic neurotransmission through the mechanism of presynaptic serotonin reuptake inhibition. It is well absorbed with oral administration regardless of the presence of food and reaches peak plasma concentrations in 5 to 10 hours following oral dosing. Steady-state concentrations are attained within 2 to 4 weeks, and a once-a-day or even once-every-2-days dosage is sufficient to maintain plasma levels once steady state has been reached. Fluoxetine has a plasma half-life of 2 to 4 days and undergoes hepatic metabolism via the cytochrome P-450 system to an active metabolite, norfluoxetine, which has an even longer half-life of 7 to 9 days. These pharmacokinetic features are important for the following reasons:

1. The prolonged half-life of fluoxetine/norfluoxetine means that should a patient discontinue this medication, a relatively longer period of time will be needed (up to 5 weeks) to ensure that full washout is complete prior to beginning other medications with potential drug-drug interactions (such as a TCA).

2. The prolonged half-life of fluoxetine/norfluoxetine means that once steady state is reached, a once-a-day or even a once-every-2-days dosage schedule can be followed. In addition, if the patient forgets to take his dose on any given day, therapeutic efficacy of the compound will not be compromised.

3. The prolonged half-life of fluoxetine/norfluoxetine may be the reason for the relative absence of withdrawal symptoms when a patient stops taking the medication. This allows for more flexibility in discontinuing the medication because a graduated tapering off may not be necessary.

4. Because fluoxetine is metabolized in the liver, patients with significant liver disease may require lower doses to achieve the clinically desired effects.

5. The association of fluoxetine metabolism with the cytochrome P-450 system means that concurrent use of other drugs metabolized by this system may lead to increased plasma levels of those drugs and potential problematic drug-drug interactions.

Side effects associated with fluoxetine use in children and adolescents are summarized in Table 9–2. Although these adverse effects are categorized as relatively common, occasional, and rare, it is important to inform patients and their parents that most people treated with fluoxetine do not

TABLE 9–2 Fluoxetine Side Effects in Children and Adolescents*

Relatively Common

Nausea	Excessive sweating
Gastrointestinal distress	Restlessness
Bloating	Agitation
Diarrhea	Nervousness

Occasional

Insomnia	Self-injury
Headache	Apathy
Sedation	Dry mouth
Disinhibition	Dream intensification
Sexual dysfunction	Hypomanic symptoms
Bradycardia of no known clinical significance	

Rare

Tremor	Mania
Allergic reactions	Dystonia
Hair loss or growth	Tinnitus
Seizures	Syndrome of Inappropriate Antidiuretic Hormone Secretion (SIADH)

*Compiled from a review of the available literature on the use of fluoxetine in the treatment of child and adolescent psychiatric disorders and the reported side effects of fluoxetine in adults. Some of these side effects (e.g., agitation, restlessness, nervousness) may be dose related.

experience any one particular side effect. For example, most patients (70 percent) do not experience nausea, and it is relatively mild in many who do experience it. Others, however, are not so fortunate, and there is no method available that can predict which patient might experience which (if any) side effect.

Some side effects that may occur at the onset of fluoxetine treatment, in particular the symptoms of restlessness and agitation, appear to be dose dependent and may be largely avoided if starting doses below 20 mg are used. Indeed, given clinical experience with the use of fluoxetine, rarely if ever is there a compelling reason to begin treatment with more than 10 mg of fluoxetine daily, and treatment initiation with 5 mg is unlikely to produce these adverse effects.

Tolerance to side effects, especially nausea, often develops within 1 to 2 weeks of continuous use. If this nausea is mild or moderate, it can often be avoided by giving the medication at bedtime. With this approach, many patients who do report initial nausea can continue taking the medication until such time as tolerance to this side effect develops.

The safety of fluoxetine in pregnancy has not been determined, although there is no clear evidence of a teratogenic effect. Prudent clinical practice includes consideration of this possibility, particularly during the first trimester, and the potential risks to the fetus must be weighed against the benefits of continuing fluoxetine over this time. A pregnancy test is indicated for females of child-bearing potential prior to initiating treatment with fluoxetine. Fluoxetine is secreted into breast milk in concentrations roughly equivalent to that found in maternal plasma. Given the lack of information about the effects of fluoxetine on the neonate, breast-feeding mothers should be advised not to continue fluoxetine treatment.

Although dose-finding studies in the child and adolescent population are currently not available, clinical experience suggests that fluoxetine therapy should be started at a low dose—5 mg daily is suggested—and increased gradually every 3 to 5 days until a total single dose of 15 to 20 mg per day is obtained. At this time, the dose should be held until the expected therapeutic response is likely to occur. The exact length of this period of time in children and adolescents has not been established, and it may take as long as 6 to 8 weeks for the full medication effect to be realized. Some initial improvements should become apparent within 2 to 3 weeks. In some cases the panic attacks are of such severity that additional pharmacologic interventions, as described later, will be necessary.

CASE EXAMPLE

H.I., an Adolescent Girl Being Treated with Fluoxetine for Panic Attacks

H.I. was given an initial dose of 5 mg of fluoxetine by mouth and tolerated it well. She reported no acute side effects and denied either drowsiness or activation. She was then advised to begin taking 5 mg of fluoxetine daily at bedtime. When seen 3 days following the initiation of the treatment dose, H.I. complained that the panic attacks were very severe and "coming as often as always." She was increasingly concerned that she might not be able to "hold on" until the medication "kicked in." She had attended a cognitive therapy session but found that when she became panicky, she could not focus her thoughts and, although she knew it would take time to "get the technique right," she worried that her panic attacks were so strong that she might never be able to learn cognitive strategies. She wondered if anything else might be done to help her in the meantime.

CASE COMMENTARY

One useful clinical strategy in cases in which the physician would like to consider an SSRI as the treatment of choice but the panic attacks are very severe and require immediate pharmacologic intervention, is to combine initiation doses of an SSRI (e.g., 5 mg fluoxetine daily) with therapeutic doses of clonazepam (1.0 to 2.5 mg daily). Once the patient has been stabilized on the clonazepam, and the SSRI has reached the initial target therapeutic dose (15 to 20 mg daily), the clonazepam can be gradually withdrawn, leaving the patient on SSRI monotherapy. This strategy is useful even in those cases in which benzodiazepine treatment would otherwise not be prominently considered, such as a family history of substance abuse.

CASE EXAMPLE

H.I., the Ongoing Saga of Treating Adolescent Panic Disorder

H.I. was informed of the possible use of concurrent short-term benzodiazepam treatment to deal with her symptoms. After discussion of the alternatives with her and her parents, it was decided that she would try clonazepam. A target dose of 1 to 2 mg was set, and a total clonazepam treatment trial of 4 to 6 weeks' duration was agreed to.

Clonazepam at a test dose of 0.25 mg was given, and no adverse effects were noted. Accordingly, H.I. was instructed to take this medication concurrently with her fluoxetine at bedtime. She was seen 2 days later and reported feeling "a bit better." Her panic attack diary showed a slight decrease in the frequency of her attacks and a decrease in the average intensity of her attacks. Her dose was raised to 0.25 mg twice daily. When seen 3 days later, H.I. reported feeling "much better" and asked, "What's in those pills?" Her dose was maintained at this level over the next 6 weeks.

On this combined treatment regime (the initial estimated therapeutic dose of fluoxetine was set at 15 mg and was reached within 1 week of beginning treatment), H.I. showed significant improvement in the frequency and intensity of her panic attacks. In addition, her anticipatory anxiety decreased from a baseline score of 8 to 3, and her phobic avoidance of situations and locations showed a similar positive change (albeit not as marked) in the identified items. Both parents and H.I. were delighted with her response to treatment, and she felt that the "medicines were helping my cognitions control my wacky brain." At the end of the 6-week trial of clonazepam treatment, H.I. stated that she did not want to stop taking the clonazepam but agreed to slowly taper and discontinue the medication with the proviso that if the fluoxetine did not maintain her remission, a return to clonazepam or an increase in the fluoxetine dose would be considered.

The clonazepam was slowly discontinued, with the morning dose being decreased from 0.25 to 0.125 mg for 5 days, followed by the evening dose being decreased from 0.25 to 0.125 mg for 5 days. The morning dose was then stopped for 5 days, followed by cessation of the evening dose. The entire medication withdrawal took 20 days, but H.I. experienced no rebound or withdrawal effects. Her symptoms remained under relatively good control.

Three weeks later, H.I. stated that she wanted to see if increasing her fluoxetine dose would lead to further improvement. She was now experiencing only one or two mild panic attacks weekly, and her anticipatory anxiety and phobic avoidance, while still present, were also much improved. She wanted to determine if she could possibly become totally symptom free. With the agreement of her parents, H.I.'s fluoxetine was raised gradually to 20 mg daily and was maintained at that dose. Four weeks

following dose stabilization at this level, she reported her first totally panic attack–free week since the onset of the disorder. A side effect scale completed at this time was unremarkable.

CASE COMMENTARY

This type of treatment response to combined fluoxetine and clonazepam treatment is not uncommon in this population. When this occurs, the clonazepam should be added in small doses for a relatively short length of time and then gradually withdrawn to avoid rebound or withdrawal symptoms. Alprazolam or diazepam should not be used together with fluoxetine because their plasma levels can be significantly increased by this combination. In some cases, clonazepam itself may be chosen by the patient and family as the pharmacologic treatment of choice.

CASE EXAMPLE

Ten-Year-Old Boy with Panic Attacks: Choosing Treatment with Clonazepam

W.K. was a 10-year-old boy who was seen at his parents' request because he was having unexplained physical symptoms and worries that were beginning to create functional impairments in school and in sports activities. His parents were concerned that he might be suffering from a "masked depression."

W.K.'s mother was a social worker employed at a children's health center. Her family psychiatric history was positive for depression in her mother and for panic attacks in an older sister. She was receiving weekly psychotherapy for anxiety and met diagnostic criteria for generalized anxiety disorder (GAD). The father was a litigation attorney who reported situational performance anxiety, usually associated with public speaking. He had been prescribed propranolol by his family physician and was able to function quite well by using this medication occasionally together with cognitive techniques he had developed over many years of dealing with the problem. There was a history of a psychotic disorder in that an uncle had been diagnosed as schizophrenic.

W.K. described "scared feelings" that he found difficult to explain that had occurred over a period of several months. These feelings seemed to come on at all times of the day and lasted for a short time. Over the previous few months they were occurring more frequently, about four to five times per week. They were usually relatively mild, although occasionally they would be quite severe. The severe sensations were often associated with feelings of tightness and pounding in his chest, and a subjective sensation that he could not breathe.

Indeed, 4 days prior to his assessment W.K.'s father had rushed him to the emergency room of a large pediatric hospital because he was hyperventilating, crying, and saying that his chest was hurting and he could not breathe properly. The emergency room nurse helped him to stop hyperventilating and no symptoms remained by the time he was seen by the physician on call. His physical examination was unremarkable. W.K. and his father were told that the chest pain was most likely due to heartburn because he had had a stomach flu earlier in the week. Treatment with an antacid was suggested if this ever happened again.

Further history elicited a description of mild generalized anxiety "for as long as I can remember, since he was little." W.K. felt that he worried more and about more things than his friends but was able to clearly differentiate these worries from the episodes described earlier, which were of relatively recent onset. He described one such episode that had occurred while sleeping over at a friend's house. On that occasion his mother had to go and bring him home, and from then on he turned down all invitations for sleepovers, although he often invited friends to stay overnight at his house. Furthermore, he described a number of episodes that occurred at school, one during a test that resulted in his not finishing it. Although his teacher had been understanding, W.K. was worried that this would happen again, and every time that a test was scheduled for class he began worrying about it, to the point that he would occasionally ask to stay home from school.

There was no history of any other psychiatric difficulty, including ADHD or mood disorder. W.K. was physically healthy, a good student, popular with his peers, and an excellent athlete. By coincidence, the consulting physician had the opportunity to witness firsthand a panic episode experienced by W.K. while he was playing baseball. During W.K.'s game he experienced an acute episode of hyperventilation, chest discomfort, and subjective feelings of being unable to get enough air. This was witnessed by the physician, who also obtained a full description of the symptoms that W.K. was experiencing. This episode was clearly a panic attack, and it was identified by W.K. and his parents as typical of the episodes that he had previously described. A tentative diagnosis of PD with a possible comorbid GAD was made.

Following completion of the assessment and education about the disorder and its potential treatments, W.K. and his parents chose treatment with the benzodiazepine clonazepam. They felt that they wanted the symptoms to come under control as quickly as possible and did not feel that addiction to benzodiazepines was likely for W.K.

Treatment of Panic Disorder: Benzodiazepines

Benzodiazepines have a relatively long and well-studied use in psychiatry, but only recently have they been evaluated in the treatment of various anxiety disorders in children and adolescents. Information from available studies and clinical experience suggests that one of the benzodiazepines, clonazepam, may be of particular value in treating children or adolescents with PD. Although other benzodiazepines such as alprazolam or diazepam may also be of benefit, the particular pharmacokinetic and pharmacodynamic characteristics of clonazepam compared with the others possibly make it a reasonable first choice for a compound when a benzodiazepine is used.

Benzodiazepines were first introduced 30 years ago when they were found to have effective sedative and anxiolytic effects without the dangers and side effects of barbiturates. Their therapeutic activity is considered to be demonstrated through their effects on the CNS benzodiazepine receptor, which is intimately linked to the gamma-aminobutyric acid (GABA) receptor–chloride ion channel complex. Although other neurotransmitters, such as peptides, neurohormones, and noradrenergic compounds, are involved in the neurochemistry of anxiety, benzodiazepines appear to enhance the affinity of the GABA-A reception site for GABA, thereby potentiating GABA's CNS inhibitory action.

As a group of compounds, benzodiazepines are generally effective anxiolytic agents with a relatively rapid onset of therapeutic effect. Although well absorbed orally, they exhibit variable rates of onset and half-life durations (Table 9–3). Other intragroup differences include potency, adverse effects, and potential for withdrawal phenomenon. Benzodiazepines belong to one of three structural groups: 2-keto-benzodiazepines (e.g., diazepam), 3-hydroxy-benzodiazepines (e.g., oxazepam), and triazalo-benzodiazepines (e.g.,

TABLE 9–3   **Clinically Useful Pharmacokinetic Characteristics of Selected Benzodiazepines***

Medication	Rapidity of Onset	Half-Life
Alprazolam	+++	9–20 hours
Clonazepam	++	20–60 hours
Diazepam	++++	20–70 hours (doubled for metabolites)
Flurazepam	++++	1–3 hours (exceedingly long for metabolites—up to 10 days)
Lorazepam	+++	8–24 hours
Oxazepam	+++	3–24 hours
Triazolam	++++	1–5 hours

*Because of a dearth of pharmacokinetic studies in children and adolescents, the rapidity of onset and half-life data are approximates developed from studies of adults.

alprazolam). In addition, benzodiazepines are metabolized differently. Some undergo hepatic oxidation (e.g., diazepam) and tend to demonstrate longer serum half-lives and active metabolites. Others are biotransformed through glucuronide conjugation and have relatively shorter half-lives. One benzodiazepine, clonazepam, is metabolized by nitroreduction.

Benzodiazepines can best be classified clinically in terms of the combination of their rate of onset and duration of action. Compounds with a rapid rate of onset are more likely to induce initial euphoric-type effects, which may then be associated with a higher potential abuse risk in those patients who exhibit this vulnerability. Compounds with a shorter half-life are associated with a greater likelihood of rebound or withdrawal effects than compounds with intermediate or long half-lives. Compounds with long half-lives, however, may be associated with an increased risk of drug accumulation over time.

Of clinical importance, the reports that increased rapidity of hepatic metabolism necessitates more frequent and higher doses be administered to children compared with adults do not necessarily reflect on the therapeutic action of these compounds. There is no evidence in the child and adolescent literature that doses higher than those used in adults are needed. On the contrary, lower doses than those used in adults often provide therapeutic efficacy, whereas higher doses seem to be associated with increased side effects without increased efficacy. The explanation for this is that developmental pharmacokinetics of the benzodiazepines do not necessarily equate with their developmental pharmacodynamic effects. Good clinical child and adolescent psychopharmacologic practice demands an appreciation of this difference.

Although relatively well tolerated and safe, benzodiazepines do exhibit a number of side effects that need to be properly monitored. Perhaps the most common side effects are those of a sedative nature, including fatigue, drowsiness, and decreased concentration. Behavioral disinhibition (including aggression, hostility, irritability, and paroxysmal excitement) has been reported and, although the data are unclear on this point, this is thought to occur more commonly in children and adolescents than in adults, particularly when higher doses of the medication are taken. Preexisting brain damage or personality styles with features of impulse and affective dysregulation may predispose to benzodiazepine-induced behavioral disinhibition.

Psychomotor impairment secondary to benzodiazepine use has best been demonstrated in studies of adult drivers, and prudent clinical practice includes advising teens being treated with benzodiazepines to avoid driving after even one alcoholic beverage because the effects of the mixture may be synergistic. Cognitive impairment has been described in adults, including visuospatial difficulties, reduced memory storage, anterograde amnesia, and sustained attention problems. Short-term memory is not likely to be significantly affected.

The applicability of those benzodiazepine side effects described in studies in chronically ill adults (many who have been taking these medications for long periods of time), in whom the anxiety disorder may itself induce impairment, to children and adolescents receiving short-term treatment with these agents is not clear. Although these side effects cannot be ignored, their presence, severity, and frequency must be carefully studied in this population as well. The only such study, on children treated with alprazolam, failed to demonstrate significant cognitive side effects during short-term treatment. Furthermore, one potentially problematic side effect of alprazolam treatment documented in adults—the withdrawal phenomenon—has not been demonstrated in studies of alprazolam treatment for anxiety in children and adolescents. While these findings cannot be said to be definitive—nor can they be extrapolated to other benzodiazepines—they illustrate that data from adult studies cannot simply be applied to children and adolescents to establish either efficacy or tolerability standards. In the clinical situation, these potential side effects must be identified to the patient and parents and must be carefully monitored throughout treatment.

Patients and their parents are often confused about the addictive potential of benzodiazepines. This is understandable, given the intensive media portrayal of these medications as addictive and the public disagreement among physicians as to the scope and nature of this problem. Debates have raged about benzodiazepine overuse, misuse, and abuse, but the available evidence does not support the view that benzodiazepines are generally addictive. Even long-term benzodiazepine use is only rarely accompanied by drug-seeking behaviors, such as illicit purchase, multiple doctoring to obtain medication, and dose escalation. Furthermore, those who do abuse benzodiazepines rarely if ever abuse only this medication. Benzodiazepine abuse usually occurs in the context of multiple drug abuse (including the use of alcohol, prescription drugs, and street drugs), in which benzodiazepines are often mixed with hallucinogens or amphetamine-like compounds to "cushion" the "crash" that occurs with drug withdrawal.

Some of the difficulties with this issue surround the meaning of the word *addiction* and the all too common equation of pharmacologic dependence (receptor sensitization with prolonged use of some compounds) with the notion of addiction. Drug abuse or addiction is a complex social, personal, and biological phenomenon. An essential feature of addiction is the use of a drug for a purpose other than that for which it is prescribed. Most often this is a euphoric or hallucinogenic effect, although other effects are possible. In addition, drug addiction is associated with addictive behaviors such as those described earlier. The fact

that discontinuation of a specific drug can lead to symptoms of "rebound" or "withdrawal" is not evidence of addiction. Withdrawal symptoms resulting from the discontinuation of a drug are in and of themselves not sufficient evidence of drug addiction or abuse.

Discontinuation of benzodiazepine treatment may result in the experience of symptoms of anxiety. This may be caused by relapse, rebound, or withdrawal. Relapse is the recurrence of symptoms that were the initial target of treatment, for example, the return of panic attacks once the medication has been stopped. Rebound can be best understood as the return of original symptoms but in accentuated form. Withdrawal can be understood as the onset of new symptoms, not present at the onset of treatment, and resulting from the pharmacodynamic effects of the medication itself.

In long-term continuous benzodiazepine treatment (usually understood as lasting more than 6 months), withdrawal symptoms can occur when the medication is discontinued. Usually these symptoms are relatively mild, but occasionally they may be severe. Although most often associated with rapid discontinuation of benzodiazepines of short or intermediate half-lives (Table 9–4), withdrawal symptoms can occur with any benzodiazepine. Some benzodiazepines, particularly alprazolam, have occasionally been implicated in serious withdrawal reactions, such as seizures. Thus, when benzodiazepine treatment is to be discontinued, gradual withdrawal of the medication is necessary.

A reasonable strategy for discontinuation of benzodiazepines is to decrease the dose by a fixed percentage at regular intervals. Dropping the dose by 10 percent to 25 percent every 7 to 10 days (depending on the amount of medication being taken—the higher the amount, the slower the taper) is recommended at first. Rebound or withdrawal symptoms are more likely to become evident in the later stages of drug discontinuation, and the

TABLE 9–4 **Length of Action and Strength of Antipanic, Anxiolytic, and Sedative Effects of Selected Benzodiazepines***

Medication	Length of Action	Antipanic Effect	Anxiolytic Effect	Sedative Effect
Triazolam	+	?	+	+++
Alprazolam	++	+++	+	+
Lorazepam	++	+	+++	+
Oxazepam	++	?	+	+
Clonazepam	+++	+++	+	+
Diazepam	+++	+	+++	++
Flurazepam	+++	?	+	+++

*The data in this table have been estimated from studies and review articles on benzodiazepines in both adult and children/adolescent samples. Developmental characteristics of individual patients differ and may produce clinical results that vary from this information.

time interval between dosage reductions may therefore need to be lengthened. If short-acting benzodiazepines are being withdrawn, switching the benzodiazepine to an equivalent amount of clonazepam and then following the schedule suggested earlier is often useful. This withdrawal protocol is most useful for alprazolam withdrawal, which should be attempted only in this manner to avoid the possibility of seizures.

It is helpful for the clinician to provide individual patients and, where appropriate, their families information about which individuals may be at a higher risk for abusing benzodiazepines than others. Few studies are available to guide the practitioner, but clinical experience and some research suggest that the following may be relevant risk factors:

1. Past history of substance abuse (including alcohol)
2. Current substance abuse (including alcohol)
3. Male child of adult alcohol abuser
4. Child of adult drug abuser (including benzodiazepines)

Because the exact clinical course of PD cannot be predicted and the long-term effects of benzodiazepines in children and adolescents are not known, it is reasonable to consider treatment with benzodiazepines as relatively short term, that is, 4 to 6 months. A similar strategy is also reasonable for treatment of this disorder with antidepressants.

CASE EXAMPLE

An Adolescent Girl with SSRI-Treated Panic Disorder: The Story Continues—How Long Should Pharmacotherapy Continue?

H.I. was doing quite well. She had experienced only one or two very mild episodes over the previous 3 months and rated her anticipatory anxiety as ranging between 1 and 2 out of a possible 10. Her phobic avoidance had generally disappeared, although this had taken much longer to resolve than the panic attacks and required the use of cognitive techniques and some exposure therapy. She was attending school and had an active social life.

H.I. and her parents met with their physician to discuss the possibility of discontinuing the medication. After discussing the course of her illness and the risks and benefits of continued fluoxetine treatment, H.I. and her parents decided to gradually stop her medication. A set of criteria for restarting medication was agreed to

before the fluoxetine was tapered off, and a schedule for tapering was instituted.

H.I.'s fluoxetine was decreased by 5 mg, and the new dose was maintained for 1 month. Because no symptoms returned, the medication was further reduced by 5 mg and again maintained for 1 month. During this month H.I. experienced two mild panic attacks, and her anticipatory anxiety increased to a value of 4. Although concerned that her disorder might return, she continued in her decision to withdraw her medication. Accordingly, her fluoxetine dose was decreased to 10 mg daily, and this was maintained for 1 month. At this level H.I. continued to experience occasional panic attacks, but their frequency increased and she reported that their severity had worsened. Accordingly, her medication was then increased to 15 mg once daily.

Following 1 month on this dose, H.I. noted that although she was still experiencing occasional panic attacks, they were very mild and she was using her cognitive techniques to deal with them. Her anticipatory anxiety was scored at 2 or 3, and she denied any phobic avoidance, although she did report that she occasionally worried when she went to a restaurant or theater. She decided that the degree of symptom control on 15 mg of fluoxetine was reasonable and wanted to stay at that level for "a few months" and "see how it goes." A bimonthly monitoring schedule was agreed to and was followed for 4 months. At this time H.I. was doing relatively well and wanted to discontinue her medication. However, when the daily dose was lowered to 10 mg, she once again experienced an increased frequency of mild panic attacks and decided to again continue her medication at 15 mg daily, with plans to try reducing it again later.

CASE COMMENTARY

The case of H.I. illustrates some common clinical aspects of treating adolescents with panic attacks. First, while fluoxetine treatment of PD can be very effective, full antipanic activity (as with other antidepressants used in the treatment of this disorder) may take a number of weeks (3 to 6 weeks, or even longer) to become evident. Improved control of panic attacks during this early phase of treatment may be improved by the careful addition of an appropriate benzodiazepine, such as clonazepam. The clonazepam can then be gradually withdrawn, with fluoxetine monotherapy continuing.

Second, given the available knowledge regarding the natural course of PD, at this time it is recommended that treatment of panic attacks with medications be reviewed on a regular basis—every 4 to 6 months—to determine whether medication treatment is still needed. In some cases therapy can be successfully withdrawn altogether. In other cases the maintence dose may be less than the initiation dose. In still other cases, however, longer-term pharmacotherapy at the dose found to provide symptom relief will be necessary. No available information can be used to predict which of these outcomes will result for any specific patient. Thus, a systematic approach using the above-mentioned scheme is a useful clinical strategy.

The third issue that this and the next case illustrate is the differential expected treatment response times for the anticipatory anxiety and phobic avoidance found in patients with PD. Often these features will take longer to resolve than the panic attacks themselves. Often patients will require additional treatments, such as exposure therapy, to deal with the phobic avoidance component in particular. A reasonable guideline if the child or adolescent has shown a good response to treatment in terms of amelioration of panic attacks is to give the anticipatory anxiety and phobic avoidance at least 1 to 2 more months to settle down. If this does not occur, and the patient is not currently undergoing cognitive or behavioral therapy, it is recommended that such active and focused psychotherapeutic interventions be undertaken to ensure that social and educational morbidity secondary to these features does not continue. If exposure treatments or other cognitive-behavioral therapies have been ongoing, the clinician should consider increasing their frequency or intensity, or should search for other factors (such as an anxious parent who needs the child at home) that might be contributing to functional morbidity.

CASE EXAMPLE

Young Boy Treated for Panic Attacks with Clonazepam: The Story Continues—How Long Should the Pharmacotherapy Continue?

W.K. had obtained an excellent response to clonazepam at a daily dose of 0.5 mg, which had been maintained for about 4 months. His anticipatory anxiety was under good control, and he exhibited no phobic avoidance. In addition, both W.K. and his parents reported that

he was much better than previously, even before his panic attacks started, in that his level of anxiety was generally much decreased. W.K. was doing well at school and in sports and had good peer relationships.

The risks and benefits of continued clonazepam treatment were discussed with W.K. and his parents, and a decision was made to gradually taper off his medication. The possibility of rebound and withdrawal symptoms was clearly discussed, and W.K. was encouraged to call his physician if any problems developed. Also, the frequency of medication monitoring via regular clinic visits was increased.

The clonazepam was reduced by 25 percent to 0.125 mg in the morning, with 0.25 mg at night for 2 weeks. Because no side effects emerged, the morning dose was discontinued and the evening dose was maintained at 0.25 mg for 3 weeks. Because W.K. was still symptom free, the evening dose was decreased to 0.125 mg for 3 weeks and then, because he continued to do well, was discontinued altogether.

W.K. reported that he was more anxious than he had been when taking the medication, but he felt much like he did prior to the onset of the panic attacks. As he put it, "It's me." He rated his anticipatory anxiety as 1 out of 10 and reported no phobic avoidance.

Three weeks later, W.K.'s mother called to report that her son had experienced another panic attack. The attack was of short duration and was very mild, but all were concerned that W.K.'s problem would return. W.K. was seen and his course reviewed. He was urged to wait and see what would happen. It was noted that his anticipatory anxiety was now increased to 3 out of 10, but there was no increase in phobic avoidance. Another appointment time was given, and his parents were given instructions to call if any further concerns arose.

W.K. was seen at follow-up 5 months later. Things were going well for him, and although he felt he still was "a little too worried," he was not seeking any further treatments.

Two months later, W.K.'s father called to say that the panic attacks had started again. When seen, W.K. reported that about 1 month previously he had experienced two or three very mild, short-lived attacks that had not returned. Two weeks prior to the phone call, however, he experienced another attack, which was more severe and of longer duration. This was followed in quick succession by a number of milder attacks (four to five over a period of 1 week). A few days before the phone call, he reported a severe attack. The mild episodes continued and he felt that he needed "the same medicine" again.

Following another baseline assessment, W.K. once again started taking clonazepam, and this time his panic attacks required 0.75 mg daily to be controlled. His anticipatory anxiety (which had climbed to 7 of 10) also decreased significantly within a week of beginning treatment again. When seen in follow-up, W.K. stated, "I'm not going to stop taking that medicine ever again."

CASE COMMENTARY

This case further illustrates some of the issues arising in the treatment of children and adolescents for PD. W.K. was successfully withdrawn from his clonazepam medication without experiencing either rebound or withdrawal symptoms. He remained symptom free from his panic attacks, anticipatory anxiety, and phobic avoidance for a significant period of time. His disorder did return, however, and the second initiation of pharmacotherapy required a slightly higher dose than the first to obtain symptomatic improvement. The problem here is deciding what further course to take. On the one hand, the long-term effects of clonazepam treatment in children are not known. On the other hand, this treatment is relatively benign (according to studies of adults), and it has been exceedingly helpful to the patient in the short term. Furthermore, the second time the treatment was initiated, the dose needed to control the symptoms was higher, suggesting that if treatment is again discontinued, even higher doses of the medication may be needed to obtain symptom control.

There are no clear answers to these questions at this time. Further therapy for W.K. and patients like him requires a solid ongoing relationship among the clinician, the patient, and the family. The answers to this type of treatment question must be arrived at in a spirit of honesty and open inquiry involving the input of all parties concerned. This clinical process of joint decision making involving the physician and the informed patient and family is the only reasonable method by which these difficult treatment decisions can be made.

SUGGESTED READINGS

AACAP Offical Action. Practice parameters for the assessment and treatment of anxiety disorders. Journal of the American Academy of Child and Adolescent Psychiatry, 32:1089–1098, 1993.

Bernstein GA, Perwien AR. Anxiety disorders. Child and Adolescent Psychiatric Clinics of North America, 4:305–322, 1995.

Coffey B. Anxiolytics for children and adolescents: Traditional and new drugs. Journal of Child and Adolescent Psychopharmacology. 1:57–83, 1990.

Hallström C (ed). Benzodiazepine Dependence. Oxford: Oxford University Press, 1993.

Kutcher S, Reiter S, Gardner D. Pharmacotherapy: Approaches and applications. In JS March (ed): Anxiety Disorders in Children and Adolescents. New York: Guilford Press, 1995, pp 341–385.

Kutcher S, Reiter S, Gardner D, Klein R. The pharmacotherapy of anxiety disorders in children and adolescents. Psychiatric Clinics of North America, 15:41–74, 1992.

Moreau D, Follett C. Panic disorder in children and adolescents. Child and Adolescent Psychiatric Clinics of North America, 2:581–602, 1993.

Task Force Report of the American Psychiatric Association. Benzodiazepine Dependence, Toxicity, and Abuse. Washington, DC: American Psychiatric Association, 1990.

Wilkinson G, Balestrieri M, Ruggeri M. Meta analysis of double-blind placebo-controlled trials of antidepressants and benzodiazepines for patients with panic disorders. Psychological Medicine, 21: 991–998, 1991.

CHAPTER 10

Psychopharmacologic Treatment of Other Anxiety Disorders

Anxiety disorders of childhood and adolescence, when taken as a whole, may well be the most common group of DSM-IV Axis I illnesses found in this population, except for disturbances of conduct. Although these disorders are associated with significant morbidity and a decreased quality of life, adolescents and children with one of the nonpanic anxiety disorders often do not present for pharmacologic treatment. This may be because children and adolescents with anxiety disorders are not always recognized as requiring psychiatric help. Alternatively, nonpharmacologic methods may be preferentially applied, although scientific evidence for their therapeutic efficacy in many of the anxiety disorders, except for specific phobia and obsessive compulsive disorder (OCD), is essentially lacking. Given the available treatment literature for the anxiety disorders in children and adolescents, both psychological and pharmacologic interventions should be considered from the onset of treatment.

Studies evaluating the psychopharmacologic treatment of child and adolescent anxiety disorders range from the relatively well-developed investigations into OCD to few if any studies on social phobia. Recent publications of increasing numbers of case reports and open clinical trials, however, when combined with extensive clinical experience, do provide a reasonable body of knowledge about pharmacologic interventions in these disorders. The potential uses of various psychopharmacologic agents in child and adolescent anxiety disorders are outlined in Table 10–1.

It is important to note that there are compounds that in the past have been used to treat anxiety disorders in this population but for reasons of safety, lack of specific anxiolytic activity (e.g., antihistamines may appear to show efficacy in some anxiety states, but this is primarily a sedative and not an anxiolytic effect), or the availability of more effective and less potentially toxic preparations can no longer be advocated for routine clinical use in treating these disorders. These medications are antihistamines, barbituates, neuroleptics, and propanediols.

Like other psychiatric disorders of children and adolescents, the anxiety disorders may present with variable degrees of severity. At times the symptomatic distress is mild to moderate, and functioning is only somewhat impaired. In other cases symptomatic distress can be considerable, and often this is associated with a significant degree of functional impairment. Although pharmacotherapy should be considered for the entire spectrum of severity in anxiety disorders, in some mild cases treatment with medications may be postponed to determine whether other nonpharmacologic interventions will by themselves provide effective relief of symptoms and functional improvement. In these situations psychopharmacologic treatment may be considered an augmentation to those psychosocial interventions that prove partially or completely ineffective.

The alternative argument to the view of intervention that underlies the practice of treating with the least intrusive method (usually considered, for no valid reason, to be a psychotherapeutic strategy) may be more compelling. This viewpoint argues that maximal early intervention with optimal treatment strategies (psychotherapy combined with pharmacotherapy) will not only lead to a more rapid and greater resolution of current symptoms but also might prevent the development of maladaptive psychological, social, or neurobiologic functioning, which can itself become a risk for further disturbance. From this perspective, appro-

TABLE 10-1 **Medications of Potential Utility in Treating Child and Adolescent Anxiety Disorders***

Medication	GAD	ASD	OCD	PTSD	SoP	SP	SAD
TCA	×						
SSRI	×		×	×	×		×
Benzodiazepine	×	×	×		×	×	×
RIMA					×		
Buspirone	×				×		
Beta-blocker				×	×		
Clonidine				×			

*This table is a synthesis of the currently available literature on the pharmacologic treatment of child and adolescent anxiety disorders and clinical experience. It will have to be modified as new information becomes available.

GAD = generalized anxiety disorder, ASD = acute stress disorder, OCD = obsessive compulsive disorder, PTSD = posttraumatic stress disorder, SoP = social phobia, SP = simple phobia, SAD = separation anxiety disorder.

priate pharmacotherapy should be initiated early on in the treatment of all degrees of disorder.

In some cases anxiety disorders will present with a pressing need for urgent intervention. These are usually situations in which symptom distress or functional impairment (or both) is severe, such as suicidal tendencies associated with severe and frequent panic attacks or school refusal—agoraphobia with OCD. In these cases immediate optimal interventions are necessary, and there is no reason, theoretical or otherwise, to delay pharmacotherapy.

The goals of treating anxiety disorders with medications are as follows:

1. Amelioration of symptoms
2. Improvements in quality of life, including interpersonal and social functioning
3. Prophylaxis against further difficulties

Each of these goals taken alone is a reasonable target for pharmacotherapy. In most cases, however, all of these goals will be addressed.

A variety of medications are available for the treatment of anxiety disorders (see Table 10-1). In selecting any one compound as the medication of choice for initiating treatment, the clinician must ask the following questions:

1. Which of the compounds available has demonstrated treatment efficacy in children and adolescents with the same disorder as the patient I am about to treat?
2. If more than one medication shows some degree of efficacy, which evidence is stronger, and have any comparisons among these various possible medications been conducted?
3. Which medications are the least likely to cause serious life-threatening adverse events?
4. Which medications are the least likely to cause annoying or distressing subjective adverse events?
5. Which medications require additional laboratory or other physiologic monitoring (electrocardiogram, serum levels) to ensure their safety or therapeutic efficacy?
6. Which medications are less expensive, or are available in a generic form?

The answers to these questions will lead the clinician to recommend a number of medications for the patient and family to consider. The choice of the compound for treatment initiation can then be made jointly. A list of suggested first-choice medications following from the conceptual approach just described is found in Table 10-2.

Medical Considerations in Anxiety Disorders

Of importance is the recognition that many medical illnesses can present with some of the somatic symptoms found in anxiety disorders. Too often, however, children and adolescents with clear-cut primary anxiety disturbances undergo unnecessary, costly, and at times painful medical investigations for possible but highly improbable medical disorders. A relatively common illustration of this is the child or adolescent who complains of chest pains, which leads to a cardiac workup, including cardiac enzymes, electrocardiograms, echocardiograms, or other more extensive investigation. This type of approach is to be discouraged because not only does it inconvenience and disturb the patient needlessly, but it often leads to a delay in proper treatment and allows for the further development of a point of view in which a medical or surgical approach, rather than psychiatric intervention, is perpetuated. A careful psychiatric-medical history and physical examination, followed by judicious use of diagnostic laboratory evaluations (as discussed in Section Two) are preferred.

Generalized Anxiety Disorder

Children and adolescents with generalized anxiety disorder (GAD) exhibit developmentally inappropriate or excessive worries, doubts, fears, and anxiety that persist over prolonged periods of time. These symptoms are trait and not state characteristics and lead to functional impairment within one or more domains, including but not limited to academics, interpersonal, family, and social functioning. In many of these children and teenagers, GAD can occur in a comorbid form, particularly with other anxiety disorders, major depression, dysthymia, attention-deficit hyperactivity disorder, drug and alcohol abuse, or tic disorder. Furthermore, even in the absence of comorbid states, symptoms of GAD may complicate the clinical picture of many psychiatric disturbances or may overlap with those of other disorders, such as major depression.

For this reason children or adolescents presenting with anxiety symptoms must be carefully evaluated for the presence or absence of another psychiatric disorder, especially a depressive syndrome. GAD or nonsyndromal anxiety symptoms often precede the development of a major depression or dysthymic disorder. At times the depressive episode may be a so-called secondary depression, in which a true depressive syndrome arises following a primary GAD. On the other hand, the dysphoria or demoralization that often follows from the original GAD may be mistaken for a depression. This may occur particularly if the patient's subjective experiences are incorrectly labeled by the clinician. For example, the psychiatrist in search of a mood disorder may incorrectly label as a primary depression the child's sense of frustration and unhappiness with his or her lot in life that has developed out of functional impairment secondary to anxiety symptoms.

Thus, diagnostic evaluation of the patient with significant anxiety symptoms should include consideration of the possibility of both comorbid states and other psychiatric disorders that present with anxiety symptoms, especially the depressive disorders. This special care in diagnostic ascertainment is vital because the treatment of patients with a primary diagnosis of GAD who also exhibit symptoms of dysphoria and demoralization (which may incorrectly be identified as depression) differs from the pharmacologic treatment of patients who present with a depressive disorder that either is initially identified as anxiety or arises secondary to a primary GAD.

CASE EXAMPLE

Adolescent Girl with GAD: "Life is no fun this way."

K.E. was a 14-year-old girl who was referred by her school counselor because of "depression" and concerns that she was "talking about suicide." When seen, K.E. described a feeling of unhappiness with how her life was going. She was having difficulties talking to boys, was too anxious even to go out to an afternoon movie with a boy (even though her parents approved), and felt left out of much of the gossip and conversations that her girlfriends were having about these and similar topics. She reported no previous unpleasant experiences with boys or any issues regarding sexual abuse that may have accounted for these problems.

In addition, she was constantly worrying

TABLE 10–2 **Suggested First-Choice Medications in the Treatment of Child and Adolescent Anxiety Disorders***

Disorder	Drug Choice	Alternate	Alternate
Generalized anxiety disorder	Buspirone	Clonazepam	
Obsessive compulsive disorder	Fluoxetine	Clomipramine	Sertraline
Social phobia	Fluoxetine	Moclobemide	Buspirone
Post-traumatic stress disorder	Fluoxetine	Propranolol	Clonidine
Separation anxiety	Fluoxetine	Clonazepam	
Performance-specific anxiety	Propranolol	Atenolol	
Selective mutism	Fluoxetine		

*This information was obtained from clinical experience and the currently available literature on the use of medications in treating child and adolescent anxiety disorders. This information was reviewed and then evaluated using the six questions described previously to arrive at the above first-choice and alternate suggestions. Note that in many instances fluoxetine is the only compound of the available serotonin-specific reuptake inhibitors (SSRIs) for which reported studies can be found. As new information regarding the use of other SSRIs becomes available, the role of fluoxetine will need to be re-evaluated.

about whether her friends really liked her and described severe problems making decisions about minor items, such as what clothing to wear to school and who to sit with at lunch. She constantly changed her mind and worried incessantly that she might make the wrong decision. She ruminated so much about what she had or had not done on any one particular day that she felt "tied up in knots" and often had difficulty falling asleep.

With regard to schoolwork, K.E. was actually doing quite well, getting mostly As and occasional Bs, but she felt that she was "not doing well enough." She worried constantly that her grades might drop. Although she prepared extensively for tests and examinations, she invariably experienced an upset stomach and "butterflies" for days before she was due to take a test. At times she was so "sick with worry" about upcoming examinations that she vomited, other times she refused to go out socially because she felt she needed to study more. Then she would worry that her friends might not like her because she was not going out with them as often as they expected her to.

K.E. clearly identified herself as "a worrier." As she put it, "I worry so much about so many things. It seems that I worry about everything. Nobody worries as much as I do. Life is no fun this way."

K.E. reported feeling "depressed." Her score on the Beck Depression Inventory (BDI) was 14. Her score on the Hamilton Depression Rating Scale (HDRS) was 10. However, most of the HDRS score came from her endorsement of the anxiety symptoms found in that scale. Careful questioning elicited not depression but dysphoria and demoralization. She was frustrated about her lack of social ease and constant worries about her friends and schooling. Furthermore, she had tried "everything that I can think of" to help herself stop worrying, with no success. Occasionally these frustrations led her to suicidal thoughts.

Direct questioning elicited description of a variety of physical symptoms of anxiety that were frequently present and that increased in stressful situations. She had no obsessions or compulsions and denied having any panic attacks, although she stated that she could become "panic stricken" if a teacher "pulled a surprise test."

Her past history was positive for long-standing and severe anxiety symptoms and included periods in which she refused to go to school. She had undergone a number of invasive medical investigations for "stomach problems" and at one time had been seen by a pediatric gastroenterologist to "rule out a bowel disease." K.E. and her parents were apparently told that she had a "nervous stomach," and she was advised to "relax more." Although there was no previous history of any other psychiatric disorder, she had gone through a period in which she demonstrated occasional unilateral facial tics 7 years prior. These had remitted and had never reappeared.

K.E.'s family history was instructive in that her mother noted that she "came from a long line of worriers," although no one had ever been diagnosed with or treated for any psychiatric disorder. K.E.'s mother herself described a number of specific phobias, including a fear of airplane flights, which limited the family's vacation travel. K.E.'s biologic father was not present for the assessment and had not been able to attend because he lived in another city 500 miles away. As far as K.E.'s mother was aware, there were no identified psychiatric illnesses in his family, but she noted that "his brothers and father drank an awful lot."

A provisional diagnosis of GAD was made, and K.E.'s family physician was contacted to provide a detailed medical history.

CASE COMMENTARY

This case illustrates a number of the previously outlined points regarding the diagnosis of GAD. Specifically, it points out the importance of differentiating GAD and its often resulting demoralization phenomenon from depressive disorders. Furthermore, it demonstrates how individuals with an anxiety disorder who are assessed using rating scales designed for depressive disorders can score within what are often accepted as usual ranges for patients who are experiencing a primary depressive syndrome. This is because both the scales in this case (BDI, HDRS) here are symptom-rating scales designed to measure severity and are not diagnostic instruments. Because significant anxiety symptoms often occur within the constellation of depressive disorders, these "depression" rating scales may produce relatively high scores in anxious patients who are not clinically depressed. It is imperative that the clinician not confuse a severity score on such scales with a symptom threshold score used in diagnosis. Finally, this case illustrates how children or teenagers with anxiety disorders are often referred for unnecessary and at times intrusive medical investigations.

Initiating Psychopharmacologic Treatment

Medications most commonly used in the treatment of child or adolescent GAD are buspirone, benzodiazepines, and antidepressants (Table 10–3). If the patient has a comorbid or secondary depression, then the initial pharmacologic treatment should be the same as for a depressive disorder. The pharmacologic treatment of depressive disorders is discussed fully in Chapter 11.

Baseline Evaluation
Medical Considerations

Medical considerations are outlined in Section Two. Of particular importance is the evaluation of those physical parameters that may be affected by pharmacologic treatment. Because expected treatment will often begin with either buspirone or a benzodiazepine, the standardized baseline physical assessments suggested are Medication Specific Side Effect Scales (MSSES) (see Appendix IV for scales for buspirone and benzodiazepines). The patient should be assessed at every visit for the presence of side effects, and the appropriate scales should be appended to the patient's clinical record.

Laboratory Considerations

Laboratory investigations should assess those physiologic parameters that pharmacologic treatment may affect both in the short term and, because chronic treatment may be indicated, in the long term. As no such physiologic changes are expected with buspirone or a benzodiazepine, no specific laboratory investigations are indicated.

Psychiatric Considerations

Baseline evaluation should assess those symptoms that are the target of pharmacologic treatment.

The following baseline measurement tools are suggested:

1. Hamilton Anxiety Rating Scale (HARS). As described in Section Two and Appendix VI, the HARS provides a useful clinician-administered rating scale for the evaluation of anxiety symptoms in both children and adolescents.
2. Beck Anxiety Inventory (BAI). As described in Section Two and Appendix VI, the BAI provides a useful self-rating scale for the evaluation of anxiety symptoms in adolescents.
3. State-Trait Anxiety Inventory for Children (STAIC). As described in Section Two and Appendix VI, the STAIC provides a useful rating scale for the evaluation of anxiety symptoms in children.
4. Revised Children's Manifest Anxiety Scale (RCMAS). As described in Section Two and Appendix VI, the RCMAS provides a potentially useful rating scale for the evaluation of anxiety symptoms in children or adolescents.

The clinician should select the scale(s) most useful for the patient and complete it prior to beginning treatment. These same scales should be repeated weekly during the acute phase of treatment. The expected time for significant change in the various measures depends on the anxiolytic chosen. For example, clinical improvement in anxiety symptoms will be more rapid if clonazepam is chosen and is not expected to occur for 2 to 3 weeks following the onset of treatment if buspirone is chosen.

Various 10 cm Visual Analogue Scales (VAS) can be used to monitor other target symptoms that may be the focus of treatment. These are of particular value in evaluating those social, family, academic, or interpersonal features that have been identified as specific problems for the patient.

TABLE 10–3 **Suggested Medications for Treatment of Children and Adolescents with Generalized Anxiety Disorder***

Medication	Test Dose	Starting Dose	Target Dose Range (total daily dose)
Buspirone	5 mg	5 mg	Children: 15–30 mg Teens: 30–60 mg
Clonazepam	0.25 mg	0.25 mg	Children: 1.0–2.0 mg Teens: 1.5–3.0 mg
Fluoxetine	5 mg	5 mg	Children: 5–20 mg Teens: 10–40 mg

*Medication suggestions and dosage guidelines are based on clinical experience and on a review of currently available literature on the pharmacologic treatment of GAD in children and adolescents. This table is to be used as a guideline only because individual response (therapeutic and adverse) will vary. Doses should be adjusted as clinically indicated.

CASE EXAMPLE

K.E. Chooses an Anxiolytic as Part of Her GAD Treatment

After obtaining additional information from K.E.'s family physician and further education about GAD and its potential treatments, the clinician suggested a treatment program including cognitive psychotherapy and buspirone. Benzodiazepines were not chosen because K.E. and her mother were concerned about possible withdrawal and dependence phenomena with compounds from this class of medications. In addition, the family history was positive for alcohol abuse, suggesting an increased risk for potential misuse of benzodiazepines.

An HARS score completed prior to beginning treatment was 33. Four different VAS scores were obtained, including feeling comfortable with friends, going out socially, feeling comfortable at school, and having trouble falling asleep. The MSSES score for buspirone at baseline was 25.

Buspirone

Buspirone is an azapirone, recently introduced as an anxiolytic agent, that has shown efficacy in studies of adults and more recently in children and adolescents. In addition to its anxiolytic effects, which are comparable with those produced by benzodiazepines in treatment-naive patients, buspirone has also shown potential as an antidepressant, in the treatment of self-injurious behavior or organic-induced aggression, and in some behavioral symptoms in autistic patients. Although it has no demonstrated antipanic activity, buspirone provides an important advance in the treatment of GAD with a positive risk-benefit ratio. Its use demonstrates no evidence of withdrawal reactions, causes no memory or psychomotor impairments, and has no demonstrated potential for abuse. As such it may be of particular benefit for use in those children and adolescents in whom family histories of drug or alcohol abuse may raise concerns about the wisdom of benzodiazepine treatment.

Buspirone undergoes extensive first-pass metabolism with a bioavailability of only about 5 percent. It is best taken between meals to increase its rate of absorption. Most of the oral dose is excreted in the urine, and to date 12 metabolites have been identified in humans, only one of which [1-(2-pyrimidinyl) piperazine or 1-PP] is active, but with no well-defined clinical effects. Buspirone is highly bound to plasma proteins, and

peak plasma levels are found $\frac{1}{2}$ to $1\frac{1}{2}$ hours following oral intake. Its elimination half-life is quite variable, ranging from 1 to 10 hours, and thus multiple daily dosing is necessary. Unlike the benzodiazepines, which show rapid onset of anxiolytic effects, the anxiolytic effect of buspirone may take 2 to 3 weeks to maximize at an adequate daily dose.

The anxiolytic effects of buspirone are thought to derive primarily from its agonist binding to the postsynaptic serotonin receptor, 5HT1A, although its 5-HT2 and dopamine (D2) effects may also be implicated in this action. Chronic administration of buspirone is known to cause downregulation of 5-HT2 receptors, although the exact relationship of this phenomenon to the onset of effective anxiolytic activity has not been worked out. Unlike the benzodiazepines, buspirone does not influence the GABA–chloride ion channel receptor complex. Furthermore, buspirone does not demonstrate significant sedative, hypnotic, muscle relaxant, or anticonvulsant properties.

Buspirone has a relatively benign side effects profile. Although some potentially significant drug-drug interactions may occur (Table 10–4), buspirone is not known to impair cognitive functioning or to adversely affect psychomotor functioning. In many cases side effects are similar in frequency to those reported with placebos, and include headache, dizziness, fatigue, nervousness, gastrointestinal (GI) upset, and various paresthesias. While buspirone does affect dopamine receptors, there is no clear evidence of its causing tardive dyskinesia, and indeed some reports have suggested that its use in higher doses may actually improve neuroleptic-induced tardive dyskinesia. Occasional extrapyramidal symptoms have, however, been reported. Buspirone is not toxic in overdose and, although no specific teratogenic effects have been identified with its use, its safety in pregnancy has not been fully determined.

The potential anxiolytic efficacy of buspirone and its relatively benign adverse effects profile

TABLE 10–4 Potential Drug-Drug Interactions with Buspirone

Class of Drug	Possible Interaction Effect
MAOI	Elevated blood pressure
Benzodiazepine	Increased benzodiazepine serum levels
Neuroleptic	Increased neuroleptic serum levels
	Possibly increased extrapyramidal effects
SSRI	?Seizure risk

make it an attractive first-choice medication in the treatment of GAD for children and adolescents. Because some evidence exists that buspirone may be less anxiolytic in those patients who have undergone previous benzodiazepine treatment, it is suggested that buspirone, rather than benzodiazepines, be considered as first-line therapy in children and adolescents with GAD.

CASE EXAMPLE

K.E. Begins Her Buspirone Treatment: "When will this stuff work?"

Following an initial test dose of 5 mg, K.E. began taking buspirone at a dose of 5 mg three times daily. When seen 3 days following the onset of treatment, she reported no side effects and no change in the severity of her symptoms. The dose was increased to 10 mg three times daily. At her next visit, K.E. complained of feeling a little sick to her stomach and stated that she was getting diarrhea. She also complained of stomach cramps and dizziness.

A review of her baseline MSSES scores, however, did not substantiate the concern that these symptoms were treatment emergent, and after reviewing this with the clinician, she agreed. She did complain that she was not feeling any better, asking, "When will this stuff work?" These concerns necessitated a review of her symptoms and the expected time of onset of buspirone's therapeutic action. She agreed to "wait it out." In the meantime, she was still hoping to begin cognitive therapy "as soon as the doctor has an opening."

When next seen, 10 days following the onset of buspirone treatment, K.E. reported feeling "a little bit better." She stated that she was "not worrying so much as before." Her HARS score was now 26. There was no significant change in her VAS scores for any of her functional concerns. Her MSSES score was 19. She was asked to continue with the same medication dose, and a further appointment was set for 1 week later.

At K.E.'s next appointment she reported feeling better than before. Her HARS score was now 15 and her MSSES score was 14. Her VAS scores, however, were not significantly changed. She was looking forward to her first appointment with her cognitive therapist.

When seen 2 weeks later, K.E. reported that she was "doing OK." Her HARS score was 14, and her MSSES score was 16. Her "trouble sleeping" score had dropped from a baseline of 8 to 4. The other VAS scores showed little or no change. She had begun cognitive therapy and reported that she thought it was "weird." A discussion with K.E. and her parents identified a plateau phase in her improvement. Because she had just begun psychotherapy, it was decided to wait and see whether there would be future symptomatic improvement without an increase in the buspirone dose. A period of 3 weeks was chosen as a reasonable time frame for re-evaluation.

When next reviewed, K.E.'s HARS score was 12 and her MSSES score was 14. Her "trouble sleeping" score was now 3, and her other VAS scores had shown an average drop of 2 points from baseline. Although she was less anxious and felt she was coping better, she did agree that she was still symptomatic and not doing as well as she had hoped. Accordingly, her buspirone was raised to 15 mg three times daily, and a follow-up appointment was scheduled for 2 weeks. She was continuing her weekly cognitive therapy sessions.

Two days later, K.E.'s mother called and reported that K.E. was complaining about an upset stomach. She was concerned that the increase in medications was making K.E. nauseated and crampy. A review of K.E.'s course to date and further discussions about the possibility of side effects and the presence of somatic symptoms as a part of anxiety itself led to the decision to maintain the medication at its present dose for another 3 days, with a telephone check-in at that time. Three days later, K.E.'s mother called again, reporting that K.E. was "better."

When next seen, K.E. was in good spirits. She stated that she was "a lot better." Her HARS score was now 7 and her MSSES score was 4. All four VAS scores had improved 50 percent or more. She felt her cognitive therapy was going well. K.E., her parents, and the physician were unable to determine whether her improvement was because of the increased buspirone dose, or the cognitive therapy "kicking in." Her therapist identified K.E.'s improved ability to use cognitive techniques and relayed an impression that "she is improving." It was decided that a follow-up medications appointment in 2 months would be the strategy to pursue and that she should continue with the buspirone treatment at least until then.

CASE COMMENTARY

This case illustrates a number of common features found with buspirone treatment of GAD in teenagers and children. First, the medication can be rapidly increased to the expected effective target dose of about 30 mg daily for teens and 15 mg daily for prepubertal children. Maximal doses have not been adequately identified in children or adolescents but should be determined using clinical criteria of outcome and side effects. In most cases, initial target dosage ranges similar to those suggested for adults (30 to 60 mg daily) will be sufficient for adolescents. For prepubertal children, the initial target dose range may be more cautiously set at 15 to 30 mg daily.

Second, the onset of buspirone's anxiolytic activity at an effective total daily dose is somewhere between 2 and 3 weeks. In the case of K.E., this occurred at about $2\frac{1}{2}$ weeks at 30 mg daily. Anxious patients (or their parents) are often concerned that their symptoms are not getting better and need physician support to be able to tolerate this waiting period.

Third, a plateau of the anxiolytic response can occur, especially at the lower range of the potentially effective dose. The clinical approach is to allow sufficient time to pass to identify the pattern of response as an actual plateau and then to gradually increase the medication in a stepwise manner, allowing sufficient time between dose increases to be able to ascertain a potential therapeutic effect.

Fourth, the timing of monitoring visits was much less frequent in K.E.'s case than that described in other disorders using different medications. This is because the expectation of efficacy and emergence of side effects should govern the visit schedule. In the case of a child or teen with GAD treated with buspirone, visits spaced 2 weeks apart may be sufficient if telephone contact is available.

Fifth, the onset of pharmacologic treatments often coincides with the beginning of psychotherapeutic intervention. When this occurs, it is sometimes difficult to tell which agent is responsible for improvement. A sit and wait strategy, as described in K. E.'s case, in which the medication is kept constant for a period of time to assess potential further symptomatic improvement, is a reasonable procedure to follow. Should significant improvement occur while the medication dose remains stable, there may not be a need to increase the dose. However, if improvement does not continue when the dose is maintained at a stable level over a reasonable period of time, the dose can then reasonably be raised.

Sixth, the monitoring of MSSES scores will often show an improvement over time, similar to that found with decreases in the severity of anxiety symptoms. This is because many of the physical symptoms endorsed by the patient are part of the anxiety disorder itself and are not caused by medication treatment. Finally, measures of functioning may take longer to show improvement than measures of symptom severity. In many cases a symptom reduction threshold of 50 to 60 percent from baseline is necessary before measurable improvement in functioning is seen. Often the addition of psychotherapeutic strategies, such as cognitive or behavioral therapy, can assist in the reduction of functional impairment beyond what can be obtained by medication alone.

CASE EXAMPLE

"It's 3 months later. Now what, doc?"

K.E. was reassessed 3 months following her improvement. Although she was not entirely symptom free, she reported "feeling fine" and "doing good." She was much less anxious around her friends, had an active social life, was doing well at school and worrying less about her tests, and had begun to go out on group dates. Her HARS score was 6 and her MSSES score was 4. Her four VAS scores continued to show a greater than 50 percent improvement over baseline. The question arose as how to proceed.

Because she was not entirely symptom free, one option was to again increase the buspirone to see if that would be helpful. Another option was to maintain the dose at the same level for another period of time and see how she did. A third option was to decrease the medication dose and then increase it again if her symptoms reappeared.

K.E. did not wish to increase her medication. Her mother wanted the medication to remain stable, but K.E. wanted to "stop the pills." K.E. was confident that her disorder would remain under control. After a spirited discussion, her mother agreed to her request, and a signs and symptoms anxiety checklist for relapse identification (see Appendix II) was developed for K.E. to monitor herself. Her dose was then decreased to 10 mg three times daily, and she was scheduled to be seen in 1 month.

When next seen, K.E. was still doing well. However, with her mother's approval she had increased her dose of buspirone to 15 mg three times daily because she had found that 10 days after the medication decrease her anxiety had started to increase. She was now willing to continue at the same dose for another 3 months "or so."

CASE COMMENTARY

This continuation of K.E.'s case illustrates two common questions in the treatment of GAD: What is the optimal pharmacotherapy of GAD? In other words, how do I know when to stop increasing the medication? And what is or what should be the duration of pharmacologic treatment of GAD? At this time, there are no scientific data that can provide clear answers to these questions, and good clinical intuition plus the application of some general principles regarding pharmacotherapy can be used as guidelines.

To decide when to stop increasing the medication dose when treating children or teens, the clinician can use these questions to provide helpful guidelines:
1. Is the patient fully symptom free?
2. Does the patient still show functional impairment attributed to the disorder?
3. Is the patient experiencing adverse effects from the medication that are causing significant distress?
4. What are the available published guidelines for dose ranges with the medication?
5. Did I wait long enough for the medication to establish its full therapeutic efficacy?
6. What potential problems will arise if the medication dose is raised?
7. What are the patient's (and parent's) feelings about all of the above?

Answering these questions and discussing them with the patient and parents will not provide the clinician with a simple answer but should help in the decision-making process.

The second issue is: What should be done if the patient is feeling and functioning relatively well and does not want to try to maximize the outcome pharmacologically? How long should pharmacotherapy for GAD be continued? As discussed in Section Three under continuing and discontinuing pharmacotherapy, the guidelines in Chapter 7 could be applied. It is suggested that the same dose that was used to provide symptom remission be continued for 6 months.

In the case of K.E., she did not want to follow that strategy, and the physician instituted a gradual dose-lowering strategy to determine whether a lower total daily dose would provide a sufficient maintenance effect. Because buspirone decrease or discontinuation is not known to be associated with withdrawal or the rebound phenomenon, the onset of symptoms occurring during discontinuation may more easily be identified as an impending relapse, and the medication may be increased to its previous dose when this occurs. When a discontinuation strategy is chosen, with buspirone it is nevertheless useful to decrease the daily dose by not more than one third and then to monitor the effect of this dosage decrease on symptom expression. Clinical experience suggests that a time frame of 4 to 6 weeks between steps in dosage decrease is a reasonable length of time in which to assess the possibility of symptom re-emergence.

Treatment resistance to buspirone's anxiolytic effects may be defined as an adequate trial with minimal or no symptom improvement. This consists of a minimum of 4 weeks at a maximal oral dose (60 mg or more per day, as limited by tolerability in teens, and 30 mg or more per day in children) with good compliance. In addition, the patient should have undergone concurrent psychotherapy of proven or suggested efficacy for GAD. Unfortunately, sufficient good evidence for the efficacy of one or more particular psychotherapies in GAD is not available, although studies of cognitive self control combined with relaxation therapy suggest that this may be of benefit.

If treatment resistance is demonstrated, the first step should be diagnostic reassessment, with particular attention paid to the presence of comorbid psychiatric or unrecognized medical conditions. Careful review of potential drug abuse, particularly with compounds not often considered, such as diphenhydramine, should be conducted, including urine testing. A second opinion is also of value. Should the diagnosis of GAD be upheld, consideration should be given to initiating treatment with either a benzodiazepine or an SSRI.

Obsessive Compulsive Disorder

OCD in children and adolescents is characterized by a symptom profile essentially identical to that found in adults. The estimated lifetime prevalence of OCD is 1 to 2 percent. In addition to experiencing recurrent obsessive thoughts and intrusive images, or compulsive behaviors, patients with OCD often experience moderate to severe functional impairment. Symptoms wax and wane over the course of the illness, and various obsessions or compulsions may disappear, only to reassert themselves at a later date or to be replaced by others. Many children and adolescents are secretive about their symptoms, often fearing that if they share their often bizarre ideas others will think that they are "crazy." The placebo response rate in patients with OCD, unlike that in patients with many of the other anxiety disorders, is reported to be quite low, less than 5 percent in many estimations, and both pharmacologic and behavior interventions have demonstrated utility.

To date a variety of medications (perhaps more than in all the other anxiety disorders in this age group combined) have been studied in children and adolescents with OCD. Evidence suggests that drugs that demonstrate serotonin reuptake inhibition may be effective anti-OCD agents. In addition, some studies suggest a clinically useful pharmacologic augmentation strategy in those patients who demonstrate only partial response to initial pharmacologic treatment. Psychosurgery, a subject beyond the scope of this book, is available for selected patients who have demonstrated resistance to optimal pharmacologic and psychological treatments. Behavior therapies (stopping offending thoughts, exposure, response prevention) are useful in treating OCD. Furthermore, although the needed studies have not yet been reported, clinical experience and data from studies in adults strongly suggest that the optimal treatment of child and adolescent OCD is obtained with combined pharmacologic and behavioral treatments.

CASE EXAMPLE

The Girl Who Couldn't Stop Counting: Childhood OCD

M.K. was an 8-year-old girl referred for treatment to an outpatient clinic in a small rural hospital. She had been tentatively diagnosed as having OCD by her family physician. M.K. reported a 2-year history of excessive counting and ordering rituals. Her parents considered her to have been "careful, ordered, and especially clean" since her earliest years, but she began to exhibit problems getting to school on time, playing with her friends, and relating to other family members because of her "plans." These plans had onset 2 years previously and had gradually become more complex and time consuming. At first her parents had considered them "cute," but they had rapidly tired of "going along with her," particularly when her demands became more insistent and forceful around the time her grandmother died.

Her compulsive symptoms included counting and cleaning rituals, and she exhibited lit-

tle if any control over this behavior. For example, she would fastidiously tidy her bedroom prior to leaving for school in the morning. If any book, paper, stuffed animal, hair brush, or other special object was not exactly in its place, she could not leave the room. At times it took her 15 to 30 minutes to make sure that everything was in its properly assigned location. She would then count all the telephone poles on the way to school. If she thought that she might have missed one, she became very distraught and demanded that she be taken home to start all over again. This had become so problematic that she had been taken off the school bus for "behavior problems," and her mother was pressed into taxi service. This arrangement was also unsatisfactory. M.K. would often demand that her mother return home so that the telephone pole counting could begin anew, her mother would refuse, and at times severe altercations would break out because, according to her mother, M.K. would "become hysterical." As a result of these symptoms, M.K. was often late to school or missed it.

At school she attended to various other rituals. One of these included walking in and out of the door four times every time she entered or left a classroom. Another included meticulous attention to her spelling words to make sure that all the letters were exactly the same height. If they were not, she would erase the entire word and try again. She rarely completed any writing tasks and would often erase the same word so many times that she would tear her work page.

In addition to these and many other rituals, M.K. reported many obsessive thoughts. The two that she found most distressing were "that my daddy has got run over by a truck" and "that my baby brother drowned." On arriving home from school every day, she would check to make sure her father and brother were indeed safe. She insisted on being present whenever her younger brother was being bathed, and if her father was not home at her appointed bedtime, she would try to stay awake until he returned.

M.K.'s family history was positive for depression on her father's side. Her paternal grandmother had received electroconvulsive therapy treatments on at least two occasions. Alcohol abuse was identified on her mother's side, involving her maternal grandfather and an uncle. A maternal aunt had committed suicide as an adolescent, although little was known about her mental status prior to that event.

No comorbid psychiatric conditions current or past were found for M.K., and neither parent described a diagnosable psychiatric disorder, although the father admitted to being "a perfectionist" and reported that the neighbors joked about how neat and clean his workbench and garage were. He was also very concerned about how clean his truck was and would wash and vacuum it at least two or three times a week. He kept the truck seats covered with a dark blanket, which he washed every other day to protect them from "dust." He denied any other behaviors that could possibly be rituals and denied having any obsessive thoughts.

M.K. was experiencing increasing difficulties at school and with her peers. Her teachers felt that she was avoiding her work, and her grades were poor. Other children made fun of the way she walked in and out of classrooms, and she had been involved in a number of altercations as a result of teasing she had experienced because of her behavior. The school authorities designated her a "behavior problem" and labeled her as "showing emotional problems" that they believed were secondary to her grandmother's recent death.

CASE COMMENTARY

This case illustrates a number of common features of child and adolescent OCD. First, the young girl in this instance was clinically symptomatic for a relatively long period of time prior to the initial diagnosis. Second, she exhibited significant functional impairment in school, and in family life; most of this was felt to be secondary to the OCD. Third, family difficulties associated with her OCD symptoms had arisen. Fourth, although she had been identified as a child with "problems," the nature of her difficulties had not been adequately characterized, and a simplistic stress-diathesis model was evoked to explain her behaviors. She was actually quite fortunate that her primary care physician recognized both the nature and severity of the disorder and referred her for immediate treatment.

Initial Pharmacologic Management

Medications that may be useful in the pharmacologic treatment of OCD in children and adolescents are listed in Table 10–5. It is recommended that in all cases their use be combined with cognitive-behavioral treatments, such as exposure and response prevention strategies. Family inter-

TABLE 10–5 Potentially Useful Medications in the Treatment of Child and Adolescent OCD*

Medication	Initiation of Treatment	Augmentation of Treatment[†]
Clomipramine	×	
Fluoxetine	×	×
Sertraline	×	×
Fluvoxamine	×	×
Trazadone		×
Clonazepam	×	×
Buspirone		×
High-potency antipsychotics (in low dose)		×

*The information in this table was compiled from clinical experience and the available current literature on the pharmacologic treatment of child and adolescent OCD.

[†]Some evidence suggests that combined clomipramine and fluoxetine treatment may be an effective initial treatment for OCD. However, given the potential medical complications of treatment with this combination, this approach should be reserved for either augmentation or treatment-resistant cases.

ventions are also usually indicated for optimal interventions in this disorder.

Because OCD in children and adolescents may occur comorbidly with other psychiatric disorders, particular attention must be paid during the diagnostic process to identify potential comorbid states. These may commonly include major depression, dysthymia, Tourette's syndrome, conduct disorders, and substance abuse. Learning disabilities may affect up to one fifth of OCD children and adolescents, but the relationship between specific types of learning problems and OCD has not been clearly elucidated. Soft neurologic signs may appear in a substantial number of these patients, and there is some evidence that their presence may possibly predict a poorer response to initial clomipramine treatment. There is no clear evidence, however, for any specific clinical or biologic characteristics to serve as indicators for either the selection of initial pharmacologic treatment or the prediction of outcome for any particular medication treatment.

A reasonable first approach is to select one of the above-mentioned selective serotonin reuptake inhibitors (SSRIs) such as clomipramine, fluoxetine, sertraline, or fluvoxamine (see Table 10–6). In some cases an earlier and perhaps increased initial response can be obtained by the addition of a low dose of clonazepam (0.25 to 0.5 mg given by mouth, twice daily) to initial SSRI treatment. Although clomipramine has been studied more than any SSRI in child or adolescent OCD, there is no

TABLE 10–6   **Suggested Medications for Initial Treatment in Child or Adolescent OCD***

Medication	Test Dose	Starting Dose	Target Dose Range (total daily dose)
Fluoxetine	5 mg	5 mg	Children: 5–40 mg Teens: 10–60 mg
Clomipramine	10 mg	10 mg	Children: 75–150 mg Teens: 100–200 mg
Sertraline	25 mg	25 mg	Children: 50–100 mg Teens: 50–200 mg
Fluvoxamine	25 mg	25 mg	Children: 50–200 mg Teens: 150–300 mg

*The information in this table was compiled from clinical experience and the available current literature regarding the pharmacologic treatment of child and adolescent OCD. Individual patients will demonstrate differing therapeutic and adverse responses to treatment, and doses must be clinically titrated. In some cases higher daily doses may be necessary to optimize outcome.

clear evidence that any one of these medications is clinically superior to another. Side effects, however, may be expected to differ, with clomipramine demonstrating a higher rate and severity of various side effects (particularly of the anticholinergic variety) than fluoxetine or sertraline. Deciding which medication should be the choice for treatment initiation of this disorder then rests very much with patient preference, often expressed as comfort in using a medication that has been studied more or in using a medication that is less likely to cause side effects.

Applying the questions discussed previously to the issue of suggested medications for OCD, the clinician can make the suggestions given in Table 10–6 for consideration by the patient and family.

Baseline Evaluation

Medical Considerations

Medical considerations are outlined in Section Two. Of particular importance is the evaluation of those physical parameters that may be affected by pharmacologic treatment. If treatment includes clomipramine, the standardized baseline physical assessments suggested are heart rate and blood pressure (standing and sitting), and MSSES (See Appendix IV). If one of the SSRIs is used, the suggested assessment is the MSSES. The patient should be assessed at every visit for the presence of side effects, the nature and management of which are described more fully later. Completion of MSSES at every visit will allow for a comprehensive monitoring and documentation of the patient's medical state.

Laboratory Considerations

Laboratory investigations should assess those physiologic parameters that pharmacologic treatment may affect both in the short term and, because chronic treatment may be indicated, in the long term as well. If initial treatment is with clomipramine, baseline laboratory measures suggested are (1) a pregnancy test for sexually active females, (2) an ECG, and (3) CBC and liver function tests. The routine monitoring of CBC and liver function tests are not necessary and should only be done when clinically indicated. These measures are obtained at baseline in the unlikely event that a patient may develop hematologic or hepatic difficulties during treatment with tricyclics. In this case having baseline values on hand will allow for a more accurate evaluation of these laboratory values if obtained later. For example, a mildly elevated bilirubin obtained after 10 weeks of clomipramine treatment is of little use in clinical decision making unless a baseline bilirubin was obtained. With a baseline measure the clinician can determine whether the bilirubin level is rising, staying the same, or maybe even falling.

Whether to use ECG monitoring is a difficult issue to resolve, particularly in light of reports of sudden death occurring in children treated with a tricyclic, albeit not clomipramine. These concerns have clinical implications, even though a causal link between tricyclic use and sudden death has not been clearly established. However, a recent report of a study using a rare events epidemiologic paradigm has suggested that a small increased risk of sudden death may be associated with desipramine use. On the other hand, extensive investigations of the effect of desipramine on cardiac function in children and adolescents with attention-deficit hyperactivity disorder and major depression have not found that desipramine use in generally recognized therapeutic doses is associated with evidence of clinically significant cardiotoxicity. The relationship of these findings to tricyclic-associated sudden death is not known because sudden death may not be related in any way to readily identifiable or clinically significant cardiovascular disturbances.

Furthermore, the relationship between findings obtained in the study of desipramine-associated cardiovascular disturbances and clomipramine-associated cardiovascular disturbances is not clear. Desipramine-associated cardiotoxicity may be primarily related to its 2-hydroxy metabolite, 2-OH-DMI. This metabolite is not present if clomipramine is used, and thus clomipramine may be less likely to demonstrate clinically significant cardiovascular toxicity than desipramine. Both short-term and long-term studies of clomipramine treatment in child and adolescent OCD have not identified clinically significant clomipramine-induced cardiotoxicity. However, current literature recommendations suggest that clinicians routinely use ECG monitoring whenever tricyclic medications are used.

There is no evidence that routine ECG monitoring will in any way decrease the risk of sudden death in children treated with tricyclic antidepressants (TCAs). When ECG monitoring during TCA treatment in children and adolescents is conducted, asymptomatic increases in heart rate are commonly found. Although recommendations from investigators vary, it is generally held that if heart rates approach 120 beats/min in children or 110 beats/min in adolescents, clinical concerns may arise. Slight increases in PR and QRS intervals are also quite commonly found with TCA treatment, but prolonged PR or QRS intervals may be associated with the onset of cardiac arrhythmias (Table 10–7).

Preexisting minor cardiac abnormalities, such as sinus tachycardia and incomplete right bundle branch block, are relatively common in healthy prepubertal children, occurring in approximately 10 to 20 percent of the population. The clinical significance of these findings as they pertain to treatment with a tricyclic medication is unknown. If they are identified in children in whom clomipramine treatment is being considered, a cardiologist should be consulted prior to initiating treatment. Those OCD children with preexisting cardiac disease, such as rhythm disruptions, hypertension, congenital heart disease, or murmurs, should probably not be considered as candidates for TCA treatment, particularly because medications with potentially less cardiotoxicity (the SSRIs) are now available.

Some earlier evidence suggested that cardiotoxic effects may be more frequently associated with peak TCA plasma levels, especially when daily doses approaching 5 mg/kg are utilized. More recently, total daily doses in the range of 2.5 to 3.0

TABLE 10–7   Potentially Problematic Cardiovascular Parameters in TCA-Treated Children and Adolescents*

Parameter	Measurement Value
PR interval	≥ 0.20 s
QRS interval	> 0.12 s or shows an increase of 50% or more from baseline
Corrected QT interval	≥ 0.47 s
Resting heart rate	≥ 110 beats/min in children < 10 yr or > 100 beats/min in children over 10 yr
Sitting, *resting* blood pressure	> 140 mmHg over 90 in children under 10 yr
	> 150 mmHg over 95 in children over 10 yr
	Persistent elevations of systolic values of 15 mmHg or diastolic values of 10 mmHg over baseline may also be an indication for TCA dosage reduction (a cardiology consultation is suggested in this case)

*This table has been adapted from the cardiovascular guidelines for TCA use in children and adolescents developed by Dr. B. Birmaher and Dr. J. Zuberbuhler at the University of Pittsburgh Medical Center, with permission.

Note: Patients whose ECG evaluations show *one or more* of the following criteria should have their TCA medication dose reduced.

mg/kg have been considered to show this effect. Thus, giving clomipramine in divided daily doses (and not exceeding 3.0 mg/kg per day as a total daily dose) for prepubertal children is suggested. Adolescents, however, may potentially safely take most TCAs, including clomipramine on a single daily dose schedule, although the exact age at which this changeover effect occurs is not known. Prudent clinical practice thus suggests the use of divided dosage in adolescents as well.

Given the above-mentioned uncertainties and the very real concerns about the cardiotoxic effects of TCA medications, careful cardiovascular monitoring is necessary when clomipramine is used. Resting heart rate and blood pressure (sitting and standing) should be obtained at every clinic visit. ECGs should be obtained at baseline and within 3 to 4 days of every dose increase. Table 10–7 should be used as a guide for dose reduction. However, the experience of many clinicians and researchers suggests that resting heart rates and blood pressures are quite variable in the child population and that the *method* by which routine clinical cardiac monitoring occurs can significantly influence heart rate and blood pressure recording. It is suggested that the following procedure be used whenever resting heart rate and blood pressure are obtained:

1. Conduct this procedure in the same location using the same staff as much as possible.
2. Provide a comfortable place for the child to sit and wait before the procedure begins.
3. Allow for 5 to 10 minutes of settling in before the procedure begins.
4. Begin the procedure by having the child lie quietly on a comfortable bed, not an examining table, if possible.
5. If using an ECG, conduct a pulse rate measure first (see item 7).
6. Use only those ECG leads needed to obtain a rhythm strip.
7. Wait 5 to 10 minutes after attaching the ECG leads before taking the rhythm measurement. During this time the staff speaks quietly to the child about non–anxiety-eliciting subjects. If the pulse rate is being used to monitor the heart rate, complete a similar procedure but leave the hand on the child's wrist for 2 to 3 minutes prior to beginning the timed count. Record the pulse rate over 2 to 3 consecutive minutes and divide the total number of beats recorded by the recording time to obtain the heart rate.
8. Take the blood pressure reading after the ECG strip or pulse rate reading is completed, making sure that a properly sized cuff is used.

Many clinicians believe this procedure, although desirable for obtaining a correct resting heart rate and blood pressure, is so cumbersome and time consuming as to make routine office monitoring unrealistic. Because these concerns are justified and proper cardiac monitoring of TCA is necessary, it is suggested that, whenever possible, alternative medication choices to TCAs be considered as initial treatments to ensure as much as possible, patient safety, compliance, and comfort. When TCAs are clearly indicated, parents should be taught how to properly monitor their child's resting heart rate, and this can be done at home and the results reported at each clinic visit. It is still advisable to conduct resting heart rate and blood pressure monitoring in the clinic, even if the parents are reliably doing so at home.

If the pretreatment ECG is unremarkable, further ECG monitoring may be limited to rhythm strip determinations. Current recommendations suggest that ECG rhythm strips be obtained before each TCA dose increase and 3 to 5 days following each increase, when a new steady-state plasma level has been reached. The optimal intervals for resting heart rate monitoring during maintenance treatment with TCAs is not known, although re-

peating the ECG at 4- to 6-monthly intervals has been suggested. The utility of this practice has not been established, and it is of doubtful predictive or clinical value. It must be remembered that routine ECG monitoring has no demonstrated role in preventing sudden death associated with tricyclic use, and the patient and parents should be informed of this.

Psychiatric Considerations

Baseline psychiatric assessments should include the following measures:

1. Yale Brown Obsessive Compulsive Scale (YBOCS) for symptom severity measures
2. VAS for measurement of specific functional difficulties
3. Other instruments, as outlined in Section Two, depending on the treatment goals identified

Measures should be completed at baseline and at specific times during treatment. Because symptom change in OCD can be expected to occur relatively slowly (in 8 to 12 weeks), symptom severity and functioning measures can be used approximately every 2 weeks during the acute treatment phase. Once maintenance treatment has begun, these measures can be taken less often. However, it is suggested that they be repeated once every 6 to 8 weeks during long-term treatment to provide continued objective evaluations over time.

CASE EXAMPLE

"We want a medicine that is tried and true."

After considering possible alternatives, M.K.'s parents decided that they would prefer her to begin treatment with clomipramine, largely because they felt that more was known about that medication than about either fluoxetine or sertraline. They also decided that they did not want her to be treated with concurrent low-dose clonazepam during the early phases of treatment because they were concerned that she would become addicted to it.

Because this was a reasonable choice (although not the clinician's first choice), after the appropriate baseline measures had been obtained, clomipramine was begun at a dose of 50 mg/day in equally divided doses. A follow-up appointment was scheduled for 2 weeks, and the physician instructed M.K.'s parents to increase the clomipramine dose to 100 mg on the third treatment day. On day 7, following the physician's instructions, the dose was increased to 150 mg, with 50 mg being given in the morning and 100 mg at bedtime. On day 8, M.K.'s mother called to report that her daughter was complaining of dry mouth, blurry vision, and constipation. In addition, she felt that M.K. was groggy and "not herself." The physician reassured her that these effects would soon wear off and confirmed M.K.'s appointment for a week hence.

Three days later M.K. was seen in the hospital emergency room, where she was found to be suffering from severe anticholinergic side effects. Her heart rate was 130 beats/min and her blood pressure was obtained at 140/90 mmHg. There was no history of overdose, and she had not taken any other medications. A serum clomipramine level obtained at that time was reported as 1475 nmol/L. She was admitted to the hospital for overnight observation and placed on cardiac monitoring. Her clomipramine was discontinued. The next day she was feeling better, and her vital signs had improved.

CASE COMMENTARY

This case illustrated some of the problems that may arise with clomipramine treatment. First, the dose was initiated at too high a level. Second, the dose was raised too quickly. Third, inadequate monitoring of the pharmacotherapy was performed, and the physician did not react to M.K.'s mother's reports by seeing the patient and decreasing the dose. None of these "errors" should be made in proper pharmacologic care.

Understanding the issues regarding medication initiation and monitoring are key to proper psychopharmacologic treatment and cannot be ignored with any medication. In this case the physician also failed to consider—and had neglected to inform the patient's parents about—the possibility of slow hepatic hydroxylation of TCAs, which may be present in up to 10 percent of the population. This can lead to a longer half-life and increased serum levels of the medication. The high clomipramine plasma level found at hospital admission suggests that this may have been the case for M.K.

Clomipramine

Clomipramine undergoes extensive first-pass hepatic metabolism using the P-450 2D6 enzyme system and has an elimination half-life of 15 to 30 hr. Although the usual route of application is oral, the use of intravenous clomipramine has been reported in treatment of OCD. This approach is not recommended outside of specialty clinical-research units and is considered to be experimental.

The usual total daily dose of clomipramine in children is 2.5 to 3.0 mg per kg (75 to 150 mg daily), although with careful cardiovascular and serum level monitoring, amounts up to 5.0 mg per kg, that is, 150 to 300 mg per day in adolescents, can be used if tolerated. Medication is usually given with meals, in divided amounts, with one third of the daily dose being administered in the morning and two thirds at bedtime to decrease the experience of peak plasma-level–associated side effects. A relationship between clomipramine serum levels and therapeutic response in OCD has not been clearly established. Some patients demonstrate slow hepatic metabolism of TCAs. This will lead to an increased serum half-life. Others may be rapid metabolizers. Thus, individual variability of serum levels at any one dose can be considerable, and side effects need to be monitored carefully.

Clomipramine has a number of side effects that can be uncomfortable, can limit total daily dosage to below expected therapeutic amounts, and can adversely affect compliance. The most common of these are listed in Table 10-8.

Other important considerations pertaining to the side effects of tricyclic medications should be kept in mind if clomipramine treatment is used for OCD. Rapid dose increases in pediatric populations may be associated with seizure induction, particularly if the patient has a seizure disorder under only moderately good control.

In addition, abrupt withdrawal from high doses may be associated with a tricyclic withdrawal syndrome, the characteristics of which include anxiety, sweating, myalgia, nausea, dizziness, restlessness, and fever. All TCAs can be fatal in overdose;

TABLE 10–8   Common Side Effects of Clomipramine

Increased resting heart rate
Orthostatic hypotension
Dry mouth
Constipation
Delayed micturition
Blurry vision
Excessive sweating
Weight gain
Drowsiness
Tremor
Loss of appetite
GI upset
Rash
Dizziness
Headache

thus the clinician must be careful to prescribe only limited amounts of medications at a time and to carefully evaluate the suicidal potential and impulsivity of the patient at each visit. Parents must also be advised of this and encouraged to store TCA medications in a safe location to decrease the possibility of accidental self-poisoning, particularly if there are young children in the house who might gain access to the medications.

The possibility of inducing manic or hypomanic mood states in vulnerable individuals with clomipramine treatment exists. Unfortunately, no clear-cut predictors are available to identify which children or adolescents are most likely to experience this relatively rare yet problematic effect, although a premorbid history of cyclothymia or a family history of bipolar disorder may be informative. Thus, it is necessary to inform the patient and parents of this possibility and to educate them about the signs and symptoms of a possible mood swing, including the presence of significant irritability and mood lability.

Monitoring clomipramine serum levels may be of value in clomipramine treatment. A serum level can be obtained early on in the treatment process after the initial steady state has been reached. This information can then be used to direct further dose increases. Once the treatment maintenance phase has begun, clomipramine serum levels are not routinely necessary but may be obtained if concerns are raised about compliance or if other medications, which may potentially increase serum clomipramine levels (e.g., neuroleptics), are concurrently used. The issue of therapeutic drug monitoring is discussed in Section Three.

Clomipramine drug-drug interactions associated with commonly prescribed compounds are as follows:

Antiepileptics
TCAs
SSRIs
Neuroleptics
MAOIs
Quinidine
Moclobomide

Of further importance, two commonly used antihistamines, astemizole (Hismanal) and terfenadine (Seldane), which in some locations may be available over the counter, may cause cardiac problems if taken in high doses or combined with other potentially cardiotoxic medications such as a TCA. Patients and their parents should be advised to avoid these compounds if the potential for a drug-drug interaction exists. A good guideline to follow is to have the patient or parent contact the prescribing physician if *any* new medication is to be introduced.

CASE EXAMPLE

A Young Teenager with Partial Response: "I'm better, but . . . "

S.D. was a 13-year-old boy with OCD and learning problems who had begun clomipramine treatment. At treatment onset, his YBOCS score was 32. His medication was started at 25 mg daily and increased to 25 mg twice daily after 1 week. Further weekly increases of 25 mg/day, combined with proper medical and psychiatric monitoring, resulted in a total daily dose of 150 mg given one third in the morning and two thirds at bedtime. Side effects were relatively mild and included dry mouth, sweating, and an increased resting heart rate (108 beats/min). S.D. tolerated these well and compliance was excellent. A course of behavioral therapy using exposure and response prevention, begun before the onset of clomipramine treatment, continued.

On this regime, S.D. experienced some symptomatic relief and improved social functioning. He remained symptomatic, however, and after 6 weeks of 150 mg per day of clomipramine treatment, his YBOCS score was still 22. A meeting with S.D., his father, and his behavioral therapist led to a decision to attempt to try to deal with his "resistance" to pharmacotherapy.

CASE COMMENTARY

This case example illustrates a commonly encountered issue in treating the patient who demonstrates a partial response or nonresponse to initial pharmacologic intervention. When does the clinician consider that currently ongoing pharmacotherapy needs to be changed to maximize results? As described in Section Three, the clinician needs to consider a number of issues before changing the ongoing initial pharmacologic treatment. The essential issue is whether the current treatment has been adequate (an optimal dose over a sufficient period of time). In this case neither criteria had been met.

First, the time period was inadequate. It may be necessary to maintain a clomipramine dose of 150 mg daily for 8 to 12 weeks before sufficient symptomatic improvement occurs in OCD. Once the adequacy of the length of treatment has been established, the clinician can consider the second component of the equation: the adequacy of the dose. In determining this, the clinician should gradually increase the dose from the initial target dose to a reasonably higher target dose, using side effects as a guideline. This new dose should then be continued for a sufficient length of time (usually another 8 to 12 weeks) to allow therapeutic effect to occur. The physician cannot consider treatment resistance to have been demonstrated if the optimal total daily dose (as determined by tolerability) has not been continued for the necessary length of time.

CASE EXAMPLE

"I know how to approach this problem."

The clinician reviewed the expected time course for improvement with S.D. and his family, and they all waited 4 more weeks. Although behavior therapy with good compliance had continued throughout, at this time the YBOCS score was 20 and a dose-augmentation strategy was determined. Accordingly, a new target dose was set (200 mg daily), and the clomipramine dose was increased by 25 mg. This, however, was accompanied by a significant increase in side effects that S.D. found very difficult to tolerate, and the dose was again dropped to 150 mg daily.

Following this, augmentation strategies were attempted. From the choices available S.D. chose clonazepam as the initial augmentation agent. The medication was begun at 0.25 mg and was gradually increased. At a total dose of 0.75 mg given in equally divided amounts, S.D. experienced daytime sedation and dizziness, which he was not prepared to tolerate. Accordingly, this treatment was gradually discontinued and buspirone treatment was initiated. Although buspirone augmentation reached 60 mg daily, a level reached gradually over a number of weeks, it was unremarkable in terms of side effects. Unfortunately, it was also unremarkable in terms of increased symptom reduction. Eventually fluoxetine treatment was begun. At a fluoxetine dose of 10 mg daily, continued over 6 weeks, S.D. experienced further significant symptom improvement with tolerable side effects, and, although all his symptoms did not remit, his YBOCS score dropped to 13 and his functioning improved.

CASE COMMENTARY

This case illustrates some of the difficulties that can be experienced in optimizing pharmacologic treatment of OCD. Such treatment is difficult and the clinician must persist in attempts to optimize outcome. Although a number of augmenting agents are available (see Table 10–5), the superiority of any one agent has not been clearly demonstrated, and a trial-and-error approach is necessary. Published studies are unavailable to provide confirming evidence, but some "clinically reasonable" guidelines as to a first-choice of augmentation medication are as follows:

1. When there is a premorbid or family history of a mood disorder, an SSRI might be a reasonable first choice.
2. When there is a premorbid or family history of panic disorder, clonazepam might be a reasonable first choice.
3. When a premorbid history of tics, current tics, or a family history of Tourette's syndrome is present, a low dose of a high-potency neuroleptic, such as haloperidol or pimozide, might be a reasonable fist choice. Alternatively, the new "atypical" neuroleptic risperidone (in low doses) may be considered.

This process may be quite time consuming because each augmenting agent must be allowed sufficient time (usually 8 to 12 weeks) at a specific dose to determine whether a positive effect will indeed occur. Furthermore, whereas an augmentation strategy may be associated with improved symptom control, it is not always clear that improvement resulted from the medication and not the natural waxing and waning course of the disorder itself. Finally, in many cases a 50 percent reduction in symptoms is all that might be expected; hopefully, this improvement will be associated with functional improvements as well. This does not mean that when the patient achieves a 50 percent reduction in symptoms the clinician should simply continue with the treatment as is. On the contrary, the physician should consider the issue of maximizing pharmacotherapy and ask the necessary questions to direct this endeavor (see Section Three).

Continuation or maintenance treatment provides its own challenges as well. Clinical experience suggests that compliance is rarely a major problem in this population, particularly if significant symptom reduction has been obtained. Relapse when medication treatment is withdrawn is exceedingly high, and it is suggested that long-term treatment is necessary. A reasonable guideline is that once OCD symptom control has been optimized, treatment should continue for at least 1 year before any decrease in medications is considered. Many patients with OCD may need to face the possibility of lifelong pharmacologic treatment.

Post-Traumatic Stress Disorder

Post-traumatic stress disorder (PTSD) arises in some children or adolescents who have been exposed to trauma outside the range of usual human experience. Although its symptoms in this population are generally similar to those of adults, some developmentally specific differences may arise. In addition to displaying the symptoms used to define the disorder, children and adolescents with PTSD also demonstrate signs and symptoms that overlap with GAD, panic disorder, and depressive disorders.

Research into pharmacologic treatments for PTSD is in its earliest stages, even in adults. At this time psychotherapeutic interventions, although lacking in controlled studies to support their use, are generally considered to be the treatment of choice for children and adolescents with PTSD. Pharmacologic treatments, however, may be of value if significant depressive or anxiety-type symptoms are present, and some recent evidence, mostly from studies in adults, suggests that antidepressant medications, such as fluoxetine or clomipramine, may decrease the severity of the core symptoms of the disorder. In other cases, propranolol may reduce symptoms of autonomic hyperarousal, and clonidine may be useful in decreasing impulsivity and startle responses. These medications are discussed in Chapters 16 and 17 respectively. Benzodiazepines are probably not indicated for treatment of PTSD, and other medications that have been only minimally investigated in adults (such as carbamazepine and lithium) are unlikely to show significant advantages over the better tolerated and less complicated compounds, such as fluoxetine or sertraline.

If psychopharmacologic interventions are being contemplated to treat PTSD, a similar process of baseline assessment, education, and evaluation as described for the other anxiety disorders already discussed should be followed. The optimal choice of compounds cannot at this time be adequately addressed although suggestions can be made, given the available information (see Table 10–1.) No substantive guidelines for directing either short-term or long-term pharmacotherapy of PTSD in children and adolescents is possible at this time, given the paucity of good data available.

Social Phobia

A relatively large number of children and adolescents may have social phobia. In previous diagnostic classifications (prior to DSM-IV), many of these individuals may have been identified as having avoidant personality disorders or avoidant disorder of childhood. These children and adolescents tend not to be referred for psychopharmacologic treatments, and a variety of psychotherapeutic strategies (albeit without evidence of efficacy) are frequently applied.

Studies of pharmacologic treatment for social phobia in child and adolescent populations are essentially lacking, but those that are available suggest that fluoxetine, buspirone, or short-acting benzodiazepines may be of value. Clinical experience suggests that when these agents are used together with some behavioral therapies, a reasonable success rate may be realized. Unfortunately, there are no controlled studies of behavior therapies in this disorder. Clinical experience suggests that other types of individual psychotherapies (such as insight-oriented dynamic psychotherapy) are unlikely to be of substantial benefit.

Pharmacotherapeutic studies of social phobia in adults suggest a potential role for monoamine oxidase inhibitors (MAOIs) (especially the typical MAOI phenelzine), high-potency benzodiazepines (e.g., clonazepam and buspirone), or the SSRIs (fluoxetine and sertraline) in the acute treatment of social phobia. Reliable data about long-term treatment are unavailable.

Given the available information, if pharmacologic interventions are used, they should follow the process of baseline assessments, education, and treatment evaluation that has been outlined for other anxiety disorders. The patient and parents should be informed about the experimental nature of the treatment, and appropriate psychotherapies (such as systematic desensitization, graduated exposure, or participant modeling) should always be included.

The SSRIs such as fluoxetine or sertraline may be a reasonable first choice of medication for children and adolescents with social phobia because they are relatively safe and reasonably well tolerated, and compared with other possibilities, more is known about their use with children and adolescents, albeit often from studies and clinical experience with these agents in other disorders. Alternatively, buspirone may be considered. The MAOI phenelzine is not recommended because of the dangers of the "wine and cheese" (tyramine) reaction associated with its use and the high prevalence of orthostatic hypotension found in younger patients treated with this compound. An alternative to consider is the reversible inhibitor of monoamine oxidase A (RIMA), moclobomide. Studies of its use are currently ongoing in adults, and available clinical experience suggests that it may be potentially helpful in a number of socially phobic youngsters. In studies of adults, adverse events attributed to moclobomide are generally not significantly different from those obtained with a placebo. This tolerability profile is consistent with that observed with its limited clinical use in children and adolescents and there appears to be a low prevalence of treatment-emergent side effects.

CASE EXAMPLE

"He just won't go anywhere or do anything. He's more than shy."

S.I. was a 13-year-old boy who was referred for psychiatric assessment and treatment because of suicidal ideation. He admitted to occasional demoralization and dysphoric feelings but did not meet criteria, either present or past for a mood disorder. He did give a history of excessive shyness and severe social inhibition. He had one close friend with whom he spent most of his social time, but recently they had been seeing less of each other because the friend was beginning to take more of an interest in girls and was spending more time "hanging out" with groups of boys and girls. Although S.I. did not feel that the group was excluding him, he did not feel comfortable with them and he worried that he would say the wrong thing, do something embarrassing, and begin blushing. He refused to accompany his friend when he went out with the group, and as a result was spending more time alone. His fleeting suicidal ideation arose from the feelings of frustration and loneliness.

S.I.'s past history was characterized by excessive shyness and behavioral inhibition. As his mother put it, "He was born shy." An only child whose father had left the family, he had essentially been raised by his maternal grandmother because his mother worked outside of the home. He had experienced difficulty fitting in when he attended school for the first time and had always had problems speaking out in class. He always hung back when his class was involved in sports or recreational activities, and he tended to engage in solitary play during recess and at lunch hour. In spite of this excessive shyness, he was well liked by his classmates and was not subject to excessive teasing,

except for a few instances in the school gym locker room when he refused to change into his gym shorts.

The family history was positive for depression on S.I.'s father's side, and his paternal grandmother had been hospitalized for treatments that had included electroconvulsive therapy. S.I.'s mother was herself shy but had forced herself to overcome her social fears when she needed to obtain employment after her divorce. She reported that she never drank alcohol because she knew that it would ease social anxiety and was worried that this effect would cause her to become dependent on it. Although she did date occasionally and attended work functions, she described feeling anxious in social situations, especially when she did not know the other people well. Even at work-related functions, she tended to "hang on the fringe."

A preliminary diagnosis of social phobia was made for S.I., and after a full discussion about treatment alternatives, a referral to a therapist who specialized in cognitive-behavioral treatment was initiated. However, S.I. was not able to obtain an appointment for 4 months and no other resources were available to him. Because both he and his mother felt this was too long to wait, they explored alternative treatments that could be implemented in the meantime. After discussing it further and reading about a variety of potential medication treatments, they chose moclobomide pharmacotherapy combined with cognitive techniques that would be taught by the clinician. A notation was made in the clinical record regarding the experimental nature of this treatment.

CASE COMMENTARY

The difficulties with choosing a best first-choice medication in this disorder are clear. In S.I.'s case moclobomide was chosen over fluoxetine because his mother was concerned about the effect the latter might have on her son's suicidal ideation. S.I. thought that the side effects profile for moclobomide was more to his liking then that of fluoxetine. The clinician, who was experienced in the research and clinical use of this medication, was willing to support this decision on the grounds that this would be an experimental trial and that the patient's clinical condition was such that it was not appropriate to withhold potentially useful, albeit scientifically unstudied, therapy.

In child and adolescent psychopharmacologic treatment such decisions may at times need to be made. When this is the case the clinician should clearly communicate to the patient and parents the experimental nature of the treatment. This should also be written on the patient's chart, along with an explanation of why the clinician thought it was reasonable to go ahead with this treatment at this particular time.

Baseline Evaluations

When moclobomide is chosen, no specific medical or laboratory investigations are necessary. The usual baseline medical examination and an MSSES should be completed. Given the lack of suitable evaluation instruments for social phobia, a HARS combined with a number of symptom-specific VASs can be used to evaluate the outcome.

CASE EXAMPLE

"Well, let's go ahead."

S.I. was given an initial dose of 100 mg of moclobomide by mouth at noon. Because he tolerated this dose well, it was increased to 100 mg given in the morning after breakfast and in the evening after dinner. On this schedule, he experienced some mild agitation and difficulty sleeping, but this wore off after about 4 days on continued treatment. S.I. was maintained on this dose for 4 weeks. At the end of this time, his VAS ratings showed a slight symptomatic improvement, and his HARS score had decreased. It was decided to increase the dose by 100 mg given after lunch. This dose (300 mg daily) was maintained for an additional 4 weeks.

At the end of the second month of treatment a symptom review showed a decrease of 50 to 70 percent on most of the VAS ratings. The HARS showed a decrease in total score of about 60 percent from baseline. In addition, S.I. reported that he felt more confident with his classmates and had begun to speak out somewhat in class. Of more importance to him, however, was his ability to go with his friend to the mall and "hang out" with other adolescents (including girls) without always worrying about making a fool of himself. He was a long way from being the "life of the party" but was very happy with his improvement. His MSSES was unremarkable and he was tolerating the medication well. His only complaint was that taking the medication three times daily was "a pain."

Two months later he began cognitive-behavioral treatment with a therapist. With the combined approach, he showed further behavioral improvements and responded to discussions about stopping his medications with the comment that he wanted to keep taking it for at least another year.

CASE COMMENTARY

As illustrated in this case, this experimental pharmacotherapy was successful and became increasingly so when further psychotherapies were added. Although the treatment was experimental, it was entered into carefully, with full informed consent, and it was properly monitored throughout. These characteristics of appropriate pharmacotherapy apply equally well to novel or well-established interventions.

Moclobemide

Although at this time not specifically indicated for the treatment of social phobia, moclobemide may be a potentially useful medication for children or adolescents with this condition. This medication may be of further value when social phobia is complicated by major depression or panic disorder, although this also awaits proper study.

Moclobemide is a reversible inhibitor of monoamine oxidase A, a benzamide derivative that is chemically distinct from the irreversible MAOIs such as phenelzine and tranylcypromine. Whereas it inhibits the central activity of MAOI-A, thus affecting serotonin, norepinephrine, and dopamine activity, it has little effect on alpha-adrenergic, histaminergic, or cholinergic receptors. Taken orally, moclobemide is rapidly absorbed and relatively poorly protein bound (50 percent); it undergoes oxidative metabolism apart from the cytochrome P-450 system. These features figure prominently in its relatively benign side effects profile and its low potential for serious drug-drug interactions.

In studies of adult depressives side effects of moclobemide have often been reported as not significantly different from those of placebos in both structured clinical trails and extensive review of clinical practice. Reported rates of most side effects generally fall between 2 and 10 percent (Table 10–9). Mild to moderate side effects may occur at the onset of treatment and can be managed by beginning the dose at 100 mg daily and gradually increasing it to expected therapeutic daily doses, which can range from 150 to over 600 mg, given in divided amounts. In addition, clini-

TABLE 10–9 Relatively Common Adverse Effects of Moclobemide*

Dry mouth	Restlessness	Nausea
Dizziness	Insomnia	Anxiety/agitation
Headaches	Rash	Sedation

*These usually occur in less than 10 percent of patients. This information is based on reported studies in adult patients and limited clinical experience with children and adolescents. The frequency and nature of side effects in children and adolescents may differ somewhat, and careful clinical monitoring is necessary.

cal experience shows that these side effects, if they do occur, will often show substantial improvement after 2 weeks of continued treatment. Giving the medication 1 hour after meals will decrease the risk of headaches, and if insomnia is a problem, giving the last daily dose before 5 o'clock in the afternoon may be helpful.

Dietary constraints that are necessary with the irreversible MAOIs are not thought to be necessary with moclobemide. Although excessive ingestion of tyramine can be associated with increases in blood pressure, even with this compound, this would need to be an amount ≥ 100 mg of tyramine taken as a single dose. Because this is approximately three times the amount of tyramine found in an average meal, this is generally not a likely possibility. However, prudent clinical practice suggests that patients and their parents be fully informed of this concern and instructed to avoid those few foods that have very high levels of tyramine. These foods include Marmite, Vegemite, very ripe bananas, and aged cheeses, which are unlikely to be high on the dietary list of most children and adolescents. Beer, if consumed by older adolescents, should be bottled nondraft beer.

Other medications that should be avoided or used with caution are the following:

Antiparkinsonian drugs
TCAs
SSRIs
Irreversible MAOIs
Buspirone
L-Tryptophan
Sympathomimetic amines
Cimetidine
Lithium
Narcotics
Sumatriptan
MAO-B inhibitor (L-deprenyl)
Ibuprofen

Generally, careful clinical practice suggests that patients and their parents check with the prescribing physician before taking any other medications. Over-the-counter sympathomimetics including most cold remedies and weight-reducing agents, should be avoided. If these are used, they should be monitored by the prescribing physician. Clomipramine, meperidine, and dextromethorphan are contraindicated, and if moclobemide is being used following either TCA or SSRI treatment, a withdrawal period of 4 to 6 half-lives (usually about 2 weeks) is needed before commencing moclobomide treatment. An exception to this rule is fluoxetine, for which a washout period of 5 weeks is recommended to avoid potentially problematic side effects. Moclobemide has reportedly been used safely concurrently with a number of SSRIs in a small series of adult patients. However, this practice is not routinely recommended, and if undertaken requires very careful clinical monitoring and the initial use of low doses of both compounds.

Phobic-Type Disorders and Acute Stress Disorder

Simple phobias such as claustrophobia and arachnophobia are perhaps best treated with various behavioral therapies. Although no reasonable studies are available, clinical experience suggests that small doses of a high-potency benzodiazepine (such as clonazepam 0.25 mg twice daily) or diazepam (2.5 to 5.0 mg daily) may be a useful short-term intervention as an adjunct to ongoing behavior therapy. If this is clinically indicated, the duration of treatment should be 3 to 6 weeks with a carefully defined onset and offset, including a prolonged discontinuation phase to avoid rebound and the withdrawal phenomenon.

If specific phobic-type situations such as various situational anxieties (fear of flying, fear of boats) are the focus of treatment, either propranolol or low-dose, high-potency benzodiazepines are the medications of choice. Performance anxiety is perhaps best treated with propranolol at doses of 10 to 40 mg given 30 to 45 minutes prior to the time of the expected situation occurring. It is essential to remember to test out this treatment and establish a potentially useful dose prior to using the medication for the first time during actual performance. This is illustrated in the following case.

CASE EXAMPLE

The Adolescent with Stage Fright; Butterflies on Parade

G.O. was an 18-year-old boy who was self-referred because a friend of his had been treated for "stage fright" with propranolol. G.O. was a pleasant young man with no other psychiatric or medical problems and an unremarkable family psychiatric history. Although he was an excellent pianist, he would often experience severe stage fright just before performing. His symptoms would include dry mouth, a racing and pounding heart, "butterflies," and lightheadedness. At times he would feel "so worked up" that he would vomit. Once the performance started however, he usually improved quickly and managed to satisfactorily complete his performance as long as he forced himself to ignore the audience. He was extremely distressed by his anxiety and felt that it negatively affected his playing. He was becoming anxious about upcoming performances and was scheduled to play at a number of school functions over the next month, culminating in a major citywide piano competition.

His medical history was negative and he decided to try propranolol. He had three "little concerts" coming up over the following 2 weeks. It was decided that these would be experimental runs for his medication treatment—to try to find an effective dose prior to the major competition. A dose of 10 mg was chosen as the initial dose, and he was instructed to take it 1 hour prior to his performance.

When next seen, he reported that the medication had not made any difference in his symptoms and the objective symptom-specific rating scales (using the VAS technique) that he had completed at the end of the concert were unchanged from baseline. He did not report any side effects. Accordingly, his preconcert dose was raised to 20 mg for his next performance. At this dose, he reported feeling "better" but still described significant symptoms. He decided to try 30 mg prior to his major concert performance. On this dose, G.O. reported a noticeable improvement in his symptoms and no side effects. Although he still had felt tense prior to going on stage and did not win the piano competition, he felt that he had performed as best as he could and was very pleased that his performance anxiety had been somewhat controlled.

CASE COMMENTARY

This case illustrates the successful use of propranolol in treating performance anxiety. If this medication is to be used, careful screening for a variety of medical conditions such as diabetes, asthma, and cardiac problems should be

undertaken. This is discussed in more detail in Chapter 16. The evaluation of medication treatment in performance anxiety is reasonably conducted using a VAS. Because dose requirements for therapeutic effect cannot be predicted in advance, dry runs, as were used in this case, are a useful strategy.

Benzodiazepines are probably not indicated in the treatment of performance anxiety because of their potentially sedative-hypnotic effects. However, they may be useful in other situational anxieties such as airplane travel. In this case lorazepam taken sublingually at a dose of 1 mg about 15 minutes to $\frac{1}{2}$ hour prior to boarding the plane is suggested. Again, it is important for the patient to try out the medication prior to using it for the first time on the airplane flight, just to ensure that he or she does experience an anxiolytic effect and that no unusual or unexpected side effects, such as behavioral excitation, occur. The use of guided imagery techniques to evaluate symptom response prior to actually using the lorazepam on the flight is clinically quite useful and can be practiced by the patient at home for a few days prior to leaving.

Anxiety states associated with anticipated traumatic events, such as preoperative anxiety, often respond to reassurance and familiarization of the child with the setting in which the procedure will take place. In some cases, however, the level of distress may be so high that pharmacologic interventions may be indicated. In these situations the use of low doses of high-potency, relatively short-acting benzodiazepines such as alprazolam (1 to 2 mg orally) or lorazepam (1 mg sublingually) given 45 to 60 minutes prior to the procedure may be of value. Some clinicians with expertise in this field suggest the use of low doses of midazolam during a long and potentially painful medical procedure. This may be considered if feasible because it apparently has the benefit of reducing anticipatory anxiety.

The use of single low doses of these compounds is unlikely to be associated with any significant side effects, although some mild behavioral disinhibition might occur. Crushing and swallowing the tablet or using sublingual lorazepam can be expected to increase the rate at which the anxiolytic effect occurs.

School Refusal and Separation Anxiety Disorder

School refusal is not an anxiety disorder. It is a symptom of a host of potential underlying possibilities, including mood disorders, various anxiety disorders, and a variety of psychosocial difficulties. Successful intervention for this symptom begins with a full diagnostic assessment to determine whether an Axis I syndrome is present. If that is the case, then pharmacologic treatment should be directed toward amelioration of that disorder. In the absence of an Axis I disorder, initial treatment of school refusal usually relies on behavioral applications. Pharmacologic interventions may be considered for the child or adolescent with school refusal in the following situations:

1. When significant anxiety symptoms complicate the picture
2. When an Axis I disorder, such as separation anxiety disorder (SAD) or major depression, is felt to underlie the school refusal
3. When optimal psychosocial treatments by themselves either are ineffective or elicit only a partial response

In the latter case, pharmacologic intervention becomes an augmentation strategy for psychological treatment.

Studies on pharmacologic treatment of school refusal have evaluated the use of tricyclic medications and benzodiazepines (Table 10–10). Initial reports of the potential utility of the tricyclic imipramine have not been subsequently replicated, and no other tricyclic medication has demonstrated value in treating this symptom. Reports evaluating the potential utility of high-potency benzodiazepines in treating school refusal have suggested that alprazolam and possibly clonazepam may be useful, particularly in those children with significant symptoms of anxiety or a diagnosis of SAD. Although of potential utility, buspirone and the SSRIs await systematic evaluation.

Given the available information regarding the potential therapeutic efficacy and the potential severity of adverse events of medications for treating school refusal in the absence of an Axis I disorder, it is suggested that clonazepam (0.5 to 2.0 mg daily) might be a reasonable first-line medica-

tion if psychotherapeutic attempts are not successful. If this is instituted, short-term (3 to 4 week) use accompanied by maximal behavioral interventions is suggested.

Separation Anxiety Disorder

SAD is commonly seen in outpatient clinical practice and is estimated to occur in 2 to 4 percent of children and adolescents. It is often accompanied by school refusal and may be associated with parental anxiety or depressive disorders. More recently, some evidence has suggested that a number of children with SAD may be demonstrating early signs of panic disorder (see Chapter 9). Family issues, although not necessarily pathoetiologic in many children with SAD, often complicate the clinical picture.

CASE EXAMPLE

"She's tied to us by apron strings."

V.T. was a 7-year-old girl who was seen to determine whether a psychiatric disorder was the cause of her refusal to attend school. A psychiatric history identified a 2-year duration of symptoms, consistent with a diagnosis of SAD that had intensified over the previous 6 months. V.T. demonstrated "clingy" behaviors at home (following her mother or father around the house) and outside (refusing to leave her mother's side in stores and refusing to attend school). She spontaneously reported worries about her parents, including that they might die in a traffic accident. She was worried that she might get kidnapped or lost if she ever strayed away from them. V.T. reported numerous somatic complaints, mostly headaches and stomachaches, that prevented her from leaving the company of one or other of her parents and intensified whenever she felt that she might be separated from them. Recently she had also begun to exhibit "uncontrollable" temper tantrums if her mother and father wanted to go out together. These would only remit if one of her parents agreed to stay home. This behavior was seen by both parents as putting an unhealthy strain on their relationship.

The family history was positive for social phobia and OCD in V.T.'s mother's family. Her mother was being treated for panic disorder (with cognitive therapy and low-dose fluoxetine), which was under good control. V.T.'s father reported no psychiatric disorder in himself or his immediate family.

TABLE 10–10   Medications of Potential Benefit in Treating School Refusal*

Medication	Estimated Risk (?)/Benefit (+) Rating[†]
Imipramine	???/+
Alprazolam	?/+
Clonazepam	?/+

*In the absence of an Axis I disorder.
[†]Rated as risks (shown as ?) versus benefits (shown as +).

V.T. was an only child, as were both her parents. V.T.'s parents disagreed strongly on how to deal with her behavior. Her father believed she should not be forced to do things she didn't want to do. Her mother tried to force her to go out and was usually left at home in the morning to deal with the school refusal while the father went out to work. V.T.'s maternal grandmother, who lived just three houses away, often became involved. Usually she would come to the house in the morning as the mother was attempting to get V.T. off to school and would intercede on V.T.'s behalf. As expected, V.T.'s mother became extremely annoyed at this interference but could not bring herself to disagree openly.

CASE COMMENTARY

This case shows the complexities of behavioral, social, and family problems that often accompany SAD. Effective treatment of this disturbance can be expected to include psychological interventions such as behavioral and family therapy as well as medication. V.T.'s problems had reached a crisis, and urgent maximal intervention using all available treatment modalities was thought to be necessary.

Sufficient valid studies of pharmacologic treatments for SAD are lacking. Those that are available suffer from a focus on the symptom of school refusal as opposed to SAD itself. Nevertheless, some useful clinical studies and one or two open studies can be used to guide pharmacologic treatment. Given this information, it is reasonable to begin with the medication choices identified in Table 10–1.

If fluoxetine is chosen, the guidelines for its use (Chapter 9) should be followed. Beginning doses of 5 mg daily, increased gradually to an initial target dose of 10 to 15 mg daily for children and 15 to 20 mg daily for adolescents, is suggested. Occasionally a child may show an improved rate of response if a small amount of clonazepam (0.25 to 0.5 mg daily) is added at the onset of treatment. This can later be discontinued gradually when the projected effective target dose of fluoxetine has been reached and maintained for 3 to 4 weeks. Intensive behavioral and family therapy should be prescribed.

Strategies for maximizing response to medication and deciding about treatment duration should be made following the guidelines described in Section Three. Monitoring the efficacy of treatment can best be accomplished using a number of specific VAS scores that report on both behavioral and cognitive symptoms.

Selective Mutism

Research into the basic aspects of this seemingly relatively rare disorder is essentially just beginning, and it has only recently been considered a type of childhood-onset anxiety disorder. As a result, few if any valid treatment guidelines can be offered with any degree of certainty.

Pharmacologically, only a few reports from small samples are available, and most clinicians do not see sufficient numbers of these children and adolescents to have developed great experience in the psychotherapeutic or pharmacologic treatment of this disorder. What literature is available suggests that behavioral or family interventions combined with either fluoxetine or phenelzine pharmacotherapy may be of value. Although earlier pathoetiologic models focused on presumed intrapsychic conflicts leading to speech refusal, neither these nor the dynamic treatments derived from them have stood the test of time. Parents may find the Foundation for Elective Mutism useful in terms of support and information about this disorder.

The suggestion for the use of fluoxetine as the medication of choice in selective mutism is made on the basis of all published studies on this topic and discussions with clinicians who have expertise in treating this disorder. Although the MAOI phenelzine may be considered in cases that do not respond to fluoxetine, this should be done only with careful and reliable parental supervision accompanied by the necessary medical (including the appropriate MSSES) and psychiatric monitoring. No rating scales of demonstrated utility in this disorder are available to monitor treatment outcome, so the clinician may need to develop his or her own scale. A reasonable evaluation package can be put together using a VAS and a Kiddie-Global Assessment Scale.

The guidelines described in Section Three should be followed with regard to the initiation, maximization, monitoring, and duration of pharmacotherapy. Information regarding the use of fluoxetine can be found in Chapter 9.

SUGGESTED READINGS

Allen AJ, Rapoport JL, Swedo SE. Psychopharmacologic treatment of childhood anxiety disorders. Child and Adolescent Clinics of North America, 4:795–818, 1993.

Coffey BJ. Anxiolytics for children and adolescents: Traditional and new drugs. Journal of Child and Adolescent Psychopharmacology, 1:57–83, 1990.

Dubovsky SL. Approaches to developing new anxiolytics and

antidepressants. Journal of Clinical Psychiatry, 54 (Suppl): 75–83, 1993.

Kutcher S, Reiter S, Gardner D, Klein R. The pharmacotherapy of anxiety disorders in children and adolescents. Psychiatric Clinics of North America, 15:41–67, 1992.

Leonard H (ed). Child and adolescent anxiety disorders. Psychiatric Clinics of North America, 4:563–818, 1993.

March J (ed). Anxiety Disorders in Children and Adolescents. New York: Guilford Press, 1995.

Popper CW. Psychopharmacologic treatment of anxiety disorders in adolescents and children. Journal of Clinical Psychiatry, 54(Suppl):52–63, 1993.

CHAPTER 11

Psychopharmacologic Treatment of Depressive Disorders

Depressive disorders, e.g., major depression (MDD) and dysthymia (DYS) may onset during childhood, and their prevalence increases dramatically in adolescence, reaching close to adult levels in the late teenage years. These disorders are characterized by a prolonged course and repeated episodes. DYS is predictive of future major depressive episodes, and MDD in adolescence is a substantial risk factor for repeat occurrence in adulthood. These illnesses are associated with a variety of functional disturbances, some of which may continue in some form after the acute episode has remitted. Problems in academic, social, interpersonal, and family functioning have been well described in depressed children and adolescents. Suicide is a particularly dramatic outcome of depression, and its epidemiologic profile parallels the rise in the prevalence of depression over the adolescent years, a disorder to which it has been clearly linked.

The diagnosis of MDD and DYS in children and adolescents has now been well established, and there is no reason for the practitioner to resort to earlier unvalidated constructs, such as "masked depression," "depressive equivalent," or "depressive reaction." Even the tentative diagnosis of "adjustment disorder with depressed mood" should be considered to signal the potential presence of either MDD or DYS. There is no excuse for clinicians to still consider a depressive disorder as a part of "expected adolescent turmoil" or a "normal" psychological response to physical, social, or cognitive development.

A depressive disorder onsetting in childhood or adolescence can best be understood as a serious psychiatric condition that may quite possibly become a chronic psychiatric illness. Therefore, the treatment of this disorder is undertaken with two goals in mind. The first is the acute goal, the rapid and effective resolution of the current episode.

The second goal is the effective long-term treatment of the child or adolescent to attempt to prevent future episodes or to reduce their morbidity if they recur. In this treatment framework, pharmacotherapy can play a useful role. However, given the nature of these disorders and the available knowledge of other potentially beneficial forms of treatment, medications should not be prescribed as the only intervention. Psychopharmacologic treatments must be used in conjunction with interventions designed to improve interpersonal, social, and academic functioning. In all cases, every attempt to assist the child or adolescent in the maintenance of their expected developmental trajectory must be made.

Compared with available systematically conducted, scientifically based, research-derived information about pharmacologic interventions in many child and adolescent psychiatric disorders, study regarding the psychopharmacologic treatment of MDD in children and teens has been relatively well conducted. However, a great deal of research remains to be done and is currently underway. Furthermore, the study of pharmacologic interventions in DYS or in combined DYS and MDD (so-called double depression) is less well developed than similar studies in MDD. At this time it is unclear if similar psychopharmacologic treatment strategies can be applied to dysthymic children and adolescents as well to those with MDD. Clinical experience and extrapolation from the adult treatment literature suggest that pharmacologic interventions that prove to be successful in MDD are often found to be helpful in DYS as well. This observation, still hypothetical, requires further testing. With this important caveat in mind, the clinician can apply the information presented in this chapter to both MDD and DYS in children and adolescents.

CASE EXAMPLE

"Mommie, I just feel sad."

K.F. was an 8-year-old girl who presented to an outpatient child psychiatric service in referral from her family physician who suspected a depressive disorder. A detailed psychiatric evaluation, which included the application of a semistructured diagnostic interview, (see Section Two), revealed that she met criteria for MDD of 11 months' duration. This episode was her first depression, although she was described as a child who was "always anxious," and indeed, she also met DSM-IV diagnostic criteria for generalized anxiety disorder (GAD) as well.

Functionally, K.F. was experiencing academic difficulties; her grades were lower than her teacher believed they should be. She was described by her current teacher as "working below potential," "tending to daydream," and "an unenthusiastic participant in classroom activities." K.F., who had done quite well in previous grades, now felt that she was a failure as a student and had begun to call herself "stupid." She also had started to experience stomach pains and headaches that seemed to be so severe that she often felt she could not attend school. Indeed, although no organic etiology had been found for these complaints, they led to noticeably decreased attendance, which in turn made it difficult for her to keep up with her academic demands.

Socially, she maintained her friendships with one or two close friends, but her interest in initiating or pursuing activities with them had dropped off considerably. She would spend hours in front of the television or "just resting" and often needed parental encouragement to "go outside and play." She would often say that playing with her friends was "not a lot of fun," and she occasionally complained that they seemed to be "picking" on her. In addition, her appetite and weight had increased, and she had begun to refer to herself as "fat" and "ugly." These features were quite different from K.F.'s previous functioning in which, although she had often been shy about new situations, she would spontaneously initiate play activities and enjoyed going out with her friends.

Family functioning was described as becoming "more difficult." Both parents had noted increased irritability and conflict. Fighting between K.F. and her older sister had increased

noticeably, with the usual outcome leading to tears and withdrawal on K.F.'s part. K.F. appeared to be sullen and unhappy to her parents.

The family history was positive for depression on K.F.'s mothers' side, with both her mother and maternal grandmother having been treated for depression. K.F.'s mother had received antidepressants (amitriptyline) on two separate occasions, each time with good results, and she saw a therapist "every few weeks or so." K.F.'s grandmother had been hospitalized for depression a number of times and had received three courses of electroconvulsive therapy (ECT). K.F.'s father reported problems with alcohol abuse that had required admission to a treatment facility as part of an alcohol treatment program. He was still attending outpatient follow-up and was an active member in the local Alcoholics Anonymous group. One of his brothers had committed suicide at age 20, but little else was known about K.F.'s uncle's psychiatric history.

Both parents had considered that K.F. might be depressed, and their family physician had agreed with their assessment. Both parents wanted her to be "treated."

CASE EXAMPLE

A Bad Egg or a Sad Egg?

P.B. was a 17-year-old boy who was referred for psychiatric assessment by his school social worker after his teacher became concerned about his "morbid stories about death and suicide." He attended the clinic interview accompanied by his mother, who expressed her concerns about his "bad" behavior. According to P.B.'s mother, he had begun to "run with a bad crowd" and was now drinking, smoking, and getting in trouble. Recently he had been arrested for "theft" after another teenager's jacket had been stolen by a group of boys. P.B. had not been prosecuted because it could not be established that he had actually taken part in the episode as opposed to viewing it.

P.B.'s mother described herself as overwhelmed with taking care of three children—ages 17, 13, and 11—while she held down a full-time job. P.B.'s father had left the family 4 years earlier and now lived in another city and provided no child support. She complained that P.B. hardly ever helped her out and would respond to her requests for assistance with short-lived angry outbursts. She was concerned that he would end up "dead in an alley someday" and felt that he needed "to be straightened out."

When seen individually, P.B.'s initial "cocky" mood subsided during a gentle exploration of what was happening in his life. He admitted to feeling depressed and irritable, and he described suicidal ideation. He exhibited the classic negative triad of depressive cognition and described numerous vegetative symptoms, including loss of appetite, difficulty falling asleep, early morning waking, daytime fatigue, and sleepiness. He reported a marked decrease in interests and was anhedonic. He described his "crowd" activities as a way to keep his "mind off my problems" and noted that he drank alcohol because "everyone else did." He denied drug use but noted that "smoking makes me feel better."

These symptoms had come on gradually over 9 months and according to P.B. were at their worst currently. He described a similar episode of shorter duration and less intensity 4 years previously that had occurred about 6 months after his father had left the family. This episode had not been identified as a potential problem, although his teacher had noticed that he was withdrawn at school and his grades had dropped.

P.B.'s family history was positive for a number of psychiatric disorders. His paternal grandmother was reported to have been depressed, although she had never been treated for this. His father was described as "unstable" and "with a drinking problem." One of his father's sisters had been hospitalized for "emotional problems," although it was not clear exactly what these were. P.B.'s mother had experienced a postpartum depression after the birth of her second child and had been treated with "sleeping medicines." She had also become "depressed" for 4 months after P.B.'s father had left but had not sought help because she felt that this was "normal." In addition, she described long-standing low-grade dysphoric symptoms that seemed to have begun in early adolescence. Her father had died in an automobile accident after a bout of heavy drinking, and she felt that he might have been an alcoholic.

CASE COMMENTARY

These cases identify common presentations of a depressive disorder in children or adoles-

cents. In both cases, a family history of a mood disorder or alcohol abuse was present. This frequently characterizes the family histories of patients in whom depressive disorders onset in childhood or adolescence.

In both cases, the child's disorder was characterized not only by depressive mood but also by irritability and temper outbursts. These are well recognized but too often overlooked features of depression in children and adolescents. In some cases, these disturbances of mood can lead to family difficulties because the irritability and temper outbursts are often expressed within the family context.

The child in the first case presented with a history of anxiety symptoms, with the depressive episode arising later in the developmental process. This may commonly be seen in this population. In the second case, no anxiety disorder was present, but the depressive episode was accompanied by behavioral disturbances, which may have too easily led to a primary diagnosis of conduct or oppositional disorder. This is particularly problematic if only parental or external information is considered because in cases such as P.B.'s many parents or other authority figures may not be aware of the adolescent's inner state and are only too painfully aware of the external behaviors.

In the first case, the child was fortunate to have parents who were well educated about the disorder and who had taken positive steps in the identification of their child's difficulties. In the second (and perhaps the more common of the two), the family is either not aware of or else not anticipating the possibility of a depressive disorder. In some cases this may manifest itself as anger at the child or may be expressed as a parental response to only the behavioral pattern that the child or teen is exhibiting. In the latter case, the clinical use of a semistructured interview can assist both in the diagnosis and the subsequent education about the disorder. This is further discussed later.

Initial Pharmacologic Management

The available evidence suggests that tricyclic antidepressants (TCAs) have not demonstrated clinical utility in the treatment of child and adolescent depression. In addition, side effects are common with their use, including cardiovascular complications. Thus, there is generally little benefit to be derived from treating the child or adolescent whose primary diagnosis is a depressive disorder with a tricyclic medication, although some investigators will consider imipramine in the treatment of a depressed child who exhibits concurrent enuresis.

Similarly, there is little evidence (albeit many fewer studies) that the typical monoamine oxidase inhibitors (MAOIs), e.g., tranylcypromine or phenelzine, are by themselves an effective first-line treatment for depressed children or adolescents. The dangers of traditional MAOIs are well known, and the special dietary requirements that accompany their use make their application in children difficult and in adolescents problematic. Thus, it is not advised that these medications be considered as standard first-line treatment in depressed children and adolescents.

The clinician is then left with a number of potential medication choices. These include serotonin-specific reuptake inhibitors (SSRIs), reversible inhibitors of monoamine oxidase-type A (RIMAs), the monocyclic antidepressant bupropion, the azaspirodecanedione buspirone, and serotonin norepinephrine reuptake inhibitors (SNRIs). These are listed in Table 11–1.

Baseline Evaluation

Medical Considerations

Medical considerations are outlined in Section Two. Of particular importance is the evaluation of those physical parameters that may be affected by pharmacologic treatment. As expected treatment will include one of the medications listed in Table

11–1, the following baseline medical measures are suggested:

1. Medication-Specific Side Effects Scales (MSSES)
2. Physical examination for extrapyramidal symptoms
3. Blood pressure and heart rate

These measures should be completed at every medication monitoring visit. Dosage increments should be titrated against data obtained from these scales and the rate of symptom improvement, as elicited later.

Laboratory Considerations

Laboratory considerations should assess those physiologic parameters that pharmacologic treatment may affect in both the short and long term. As expected treatment will include one of the medications listed in Table 11–1, the suggested baseline laboratory investigations are (1) complete blood count (CBC), (2) liver function tests, (3) pregnancy test for females, and (4) electrocardiogram (ECG). These measures need to be repeated only if the patient complains of treatment-emergent symptoms (see earlier under MSSES) that involve the physiologic system previously evaluated. The routine repetition of these laboratory measures in the absence of clinical signs and symptoms is not indicated.

If the physical examination or functional inquiry elicits significant neurovegetative symptoms, the following screening tests may be indicated: (1) thyroid-stimulating hormone (TSH), (2) cortisol, and (3) serum electrolytes. The routine repetition of these laboratory screening tests, if they have been previously noted to be negative, is not indicated.

Psychiatric Considerations

Baseline evaluation should include those symptoms that are the target of pharmacologic treatment. The following baseline measures are suggested:

1. A subjective rating scale of mood: Beck Depression Inventory (BDI), Child Depression Inventory (CDI), or Self-Rating Depression Scale (SDS)
2. An objective rating scale of mood: Hamilton Depression Rating Scale (HDRS) or Montgomery Asberg Depression Rating Scale (MADRAS)
3. An overall or global rating: Clinical Global Impression Scale (CGI)

These rating scales should be repeated weekly during treatment of the acute phase of the illness.

TABLE 11–1 Antidepressant Medications of Potential Benefit in Children and Adolescents

Class	Medication	Evidence (? to ++++)*
SSRI	Fluoxetine	+++
	Fluvoxamine	++
	Paroxetine	++
	Sertraline	++
Monocyclic	Bupropion	+
Azaspirodecanedoine	Buspirone	?+
RIMA	Moclobomide	?
SNRI	Venlafaxine	?

*The information upon which the evidence rating is based includes data published, presented, or in press plus clinical experience with children and adolescents.

RIMA, reversible inhibitor of monoamine oxidase-type A; SNRI, serotonin norepinephrine reuptake inhibitor; SSRI, serotonin-specific reuptake inhibitor.

Some symptom score changes (10 to 20 percent decrease from baseline) should be noted in the subjective or objective rating scales by the third or fourth treatment week. Significant changes (50 percent or more from baseline) may not become evident until the sixth to eighth treatment week.

In addition, a number of measures useful in evaluating a variety of functional areas may be of use. These include the following:
1. The Adolescent Autonomous Functioning Checklist (AAFC)
2. School and Social Disability Scale (SSDS)
3. Children's Global Assessment Scale (C-GAS)

These rating scales should not be repeated weekly because they are not expected to be sensitive to the degree of change that can occur over that length of time. They are best repeated at the end of the initial treatment trial (discussed later) 6 to 8 weeks after a putative therapeutic dose of medication has been obtained and continued for an appropriate length of time.

Visual Analogue Scales (VAS), however, are of clinical utility if repeated on a more frequent basis—once every 2 weeks is reasonable. These will provide information about the child or adolescent's functioning that may help in directing other therapeutic modalities that are being used concurrently with medications. Some useful items that lend themselves to VAS monitoring include the following: (1) temper outbursts, (2) getting along with family, (3) getting along at school (academic), and (4) getting along at school (social).

Other items may be identified for an individual patient and should be used by the clinician to monitor treatment. With the VAS it is useful to have the child or adolescent and the parent each complete the pertinent VAS independently of each other. Major discrepancies (such as the child scores 2 and the parent scores 8) will need to be clarified and may identify important issues that will need to be addressed psychotherapeutically.

Once the diagnosis has been clearly established, it is necessary for the clinician to engage the patient and family in a discussion of the disorder and its possible treatments. Education about the illness and the various available treatments is necessary for the patient and family both to understand the problem and to make informed choices about treatment options that are open to them. These issues, discussed more fully in Section Three, are of particular importance in child and adolescent depression, in which nonpharmacologic treatments may be of benefit in and of themselves, eliminating the need for pharmacologic interventions. However, the opposite is also true. Honest and open discussion of what is known and what is not known about the efficacy of various psychological treatments in depressed children and teenagers is necessary to help the patient and family select their treatment choice with the facts in hand. It must be remembered that unequivocal evidence for most psychological treatments in child and adolescent depression is lacking, and patients should not be denied potentially effective pharmacologic treatments because the clinician fails to inform the patient and parents of this.

If the patient's condition does not require beginning pharmacologic intervention immediately (such as would be required in a psychotic depression), it is reasonable to suggest that the patient and family research the area of treatment for depression on their own and meet with the clinician in 2 or 3 days following the diagnostic interview for further discussions. At this time a comprehensive treatment plan can be developed based on the patient's and family's choices with the informed guidance of the physician. The clinician can assist in this process by directing the patient or family to appropriate educational materials.

Choosing a First-Line Medication

The current understanding of the biologic pathoetiology of depression highlights the role of serotonin neurotransmitter systems in this disorder, and the neuroendocrine evidence available in depressed children and adolescents tends to support this view. Given the available medications for first-line use in child or adolescent depression and the evidence for their efficacy and tolerability, the clinician may reasonably select one of the SSRI compounds for initial use.

Generally, the SSRIs are thought to produce their antidepressant effects through selective blockade of serotonin reuptake. This tends to increase serotonin concentrations in the synapse and results in desensitization of presynaptic serotonin autoreceptors, with an outcome of enhanced serotonin neurotransmission. Other less firmly established evidence suggests that SSRIs may affect intracellular second messenger systems and even enhance the maintenance of cellular structural integrity, although the relationship of this to clinical improvement in depressive symptoms has not been determined. Somewhat similar explanations have been proposed to explain the efficacy of these compounds in treating other psychiatric disturbances such as obsessive compulsive and panic disorders. The SSRIs are a group of structurally diverse compounds that share the common feature of potent and selective serotonin reuptake inhibition. The commonly available SSRIs are currently fluoxetine, sertraline, paroxetine, and fluvoxamine.

Fluoxetine

Fluoxetine is well absorbed with oral dosing and its pharmacokinetics are thought to be nonlinear in that higher doses result in disproportionately higher plasma concentrations. Peak plasma concentrations following an oral dose occur in 4 to 8 hours. Fluoxetine has a half-life of 1 to 3 days. Norfluoxetine, the major active metabolite of fluoxetine, extends the pharmacologic activity significantly on account of its long half-life of up to 14 to 15 days. With multiple dosing, this half-life increases, so that patients undergoing antidepressant therapy with this compound can expect an effective serum half-life of 3 weeks. This feature allows for a longer dosing interval when steady-state levels are reached but also means that significant amounts of active serotonin uptake inhibition remain for a number of weeks following drug discontinuation, increasing the potential for problematic drug-drug interactions with other medications that affect serotonin system functioning. Fluoxetine is metabolized through the hepatic P-450 system and interacts with other compounds undergoing similar metabolism.

Sertraline

Sertraline is best absorbed when given together with meals, and peak plasma concentrations occur 6 to 8 hours after oral dosing. The elimination half-life varies from 20 to 28 hours, allowing for once-daily dosing. Using this dosing schedule, steady-state plasma concentrations of sertraline can be expected to be achieved within 1 to 2 weeks of initiating treatment. Bioavailability and elimination of sertraline tablets are not influenced by time of day or concomitant food use and thus can be taken at any time of day, with or without food. However, some evidence suggests that sertraline capsules should be taken with food. Unlike other SSRIs, sertraline undergoes metabolic hydroxylation. It has a long-lasting (60 to 70 hour half-life) desmethyl metabolite that shows some limited selective serotonin reuptake inhibition but is unlikely to be of clinical significance.

Paroxetine

Paroxetine is considered to be the most specific of the SSRIs, although the clinical significance of this is not clear. It is well absorbed orally and has a half-life of about 20 to 25 hours, reaching steady state within 1 to 2 weeks. Paroxetine has a marked interindividual variability in its dose to plasma level relationship, and plasma levels are not predictive of clinical response. It is metabolized through the hepatic P-450 cytochrome system and interacts with other compounds that use a similar route.

Fluvoxamine

Fluvoxamine is well absorbed orally, and this process is not significantly affected by the presence or absence of foods. Peak plasma levels occur 2 to 8 hours after oral dosing, and the elimination half-life is about 14 to 18 hours. Individual dose-to-plasma level ratios are quite variable, and there is no generally accepted plasma level/response relationship.

Taken as a group, these compounds may be equally effective and generally exhibit a similar side effect profile (Table 11–2). On the whole, they are much better tolerated than the TCAs, and they present minimal cardiovascular dangers in overdose, which makes them particularly attractive for use in depressed adolescents, who may present a considerable suicide risk.

Because there is probably no difference in ther-

TABLE 11–2 **Side Effects of SSRIs in Children and Adolescents***

Relatively Common Side Effects	Relatively Uncommon Side Effects
Dizziness	Delayed micturition
Sweating	Blurred vision
Diarrhea	Hypomanic symptoms
GI distress	Tachycardia
Sexual disturbances	Seizures
Headaches	Skin rashes
Fatigue	Hypersomnia
Restlessness	Sexual dysfunction
Initial insomnia	Dry mouth
Weight gain	Tremor
	Constipation
	Frontal lobe amotivational syndrome

*The classification of side effects into relatively common and relatively uncommon is made on the basis of available published and unpublished data for this age group and clinical experience with this population. Any individual patient can experience one or more of the above side effects with SSRI treatment. Restlessness and seizures are thought to be dose related. Data from studies in adults suggest that there may be some differences in the frequency of side effects among the various SSRIs. Insufficient data regarding this issue are available for children and adolescents. The clinician should consult the suggested readings at the end of this chapter.

apeutic efficacy among the various SSRIs, the choice among the potentially useful preparations will usually be guided by one or more of the following criteria:

1. Potential specific side effect profile (comparing one SSRI to another)
2. Potential drug-drug interactions (if the patient is currently taking another medication)
3. Specific pharmacokinetic features of a particular SSRI compared with others
4. Specific demonstrated efficacy of one SSRI compared with others for particular clinical presentations (does the patient have a specific subtype of depression or clinical picture that will predict which SSRI will be most useful?)

Potential specific side effects profiles among the various SSRIs may be considered in the selection process, although it is not possible to predict which side effect, if any, a particular patient may experience. Additionally, many experienced clinicians find that side effects profiles of the various SSRIs are quite similar. Nevertheless, clinical experience and the available information suggest the following SSRIs in Table 11–3 may be associated

TABLE 11–3   Selected Side Effects of SSRI Compounds in Children and Adolescents*

SSRI	Side Effect
Fluoxetine	Initial restlessness, akathisia-like symptoms; may be dose related and usually do not appear if the medication is started at 5 mg daily; headaches may also be more common and be dose dependent
Sertraline	Dry mouth and gastric upset, including nausea and diarrhea, may occur at dose initiation and with subsequent dose increments; these symptoms are usually mild and will often subside after 2 or 3 days
Paroxetine	No specific side effects of any greater frequency than any of the other SSRI compounds, although there is some suggestion that muscarinic-type side effects (such as dry mouth) may be more common with paroxetine; some clinicians report increased weight gain with paroxetine vs. other SSRIs
Fluvoxamine	Dry mouth and gastric upset, including nausea and diarrhea, may occur at dose initiation and with subsequent dose increments; these symptoms are often mild and tend to subside over 2 to 3 days

*The information regarding these comparative side effects has been obtained from published and unpublished data and clinical use of these compounds in this population.

with more particular side effects in this population.

Although often under-reported and under-recognized, sexual dysfunction induced by SSRIs can significantly complicate treatment, particularly in adolescent boys. Clinicians should be aware of this and inquire openly about this when monitoring side effects. Additionally, recently some clinicians have reported the occurrence of a frontal lobe amotivational syndrome associated with SSRI use. This is characterized by subjective feelings of being cut off, loss of initiative, and complaints about memory. This resolves if the medication is discontinued or decreased.

Another consideration regarding the choice of a particular SSRI in an individual patient is the possibility of drug-drug interactions. Most of the SSRIs undergo hepatic metabolism by the cytochrome P-450 system and will inhibit the metabolism of other compounds that also use this system. Sertraline is unique among the SSRIs in essentially avoiding this metabolic pathway, although there is some suggestion that high doses (>200 mg daily) may affect P-450. Thus, if the patient is currently being treated with one of the medications listed in Table 11–4, caution should be taken in prescribing an SSRI. In cases in which treatment with an SSRI is clinically indicated, the physician can either choose to use sertraline as the SSRI of choice or else use one of the other SSRIs and carefully monitor the patient for potential drug-drug interactions. Because many of the SSRIs are known to increase the serum concentration of other drugs, serum levels available for concomitantly used compounds (such as valproate, carbamazepine, or TCAs) should be obtained prior to initiating treatment with an SSRI and should be closely monitored thereafter to guide dosage requirements of the non-SSRI compound.

Genetic polymorphism regarding the cytochrome P-450 IID6 isoenzyme may lead to differential metabolic rates among the SSRIs using the hepatic P-450 system. Paroxetine and fluoxetine seem to be the two SSRIs most commonly affected because both rapid and slow metabolizers may be found. The exact prevalence of this effect has not been fully established. Clinically, this may result in specific patients requiring total daily doses that fall outside the expected ranges.

Serotonin Syndrome

The *serotonin syndrome* is a descriptor of a group of adverse events associated with the use of medications that have the effect of enhancing central serotonin activity. The precise incidence of the serotonin syndrome is not known, and it appears

TABLE 11–4   **Some Common Potential Drug-Drug Interactions with SSRIs in Children and Adolescents***

Class of Compounds	Potential Difficulties
Anticonvulsants	Increased plasma levels of anticonvulsants, decreased or increased plasma levels of SSRIs
Anticoagulant	Increased plasma levels of warfarin; may lead to bleeding
Antidepressants	Increased plasma levels of antidepressants; may create a serotonin syndrome
	Fluoxetine may increase bupropion levels to seizure-induction amounts at otherwise moderate total daily dose ranges
Benzodiazepines	Increased plasma levels of some benzodiazepines by fluvoxamine
Cimetidine	Increased plasma levels of SSRIs
Lithium	Potential for serotonin syndrome, increased lithium side effects
Neuroleptics	Increased serum levels of neuroleptics, increased neuroleptic side effects
Propranolol	Very high propranolol levels with fluvoxamine
Sulfonylurea	Increased hypoglycemic effect
Other serotonin-active agents	Increased serotonergic effects, possible serotonin syndrome

*This table is not a comprehensive listing of all possible drug-drug interactions with each SSRI. For many of these and other potential drug-drug interactions, the necessary specific data are not available for children and adolescents. If you are not sure about any particular drug-drug interaction, please consult a specialist or psychopharmacologist. Most pharmaceutical companies will also provide you with the information that they have on file on request.

to demonstrate a variable clinical picture, ranging from mild to severe symptoms. The use of SSRIs with other serotonergic agents may result in symptoms such as agitation, excitation, nausea, vomiting, diarrhea, chills, muscle twitching, fever, confusion, diaphoresis, and dizziness. In severe cases this may lead to delirium, coma, or seizures. Treatment of this side effect begins with an awareness of its seriousness and early recognition. In most cases, simple discontinuation of the offending compound will lead to symptom resolution. In more severe cases, hospitalization for observation may be needed, with supportive measures or direct interventions for specific symptoms (such as anticonvulsants for seizures) used as necessary. Although this phenomenon has not been frequently described in children and adolescents, its possibility requires consideration whenever serotonergic polypharmacy is contemplated.

Pharmacokinetic Differences

Pharmacokinetic differences among SSRIs may be of importance in the selection of an initial treatment agent. Fluoxetine has a long therapeutic half-life compared with the other SSRIs. In some cases this may be a disadvantage. For example, if the patient does not respond to treatment and an alternative pharmacologic intervention is planned, the clinician may need to wait 4 to 5 weeks before initiating further psychotropic therapy. In some cases this may be an advantage. For example, once steady state is reached, patients can be maintained on once every 2 to 3 day dosing. Alternatively, if a patient tends to "miss doses," the use of fluoxetine

will provide adequate serum levels over a longer period of time than a compound with a shorter half-life. The clinician and the patient must together identify if the choice of a long half-life compound will produce a potentially problematic or positive effect.

Although the marketing strategy employed by some manufacturers of the SSRIs suggests that one or another SSRI may be more effective in a particular clinical situation, little scientifically valid evidence supports the notion that one SSRI is better than another for a specific depressive subtype. Thus, patients with atypical depression or melancholic depression most likely will show similar responses to all the SSRIs. One type of depression, psychotic depression, will require additional pharmacologic interventions, specifically the concurrent use of neuroleptics, for its treatment.

Suicide and the Use of SSRIs

Suicide is a well-recognized outcome of untreated depression. Additionally, some patients treated with antidepressants may undergo a period of time early in the treatment course in which the activation provided by antidepressants may increase the risk of suicide. However, there is no valid evidence that SSRIs in general and fluoxetine in particular may specifically cause suicidal activity. Although this effect has been reported in some cases, detailed analyses of the SSRI treatment literature fail to identify such a general phenomenon. Furthermore, ongoing studies of this phenomenon and extensive clinical experience with large numbers of depressed children and adolescents treated with SSRIs fail to support a causal link between SSRI treatment and suicidal actions. This does not mean that the clinician should take lightly the risk of suicide in the adolescent patient being treated with an SSRI medication. The possibility of suicide is a very real problem in the treatment of any depressed child or adolescent, and suicidal potential must be carefully monitored during the entire duration of treatment.

CASE EXAMPLE

Child Depression: "We must use the medicine that helped me."

K.F. and her parents agreed to a treatment plan for her depression that included individual psychotherapy and a medication. Because K.F.'s mother had obtained a good antidepressant response to amitriptyline with her own depression, she felt quite strongly that K.F. would experience a similar effect. Although the physician carefully reviewed the evidence regarding the efficacy and tolerability of tricyclics in general and amitriptyline specifically in depressed children and adolescents, K.F.'s mother persisted in her opinion. Additionally, she asked her own therapist about the likelihood that "what worked for me should work for my daughter as well" and was told that this was a valid method of predicting clinical response and that amitriptyline was, as far as the therapist knew, a good medicine for treating depression.

Against the physician's best judgment, a trial of amitriptyline was initiated. This resulted in little or no therapeutic response at 8 weeks and multiple side effects, including dry mouth, daytime somnolence, dizziness, and sinus tachycardia. Eventually this treatment was discontinued and an SSRI medication was begun. Eight weeks later K.F. was feeling "much better." Her HDRS and BDI scores had decreased significantly, and, although her grades had not yet improved, she was doing her schoolwork more enthusiastically and spending more time with her friends.

CASE COMMENTARY

"What helped you will not necessarily help your child."

One of the most common myths in psychopharmacologic treatment of children and adolescents is that the same medication that was helpful for the parent or other family adult will be also helpful for the child. There is little if any reasonable evidence to substantiate such a view, yet it still persists, perhaps because of practitioner uncertainty. In this case the physician was informed of the lack of demonstrated efficacy of amitriptyline in treating childhood depression and its generally poor tolerability in this age group. More effective and less toxic alternatives were available. Nevertheless, pressure from the child's parent and the support of that viewpoint by another physician led to a therapeutic intervention that was unlikely to provide any positive benefit and was likely to result in significant, if only unpleasant, adverse events.

In this case, a more useful approach may have been to speak directly with the mother's therapist about the issue of pharmacologic intervention for the child. The other physician may have been well meaning but simply uninformed about newer developments in the pharmacologic treatment of child depression. Establishing therapeutic boundaries, which in this case was also an important issue, would have been helpful. Another strategy would have been to obtain a third-party consultation about the specific pharmacologic treatment issue. Once this was done, it would have then been useful to identify the psychodynamics of the decision making process in the context of this family, to attempt to psychotherapeutically deal with any problems.

The physician's decision in this case to prescribe a pharmacologic treatment that he knew was likely to be ineffective and potentially problematic was not a reasonable intervention. Had other methods been used to explore the psychological issues involved in the pharmacologic treatment decision making process, one would expect that this would not have occurred. However, it is possible that such a situation cannot be easily resolved. In such a scenario the physician's responsibility to provide reasonable treatment outweighs the wish to provide any treatment. These and related issues are discussed more fully in Section Three.

CASE EXAMPLE

Adolescent Depression: "OK, I need some help but I don't want any pills."

Following a full diagnostic assessment and education about the disorder, P.B. and his mother both agreed that he most likely was depressed, and she was also made aware of her own mood difficulties. She agreed to seek assistance in this matter, and an appropriate referral was provided. P.B. agreed that he needed "help with the depression" but was adamant that he was "not going to use any of those pills." He was very concerned about the possibility of side effects and also felt that he would become "an addict," even though he professed to understand that antidepressant medications were not drugs of abuse. He did, however, agree to individual psychotherapy using an interpersonal paradigm, and fortunately this was available for him within a reasonable length of time.

A meeting that included P.B., his mother, his therapist, and the physician was held to review the diagnosis and treatment plan. A time frame of 10 weeks was set for evaluation of efficacy. It was decided, with P.B.'s approval, that if he were not significantly better by that time, the issue of pharmacotherapy would be reconsidered. A suicide identification and prevention plan was constructed, and all parties agreed to it. A midpoint for treatment review was scheduled, and P.B. was assured that if at any time during his treatment he wished to consider medications, he could do so without loss of face or without interrupting his psychotherapy.

CASE COMMENTARY

Support a Reasonable Choice but Provide the Evaluative Structure

In this case, the patient chose not to accept pharmacotherapy for his depression but opted instead for a first-line psychological treatment instead. The decision may not have seemed rational to the physician, particularly P.B.'s concern about addiction, but the choice of treatment was reasonable. Thus, the physician was able to support the patient's decision.

However, the clinician in this case provided more than just assessment and triage. He helped the patient to obtain good psychotherapeutic care (in some cases, the physician is skilled enough to be able to provide this care himself or herself) and, by collaborating with P.B.'s therapist, helped set up a structure that would allow for a systematic evaluation of P.B.'s treatment. In addition, a midpoint mini-review was scheduled, which allows a clinician to make, or a patient to request, changes or alterations in treatment if problems with the initial treatment plan are encountered. P.B.'s autonomy and self-respect were recognized (an essential point in treating adolescents), and he was given a safe route by which to change his mind without losing face.

CASE EXAMPLE

Adolescent Depression: The Saga of P.B. Continues

P.B. began his psychotherapy but 4 weeks later the physician received a phone call from the therapist. P.B. had not been keeping up his sessions, and the therapist expressed concern that P.B. was becoming increasingly depressed and was beginning to drink heavily. Three days later, P.B.'s mother called to tell the physician that P.B. had been admitted to the hospital following a serious suicide attempt by carbon monoxide asphyxiation.

The physician and therapist arranged to visit P.B. while he was in the hospital and spoke at length with the hospital physician about the appropriate treatment course. P.B. was profoundly depressed and expressed significant suicidal intent. He wanted to leave the hospital but was persuaded to stay as a voluntary patient. Individual psychotherapy was again begun while P.B. was an inpatient, and a trial of antidepressants was suggested. P.B. agreed to this course of action and after considerable discussion he decided to try fluoxetine. The physician supported this choice because of the relative safety of fluoxetine in overdose and because of the concerns about P.B.'s compliance with treatment that his therapist had raised. It was believed that the long half-life of fluoxetine would be of benefit in this case because all clinicians involved in his care expressed concerns about his compliance.

CASE COMMENTARY

"This is sometimes how it goes."

In spite of the best treatment plans and the provision of reasonable interventions, P.B. remained depressed and even made a serious suicide attempt. Hospitalization and a review of the treatment plan are necessary in such a case. The physician and therapist continued to work together with P.B. and were joined by the hospital treatment team. Such consistency and joint purpose are essential in the treatment of an adolescent patient who may too often slip between the cracks.

P.B. chose to try an antidepressant in addition to his psychotherapy. The choice of fluoxetine was reasonable, given the risks and benefits of that treatment. The medication was prescribed only in the context of a comprehensive treatment program.

Initiating Treatment with an SSRI: General Principles

As with many psychotropic interventions, initiating SSRI treatment follows a relatively predictable and pragmatic process. This is summarized as follows:

1. *Begin with "test" dose of medication.* Although it is unlikely that a patient will experience a serious allergic reaction to an SSRI, using a test dose approach allows for the immediate recognition of such a problem should it occur. This also provides both reassurance for the patient and family that the treatment is being taken seriously by the physician and underscores the importance of the need to be careful and conscientious about medication use. As one youngster put it, "It's not candy, you know."

2. *Use a small daily dose to start.* Beginning SSRI treatment with high daily doses is not likely to lead to earlier improvement in symptoms but is quite likely to result in adverse events early on in treatment, which may then lead to problems with compliance or discontinuation of what would have been a potentially useful therapy. Suggested SSRI initiation doses are found in Table 11–5.

3. *Identify a reasonable initial daily target dose.* Dose-response occurs over a wide range, and there may be a great deal of interindividual variability in optimal total daily dose. Because there is no method of determining a priori what the optimal total daily dose will be for any one individual, and because that yet-to-be-determined total daily dose will need to be taken for a sufficient time after steady-state levels are reached, it is not reasonable to titrate each patient to every point on the expected range of target doses. It is more reasonable to identify a target dose within the average or midpoint of the expected range and to treat to that goal. Adjustments to that dose (up or down) can be made either on the basis of adverse events experienced by the patient or the degree of therapeutic efficacy obtained after a sufficient treatment time for therapeutic efficacy to be evaluated has passed. Suggested initial target doses and expected dose ranges for SSRIs are found in Table 11–5.

4. *Identify an expected treatment duration prior to evaluation.* A treatment duration is important for the patient and physician to know and will depend on the expected time of therapeutic effect in depression and possibly on the pharmacokinetics of the specific SSRI. Because it is generally considered that steady-state levels of an antidepressant should be maintained over a specific length of time, it is possible that the timing of the therapeutic response may be associated with the length of time the treatment is continued following the attainment of steady-state drug levels. Thus medications that may take longer to achieve steady-state levels may be expected to have a longer latency of onset from the time that treatment is first initiated. Although this is not always the case, it is reasonable to err on the side of the longer expected time frame so as not to premature-

TABLE 11–5 **Suggested Initiation Doses, Initial Target Doses, and Expected Dose Ranges for SSRIs in the Treatment of Depressed Children and Adolescents***

Medication	Initiation Dose	Initial Target Dose	Expected Dose Range
Fluoxetine	Children: 5 mg Teens: 5 mg	Children: 20 mg Teens: 20 mg	Children: 5 to 40 mg Teens: 10 to 60 mg
Sertraline	Children: 25 mg Teens: 50 mg	Children: 50 mg Teens: 50 mg	Children: 50 to 150 mg Teens: 50 to 200 mg
Paroxetine	Children: 10 mg Teens: 10 mg	Children: 20 mg Teens: 20 mg	Children: 10 to 30 mg Teens: 20 to 40 mg
Fluvoxamine	Children: 25 mg Teens: 50 mg	Children: 150 mg Teens: 200 mg	Children: 50 to 200 mg Teens: 100 to 300 mg

*These doses are guidelines only. They are derived from published and presented data and clinical experience with these medications in children and adolescents. Individual patients may show variable therapeutic efficacy and adverse reactions to these doses. Total daily doses must be titrated to an individual patient's clinical response. In many cases, extending the treatment assessment time (e.g., from 10 to 12 weeks) instead of increasing the total daily dose will identify a reasonable therapeutic response.

ly discontinue a potentially effective treatment. Expected treatment duration to efficacy for SSRIs in depressed children and adolescents (taken from the time the medication is begun) is generally about 6 weeks for initial improvements and may take 8 to 12 weeks for substantial improvement.

5. *Titrate initial dose increments to the expected target dose and the treatment-emergent adverse events experienced by the patient.* Therapeutic efficacy in antidepressant treatment of depressed children and adolescents is not immediate and will often take up to 6 weeks to show initial improvements, with 8 to 12 weeks needed to identify substantial improvements. Treatment-emergent side effects, however, will make themselves known early on. Thus dose titration over the initial treatment phase will be directed by two considerations. First, the target dose established and, second, the side effects experienced or expected as the patient is titrated to that target dose. During the titration phase, patients should be seen frequently to evaluate adverse effects and should be able to contact the physician or a reasonable substitute (clinic nurse, other physician providing coverage) immediately if any problems arise. This process is more fully described in Section Three.

Prior to initiating treatment with an SSRI, the clinician must ensure that the baseline medical, laboratory, and psychiatric measures have been completed. These are then repeated as described earlier during the course of treatment. The information obtained from these measures is used to identify adverse events and to provide a reasonable database from which to make decisions as to the efficacy of pharmacotherapy at the time selected for treatment evaluation.

CASE EXAMPLE

Childhood Depression: The Trials and Tribulations of Medications

K.F. and her parents chose to use paroxetine as the medication part of her treatment for depression. Baseline psychiatric evaluations included an HDRS, a BDI, and an MSSES for paroxetine, each completed independently by K.F. and her mother. Baseline medical and laboratory evaluations were unremarkable, and paroxetine was started with a test dose of 10 mg, given at noon on a weekend day when K.F.'s parents could observe her. She was seen by her physician on the first following week-

day. At this time, paroxetine was started at a dose of 10 mg daily, given in the morning, and she was again seen 3 days later.

At this visit, K.F. reported no adverse events, but her parents considered her to have increased headaches, gastrointestinal (GI) distress, and sleepiness. A review of the baseline MSSES showed that both child and parent ratings of headaches had actually decreased and the items regarding GI problems were unchanged. The items that measured daytime sleepiness, however, were increased. As a result, K.F.'s medication was switched to an evening dose, and her parents were asked to contact the physician by telephone over the next 2 days to discuss the effect of altering the timing of the medication dose on K.F.'s side effects. This occurred as planned, and a decrease in her daytime sleepiness was identified.

When next seen (1 week after initiation of treatment, visit no. 3), K.F.'s medication was increased to 20 mg daily, the expected target dose, and she was again seen 3 days later. At this visit K.F. complained of nausea and constipation. Scores for both of these symptoms were significantly elevated from baseline. It was decided to alternate 10 mg with 20 mg doses over the next 4 days to determine if this dosage modification and time would lead to a decrease in these adverse events. When next seen, both K.F. and her parents reported no significant adverse events, and her dose was then raised to the identified target dose of 20 mg daily.

At her next visit, K.F.'s MSSES showed an overall, albeit slight, decrease in score from baseline, and no new adverse events were identified. Because she had reached her target dose, the medication was maintained at this level, and her medication and symptom monitoring were changed to once weekly. She and her parents were encouraged to telephone the physician or clinic nurse should any concerns arise about medication treatment between visits.

CASE COMMENTARY

Dealing with the Side Effects

As this case illustrates, handling the adverse events of medications is exceedingly important and particularly so during periods of medication induction or increments. The importance of careful baseline symptom measurements, as identified by the child and parents, is also well illustrated. When treating a child with psychotropic medication, it is advisable to obtain both the child's and a parent's assessment of somatic symptoms independently prior to initiating treatment. This is done to ensure that both child and parental observations are considered when evaluating treatment-emergent side effects.

In this case, K.F.'s parents were concerned that the medication was causing side effects. Because K.F.'s initial clinical presentation included a number of somatic complaints, without a proper baseline assessment of all these complaints, true treatment-emergent side effects could not have been adequately differentiated from the initial somatic symptoms. In K.F.'s case, as commonly occurs, some of the identified concerns were not explicable on the basis of treatment-emergent side effects, while others clearly were. Identifying true treatment-emergent adverse effects can lead to a reasonable intervention (such as changing the timing of the dose), which can be directed toward the specific events identified. Not all intervention strategies are similar, and some are more useful with certain side effects than with others (e.g., daytime sleepiness will usually respond to a change in dose timing, whereas severe headaches may often require dose decrements). In K.F.'s case, it was important to determine which of the somatic symptoms were actually treatment emergent because the management of these may have differed had the physician considered that all the complaints were caused by the initiation of medication treatment.

Similarly, the dose increment was associated with the emergence of adverse events, which were able to be so identified. The strategy taken to deal with them was appropriate but could only be properly instituted because the physician was clear about the treatment-emergent nature of the symptoms.

The timing of the patient-monitoring visits also changed depending on the course of the treatment. Once steady-state drug levels had been established and it was clear that no significant increases in side effects were occurring, the physician could decrease the frequency of patient monitoring without increasing the risk of missing problems. The patient and family, however, knew that they could contact the physician by telephone at any time should a concern arise. This availability is essential for the conduct of good pharmacologic treatment because it provides a safety net for the patient and family, and emphasizes the care in medication monitoring that the physician expects (see Section Three).

CASE EXAMPLE

Adolescent Depression: "It doesn't always go so smoothly."

P.B. decided to accept treatment with fluoxetine while still an inpatient. A baseline psychiatric assessment, which included the HDRS and BDI, was completed, and a baseline medical and laboratory investigation was unremarkable. Fluoxetine treatment was initiated with a dose of 5 mg daily.

The attending physician ordered a dose initiation schedule for fluoxetine that was to be administered by the hospital nursing staff. Two days later, P.B.'s fluoxetine dose was raised to 10 mg daily and after a similar time frame was once again raised, this time to a total daily dose of 30 mg. Two days following this last increment, P.B. was noted to be restless and irritable. He complained of feeling "jumpy" and was observed by hospital staff to have difficulty sitting still. No changes in the medication treatment were made, and over the next day P.B. became increasingly restless and complained of headaches, diarrhea, and sweating. Because it was now the weekend, P.B. was seen by the physician on call, who prescribed lorazepam at a dose of 1 mg to be given twice daily. The effect of this intervention was to decrease the restlessness somewhat but at the expense of complaints about headaches.

Following the Monday ward round, the fluoxetine was discontinued and the lorazepam tapered for discontinuation. The symptoms remitted over the next 3 to 4 days. P.B. vowed never to take "that medicine again. It almost killed me."

CASE COMMENTARY

Monitor Properly and Follow the Guidelines for Initiating Treatment

This case illustrates a problem that should never have occurred. The initiation of the chosen SSRI treatment began reasonably, but it was not monitored properly. Even though the dose of the medication was initially slowly increased, the attending physician did not conduct a careful review of the patient's tolerability of this schedule while it was being implemented. Good clinical practice demands that the effect of dose increments be established before proceeding to further dose increases. Furthermore, the physician must take individual responsibility for medication monitoring. It is not reasonable to establish a dose initiation schedule and then ask others to implement it.

In addition, one of the dose increments was excessive. The patient's total daily dose was effectively raised by 200 percent at one time. Such a dose increment would be expected to lead to significant side effects, and it did. To further complicate matters, the lack of careful assessment for treatment-emergent side effects led to an unnecessarily long period of time before appropriate action was taken. It is almost a clinical truism that significant changes to a hospitalized patient's medication (unless it is an emergency situation) should not be made prior to a weekend. This case clearly illustrates why.

If significant medication changes are made prior to times when staff unfamiliar with the child or adolescent patient are covering, the attending physician should discuss the nature of these changes and potential problems arising from them with the covering clinician. Better still, should such medication changes be deemed necessary, they signify that the patient is severely ill, and in such a case it may be reasonable for the attending physician to perform his or her own weekend review of the patient's condition. Although in this case a medically serious negative outcome did not occur, the effect of less than optimal care led to unnecessary discomfort for the patient and to the patient's understandable refusal of a treatment that might have proven beneficial to him.

Initiating Pharmacotherapy for Depressed Children and Adolescents: Time to Evaluation of Outcome

The period from the initiation of pharmacotherapy (the first 1 to 2 weeks) to the first outcome evaluation review is approximately 8 weeks. During this time, the patient will usually be on a tolerable dose of medication at steady-state levels. This phase is characterized by fewer problems with treatment-emergent side effects, but these can occur. Often the patient and family will experience "therapeutic impatience" as they wait for improvement.

During this period, active psychotherapeutic interventions should be taking place. Often these are directed at helping the patient deal with interpersonal issues at home and at school, or with his or her friends. If available, cognitive behavior therapies should be well underway. Education about the illness and such family interventions as are necessary should also be ongoing.

From the pharmacologist's perspective, the goals of this phase of treatment are as follows:

1. Optimize pharmacotherapy by encouraging compliance.
2. Provide careful and systematic monitoring of side effects and symptoms.
3. Continue education about the illness and its treatment.
4. Provide appropriate support to the patient and his or her family.

In many cases, the clinician who is prescribing the medication will be engaged in one or more of the following psychological interventions: individual psychotherapy, family counseling, and/or child-adolescent advocacy (e.g., with a school). If this is the case, it is essential that he or she not cut corners on the proper monitoring of side effects and symptoms. A suggested format for patient visits is to allow for a short time of initial settling in at the beginning of every visit and then proceed to the review of side effects and symptoms. Subjective ratings such as the BDI can be completed by the patient while waiting for the appointment. Often important psychotherapeutic issues will arise from the process of symptom review. If they do not, these issues can then be comfortably addressed over the remaining time of the interview.

This structure has the advantage of ensuring that proper medication monitoring occurs. Concurrently, it gives the patient and family the assurance that the physician is serious and careful about the pharmacologic treatment. Additionally, it allows for family input to occur (often a parent may accompany the child or teenager to that part of the interview in which side effects and symptoms are assessed), while at the same time preserving the privacy necessary for individual psychotherapy (the child or adolescent will have additional time alone with the physician to discuss issues of personal importance).

In some cases, the physician prescribing the medication will not be the same person who is conducting other therapeutic interventions. If this is the case, it is the responsibility of the physician to keep in close contact with other treatment providers about how they see the patient progressing and about any issues that are arising in either individual or family treatment that may impact on the psychopharmacologic intervention. Weekly telephone contact is usually sufficient for this, but occasionally treatment conferences may be necessary if significant problems occur. Patient and family education about the illness and its pharmacologic treatment and supportive therapy for the patient and family should still be carried out by the prescribing physician. In many cases, it will be useful to follow a similar structure to that described earlier at each interview.

In some settings, a medications clinic model may be used. This has many advantages for the effective and efficient conduct of pharmacotherapy. If this is the case, some of the above-mentioned procedures can be taken on by members of the clinic team. However, in all cases it is essential that the responsible physician spend sufficient time with each patient and family to ensure that the monitoring and treatment process is proceeding as planned. Furthermore, it is essential that the physician be available for discussions with a patient or a family member when such requests are made. The structure of a psychopharmacology clinic for children and adolescents is described in Section Three.

Outcome Evaluation Phase

At the predetermined time, usually about 8 weeks following the onset of antidepressant treatment, the outcome evaluation should take place. The data obtained from the assessment instruments should now be used to assist in the evaluation of treatment outcome by comparing the current symptom scores to baseline. Additionally, reapplication of the depression section of the K-SADS or a DSM checklist is useful to determine if the patient still meets diagnostic syndromal criteria for depression. The goals of this phase are (1) to determine the degree of efficacy of current treatment and (2) to decide on the next course of action. The second goal follows from the first. If pharmacologic treatment has been effective, that is, the symptoms of depression have improved by 70 to 80 percent or more from baseline and the medication is well tolerated, the goal should be optimizing treatment outcome prior to continuation treatment.

Outcome criteria for depression are often derived from clinical research studies designed to show whether a specific pharmacologic treatment is or is not generally effective. Although useful as guidelines, these criteria should not be accepted uncritically as optimal for any individual patient. It is important that the physician attempt to optimize outcome for each patient, not just approximate a predetermined "good enough" response. Pharmacologically, this goal can be achieved by one of the following methods:

1. Continue medications at the same dose for a longer period of time and then re-evaluate.
2. Change the dose of the medication and establish another outcome evaluation point.

If pharmacologic treatment has been partially effective, that is, either the symptoms of depression have shown between 50 and 80 percent improvement from baseline or, if the medication is not well tolerated, the second goal should be deciding on one of the six following courses:

1. Continue the same treatment for a longer period of time.
2. Increase the medication dose.
3. Decrease the medication dose.
4. Substitute another medication.
5. Augment the initial treatment.
6. Consider combination treatment.

However, prior to choosing one of these options, the physician must address both of the following issues:

1. Compliance evaluation. Has the patient been taking the medications properly? In some cases, therapeutic drug monitoring will be useful in this situation (see Section Three).
2. Assessment of other factors that may be associated with a suboptimal response to pharmacotherapy, including medical, personal, and environmental (a blood and urine sample for drugs and alcohol may be useful).

Once the physician is satisfied that one of the above-mentioned items does not account for the partial treatment response, he or she should go on to pursue one of these six options.

If pharmacologic treatment has not been effective—that is, the symptoms of depression have not improved beyond 50 percent from baseline—the second goal should be reviewing both of the possible issues potentially associated with the negative outcome described earlier and then deciding on one of the six courses identified under partial improvement. However, the physician should also include diagnostic reassessment. Was the initial diagnosis correct? Is the patient psychotic as well as depressed? Could the disorder be part of a prodrome of a schizophrenic illness? Following such a thorough review, the physician should consider one of the six possible strategies described earlier. A review of the general approach to inadequate therapeutic response to pharmacotherapy is found in Section Three.

CASE EXAMPLE

Childhood Depression: "This one went relatively smoothly."

Four weeks after starting pharmacotherapy, K.F.'s HDRS showed a drop of about 20 percent from baseline. A similar profile was identified in her BDI scores. She was experiencing minimal side effects from her medication, and her target dose was continued until her treatment evaluation review.

A treatment evaluation review was held at the end of the 10th treatment week. At this time K.F's symptom rating scales showed a decrease of 70 (BDI) to 85 (HDRS) percent from baseline. Her MSSES score had dropped by 55 percent from baseline, and she was tolerating her medications well. VAS scores pertaining to her school effort, school performance, relationships with the family, and involvement with her peers also showed improvements ranging from 30 to 70 percent of baseline. K.F. felt that she was "getting better," and her parents felt that she was "almost back to her usual self." It was decided to continue with her medications for another 4 weeks and then to reassess.

CASE COMMENTARY

"This actually does occur."

In many cases like this, a relatively smooth pattern of improvement is found. In this particular case, all parties—the child, family, and physician—agreed as to the amount of improvement, so that this could be considered a treatment success. However, it was felt that the patient, although clearly much improved, was still not "back to her normal self." In this situation, clinical wisdom takes precedence over statistical data. Although "statistically" the patient met the criteria for successful treatment, this did not equate with optimization of treatment. In her case the physician believed that further improvement could occur.

After a thorough discussion of the various options and their risks and benefits, the physician, patient, and family decided to simply extend the length of the treatment trial rather than risk producing side effects by increasing the dose of the medication further. In this particular case the result was an even further improvement in symptoms and functioning without increased side effects. Had this not occurred, it would have not been unreasonable to increase the dose of the medication slightly and begin careful monitoring once again.

CASE EXAMPLE

Adolescent Depression: Wouldn't You Know It, a Partial Responder

P.B., after a few days of refusing all medication treatment, eventually decided to try fluoxetine

again. This time the dose initiation phase was properly monitored, the medications were gradually increased, and all went relatively smoothly. A target dose of 30 mg daily was obtained, and 8 weeks after treatment was initiated an outcome evaluation was conducted.

The evaluation showed an improvement of 60 percent from baseline in HDRS scores and an improvement of 50 percent in BDI scores. No significant side effects or medical-laboratory considerations were identified. Although P.B. was no longer in the hospital and not acutely suicidal, he was not functioning well at school, at home, or with his peers. Although it was recognized that the outcome evaluation may have taken place relatively early in his treatment (i.e., by waiting another 2 weeks further improvement might have been expected to occur), the treating physician believed that further delay would be counterproductive and after discussion with P.B. and his mother the dose of the medication was increased to 40 mg daily and another outcome evaluation point was identified for 1 month thereafter.

P.B. tolerated this increased dose well and the next assessment point showed some further, albeit slight, improvements in symptoms but not in functioning. Accordingly, the dose was raised to 60 mg daily. This resulted in increased side effects of headache, nausea, and a fine tremor. P.D. also complained that he was experiencing difficulties obtaining and maintaining an erection and was worried that his new girlfriend would find out about this and drop him. Although the dose was decreased to 50 mg daily, these symptoms still persisted, albeit somewhat less intensely. The tremor continued to be bothersome, and P.B. found it socially awkward. A symptom reassessment taken 4 weeks after the initiation of the 50 mg dose did not identify any significant improvement over the 40 mg dose, and P.B.'s medication was decreased to 40 mg daily, with gradual improvement in all his side effects. No significant improvements in symptoms from the initial evaluation point, however, were noticed.

After discussion with P.B. and his mother, and a review of potential pharmacologic treatment strategies, it was decided to attempt augmentation of his partial response using triiodothyronine. Accordingly, 25 µg daily was added to the fluoxetine and the patient was carefully monitored. About 2 weeks later, P.B.'s symptom scores had improved considerably and were now within the range of a 75- to 85-percent decrease from baseline. He was feeling "really OK" and reported no significant adverse events. His mother reported improved relationships within the family, felt that P.B. was "pretty well," and wondered why this "magic medicine" had not been used previously. It was decided to continue this augmented treatment for another 6 weeks and to re-evaluate at that time.

CASE COMMENTARY

Choosing a Strategy for Partial Responders

In this case, the patient clearly showed a partial response to initial pharmacotherapy with an SSRI. In this situation the physician attempted to maximize monotherapy by increasing the dose, but this was not tolerated by the patient. This then led to three different options: substitution, augmentation, or combination.

Assessment of the Partial Responder

Suggested strategies for treating depressed children and adolescents who are partial responders to SSRI therapy are as follows:
1. Evaluate adequacy of treatment—dose and duration
2. Evaluate compliance
3. Evaluate nonpharmacologic treatment
4. Review environmental factors, including possible drug and alcohol abuse

If one or more of these factors are identified and it is believed that this might reasonably be expected to contribute to the partial response, continue current pharmacologic treatment, direct interventions toward those factors, and then re-evaluate in 4 to 6 weeks. If none of these factors are identified, if it is determined that their presence is not contributing to a partial response, or if they have been previously identified and optimal interventions directed toward them have not resulted in adequate improvement, then consider the following pharmacologic strategies.

Pharmacologic Strategies for the Partial Responder

Identify a new target dose and gradually increase as tolerated to that level; maintain for 6 to 8 weeks and re-evaluate. If there is a positive response, maintain the new dose. If there is an inadequate response and the medication is well tolerated, increase the target dose, and then re-evaluate in 6 to 8 weeks. If the medication increase is not tolerated, and the SSRI has a long half-life, proceed to one of the following augmentation strategies: light

therapy, triiodothyronine, or lithium. If the SSRI has a short to medium half-life, consider a substitution strategy with moclobomide or another SSRI or proceed to the previous strategy for the long half-life SSRI. If the response is still inadequate, attempt one or two further augmentation strategies. If the response continues to be inadequate, consider the strategies described earlier for treatment nonresponse, including diagnostic re-evaluation, further consultation, combination treatment, or ECT. Whenever a positive response is seen, maintain treatment and consider optimization strategies.

Substitution is a potentially useful strategy and is well recognized in the adult depression literature, which indicates that 40 to 60 percent of patients who are nonresponders to initial pharmacotherapy may respond when switched to either an SSRI or MAOI (RIMA). In addition, substitution strategies may involve switching from one compound to another within a similar class (e.g., fluoxetine to sertraline; both are SSRIs). The success rate of a substitution strategy in switching from an initial SSRI to a RIMA or other nontricyclic antidepressant is not clear. In children and adolescents, there is no literature to suggest whether any of the possible substitution strategies are likely to be effective.

In the case of P.B., the patient was taking an SSRI with a long half-life. Switching to another antidepressant (such as moclobomide, bupropion, or buspirone), although a possible option, would have necessitated a long washout period in order to decrease the risk of a serotonin syndrome. Thus, a substitution strategy was not believed to be in the best interests of the patient, given his complicated and difficult history. This may be considered if an SSRI with a shorter half-life is being used and if the patient's history suggests that such a course of action is reasonable.

Augmentation is also a potentially useful strategy and has been described in the child and adolescent literature, particularly with the use of lithium. A list of potentially useful augmentation agents is found in Table 11–6.

In P.B.'s case, lithium augmentation was not used for two reasons. First, the patient expressed serious concerns about the possible side effects of lithium and, secondly, because he had shown significant serotonin syndrome–like side effects on SSRI monotherapy, it was considered (albeit with little evidence) that the addition of lithium might be more likely to precipitate a serotonin syndrome. The alternative choice was triiodothyronine, which in a randomized double-blind study conducted in adults was found to be equivalently effective to lithium and significantly more effec-

TABLE 11–6 Augmentation Strategies of Potential Benefit in Children or Adolescents Who Are Partial Responders to SSRI Monotherapy*

Medication	Dosage and Issues[†]
Lithium	Total daily dose usually 600 to 900 mg; may show rapid (1 week) or gradual (4 to 6 week) response
Triiodothyronine	Total daily dose is 25 to 50 µg; usually shows response in 2 to 3 weeks
L-Tryptophan	Total daily dose is 1 to 4 g given at bedtime; usually shows a response in 3 to 4 weeks and is very difficult to take in tablet form
Carbamazepine	Total daily dose determined by blood levels; SSRI medications may alter plasma levels
Buspirone	Total daily dose is 20 to 60 mg; usually shows a delayed response of 4 to 6 weeks

*The suggested augmentation strategies are derived from published and presented material and clinical experience as it pertains to children and adolescents. All the above have also been successfully used in adults. Caution must be taken in extrapolation of data from adults to children or adolescents. Individuals may experience different therapeutic or adverse events to different agents, and treatment must be individually tailored with careful monitoring.

†Many of the agents identified here, when combined with an SSRI, may potentially cause a serotonin syndrome. Informing the patient and family of this possibility and carefully monitoring the patient are necessary. Some studies in adults suggest that the beta-adrenergic blocker pindolol (SHTIA effect) may be of value. No evidence for this is available for children and adolescents.

tive than placebo. In P.B.'s case, this turned out to be a useful and successful intervention.

Combination is also a potentially useful strategy that involves adding another antidepressant medication to an already ongoing antidepressant treatment. In the case of a child or adolescent, this may involve adding the RIMA moclobomide or the monocyclic bupropion to an SSRI. Some very experienced child and adolescent pharmacotherapists have reported successful combination strategies using an SSRI and tricyclic. In general, however, although there are reported cases in which this has been successfully carried out in young adults and in older adolescents, such a treatment strategy involves a high risk of potentially serious adverse effects and is not recommended as an initial combination strategy. If used, it should be supervised by a physician who is experienced in this practice and with careful medical monitoring. An alternative is to use the new SNRI compound venlafaxine.

Successful combination of a TCA and a traditional MAOI in tricyclic refractory adolescent depression has also been described. In this report, however, dietary compliance was identified as a

problem, and a significant minority of patients experience a hypertensive tyramine-type reaction. This information, although of interest, provides little clinically useful direction for the combination of SSRIs with MAOIs. Generally, given the potential adverse effects of traditional MAOIs, their routine use in the pharmacologic treatment of child and adolescent depression is not recommended. If the physician is faced with a case in which combination treatment with an MAOI is potentially indicated, the RIMA moclobomide should be used.

If a combination strategy is used, it is recommended that it be instituted in a facility in which daily medical monitoring can occur and by practitioners who have had some experience with this method. This is not a strategy for a busy outpatient office practice.

Other Potential Nonpharmacologic Augmentation Strategies

Theoretically, some psychotherapeutic strategies may be viewed as potential augmentations for patients who are partial responders to antidepressant monotherapy. These have not been studied in children or adolescents. They might be considered if specific indications for their use apply, and there is reason to expect them to show efficacy within an appropriate length of time. A further potential nonpharmacologic augmentation strategy for antidepressant monotherapy partial responders is the use of light therapy. Light therapy has been successfully applied to the treatment of seasonal affective disorder and other depressive states in adults, but its evaluation in depressed children and adolescents is surprisingly lacking. One study suggests that it may be useful in ameliorating breakthrough depressive symptoms in adolescent bipolar patients who are undergoing concurrent thymoleptic treatment.

Because side effects from this type of treatment are minimal and therapeutic response, should it occur, may be expected within 2 to 3 weeks of initiating treatment, light therapy can be considered in the child or adolescent in whom addition of another pharmacologic agent may be problematic. A reasonable treatment course involves the delivery of 2500 lux of full-spectrum light twice daily for 2 weeks. Each treatment should last for 45 to 50 minutes, and treatment times should be between 0600 and 0800 and between 1800 and 2000 hours.

Treatment Nonresponse (Treatment Resistance)

If following a diagnostic re-evaluation and treatment review, the patient is still considered to be treatment resistant, the clinician can consider all the options described in the case commentary under partial treatment responders. In many cases, application of one or more of these strategies will lead to at least a significant, if not optimal, therapeutic response. However, if such an outcome is not forthcoming after a number of adequate treatment trials and the child or adolescent continues to be severely depressed and functioning poorly, consideration should be given to using ECT.

If ECT is contemplated, sufficient patient and family education about this form of treatment must precede its use. Fully informed written consent following all legal guidelines must be given. Prior to initiating ECT, the child or adolescent for whom the treatment is proposed should have two independent psychiatric evaluations regarding the suitability for this type of intervention. At least one of those evaluations should be by the physician who will be actually providing the treatment.

If the choice to proceed to ECT is made, anesthetic consultation must be obtained, and the treatments given in an appropriate medical setting. Although there is generally no need to discontinue SSRI treatment during ECT, other medications, such as anticonvulsants or lithium, may well need to be stopped. Post-treatment patient care should be carried out by qualified nursing staff, and successful outcome from electroconvulsive treatments should be followed by maintenance pharmacotherapy with an SSRI or RIMA.

Long-Term Pharmacologic Treatment

Depression is now known to be a chronic disorder, with episodes of illness often alternating with periods of remission across the life cycle. In some cases functioning between episodes returns relatively close to the premorbid state. In other cases, interepisode functioning becomes progressively more problematic over time and may itself become a risk factor for future episodes. In many children and adolescents, the probability of recurrence is quite high; depression is more likely than not to recur. Therefore, effective pharmacologic treatment of a depressive disorder should include not only optimal acute interventions but also a useful strategy for long-term pharmacologic care.

On the basis of current knowledge, it is useful to conceptualize long-term treatment with antidepressant medications as comprising two phases:

1. Continuation or consolidation phase
   This is the period of time over which treatment with antidepressant medications is needed to prevent relapse (the re-emergence of symptoms from the initial episode). This phase can be expected to last about 6 months following remission of the acute episode.
2. Maintenance or prophylaxis phase
   This is the period of time over which treatment with antidepressant medications is needed to prevent recurrence (the onset of a new episode). This phase can be expected to be of variable length, lasting from a year or more to lifetime, depending on the clinical history of the patient.

Continuation Treatment

Continued antidepressant treatment following optimization of outcome in the acute episode is necessary to prevent relapse. Although no specific studies are currently available for children and adolescents, extensive clinical experience and data from adult studies show that withdrawal of an effective antidepressant medication soon after the remission of an acute episode is highly predictive of relapse. Relapse is an outcome that must be avoided, therefore, the use of continuation treatment for remitted children and adolescents is highly recommended. This phase of treatment should last for about 6 months from the time of remission.

There are two alternative dosing strategies for this phase. The first strategy is to decrease the total daily dose of the antidepressant to about one half or two thirds of the total daily dose used during acute treatment. If an SSRI is being used for continuation treatment, in the absence of significant adverse events there is no clearly understood or valid rationale for such a strategy, although this approach (for unknown reasons) is often considered to be a clinical "truth." Available studies from adult populations suggest that this approach is not optimal and that another continuation strategy confers increased prophylactic effect without increased risks.

The second strategy is to maintain the same total daily dose of the antidepressant that produced remission of the acute phase over the entire continuation phase. In the absence of significant or poorly tolerated adverse events, this is a reasonable strategy and is preferred over the decrease in total daily dose option identified earlier. This strategy can be modified somewhat if the patient experiences adverse effects that prove to be somewhat problematic. These adverse effects may lead to difficulties with compliance, which would be expected to heighten the risk of relapse. In such a case, slight decreases of the total daily dose may be considered.

CASE EXAMPLE

Childhood Depression: All Better, Time to Quit the Medicine

K.F. was doing very well. Her mood was stable, her school performance had improved, she was out playing with her friends, and family interactions had returned to "normal—just the usual ups and downs." The issue of continuation treatment was discussed with K.F. and her parents. K.F. wanted to "stop the pills because I feel better." She was experiencing no side effects from the medications, and compliance did not seem to be a problem because her parents took responsibility for administering her medications. Following a prolonged discussion about the use of the medicine to "help keep you well" and a better understanding about the risks of withdrawing effective antidepressant treatment too early, both K.F. and her parents decided that she should continue taking her medications for 6 more months.

Monthly medication monitoring visits were set up, and a signs and symptoms checklist for the identification of relapse was provided—one copy for K.F. and one for her parents (see Fig. 11–1). The family was asked to contact the physician at any time with concerns about return of symptoms or if problems about the use of the medication arose. Finally, they were given a Medications Monitoring Form listing medications that might potentially interact with her SSRI. A copy of this form was also sent to her family physician with the physician's progress note.

CASE COMMENTARY

Maintain Monitoring and Help the Patient and Family Identify Possible Relapse Early

This case illustrates the important components of the pharmacotherapy in the continuation phase. These include continued education about the nature of the illness and the identification of the potential consequences of relapse if effective pharmacologic treatment is withdrawn too quickly. Patients or their families will often apply another component of the aspirin model of medical treatment to remission as well. This thinking follows along the lines of "the pain (or fever) is gone, so I don't need the aspirin any more." It is usually necessary to identify this type of thinking about pharmacologic treatment with the patient and family, and

to help them understand how this model does not apply to the pharmacotherapy of depression (see Section Three).

The pharmacologic treatment of the continuation phase continues to be a very active process. The goals of this are as follows:
1. Maintain remission
2. Ensure compliance
3. Identify relapse early
4. Intervene aggressively at signs of relapse

Maintaining Remission and Ensuring Compliance

Remission is best pharmacologically maintained by continued use of therapeutic doses of antidepressants over the entire continuation phase. Patient compliance with taking medications can often become an issue, because most people do not want to take a medication when they feel well. Furthermore, patients or their families may have concerns about the long-term effects of prolonged pharmacologic treatment. These are both understandable concerns and must be identified as such and discussed with the patient and family by the physician at the onset of continuation treatment. Furthermore, they must be reviewed at regularly scheduled times during this phase. Setting up specific and regular medication monitoring times at the beginning of the continuation treatment phase allows the physician not only to monitor the continued efficacy and tolerability of the antidepressant but also to continue to educate the family and support the necessity for compliance. The importance of this regular monitoring should be stressed to the patient and family because people do not like to go to the doctor when they are feeling well, and missed appointments should be followed up.

Identifying Early Relapse and Intervening Quickly

It is important to identify relapse, if it occurs, as soon as possible so as to intervene quickly, thereby decreasing the severity, duration, and degree of impairment of the new episode. Even with optimal continuation treatment, relapses may occur. However, it is expected that rapid intervention will decrease the severity, duration, and accompanying morbidity of the relapse.

To this end, it is important to provide the patient and parents with a tool that they can use to help them identify the symptoms of relapse. A signs and symptoms of depression checklist is helpful for this purpose (Fig. 11–1). This checklist can be individualized for each patient by reviewing with the patient and family the earliest

Depressed feelings and feeling "blue" are common; everybody has them at some time or other. Often these feelings happen because something in your life is not going right or is bothering you. Sometimes these feelings seem to come out of the blue.

You have had a clinical depression. That means that the depressed feelings that you had were not an expected part of daily life, but a problem that needed treatment. You are feeling better now, and that is good. The medicines that you have been treated with and are now taking have helped you to get better. Many people who stop taking their medicines will soon get sick again. However, if you continue taking your medicines for the next little while as prescribed by your doctor, hopefully these medicines will make sure that you stay better.

For some people, even if they take their medicines as prescribed, the depressed feelings still come back. If this happens you could get another clinical depression like the one you just had. However, if you, your parents, or your doctor find out that the clinical depression is coming back, as soon as it starts to come back your doctor can help you with treatments that will try to either stop this from happening or will stop the clinical depression from being very strong.

Clinical depression has a number of symptoms (things you feel) and signs (things that other people notice about you) that can signal it is coming back. The following is a list of those symptoms and signs. The reason that you and your parents have this list is that if these symptoms and signs begin, you can let your doctor know right away. Both you and your parents have this list because sometimes the symptoms are more easily recognized by you and the signs are more easily recognized by your parents. If either you or your parents notice these symptoms and signs, you can let your doctor know.

Because the symptoms and signs of clinical depression can often be confused with regular depressive feelings, it is important to let you doctor know about them, even if you are not sure that it is the clinical depression coming back.

These are the symptoms and signs of a possible clinical depression. If you have two or more of these, and they have been there pretty much every day for 3 or 4 days in a row, call your doctor immediately.

Trouble Sleeping:

_____ Sleeping too much and during the day
_____ Having trouble falling asleep
_____ Waking up early in the morning and feeling tired at the same time

Trouble Eating:

_____ Eating much too much, even when you are not hungry
_____ Not feeling hungry for food, even food you usually really like
_____ Eating only because you think you should

Interest and Activities:

_____ Not interested in your usual hobbies, sports, or friends
_____ Having trouble concentrating on your school work
_____ Not going out because you can't be bothered
_____ Not having your usual energy or feeling tired a lot

Feelings and Thoughts:

_____ Feeling sad, depressed, blah, or blue
_____ Feeling that most things are not fun any more
_____ Thinking that you are not a very good person
_____ Thinking about death or suicide
_____ Feeling irritable a lot or fighting with friends and family for no good reason

Other Symptoms or Signs That You Can Remember Were Happening Before You Had Your Clinical Depression:

_____ _____

_____ _____

_____ _____

_____ _____

_____ _____

Your doctor's telephone number is _____

FIGURE 11–1 Signs and Symptoms Checklist for Depression

signs of depressive symptoms as they occurred at the onset of the past episode. This process also has the added advantage of increasing patient and parent sensitivity to the early symptoms of the disorder, with the potential benefit of earlier recognition if it does recur. The family and patient should be instructed to contact the physician if they feel a relapse might be possible. It is better to have them speak to the clinician over the telephone or even be seen immediately about their concerns, even if they overcall or over-react, than to have the recognition of relapse delayed.

It is also useful to provide the patient and family with a Medications Monitoring Form (see Appendix). This can easily be compiled by the clinician and should list the medication(s) that the child or adolescent is currently taking, the dose and timing of doses, and any medications that might be expected to demonstrate drug-drug interactions. A copy of this should be sent to the child's or adolescent's pediatrician or family physician.

A relapse can occur during the continuation phase, even if the patient is taking the medication properly. Should a relapse occur, the following strategy may be helpful:

1. Review compliance, other treatments received, and the presence of possible contributory environmental factors.
2. If compliance has been problematic, return the patient to the dose that was effective in reaching the initial remission.
3. If relapse is thought to be associated with a decrease or discontinuation of an effective psychotherapy, reinstitute the psychotherapy, and at the same time consider increasing the total daily medication dose to a new target level as tolerated.
4. If environmental factors are thought to be having an impact, develop a strategy to deal with them therapeutically and at the same time consider increasing the total daily medication dose to a new target as tolerated.
5. If the depression continues to develop in spite of these interventions, consider using the strategies for partial responders described earlier.

Maintenance Phase

Although this phase is well recognized in the long-term antidepressant treatment of adults, it is unlikely to be considered by the physician treating a child or adolescent patient, often because the patient is not followed-up for a long enough period of time to identify the presence of multiple depressive episodes. In some cases, however, long-term maintenance pharmacotherapy can be considered if the child or adolescent fulfills one of the following criteria:

1. Three or more episodes of MDD
2. DYS plus two or more episodes of MDD
3. DYS of 3 or more years' duration with associated functional impairment that has shown a therapeutic response to pharmacotherapy and relapse when pharmacotherapy is withdrawn
4. Two or more clear-cut relapses occurring within 4 to 6 months of antidepressant medication withdrawal

If a child or adolescent patient meets one or more of the above-mentioned criteria, the physician should discuss the issue of long-term maintenance with the patient and family. A reasonable first strategy is to apply maintenance antidepressant treatment for a minimum of 12 to 16 months. If this leads to continued remission, one of two choices can then be entertained: the patient may wish to gradually withdraw the medication to determine if relapse will recur, or the patient may consider that the risk of relapse, based on past history, is not worth a medication-free trial. If this option is chosen, it is reasonable to set another target date of 12 to 16 months later for this issue to be reviewed.

Similar to during the continuation phase, the patient should be seen on a regular basis, once a month is reasonable, and the early identification of relapse monitoring, as previously described, should continue. For the few patients who may follow this course, it may be useful for the physician to provide longer follow-up than is usually considered proper by clinicians who treat children and adolescents. It is not unreasonable to provide continuity of care into early adulthood, at which time the patient can be understandably transferred to a colleague who treats adults.

Withdrawal of Antidepressant Medications

At some point in time, hopefully at the end of a successful continuation phase, the withdrawal of antidepressant medications will need to be considered. If the patient does not meet criteria for long-term maintenance treatment (see earlier), the withdrawal of medications can be undertaken 6 months after remission. The following considerations would lead the physician to propose a prolonged period (12 to 16 months) of pharmacotherapy—an extended continuation phase:

1. The patient has already experienced two episodes of depression.

2. The patient's depressive symptoms have remitted but significant functional deficits (social, academic, interpersonal) remain.

3. The patient is in a vulnerable phase of the life cycle, in which the onset of another depressive episode is certain to result in significant disruption of the normal developmental process (such as a secondary school student who is preparing to write college entrance examinations).

4. There is a strong history of multiple severe depressive episodes in a first-degree relative.

5. The patient has had a difficult and prolonged treatment course (such as requiring augmentation or combination pharmacotherapy, or has required ECT for remission of the acute episode).

6. The patient has made one or more serious suicide attempts while depressed.

Although these considerations are guidelines only, in cases in which these issues appear, nothing is to be gained and much potentially to be lost in rigidly adhering to a 6 month continuation treatment regime. In these clinical situations, it may well be most prudent to increase the length of the continuation period, particularly if the medication is well tolerated by the patient. Thus, the decision to withdraw effective continuation pharmacotherapy must rest on solid clinical consideration of the relative risks and benefits of such a withdrawal to the individual patient.

When a decision has been made to discontinue antidepressant treatment, the optimal approach is to select a medication withdrawal strategy that allows for a very general tapering. For no clear reason, current "clinical lore" suggests that antidepressant treatment should be discontinued over a few weeks. A more reasonable approach would be to discontinue pharmacologic treatment very gradually over 3 to 4 months, carefully monitoring for the recurrence of depressive symptoms.

Relapse is most likely to occur relatively soon after medication is discontinued. The use of a more gradual withdrawal schedule not only would avoid the potential for an antidepressant withdrawal syndrome (see later) to occur but also would allow for careful monitoring of the patient's mood as the serum levels gradually decrease. If mood instability or other symptoms of impending relapse appear during this period of higher relapse risk, it is then relatively easy to reinstitute pharmacotherapy, to the same dose as produced the initial therapeutic response. In this manner, because the patient will be already taking some medication, the patient can be more quickly returned to the initial target dose than if the medication had been totally withdrawn.

Antidepressant Withdrawal Syndrome

It is not totally clear if an antidepressant withdrawal syndrome commonly occurs with SSRI therapy, but experienced child and adolescent psychopharmacologists have noticed that it may. It has been described with TCAs and is thought to be associated with a transient muscarinic receptor supersensitivity that may occur following long-term treatment with anticholinergic agents. The signs and symptoms of this syndrome include GI symptoms (nausea, diarrhea, abdominal distress); sleep difficulties (restless sleep, frequent wakings, vivid dreams or nightmares); and psychomotor disturbances (agitation, anxiety, restlessness, tremor). Although the use of TCAs is not recommended for depressed children and adolescents, the signs and symptoms of the antidepressant withdrawal syndrome should be familiar to a physician who treats this population and might find it necessary to withdraw ineffective TCAs prior to beginning an alternative pharmacologic intervention. Additionally, when an antidepressant withdrawal syndrome with SSRIs does occur, it shows a phenomenology similar to that of tricyclics.

A difficult clinical problem may arise when the clinician is faced with the issue of terminating ineffective tricyclic treatment prior to initiating SSRI therapy. It is important to discontinue the tricyclic medication sufficiently rapidly to allow for another potentially more effective and better tolerated treatment to begin. At the same time, it is important not to discontinue the tricyclic medication so rapidly that a tricyclic withdrawal syndrome ensues.

In this case, it is reasonable to withdraw 20 to 30 percent of the initial tricyclic dose and then 5 days later withdraw 20 to 30 percent of the remaining dose. At 5 to 7 days following this, 50 percent of the remaining dose can be withdrawn, followed by complete discontinuation 1 week later. If withdrawal symptoms occur, the patient should be returned to the previous dose level, and the rate of discontinuation should be decreased by increasing the time interval between dose reductions. For example, a 5-day schedule should be changed to a 7-day schedule. SSRI medications can be started 2 to 3 days following the discontinuation of the tricyclic, with particular attention paid to the possibility of onsetting serotonin symptoms. Obviously, frequent and careful monitoring of the patient over such a switchover period is necessary, but this can be quite reasonably done in an outpatient setting if the patient and family are responsible and understand the importance of reporting significant adverse effects to the physician immediately if they occur.

Some very experienced child and adolescent psychopharmacologists, working in university teaching hospital clinics, use an alternative switch strategy. In this scheme, the TCA daily dose is lowered by an initial 20 to 30 percent. Five days later, this total daily dose is again lowered by the same percent and the SSRI medication is begun at very low doses. Thereafter, dose decrements in the tricyclic medication are paired with small dose increments in the SSRI medication. Such a strategy must be closely medically monitored and is perhaps less suitable than the first procedure described for a busy outpatient office practice, particularly if a medications clinic is not available.

Other Issues in the Pharmacologic Treatment of Child and Adolescent Depression

Issues that may frequently arise during the pharmacologic treatment of depressed children or adolescents include (1) antidepressant-induced mania or hypomania, (2) suicide management, and (3) psychotic depression.

Antidepressant-Induced Mania or Hypomania

Symptoms of mania or hypomania in adults are known to be associated with the use of a variety of antidepressants, including tricyclics, SSRIs, and others. There is no good evidence that any one type of antidepressant is less likely to be implicated in this phenomenon than any other (although some research suggests that bupropion may be less commonly associated). This phenomenon also occurs in children and adolescents. The prevalence of this problem in the younger population has not been determined, but most estimates suggest that it is less than 5 percent of the antidepressant-treated population. Nevertheless, it is an important potential adverse event that must be expected and quickly recognized because its appearance has important treatment implications.

Although it would be useful to be able to predict which children and adolescents are most at risk for this adverse event, studies of the clinical characteristics of children and adolescents who have experienced a manic or hypomanic switch have not been able to identify a clinical profile that has much predictive validity. However, clinical ex-

perience with this population and general knowledge of the child and adolescent literature regarding depression and the risk of bipolar disorder suggests that some caution should be taken with patients who have the following clinical characteristics:

1. Psychotic depression
2. First-degree relative with a bipolar illness
3. Previous episodes of hypomania (even if subclinical)

In all depressed children or adolescents, the possibility of manic or hypomanic symptoms as an adverse event of antidepressant treatment should be identified prior to initiating pharmacotherapy. If a child or adolescent has two or more of the above-mentioned putative risk factors, the clinician has two or three choices that should be discussed with the patient and family.

The first choice is to avoid the use of antidepressant medications altogether and instead attempt a course of psychotherapy, reserving antidepressant use for those patients who do not show significant therapeutic response to psychotherapy alone. The second choice is to go ahead and treat with an antidepressant, carefully monitoring for the appearance of early symptoms of mood elevation. If this course is chosen, it is particularly important not to confuse the development of hypomanic symptoms with remission of depression. Two clinically useful points of differentiation are as follows:

1. The full antidepressant effect of pharmacotherapy in this population is unlikely to be realized before 8 to 12 weeks. Antidepressant-induced manic or hypomanic symptoms often onset 2 to 4 weeks after beginning antidepressant treatment. Thus, if the patient's symptoms show significant early improvement and mood lability or euphoria is present, the clinician should consider the possibility that the phenomenon is an adverse effect of pharmacotherapy.

2. The usual course of antidepressant-induced clinical improvement is a gradual onset of symptom remission. Antidepressant-induced manic or hypomanic symptoms tend to demonstrate a rapid and global onset of "improvement." Thus a very quick resolution of all or most of the depressive symptoms suggests the possibility that this is an adverse effect of pharmacotherapy.

In addition, the clinician must be careful to distinguish the symptoms of antidepressant-induced mania or hypomania from other side effects of antidepressant treatment, particularly the restless, akathisia-type syndrome that occasionally onsets with SSRIs. Discontinuation of the medication, followed by a more gradual reintroduction, should help clarify this picture.

The third option is to cover the patient with a thymoleptic medication while the antidepressant is being started. If this course of action is taken, lithium or valproate should be started 1 week or so prior to beginning the antidepressant. The routine schedule for initiating SSRI treatment, as outlined earlier, should then be followed once the patient is on therapeutic serum levels of the thymoleptic.

Although this option may seem rational, no evidence suggests that using this approach will significantly decrease the risk of antidepressant-induced mania or hypomania. The problem that this option leads to is that once the patient is on an effective antidepressant dose, the clinician is left with having to decide whether to continue or discontinue the concomitant thymoleptic treatment. Additionally, the patient will be exposed to the possibility of side effects from the thymoleptic medication and because of potential drug-drug interactions will need to have careful monitoring of serum thymoleptic levels with the issues regarding venipuncture that this entails.

If antidepressant treatment causes clear-cut mania or hypomania, the physician should discontinue the antidepressant and consider the possibility of a bipolar disorder. Introducing thymoleptic treatments in the manner described in Chapter 12 is appropriate in this situation.

Suicide Management

Suicide remains a potential problem during the entire duration of treatment for depressed children and adolescents. Appropriate suicide risk-identification strategies and the management of suicidal ideation, intent, and actions must be part of the overall treatment strategy. The use of SSRIs as a first-line treatment for depression substantially decreases the fatality risk of overdose found with tricyclics. However, this should not lead to clinician complacency. Because many self-harm attempts in depressed teens seem to be the result of impulsive actions, decreasing the amount of medications potentially available for impulsive ingestion is a useful preventive intervention. If clinical concern about possible suicidal actions is present, prescriptions during this phase of antidepressant treatment should only be written for a week's supply of medications and parental monitoring of the patient should be initiated. This time interval between prescriptions can be increased once the suicide risk has diminished.

For children and young adolescents, a responsible adult should be identified to dispense and monitor medications. For older adolescents, although the teenager's ability to take responsibility for medication management should be respected, responsible adult supervision is usually helpful. This can be done as unobtrusively as possible and might consist of a parent or other responsible adult gently and nonjudgmentally inquiring if there are any difficulties with the medication on a regular basis. This type of monitoring, if it is discussed and agreed to at the time that the medication trial begins, is usually well tolerated by most teenagers. A common clinical error with adolescents is to over-estimate their ability to manage their own medications and thus not provide them with a monitoring structure that can be helpful yet respectful of their developing autonomy.

Psychotic Depression

A psychotic depression onsetting in the child or adolescent is a serious affective illness that requires hospitalization for optimal treatment. It should generally not be treated on an outpatient basis. Adolescent-onset psychotic depression is predictive of a future bipolar course in 20 to 40 percent of teenagers. Thus treatment of psychotic depression differs from that of nonpsychotic depression.

Combination antidepressant and antipsychotic medications are needed to effectively treat psychotic depression. Antipsychotic medications should be started first, followed by antidepressant medication 3 days later. Middle-potency antipsychotic medications are preferred to high-potency compounds, but low-potency antipsychotics may need to be used to manage behavioral disturbances. Addition of SSRIs, which are metabolized through the hepatic P-450 enzyme systems, can affect serum levels of most antipsychotics so the clinician may chose to use sertraline as the first-line antidepressant in this case. Alternatively, lower doses of antipsychotic medication (two thirds to three quarters of the usually anticipated target dose) could be used. Sertraline may be successfully combined with low doses of risperidone (1 to 3 mg daily), and this combination may be better tolerated than combining other SSRIs with the typical neuroleptics.

Treatment nonresponse to an adequate trial of SSRI combined with an appropriate amount of antipsychotic medication should lead to the consideration of ECT. Once treatment of psychotic depression has resulted in remission, it is reasonable to continue both the antidepressant and antipsychotic medication together for 4 to 6 months. Following this period, the antipsychotic medication can be gradually withdrawn, with careful monitoring of the patient for relapse of psychosis. The antidepressant alone should then be continued for another 2 to 3 months before gradual discontinuation is initiated.

This process is expected to take 6 to 8 months or longer. It should not be rushed because nothing is to be gained with rapid discontinuation of either medication. Should symptoms emerge during the discontinuation process, the doses of both medications should be raised as quickly as possible to the levels at which the initial remission occurred. Subsequent attempts at discontinuation should then proceed no earlier than 6 to 8 months later and at a slower pace than was used previously. Should manic symptoms arise during the withdrawal phase, the antidepressant should be discontinued and a thymoleptic, either lithium or valproate, introduced. Subsequent patient management should then follow that outlined in Chapter 12 on the treatment of bipolar disorder. Appropriate psychosocial interventions should be continued throughout.

SUGGESTED READINGS

DeVane CL. Pharmacokinetics of the selective serotonin reuptake inhibitors. Journal of Clinical Psychiatry, 53(Suppl. 2):13–20, 1992.

Feighner JP, Boyer WF (eds). Selective Serotonin Re-Uptake Inhibitors, Vol. 1. Toronto: John Wiley and Sons, 1991.

Freeman H (ed). Progress in antidepressant therapy. British Journal of Psychiatry, 154(Suppl. 3):7–112, 1988.

Kutcher S, Marton P. Treatment of adolescent depression. In K Shulman, M Tohen, S Kutcher (eds): Mood Disorders Across the Life Span. New York: Wiley-Liss, 1996, pp 101–126.

Kye C, Ryan N. Pharmacologic treatment of child and adolescent depression. Child and Adolescent Psychiatric Clinics of North America, 4:261–281, 1995.

Lane R, Baldwin D, Preskorn S. The SSRI's: Advantages, disadvantages and differences. Journal of Psychopharmacology, 9(Suppl):163–167, 1995.

Leonard B. The comparative pharmacology of new antidepressants. Journal of Clinical Psychiatry, 54(Suppl. 3):3–17, 1993.

Preskorn S. Clinical Pharmacology of Selective Serotonin Reuptake Inhibitors. Caddo, OK: Professional Communications, Inc., 1996.

Preskorn S, Janicak P, Davis J, Ayd F, Jr. Advances in the pharmacotherapy of depressive disorders. In P Janicak (ed): Update: Principles and Practice of Psychotherapy, Vol. 1. Baltimore: Williams and Wilkins, pp 434–465, 1993.

Shulman R. The serotonin syndrome: A tabular guide. Canadian Journal of Clinical Pharmacology, 2:139–144, 1995.

Stokes PE. A primary care perspective on management of acute and long term depression. Journal of Clinical Psychiatry, 54(Suppl. 3):74–87, 1993.

CHAPTER 12

Psychopharmacologic Treatment of Bipolar Disorder

Bipolar disorder commonly onsets in adolescence, although it may occur prepubertally. While the first affective episode is usually a depression, the first manic episode is often characterized by an atypical presentation, usually a mixed manic or rapid cycling picture. Mania is often misdiagnosed in teenagers. Severe cases may be diagnosed as schizophrenia, and milder cases may be given a personality disorder diagnosis. Because mania often presents with psychotic symptoms, the clinician should consider a diagnosis of mania in any psychotic episode onsetting in adolescence. In addition, in this age group a clinical presentation of mood instability, irritability, impulsivity, and intrusiveness, particularly in the context of a family history of mood disorder and a past history of a depression, may signal a possible hypomanic episode, which often persists for quite some time prior to the onset of flagrant mania or functional disturbances that require psychiatric consultation. The diagnostic picture can become rather clouded if attention-deficit hyperactivity disorder (ADHD), substance use, or substance abuse is present.

Mania or hypomania in children may be even more difficult to diagnose. Often it presents with a picture of persistent mood, behavioral, and cognitive difficulties. Manic children often show marked disturbances in multiple aspects of functioning. The classic onset-offset cycles seen with this disorder in adults may occur less frequently in children and, in some cases, may be absent altogether. Diagnosis is further complicated by the overlap of symptoms with the syndrome of ADHD, and a number of children with bipolar illness may be incorrectly first diagnosed with ADHD. In some cases these children experience a worsening of their clinical picture when treated with stimulants or antidepressants for their attentional problems. To make diagnosis even more difficult, ADHD and bipolar disorder may occur comorbidly with each other. The clinical use of a semistructured interview such as the Kiddie Schedule for Affective Disorders and Schizophrenia (K-SADS) (see Section Two) is of value in the diagnostic evaluation of a child or adolescent, particularly when a manic or hypomanic presentation is suspected.

CASE EXAMPLE

Adolescent-Onset Bipolar Disorder: Beyond Normal Narcissism

G.A. was a 17-year-old boy who was brought to the hospital by his parents because he was "acting strange for the last week or so." He was staying up most of the night; expressing himself in an angry manner, including "irrational" temper outbursts; changing his clothing about 8 or 10 times daily; acting rudely toward his teachers and disrupting his school classes; and playing his trumpet at all hours of the day or night, and resisting any requests to stop because it was interfering with his parent's sleep. He told his parents that he was planning to stop school and move to New York City, where he would join the orchestra on the "David Letterman Show." He called himself a "musical genius" and became irritable and verbally threatening when his parents refused to acknowledge this. He also had designed an "acoustically perfect" music hall and had written to an architectural firm asking that they pay him for his plans. A number of his close friends had called G.D.'s parents to express their concerns about how he was doing, and his girlfriend told him that she didn't want to continue going out with him because he had "gone weird." The day of his arrival at the emergency room, he had begun to cover all the windows in his room with blankets because he was convinced that his music teacher was using radio waves to steal music scores that he had composed.

According to his parents, G.A. had been well until about 7 months prior to the date of his assessment. At that time he had become depressed and had actually voiced some suicidal thoughts. This episode lasted for 6 to 8 weeks, and his parents felt that it was "just something that all teenagers go through." No other premorbid psychiatric disturbance was identified, but the father had a history of major depression, and the mother was being treated for "panic attacks."

A mental status examination showed G.A. to be irritable, grandiose, and dysphoric. His mood state changed rapidly over the course of an hour, and he would become tearful when his recent breakup with his girlfriend was discussed. He was restless, showed pressure of speech, and demonstrated a short attention span. While cognitively intact, he was delusional, believing that his "artistic genius" was unrecognized by the world; he was convinced that "teachers" from his school were trying to steal his ideas. Furthermore, he stated that he felt that his parents might be part of a plot to make sure his music hall was never built, and although he could not explain why this would be the case, he noted that the television news announcer had mentioned this on the previous evening. When he was advised to accept admission to the hospital because his mood and thinking were "a bit off," G.D. picked up an end table and threw it at the assessing physician, exclaiming, "You are part of the plot too."

CASE COMMENTARY

This case illustrates a relatively common presentation of acute-onset mania in an adolescent. The pharmacologic management described later will use this case as its treatment paradigm. Alternative scenarios during the course of treatment will be described, and other possible interventions will be suggested. Although not discussed here, it is understood that proper psychopharmacologic treatment must occur within the context of optimal clinical care, which in the acute case includes hospitalization; provision of a safe and expected environment; appropriate nursing care; academic, functional, and family assessment; personal and family support; education about the illness and its pharmacologic treatment; and careful discharge planning. (For a detailed discussion of these issues see Papatheodarou and Kutcher listed in Suggested Readings at the end of this chapter.) Outpatient treatment follows once the acute phase of the illness has come under control, and similar, although modified, psychosocial interventions continue to be a part of optimal pharmacologic care.

CASE EXAMPLE

Childhood-Onset Bipolar Disorder: Chaos Could Be a Mood Problem

R.D. was a 10-year-old boy who had a long-standing history of severe behavioral problems. He was "always on the go," had a short attention span, and was easily distracted by environmental stimuli. He was aggressive, lashing out at parents, teachers, or peers, often without provocation. As a result, he had few friends, was academically delayed, and had been placed for treatment in a special class designed to control his behavior. This intervention was largely unsuccessful. His mood was mostly that of extreme irritability, and he exhibited frequent temper outbursts. R.D. was also sexually preoccupied, had begun a collection of "adult magazines," and made frequent lewd comments to women he would see on the street or on public transport. A diagnosis of ADHD had been made and treatment with methylphenidate had been attempted. This was discontinued because R.D.'s behavior worsened, and he became frankly paranoid and started to hide knives under his mattress so that he would be able to "get those people when they come after me."

A family psychiatric history identified substance abuse and alcohol abuse in the father, who also had never been able to hold a job for any length of time and was constantly getting involved in new schemes to "get rich quick," none of which were successful. The paternal grandmother had been treated for severe depression with electroconvulsive therapy (ECT), and a paternal uncle had a history of "personality problems" and "trouble with the law." The mother had experienced a postpartum depression after the birth of R.D.'s younger brother, with psychotic symptoms that required hospitalization and treatment with antidepressants and haloperidol. She was described as "unstable" by her treating physician. The paternal grandmother had a history of alcoholism and prescription drug abuse. The history of the paternal grandfather was not known.

TABLE 12-1 **Medications Useful in Treating Child and Adolescent Bipolar Disorder***

| Medication | Acute Treatment | | Prophylaxis |
	Mania	Depression	
Lithium	+	+	+
Valproate	+	?	+
Carbamazepine	+	?	+
Neuroleptics	+	If psychotic only	+
Serotonin-specific reuptake inhibitors	−	+	−
Tricyclic antidepressants	−	?	−

*This table was developed from clinical experience and currently available information regarding the treatment of child and adolescent bipolar disorder. Light therapy and electroconvulsive treatment may also be of benefit in selected cases. These interventions are briefly discussed later in this chapter.

CASE COMMENTARY

This clinical presentation is consistent with a bipolar spectrum problem, which may often be responsive to thymoleptic treatment. It is presented here as a case to illustrate the use of thymoleptics in this population. Information regarding the use of psychotropics in this population is provided using R.D.'s case for illustrative purposes.

Initial Pharmacologic Management

The following medications should be considered for use in treating children and adolescents with bipolar disorder (Table 12–1).

In many cases, including that of the acute-adolescent manic patient described earlier, combination treatment may well be necessary in the early stages of illness. In some cases combined pharmacotherapies will also be necessary over the long term to produce a maximal prophylactic or thera-

peutic effect. In other cases, monotherapy with a thymoleptic may be sufficient. These issues will be discussed later.

In the acute adolescent manic patient described earlier, a low-potency neuroleptic, such as chlorpromazine, and a thymoleptic (either lithium or valproate) should be used (Table 12–2) in choosing a first-line medication. Because of their propensity to induce disinhibition and the lack of demonstrated antimanic efficacy in this population, benzodiazepines are not recommended. The thymoleptics lithium and valproate are discussed in this chapter. Carbamazepine is reviewed in Chapter 16. Neuroleptics are reviewed in Chapters 13 and 14.

Baseline Evaluation

Medical Considerations

Medical considerations are those outlined in Section Two. Of particular importance is the evaluation of those physical parameters that may be affected by pharmacologic treatment. As expected, initial treatment will include low-potency neuroleptics and thymoleptics. The following stan-

TABLE 12-2 **Suggested First-Line Medications for Children and Adolescents with Severe Acute Mania***

Medication	First Choice	Alternate	Alternate
Thymoleptic	Lithium or Valproate	Valproate	Carbamazepine
Neuroleptic	Chlorpromazine	Perphenazine† or Risperidone	Haloperidol or Risperidone

*This table was developed from information derived from clinical experience and currently available literature on the treatment of this disorder. Risperidone has also been used by some clinicians with good results. Its use is discussed in Chapter 13.

†In younger children who exhibit severe behavioral symptoms in need of immediate control but for whom the target dose of chlorpromazine produces severe sedative effects, a moderate-potency antipsychotic, such as perphenazine may be a more reasonable first choice.

dardized baseline physical assessments are suggested:

1. Extrapyramidal Symptom Rating Scale—to assess extrapyramidal symptoms (see Appendix III)
2. Abnormal Involuntary Movement Scale (AIMS)—to assess dyskinetic symptoms (see Appendix III; note that the Extrapyramidal Symptom Rating Scale also allows for the rating of dyskinetic symptoms)
3. Medication-Specific Side Effect Scales (MSSES)—see Appendix IV regarding specific Medication-Specific Side Effect Scales for thymoleptics and neuroleptics

During the acute treatment of severe mania, the patient should be medically assessed daily for the presence of side effects, the management of which is discussed more fully later. Additionally, weekly completion of the above-mentioned rating scales is suggested to allow for more comprehensive monitoring and documentation of the patient's medical condition.

Laboratory Considerations

Laboratory investigations should assess those physiologic parameters that pharmacologic treatment may affect both in the short term and, because chronic treatment may be indicated, in the long term as well. Because expected treatment will include low-potency neuroleptics and thymoleptics (lithium or valproate), the following baseline laboratory measures are suggested:

Lithium

1. Serum electrolytes, blood urea nitrogen, creatinine, calcium
2. Hb, Hct, WBC with differential
3. Free T4, thyroid-stimulating hormone (TSH), thyroid antibodies
4. ECG
5. Pregnancy test for sexually active females

Valproate (Valproic Acid, Sodium Valproate, or Divalproex Sodium)

1. Liver function tests
2. Complete blood count, including WBC with differential and platelets
3. Pregnancy test for sexually active females

Low-Potency Neuroleptics (Chlorpromazine)

1. Liver function tests

Other routine baseline laboratory tests are not necessary unless clozapine is being used. At this time routine use of clozapine is not recommended in the initial pharmacologic treatment of this disorder. It may, however, have a role to play in treatment-resistant cases. For information about the use of clozapine, see Chapters 13 and 14.

There is no medical indication for the routine weekly monitoring of the above-mentioned laboratory parameters during the acute treatment phase. However, if changes in the physical condition of the patient occur (e.g., fever, vomiting, diarrhea) that may indicate a medical condition, either induced by the medication (an adverse reaction) or that may complicate medication use (viral gastroenteritis in teens treated with lithium), then the appropriate laboratory tests should be obtained. Otherwise, a repeat of baseline laboratory measures at the end of 2 weeks of treatment and at discharge from the hospital (or at 6 to 8 weeks if an outpatient) should be sufficient. In adolescent patients presenting with a mixed psychotic-affective picture, a baseline serum and urine drug screen is suggested.

Psychiatric Considerations

Baseline evaluation should include those symptoms that are the target of pharmacologic treatment. The following baseline measures are suggested:

1. Modified Mania Rating Scale (MMRS)—see Appendix VI. As described in Section Two, the MMRS provides a useful rating scale for the evaluation of manic symptoms.
2. Brief Psychiatric Rating Scale (BPRS)—see Appendix VI. As described in Section Two, the BPRS provides a useful rating scale for the global assessment of severe psychiatric pathology, including affective and cognitive symptoms.
3. Overall Clinical Impression (OCI)—see Appendix V. As described in Section II, the OCI provides a useful measure of the patient's global clinical condition.

These rating scales should be repeated weekly during the acute phase of treatment. In most cases, a 10 to 20 percent decrease from baseline in the MMRS or BPRS should be noted within 1 week of initiating combined neuroleptic and thymoleptic pharmacotherapy. Further changes of an additional 10 to 20 percent should be noted within 1 to 2 weeks of attaining steady-state thymoleptic serum levels.

Additionally, various 10 cm Visual Analogue Scales (VAS) can be used to monitor symptoms that are especially problematic for the patient or are under-reported in the above-mentioned scales.

Some target symptoms may be (1) concentration, (2) hypersexuality, (3) ability to tolerate ward milieu, (4) level of agitation, and (5) hours of sleep at night.

Acute treatment should commence with low-potency neuroleptics, and these specific target symptoms should be evaluated twice daily (morning and early evening) and the dose of neuroleptic medications adjusted accordingly. Successful pharmacologic treatment should lead to relatively rapid (within 3 to 7 days) resolution of these target symptoms. The level of agitation and hours of sleep at night provide the most sensitive indicators of early response to neuroleptic medications. During outpatient treatment, other specific target symptoms may arise. These should be identified and monitored using an appropriate VAS as clinically indicated.

Pharmacologic Management of the Acute Phase

Following baseline medical, laboratory, and psychiatric evaluations, treatment should be initiated with a thymoleptic medication. Because this process may take 1 to 2 days and the patient's clinical condition may need immediate pharmacologic intervention, the use of a low-potency neuroleptic such as chlorpromazine is suggested. High-potency neuroleptics should in general be avoided because of their propensity to cause severe dystonic and other extrapyramidal effects in adolescents and young adults, and there is no place for "rapid neuroleptization" techniques using high doses of high-potency compounds in this population.

In addition, the sedative effects of chlorpromazine are often useful in the management of the severely agitated and behaviorally out-of-control manic patient. Acute cardiovascular side effects of postural hypotension are rare but may occur in some individuals. Therefore, heart rate and blood pressure monitoring should be instituted immediately preceding each dose and should be repeated 30 to 45 minutes following the dose. Patients should be instructed not to stand up suddenly from a sitting or prone position. If medication management is complicated by hypotension, a medium-potency neuroleptic such as perphenazine may be substituted. Because hypotension arising secondary to the use of neuroleptics results from antagonism of peripheral alpha^1-adrenergic receptors, epinephrine should not be used in an attempt to correct this. Phenylephrine is useful if severe acute hypotension occurs, although this is unlikely to happen in this age group.

Some clinicians use low doses of high-potency

neuroleptics (1 to 2 mg of haloperidol per day), adding small amounts (1 to 2 mg) of lorazepam for agitation. The reasoning behind this is that low doses of high-potency neuroleptics will be less likely to produce acute dystonic reactions than high doses of high-potency neuroleptics and low doses of benzodiazepines will be less likely to produce disinhibition than high doses of benzodiazepines. Although this approach is not unreasonable, use of a single medication (such as a low-potency antipsychotic) is preferred over the use of two medications. Additionally, often in spite of the best attempts to avoid the use of high doses of high-potency antipsychotics or benzodiazepines, the patient's clinical condition may be such that initial low-dose strategies of these compounds are unsuccessful. Should that occur (and it does), the clinician is faced with the dilemma of increasing the doses of these two compounds to the point that their adverse effect profiles will begin to complicate treatment. Such problems are avoided with the use of a single low-potency antipsychotic medication such as chlorpromazine.

The initial test dose of chlorpromazine should be between 75 and 100 mg by mouth for adolescents and between 25 and 50 mg for children. The patient should then be carefully observed for the effects this dose will have. Interindividual variability in the sedative effects of a single dose of chlorpromazine can be considerable; thus, the dose needs to be tailored to the patient's clinical needs. Additional dose amounts and their optimal spacing during the day should be selected on the basis of the observed clinical effect of the test dose. The all too common practice of prescribing a dose of medication to be given "stat" and repeated routinely at 4-hourly intervals is inappropriate and unsafe pharmacologic treatment. Indeed, during the first phase of acute treatment a physician must be consistently involved in the monitoring of the patient's condition. Once improvement begins and the side effects are well tolerated, the frequency of this monitoring may decrease.

A common issue in medication management of the acute phase is noncompliance. This is particularly common in teenagers. Thus, medications need to be given in the context of a personal therapeutic relationship. The physician and nursing staff should explain the purpose of the medication to the patient and obtain his or her informed consent for its use. The anticipated side effects and hoped for outcome should be made clear to the patient. This should be done in a supportive and reassuring manner. In younger children, and indeed in some teenagers, the assistance of a parent may be helpful when medication is given for the first time. In cases where a child or adolescent is not competent to give informed consent for medication treatment, this should be explained to the patient. In these cases, informed consent should be obtained as soon as reasonably possible from the parent, legal guardian, or other appropriate authority.

Even in the best of personal therapeutic circumstances, adolescents will often "tongue their pills" and file them in the toilet at a convenient later time. Because effective treatment of the acute phase depends on proper medication dosing, the use of tablets to deliver the medication should be avoided as much as possible. The medication should preferably first be given as a liquid followed by a drink of a pleasant-tasting juice. Care needs to be taken that the patient takes the full dose of the medication and does not simply transfer the liquid medication into the following drink. A useful guideline in this situation is to give the patient a small amount of juice initially, followed by more once the medication has been totally ingested. Because the use of liquid chlorpromazine may be associated with glossitis, appropriate mouth care should be instituted concurrently. Liquid medication should be changed to oral tablet form as soon as possible, usually within 2 to 4 days. In some cases, experienced nursing staff have crushed tablets and mixed them with a pleasant-tasting substance, such as jam or honey, as a method of transition from the liquid to the tablet vehicle.

In the context of careful monitoring of the patient's clinical state, early neuroleptic treatment is designed to improve behavioral functioning (to decrease agitation or aggression and modulate excitement) and to normalize physiologic functioning (sleeping, eating, etc.). In the patient with severe disturbance, to best achieve these clinical goals daily dosing should be initiated with the total expected daily dose (a reasonable initial target dose range is 100 to 300 mg daily for children and 200 to 400 mg daily for adolescents, when taken orally) divided over four periods of time. The first dose (75 to 100 mg for teens and 25 to 50 mg for children) should be given in the morning, followed by doses of similar amounts at about noon, late afternoon, and about one-half hour before bed. In addition to this daily dosing schedule, as needed (prn) chlorpromazine can be given if the patient's behavior continues to be out of control. The dose of each prn medication will need to be estimated individually for each patient, taking into account how the patient usually reacts to a particular amount of medication. Because this type of dosing regime will be accompanied by drowsiness, the patient should be informed that this is an expected and positive effect of the medicine to help him or her rest. If this is not done, the adolescent patient, particularly if delusional, may feel that he

or she is being deliberately harmed by the medicine and, as a result, this may lead to noncompliance and intensification of the disturbance.

In some cases, the patient's clinical presentation will not require this strategy of dividing the total daily antipsychotic dose. In these situations, the total or greatest percentage of the amount of antipsychotic medication can be given at bedtime. Should the patient's behavior unexpectedly change during the day, requiring additional pharmacologic intervention, a portion of the usual evening dose can be given during the day, with the appropriate modifications made to the bedtime dose as required.

Careful monitoring of the total daily dose of low-potency antipsychotic medication is essential, and when a good early response to treatment (behavior has improved and physiologic functioning has been largely restored, especially sleeping through the night) has been obtained, the total daily dosage of the neuroleptic medication may be given either as a single dose at bedtime or in two divided doses, one third of the daily dose in the morning and the remainder before bed. In some cases, a slight decrease in the total daily neuroleptic dose is possible at this time, but care should be taken not to decrease the dose too much to avoid a worsening of the patient's clinical state. Gradual discontinuation of the neuroleptic medication should take place as soon as possible and should coincide with the onset of the antimanic action of the chosen thymoleptic, as discussed later.

Although the oral route for the use of antipsychotic medications is preferred, at times the patient's clinical state is such that intramuscular (IM) neuroleptic medications are necessary. Again, it is important to remember that these too must be given within the context of a supportive therapeutic environment, and the patient must be informed of the purpose of the medicine, how it will affect him or her, and how it is to be administered. Injections should preferably be given in the upper outer quadrant of the buttocks, and at times gentle but firm face-down restraint may be necessary to allow this to occur. Orthostatic hypotension may be more common following IM compared with oral use of chlorpromazine, and the patient should be nursed in a supine or seated state until the post-dose blood pressure reading has been taken. Children and adolescents who require IM injections are often very frightened, and at times the IM injection can be avoided by "talking the patient down" and using oral medicine instead. Even when an IM is used, it is important to keep reassuring and supporting the patient before, during, and for some time after the injection.

The usual dose of IM chlorpromazine is 25 mg

in children and 50 mg in adolescents, and this treatment modality should be used as sparingly as possible. The clinician should remember that these injections are painful and sometimes can be associated with injection-site problems, including redness, swelling, and occasionally abscesses. Often, if appropriate patient monitoring is in place, the use of oral prn medication (as described earlier) as the patient's behavior begins to escalate will improve the situation sufficiently so that IM injections are not needed. In any case, IM injections of neuroleptics should not be telephone ordered by the physician. The physician should be on site to evaluate the patient's clinical state and should be present when the IM is used.

Although the use of low-potency neuroleptics is associated with fewer extrapyramidal side effects than high-potency neuroleptics, children and teenagers treated with low-potency compounds do experience extrapyramidal side effects. In some cases, when high daily doses (over 500 mg of chlorpromazine) are used (e.g., in the severely agitated manic teenager), extrapyramidal side effects can become quite disabling, even with low-potency neuroleptics. In addition, acute dystonic reactions can occur with the use of these compounds. Because treatment compliance and patient comfort are both negatively affected if moderate to severe extrapyramidal side effects or even mild dystonic reactions are experienced, it is prudent to coadminister an antiparkinsonian agent concurrently with the onset of neuroleptic treatment.

A number of antiparkinsonian agents are available for use, and each medication has its particular therapeutic and side effect profile, although there is considerable overlap (see Chapter 13). To prevent dystonic reactions and at the same time offer a relatively well-tolerated medication with a useful antitremor and antirigidity effect, procyclidine is suggested. This compound tends to have fewer anticholinergic effects than benztropine and trihexyphenidyl, and is generally quite effective and well tolerated in the child and adolescent population. The standard oral starting dose is 5 mg once daily, but 5 mg twice daily may be a more reasonable starting dose in the agitated adolescent in whom higher doses of low-potency neuroleptics are expected to be used. Doses of up to 30 mg daily may be used if clinically indicated.

Acute dystonic reactions, if they occur, will require immediate intervention. In these cases, benztropine 2 mg or diphenhydramine 25 to 50 mg can be given IM. Severe cases may benefit from diazepam, which can be combined with IM benztropine if necessary. Diazepam can be given intravenously at a dose of 5 to 10 mg (5 mg in children) by slow infusion (maximal 5 mg per minute for teens and 5 mg over 2 minutes for children). It should not be given IM.

Akathisia is a common side effect of neuroleptic use in this age group and in its milder forms is probably found in a significant number of children and adolescents undergoing treatment with antipsychotics. Manifesting itself early on in treatment, akathisia can be incorrectly identified as a worsening of the psychiatric disorder instead of a side effect of neuroleptic treatment (see Chapter 13 for a more detailed discussion). A careful clinical assessment for akathisia should be made daily during the acute treatment phase and should include a physical examination and direct questioning about such symptoms as "shaky legs," "butterflies in the stomach," "itchy muscles," and "feeling turned on inside." Conducting an interview with the patient standing quietly can often identify the restless pacing symptoms found in akathisia. This is especially important in young children or adolescents, who may not be able to verbalize what they are experiencing.

Many antiparkinsonian medications have little or no effect in ameliorating akathisia. However, a number of compounds (beta-blockers and benzodiazepines, see Chapter 13) are available that can be helpful in many cases. Of these only the benzodiazepine clonazepam has been studied in adolescents, in whom it has been shown to be quite effective. A dose of 0.25 mg given twice daily (total of 0.5 mg daily) is usually sufficient to provide adequate symptom control. In some cases, however, doses of up to 1.0 or 2.0 mg daily may be needed. Care must be taken at these higher doses to avoid inducing the behavioral side effect of disinhibition, which may be relatively common in children and adolescents treated with benzodiazepines.

The initial pharmacologic treatment of severe mania is as follows:

1. Determine diagnosis and perform necessary laboratory investigations and baseline symptom and side effect evaluations.
2. Educate patient and family about the disorder and its treatment.
3. Develop and maintain a respectful therapeutic relationship with patient and family.
4. If clinically indicated for psychotic agitation, use a low-potency neuroleptic such as chlorpromazine (avoid high doses of high-potency neuroleptics and rapid neuroleptization techniques).
5. Target behavioral control and restoration of physiologic functioning as early treatment goals.
6. Give concurrent antiparkinsonian medication, such as procyclidine for prophylaxis against severe dystonia.

7. Carefully monitor the patient's clinical condition daily, including side effects and compliance with pharmacotherapy.
8. Watch for akathisia and treat aggressively if it appears using low-dose clonazepam or propranolol.
9. Begin a thymoleptic.

Treatment of Mania Presenting with Less Severe Symptomatology

Not all manic episodes will present with the severity described in the first case example. In many cases, less severe presentations will occur. In these cases, some of the treatment suggestions made earlier may need to be altered. The clinician should consider the following questions in cases of mania presenting with less severe symptomatology:

1. Can neuroleptic treatment be avoided altogether?
2. If some neuroleptic treatment is necessary, can it be used occasionally instead of on a daily basis?
3. If some neuroleptic treatment is necessary, can a less sedating compound than chlorpromazine be used?

Modifications to the suggested management of the severe acute manic episode can then be made, given the answers to these questions.

Treating Acute Mania: Use of Thymoleptics

Thymoleptics are usually introduced within 2 to 3 days following hospital admission once the necessary diagnostic and laboratory procedures have been completed. They have a slower onset of antimanic effect compared with neuroleptics and in many cases need to be combined with neuroleptics during the initial treatment of the acute phase.

A number of thymoleptic medications are available for use, but only lithium and divalproex sodium have undergone some systematic evaluation in children or adolescents. Thus, the following discussion will be limited to these two compounds. Carbamazepine is a possible alternative thymoleptic treatment and has been the subject of a number of case reports. It may have particular utility in treating children and adolescents whose bipolar illness has onset following central nervous system trauma, and its clinical use is described in Chapter 16. A clinical consideration regarding carbamazepine's use in treating acute mania in teenagers is its potential interaction with neu-

roleptics to produce neurotoxic side effects, such as diploplia, ataxia, and delirious states.

Lithium

Lithium is well established as a treatment for acute mania and the prophylaxis of future affective episodes in adults. Its efficacy, however, is probably diminished in those patients with a previous history of a poor response to lithium treatment, and in patients in whom the manic episode is of the rapid-cycling or mixed-state type. There is also evidence that lithium may be less effective in the presence of significant medical or psychiatric comorbidity, so-called complicated mania. Alternative treatments, such as valproate, may be more useful in these clinical presentations. In adolescents, the rapid-cycling or mixed clinical picture is the most common presentation of mania and comorbid states are common. Thus, the possibly lower overall response rate to lithium in young bipolar patients, as suggested by some clinicians and investigators, is consistent with the decreased efficacy of lithium described in similar adult populations. This, however, awaits rigorous confirmation and a rich, albeit uncontrolled, literature regarding the use of lithium in children and adolescents with bipolar disorder is available.

Lithium has a number of well-described neurobiologic effects, but the exact mechanism of its efficacy in mania is not known. Its onset of action is 7 to 14 days and its full efficacy (at therapeutic serum levels of 1.0 to 1.2 mEq/L) may take 6 to 8 weeks to be appreciated in children and adolescents. This is somewhat longer than that expected for adults, in whom 4 to 5 weeks at therapeutic serum levels is more usual. Lithium is perhaps less effective as a single medication treatment of acute depressions and for the prophylaxis of future depressive episodes compared with its efficacy in the acute treatment and prophylaxis of mania.

The side effect profile of lithium presents potential problems for long-term compliance in children and adolescents, especially its dermatologic and weight gain potential. Lithium use can exacerbate acne, and teenagers treated with lithium over the long term tend to experience significant weight gain. Both these side effects may have a considerable negative impact on the body image of adolescent patients. In spite of these considerations, however, because its therapeutic and tolerability effects are well known, it remains a reasonable first choice of antimanic agent in this population.

If lithium is selected as the thymoleptic of choice, treatment should begin with an initial test dose of 300 mg. If this is well tolerated, a daily dose of 900 mg may be immediately instituted in the adolescent patient. If side effects occur, this can be given as a 300 mg three times daily strategy for 1 week and thereafter given as one dose at bedtime. Although algorithms for use in predicting total daily dose from a first-dose lithium serum measure are available, in routine clinical use they offer little significant advantage over the tried and true "reach 900 mg daily and hold it for 5 days" strategy (see Table 12–3). Further dose increments should be made to titrate to the maximal extent of the suggested therapeutic range (1.0 to 1.2 mEq/L) as side effects permit.

In children, slightly slower dosage increments may be associated with fewer side effects and will allow for closer monitoring of serum levels. In these cases, a test dose of 150 mg of lithium can be followed by a dose schedule of 150 mg given twice daily (or 300 mg given once daily) for 2 days, with an increase to 300 mg given twice daily on the next day. At that time it is reasonable to maintain the dose over 1 week, obtain a serum level, and increase the dose using the same strategy as described earlier. Once the total daily dose necessary to obtain serum levels of 1.0 to 1.2 mEq/L are obtained, the medication can be given in one evening dose. Attempts should be made to titrate the lithium dose to the maximal extent of the suggested therapeutic range as side effects permit.

Serum lithium levels must be measured at the trough in the concentration curve, which occurs 9 to 14 hours following the last dose. Because the half-life of lithium varies greatly and can last up to 24 hours or more, even with the increased clearance and shorter half-life found with this compound in children and young adolescents, serum lithium levels should only be obtained 5 days following the last dose adjustment to ensure that the steady state has been reached. More frequent lithium determinations may inadvertently lead to overdosing because the serum lithium level obtained will not reflect steady state but rather a point on the ascending lithium level curve.

Although salivary lithium levels may be available in some centers, their routine use is not recommended because of the variability of these measures and the narrow therapeutic index of lithium. An exception to this may be made for those children or adolescents in whom multiple paired determinations of lithium serum and saliva measures have been made and the range of variance has been established. This is impractical or not possible in many cases. For those children who find venipuncture very distressing, topical analgesic creams may be of value. If the practitioner elects to use salivary lithium measures, care must be taken to correlate salivary with serum levels prior to using salivary lithium levels alone as a measure of lithium concentration.

Target serum levels should be set at 1.0 to 1.2 mEq/L for acute-phase treatment and should be reached within 8 to 10 days of beginning the medication. It is suggested that the clinician attempt to target the upper rather than the lower portions of this range using side effects as a guide. When the patient's total daily dose has been stabilized, once or twice a day dosing can be used in many cases. If this strategy is employed, it is useful to give either the total or the largest percentage of the total daily dose (66 to 75 percent) of the medication at bedtime to limit the experience of adverse effects, which often coincides with the peak serum lithium concentration. If gastrointestinal (GI) side effects are a problem, a slow-release preparation may be used, in which case, if a single dosing strategy is being employed, the dose should be given 2 to 3 hours prior to bedtime. If nocturnal enuresis is a problem, a slow-release preparation may be helpful. Alternatively, giving the major portion of the total daily dose earlier in the day may be necessary.

Lithium's therapeutic efficacy should become apparent within 7 to 14 days of achieving target serum levels. If a patient is not showing improvement by this time, a review of diagnosis and treatment is indicated. If lithium serum levels are within the therapeutic target range and improvement is not noticed, particular attention should be paid to identifying possible behavioral toxicity or extrapyramidal side effects, such as akathisia arising from excessive neuroleptic use. The full therapeutic effect of lithium is unlikely to be obtained before six continuous weeks of treatment following the attainment of therapeutic serum levels, and thus de-

TABLE 12–3 Suggested Lithium Dosing Schedule for Children and Adolescents

Age Group	Test Dose	Initial Target Dose	Introduction Strategy	Serum Level (mEq/L)
Adolescents	300 mg	900 mg/day	900 mg daily, 300 mg tid if side effects	1.0–1.2
Children	150 mg	600 mg/day	150 mg bid or 300 mg qhs	1.0–1.2

cisions to alter pharmacologic therapy with lithium (given maximization of dose) in the patient who is showing only a partial treatment response should wait for completion of an adequate treatment trial (serum level 1.0 to 1.2 mEq/L for 6 weeks).

When lithium and neuroleptic treatment are combined, the risk of neurotoxic and extrapyramidal side effects may be increased. Furthermore, the physician should also be aware of a possibly increased incidence of neuroleptic malignant syndrome (NMS) with combined treatment. This is discussed more fully in Chapter 13. However, if the patient develops severe muscular rigidity or autonomic instability, as demonstrated by heart rate and blood pressure changes, it is prudent to discontinue the neuroleptic immediately and begin careful medical monitoring. The appearance of fever is often found later in the development of NMS and early aggressive intervention, as described in Chapter 13, may prevent the full expression of the syndrome.

Education about the proper use of lithium is essential (see Section Three). Lithium has a narrow therapeutic index, and a number of conditions may arise during lithium treatment that have the potential to raise lithium serum levels to toxic concentrations. Particularly problematic are situations in which excessive sodium loss occurs, such as vomiting or diarrhea. In such cases, lithium retention takes place at the renal level, and if volume depletion is also present, serum lithium levels may rise rapidly, particularly in younger children. Furthermore, patients should be instructed to always maintain adequate salt and fluid intake, and to avoid beginning any special diets without consulting their psychopharmacologist first. This is especially important in adolescent girls, who may attempt to counter lithium-induced weight gain by food restriction strategies that are of dubious nutritional value.

Patients and their families must understand the rationale behind the dosing strategy and be instructed not to double up on their lithium dose if one is missed. Possible drug-drug interactions must also be identified. Perhaps the most important of these in the child and adolescent population are the increased chance of lithium toxicity when some antibiotics, especially ampicillin, are concurrently prescribed (because of decreased renal clearance of lithium), decreased serum lithium levels that arise secondary to enhanced lithium clearance when bronchodilators such as aminophylline and theophylline are used, and decreased serum levels of lithium secondary to increased excretion following heavy use of xanthine derivatives such as coffee.

Some over-the-counter medications may also affect serum lithium levels. Compounds such as the nonsteroidal anti-inflammatory ibuprofen (often used for relief of menstruation-associated distress) or diuretics (often used by adolescent girls as a weight control strategy) should be avoided. If analgesia is needed, alternatives are available, and teenagers should be advised not to use diuretics for weight control. This is particularly important in this population because lithium is well known to lead to significant weight gain.

A medication education component to inpatient treatment, meducation (see Appendix II), is a good place to begin to educate patients and their families about lithium. In addition, a lithium-specific Medication Information Form (see Appendix II) given to patients and parents as a handout is a useful memory aid that will also come in handy during outpatient treatment.

Side effects of lithium in children and adolescents are generally similar to those found in adults, except for the increased frequency of weight gain and acne, and the decreased frequency of tremors. Although many side effects are possible, the following are much more commonly found: nausea, polyuria, weight gain, diarrhea, polydipsia, acne, abdominal distress, tremor, and headache. These side effects, particularly the GI ones, may occur when lithium treatment is initiated or when doses are increased. These can be best managed by either increasing the dose more slowly or by changing to a different preparation of lithium, such as a slow-release or liquid form. Polyuria and polydipsia may also occur, but usually at higher doses. A reduction in daily dosage will often lessen these side effects. If dose reduction is not feasible, adding the potassium-sparing diuretic amiloride may decrease urine volume without significantly increasing serum lithium levels, which may occur if thiazide diuretics are used for this purpose. A dose of 5 mg given twice daily is usually sufficient, although amounts of up to 10 mg twice daily can be used. Even with this choice of diuretic, however, it is essential that serum lithium levels be frequently monitored.

An action tremor of 7 to 16 Hz is relatively uncommon in lithium-treated children and adolescents. This can become apparent at times of increased anxiety or when activities requiring fine motor movements are required. In these cases, propranolol (at doses of 10 to 20 mg), given one-half hour prior to the expected activity, may be used. A trial run prior to the expected activity or event should be instituted if possible to determine the minimum effective dose and to ensure that no significant adverse effects from the use of propranolol occur. If action tremor is a significant ongoing problem, divided daily doses of propranolol

(20 to 40 mg daily) or atenolol (50 mg daily) can be used.

Although uncommon in the short term, the long-term side effects of lithium on the thyroid are well known, and monitoring of thyroid function should take place, as noted earlier. Although increases in TSH from baseline levels are commonly found, true hypothyroidism is quite rare, especially in children or adolescents. Elevated levels of thyroid antibodies may signify thyroid gland damage, which might predispose patients to lithium-induced thyroid dysfunction. Thus, it is suggested that thyroid antibodies be measured at baseline. Should these be abnormal, it is reasonable to provide more frequent thyroid monitoring during long-term treatment. Elevations of TSH should be followed up with T4, free T4, and T3 determinations, and if these levels are outside normal values or have decreased significantly from baseline, an endocrine consultation should be considered. It must be remembered that even frank hypothyroidism may be well managed using thyroid replacement treatment if the patient is showing an excellent long-term response to lithium.

Significant cardiac side effects (such as arrhythmias) caused by lithium in the child and adolescent population are rare, although electrocardiographic changes (T wave flattening or inversions) may be common. A clinically insignificant benign leukocytosis is common, and when it occurs it should not routinely prompt further hematologic investigations.

Dermatologic reactions, especially acne, are commonly found in teens treated with lithium. They present as monomorphic eruptions covering portions of the face, neck, shoulder, and back. These should be treated with the usual antiacne therapies, and the clinician might consider the prophylactic use of a topical antibiotic, such as clindamycin, if this is likely to be a compliance-limiting side effect in a teenager who has shown an excellent clinical response to lithium.

Weight gain may also be a problem, with some studies showing about 25 to 40 percent of adolescents (mostly females) showing a weight gain of 20 to 30 pounds with long-term (more than 3 months) lithium treatment. Although this may be a direct result of lithium's insulin-like effect on carbohydrate metabolism, often this can be related to polydipsia, in which the child or adolescent uses high calorie drinks, such as fruit juices or sodas, to quench his or her thirst. This possibility should be clearly addressed when lithium therapy is initiated, and patients should be advised to drink water or diet drinks to quench their thirst.

If significant weight gain does occur, it is important to carefully evaluate this potentially reversible fluid intake activity. A daily drink diary (maintained over 3 to 4 days) in which the patient logs the date, time, amount, and type of fluid consumed will be necessary to evaluate this phenomenon properly. Simply asking the child or adolescent to recall or estimate how much and what was drunk over the preceding 4 to 5 days usually leads to significant under-reporting. In many cases simply switching from high calorie to low calorie (diet drinks) or noncaloric (water) fluids may lead to a significant decline in lithium-associated weight gain. Although nutritional consultation is often suggested, clinical experience indicates that this rarely is effective beyond the simple measure just outlined.

Although there is some controversy about this issue, lithium may have some teratogenetic potential, with possibly an increased incidence of cardiac abnormalities in children of women treated with lithium during pregnancy. Thus, if possible, lithium should be avoided in pregnancy and a negative serum pregnancy test should be identified prior to initiating lithium treatment in adolescent females.

Renal problems secondary to long-term lithium use in adult populations have been identified, although recent studies demonstrate that in the absence of lithium intoxication and the maintenance of serum lithium levels within the suggested therapeutic range, no significant negative effect on glomerular filtration rate has been noted. Polyuria secondary to decreased urinary concentration is common. Sufficient study of this issue has not taken place in children or adolescents, although the data that are available tend to support the findings reported in adults. Prudent clinical practice suggests that monitoring of renal functioning using determination of specific gravity and a calculated creatinine clearance is reasonable.

Lithium is known to affect bone metabolism. The significance of this is not clear, and routine monitoring of serum calcium is not indicated. Adequate calcium nutrition, particularly in adolescent girls, should be actively promoted. Cognitive effects (memory and processing speed) of lithium have been described in adults in some but not all studies. None have been reported in children and adolescents, although few investigations have addressed this issue.

Lithium toxicity is a serious medical problem and should be suspected if signs of neurotoxicity, such as muscular irritability, hyperreflexia, ataxia, and dysarthria, appear. Delirium is a late manifestation and can precede stupor and seizures. Death can occur, and survivors of severe toxicity may exhibit long-term neurologic sequelae, such as cerebellar ataxia and memory impairment. If even mild toxicity is suspected, a blood sample for immediate evaluation of serum lithium level should be drawn and the medication discontinued. If serum lithium levels are over 2.5 mEq/L, aggressive medical intervention should be started and hospitalization or monitoring in the emergency room should be considered, even if the patient looks relatively well clinically. In the case of an overdose, vomiting should be induced and continuous gastric aspiration can be helpful. Saline diuresis with monitoring of electrolytes is also recommended. If serum levels approach 4 mEq/L, hemodialysis should be undertaken. If this is not available, peritoneal dialysis is useful, although not as effective. Frequent monitoring of serum lithium levels is necessary to determine when dialysis may be terminated because serum levels will rise after an initial drop because of re-equilibration from body tissues.

Because lithium toxicity can sometimes be confused with alcohol toxicity, the physician confronted with a lithium-treated child or adolescent who seems to have, or is reported to have, overused alcohol should never assume that the presentation is caused by alcohol. In all cases, serum lithium should be tested, and it is better to err on the side of caution and assume the symptoms are caused by lithium toxicity until proven otherwise. Because of its narrow therapeutic index and fatality risk in overdose, careful evaluation of a patient's suicidal potential must be made prior to and during lithium treatment. If the clinician feels that a suicide attempt is highly probable, then alternative treatments to lithium should be prescribed, either neuroleptics, valproate, or electroconvulsive therapy (ECT) (see later).

Drug-drug interactions are common with lithium. A list of the more common clinically significant interactions is provided in Table 12–4. Because the potential drug-drug interactions with lithium are so numerous, it is best to advise the patient and his or her family that no new medications, including over-the-counter drugs, should be taken without prior consultation (at least by telephone) with the prescribing physician. The use of a medic-alert bracelet is also recommended.

Lithium-treated patients should be instructed as to which side effects need to be reported immediately to their physician. Because verbal instructions are sometimes forgotten, the patient and parent should be provided with a short written form reviewing this (Figure 12–1). In some cases, the clinician may choose to add this form to the lithium-specific Medication Monitoring Form (see Appendix II) and provide both as handouts.

Valproate

Valproate is used to describe one or more of the following: valproic acid, sodium valproate, or divalproex sodium. It is relatively rapidly absorbed on an empty stomach but when given with meals (which will decrease potential side effects of nausea and vomiting) absorption is delayed and it takes up to 5 or 6 hours to reach peak serum levels. Valproate has a half-life of 8 to 18 hours and thus twice-daily dosing is indicated.

Valproate is well absorbed orally, is highly protein bound, and undergoes hepatic metabolism. None of its metabolites are known to be active in its thymoleptic effect. Unlike carbamazepine, it

TABLE 12–4   **Common Clinically Significant Lithium Drug-Drug Interactions***

Drug Class	Interaction†
Anesthetic	Increased serum lithium levels
Antibiotics	Increased serum lithium levels
Antihypertensives	Increased or decreased serum lithium levels
Benzodiazepines	Increased sexual dysfunction
Bronchodilator	Decreased serum lithium levels
Calcium channel blockers	Increased neurotoxicity, cardiotoxicity
Iodide salt	Hypothyroidism risk
Nonsteroidal anti-inflammatories	Increased serum lithium levels
Neuroleptics	Increased neurotoxicity, neuroleptic malignant syndrome
Serotonin-specific reuptake inhibitors	Increased serum lithium levels, serotonin syndrome
Theophylline	Decreased serum lithium levels
Urinary alkalizers	Decreased serum lithium levels

*This table has been adapted from Bezchlibnyk-Butler KZ, Jeffries JJ, Martin BA. Clinical Handbook of Psychotropic Drugs (6th rev ed). Seattle: Hogrefe & Huber Publishers, 1996, with permission.

†Those drug-drug interactions that increase serum lithium levels have the potential to cause increased lithium toxicity. Those drug-drug interactions that decrease serum lithium levels may lead to decreased therapeutic efficacy of lithium. If these drug combinations are used, more frequent monitoring and subsequent adjustments of daily lithium doses will be necessary.

Lithium treatment may be associated with a number of side effects. Although many of these can be uncomfortable, they are rarely dangerous and can be discussed with your doctor at your next visit. Some side effects can be a serious medical problem and need to be addressed immediately. If you experience one or more of the symptoms listed below, please contact your doctor immediately. If your doctor is not available, please contact the physician covering for him or her or go to your nearest hospital emergency room. If you will be seeing a physician other than your usual doctor, please bring your medications and a copy of this form with you.

Difficulty with balance

Confusion

Slurred speech

Severe tremors

Convulsions

Current daily lithium dose: _____

Date current lithium dose begun: _____

Concurrent medications (daily doses): _____

_____

Doctor's name: _____

Doctor's telephone number: _____

FIGURE 12–1   Side Effect Reporting Form: Lithium Treatment

does not appear to have the property of inducing its own metabolism. It has been reported to inhibit the metabolism of a number of drugs that are metabolized by the hepatic P-450 system. The common drug-drug interactions of valproate are listed in Table 12–5. Optimal serum levels to produce a thymoleptic effect have not been established, although in current clinical practice the levels determined for seizure control (50 to 100 mg/mL in both children and adolescents) is used. Saliva valproate monitoring is not appropriate for direct treatment.

Although less well studied than lithium in both acute and prophylactic treatment of mania in adults, valproate nevertheless seems to be as effective as lithium and may be relatively better tolerated. Additionally, it may be more effective in those manic states that are characterized by rapid-cycling or mixed-state clinical presentations. It has recently been assessed in open trials of manic adolescents, where it has been found to be quite effective as an antimanic agent in the short term. No long-term studies in the child or adolescent bipolar population are available, although it has been extensively used in the long-term treatment of childhood seizure disorders and in a number of adolescent bipolar patients.

If valproate is selected as the treatment of choice,

TABLE 12–5   Common Clinically Significant Drug-Drug Interactions with Valproate

Medication	Interaction Effect
Erythromycin	Increased valproate levels
Phenobarbital	Increased phenobarbital levels
Primidone	Increased primidone levels
Carbamazepine	Possible changes in carbamazepine levels
Phenytoin	Increased phenytoin levels; toxicity caused by protein binding displacement
Tricyclics	Increased TCA plasma levels
Serotonin-specific reuptake inhibitors	Increased valproate plasma levels
Alcohol or benzodiazepines	Increased sedation, possible disorientation
Cimetidine	Increased half-life of valproate
Neuroleptics	Potentially increased neurotoxicity, sedation, extrapyramidal effect
Salicylates	Increased plasma levels of valproate

Adapted from Bezchlibnyk-Butler KZ, Jeffries JJ, Martin BA. Clinical Handbook of Psychotropic Drugs (6th rev ed). Seattle: Hogrefe & Huber Publishers, 1996, with permission.

the dosage in adolescents should begin with a 250 mg test dose (see Table 12–6). If this is well tolerated, the dose should be increased to 250 mg, three times daily (750 mg per day). This dose should then be increased gradually over 2 to 3 days to obtain a total daily target dose of 1000 to 1250 mg per day given in divided doses (two or three times daily). Most adolescents will require doses between 1000 and 2500 mg per day to achieve serum levels of 50 to 100 mg/mL (350 to 700 mmol/L), which is considered to be the putative therapeutic range.

Children will require similar but lower total daily doses. In children a test dose of valproate of 100 mg should be given. Following this, treatment should begin at a dose of 100 mg given either two or three times a day. This dose should be gradually increased to obtain a total daily target dose of about 1000 to 1200 mg. Once this is reached, valproate serum levels should be obtained and further dose titrations should be determined to obtain serum levels within the 50 to 100 mg/mL range. In both children and adolescents, clinicians should try to target the upper third of the suggested serum level, as allowed by side effects. Valproate's clinical efficacy should become apparent within 2 to 3 weeks of attaining a therapeutic serum level. The maximal clinical response usually occurs at 6 to 8 weeks in children and adolescents following attainment of steady-state serum levels.

Serum valproate levels must be measured at the trough in the concentration curve, which occurs 8 to 16 hours following the last dose. Serum valproate levels should be obtained 5 days following the last dose adjustment to ensure that steady state has been reached. More frequent valproate determinations may inadvertently lead to overdosing because the serum level obtained will not reflect steady state.

Although valproate therapy may be associated with a number of side effects, many are quite infrequently seen, particularly with monotherapy. The more common side effects of valproate treatment are: sedation, thrombocytopenia, transient hair loss, nausea, weight gain, tremor, vomiting, and increased appetite. If introduction of valproate treatment is associated with the appearance of treatment-emergent adverse events, the dose increases should be slowed down somewhat. Both GI effects and excessive sedation are best managed in this manner. In many patients, these side effects seem to wear off after 2 to 3 weeks. Transient increases in hepatic enzymes are common and of little clinical significance, although hepatotoxicity should be suspected if associated signs and symptoms occur. Fatal hepatotoxicity in a small number of children under the age of 10 years has occasionally been reported, and if this medication is chosen for use in that age group it will be necessary to monitor hepatic function more frequently. Some clinicians suggest that valproate is contraindicated in children under 3 years of age.

Because neural tube defects have been reported with valproate, its use should be avoided in pregnant women, particularly during the first trimester. Thrombocytopenia and platelet dysfunction are common but rarely of clinical significance. If surgery is planned, stopping the medication 3 to 4 weeks prior to surgery may be considered, although this is not usually necessary.

In adolescents, transient hair loss and weight gain can be problematic. If it occurs, hair loss may be successfully managed using zinc supplements. Weight gain is more difficult to control and may be caused by a direct hypothalamic effect of valproate. Recent data suggest that over 50 percent of adolescent girls treated with valproate gained significant amounts of weight on this medication over a year. In anticipation of this problem, a calorie-reduced diet, especially the substitution of low- for high-calorie snacks (celery instead of potato chips) and diet drinks, plus a prescribed program of daily physical activity, may be helpful.

Drug-drug interactions with valproate are perhaps somewhat less common than with lithium. Nevertheless, the possibilities are considerable. A list of those most probably seen in a general clinical psychiatric practice with children and adolescents is found in Table 12–5.

TABLE 12–6 **Suggested Valproate Dosing Schedule for Children and Adolescents***

Age Group	Test Dose	Initial Target Dose	Introduction Strategy	Serum Level (mg/ml)
Adolescents	250 mg	1000–2500 mg daily	750 mg daily in divided doses	50–100
Children	125 mg	1000–1200 mg daily	125 mg bid or tid	50–100

*The guidelines contained in this table have been suggested on the basis of clinical and research experience and the currently available literature regarding the use of valproate in children and adolescents. Individual patients may require modification of these guidelines. Actual individual dosing will need to take into consideration the patient's unique clinical response (adverse effects and therapeutic response).

Patients and their parents will need to be properly instructed about which valproate-associated side effects should be immediately reported to the attention of their treating physician. Because verbal information is not optimally retained, providing succinct written instructions about this issue is recommended (Figure 12–2). The Side Effect Reporting Form for Valproate Treatment may be a useful attachment to the Medication Monitoring Form previously described. This package can then be used as a patient and parent handout as part of the education program regarding the illness and its treatment. Patients should also be advised to wear a medic alert bracelet.

The use of thymoleptics in the treatment of acute mania in children and adolescents can be summarized as follows:

1. Patient and family should be educated about the various choices of thymoleptic treatments and their known and expected efficacy, side effects, and course of action.
2. Either lithium or valproate (divalproex sodium) is suggested.
3. Careful monitoring of the patient's clinical condition and side effects is required.
4. Appropriate dosages, proper serum levels, and sufficient time for optimal antimanic effects (6 to 8 weeks) to occur are essential.
5. Adjunctive use of low-potency neuroleptics may be necessary at the onset of thymoleptic treatment and should be gradually tapered over time as the antimanic effect of thymoleptics develops.

Common Acute Treatment Issues

A number of practical issues arise during the treatment of mania in children and adolescents. These are addressed using the following case examples.

CASE EXAMPLE

Why Is It Taking So Long?

After 3 weeks of in-hospital treatment (including lithium, activity support, and milieu therapy along with illness, support, and medication education for the patient and his family), G.A. was showing some clinical improvement. His MMRS score was 64 (his baseline was 76), and his BPRS score was 25 (his baseline was 32). His behavior had improved, he was much less agitated, and he was sleeping and eating well. His parents were upset that he was "not getting better faster" and demanded that the treating team "change the medications or something."

Treatment with valproate may be associated with side effects. Although many side effects are not dangerous to you, even if they are uncomfortable, a number of possible side effects should be reported immediately to your doctor if you experience them. Most patients will not experience any of these side effects; however, if you do experience one or more of these, please telephone your doctor immediately. If your doctor is not available, either speak to whomever is covering for him or her or go to your nearest hospital emergency room. If you see any doctor other than your regular physician, remember to take your medication bottles and this sheet with you. This will help the doctor who you do see evaluate your condition better. If you experience the following, call right away:

Heavy bruising with minimal trauma

Spontaneous bleeding

Severe abdominal pain

Jaundice (yellow tint to your skin)

Your daily dose of valproate: _____

Date your treatment with valproate was initiated: _____

Concurrent medications (daily dose): _____

Your doctor's name: _____

Your doctor's phone number: _____

FIGURE 12–2 Side Effect Reporting Form: Valproate Treatment

CASE COMMENTARY

This case illustrates a common issue arising early on in the acute treatment of a manic teen. The early period (about 2½ to 3 weeks following the onset of lithium treatment) is often characterized by minimal or mild clinical improvement or a relative plateau in the clinical course. The lithium treatment has usually just recently resulted in the attainment of a therapeutic serum level, and the early therapeutic effects have not yet been fully realized. This "lithium doldrum" is often associated with staff or parent demands to "do something else," with the feeling that the current treatment is not working. Prior to beginning lithium treatment, both patient and family need to know this may occur and to understand the anticipated time line for clinical improvement. In G.A.'s case, clinical improvement had occurred, but more time was necessary for further improvement.

The proper management of this stage is to make sure that serum lithium levels are within the therapeutic range and to hold tight. Increased support for the patient and family are indicated, and exploration of their concerns and fears with continued reassurance, as well as a careful repeat explanation about the expected response time with lithium treatment, is necessary. Often the family will need to be seen more frequently, and daily contact with a single staff member will help provide the needed psychotherapeutic environment. Abrupt changes in treatment are to be avoided, but offering a time frame for a treatment review if the clinical state does not improve (1 to 1½ weeks is suggested) will help provide a framework for defining patient and family expectations.

CASE EXAMPLE

"He's all better, so let's cut back on the medications."

G.A. had been hospitalized for 18 days. He demonstrated an initial rapid improvement in his acute manic symptoms. G.A.'s MMRS scores had decreased from 76 at baseline to 48 at the end of the second treatment week, and his BPRS scores had dropped from 32 to 19. His serum lithium levels had been 1.0 mEq/L during the previous week. G.A., his parents, and the treatment staff were very pleased with his progress, and a review of his medications was suggested. His daily chlorpromazine dose (500 mg at bedtime) was discontinued at the staff Thursday morning case review meeting because he was doing so well that it was believed he did not need antipsychotic medications and he complained of being sleepy in the mornings. When assessed on the following Monday, G.A.'s symptoms had worsened (his MMRS was now 63 and his BPRS was 33), and everyone was worried about his "relapse."

CASE COMMENTARY

This issue identifies a classic case of discontinuing an effective treatment because it is effective. Because lithium's antimanic effect is not expected to manifest itself before 2 weeks at adequate serum levels, the patient's symptoms were mostly being controlled by the neuroleptic medication he was taking. The treatment team was overzealous in discontinuing the neuroleptic too quickly and too early in the course of treatment, thus removing the antimanic pharmacologic effects of the neuroleptic before the lithium had taken effect. Sometimes this urge to discontinue neuroleptic medications is driven in part by the mistaken belief that these compounds are only antipsychotics and that their effect in treating mania is only sedative. Sometimes this occurs because staff or family incorrectly think that taking a neuroleptic even for a short period of time will cause long-term damage to the patient.

A more appropriate response would have been to educate the patient and family about the delayed onset of the lithium effect and the antimanic properties of the neuroleptic. If morning sleepiness was a significant side effect, this could have been treated by either giving the chlorpromazine earlier in the evening (about 2 hours prior to bedtime) or by dividing the chlorpromazine dose (e.g., one third of the dose given during the late afternoon and the remainder at bedtime). Another possibility is to consider switching to a less sedating neuroleptic, for example, from chlorpromazine to perphenazine. Furthermore, when a neuroleptic is discontinued, the dose should be gradually tapered (usually by 25 percent or less every 3 or 4 days), with careful monitoring of symptoms. It is advisable not to make significant changes in medications during those times when careful patient monitoring may be more difficult (such as over weekends).

In the younger patient with manic or hypomanic symptoms, initial pharmacologic intervention may simply begin with a thymoleptic, especially if the child's behavior is not severe enough to warrant hospital admission. In this case, outpatient thymoleptic treatment can be initiated and a parent or other responsible adult can be used to provide information regarding symptom severity. If this course of action is chosen, the patient should ideally be seen every 3 or 4 days to closely monitor side effects and the therapeutic response. A parent or responsible adult must be given an emergency telephone number, which will enable him or her to reach the prescribing physician or the physician's delegate at any time if questions about side effects arise. Close monitoring is essential for adequate pharmacologic treatment in these cases.

CASE EXAMPLE

"He is not getting better; time to do something else."

R.D. was treated with lithium at a dose of 150 mg twice daily. After 3 weeks at this dose, the medication was increased to 150 mg three times daily. Four weeks later there was little improvement in R.D.'s symptoms, although his mother said that he was less of a problem at home and that he was not fighting as much. The mother was unsure about how R.D. had been doing at school. The treating physician decided to discontinue the lithium and suggested treatment with haloperidol instead because R.D. had been on the medicine long enough and was not showing an adequate response.

CASE COMMENTARY

The issue here is the adequacy of treatment, both in terms of maximizing the initial pharmacotherapy and determining treatment resistance. In this case, the clinician seemingly broke every rule that should be applied to assess "inadequate" response to treatment. These are identified in Section Three. In this case neither the adequacy of the pharmacotherapy in terms of dose nor the adequacy of the pharmacotherapy in terms of the necessary duration of treatment at a particular dose was considered. No serum lithium levels were obtained to guide dosing, and the total daily dose given (450 mg) was likely insufficient to obtain therapeutic serum levels. Although the treatment had been underway for 7 weeks in total, it is unlikely that optimally effective pharmacologic treatment had been delivered.

In addition, no symptom rating scales had been used to monitor the treatment outcome, so that the physician was unable to properly evaluate even the treatment that had been de-

livered. It is quite likely that modest but real improvements may have been missed. Finally, the physician neglected to involve the school in the treatment plan. Thus an objective and independent evaluation of outcome was unavailable for assessment of the treatment effect and an opportunity to combine behavioral-cognitive with pharmacologic methods of intervention was lost. This case illustrates the classic easy-way-out approach to the complicated issue of maximizing initial treatment and identifying treatment resistance. Unfortunately, nobody benefits from such a process.

CASE EXAMPLE

"Improvement has stopped."

G.A. had been treated with lithium and hospital milieu for 8 weeks with lithium serum levels maintained at 1.0 to 1.2 mEq/L for 7 consecutive weeks. He had shown some clinical improvement and his MMRS score was 36 and his BPRS score was 17. However, his improvement had plateaued for 2 weeks, and he continued to require small amounts of chlorpromazine to keep his behavior under control. The treatment staff were wondering what to do.

CASE COMMENTARY

This scenario represents a partial response to lithium in an adolescent manic patient. There are four possible courses to take at this point. These are discussed in Section Three and include optimization, substitution, augmentation, and combination strategies. With the treatment of acute mania, substitution treatments (e.g., changing from lithium to valproate) are unlikely to be helpful. This then leaves the other three to be considered.

One possibility is to maximize the dose of lithium. This is done by increasing the serum lithium level if side effects are such that they remain tolerable. However, it is important to remember that increasing serum lithium levels to between 1.2 and 1.5 mEq/L is pushing the upper limits of the narrow therapeutic range of the medication. This can be problematic if any conditions occur that can potentially cause an increase in the serum lithium concentration. If this course of action is taken, then a period of 2 to 3 weeks should be identified as the appropriate time course for proper evaluation of the therapeutic potential of this strategy. Another possibility is combination therapy.

This can be accomplished by adding valproate or carbamazepine to the current lithium regime. Valproate is preferable to carbamazepine on the basis of clinical experience, although either may be useful. If valproate is used, this should be initiated following the same dosage and monitoring schedule described earlier for valproate. The combination of these thymoleptics used together may provide better control than is possible by using only one agent. If this course of action is chosen, 3 to 4 weeks should be allowed after the added compound has reached putative therapeutic serum levels for evaluation of the therapeutic effect of the combination approach.

In some cases, however, this may not prove effective. Thus a third possibility (augmentation) is using neuroleptics for improved control of manic symptoms. If this course is followed, a number of issues will need to be kept in mind. With long-term treatment using neuroleptics, tardive dyskinesia may arise. Additionally, combined lithium and neuroleptic treatment may increase the risk of extrapyramidal side effects and NMS. Thus, this course of action should be considered only if either of the above-mentioned treatments prove to be unsuccessful. In some cases the use of clozapine (see Chapters 13 and 14) could be considered. Alternatively, thyroid medications, particularly levothyroxine, may be considered, although this is probably only indicated in rapid-cycling patients and should be considered to be experimental. Other agents used in adults have not been evaluated in children and adolescents, and their use is not recommended.

A fourth possibility is the use of ECT. ECT should also be considered in the treatment of the acute manic phase if little or no effect is produced from maximal doses of neuroleptics combined with thymoleptics in controlling severe manic symptoms, or if serious medication side effects limit the use of pharmacotropic agents. Suggested guidelines for the use of ECT in adolescent mania are as follows:

1. Response to optimal pharmacologic treatment has been unsuccessful.
2. Severe side effects have limited medication use.
3. The clinical picture is complicated by catatonia.
4. Extreme agitation and aggressive suicidal or homicidal actions place the patient or others at serious risk.

In cases meeting these criteria, ECT may provide rapid symptom relief, which can then be maintained with the use of a thymoleptic for prophylactic purposes.

Prior to proceeding with ECT, the following should be completed:

1. The patient's competency to make decisions about his or her treatment with ECT must be determined and patient permission to use ECT should be obtained in writing.
2. Permission to use ECT should be obtained from both parents or a legal guardian, even if an adolescent patient is legally able and competent to give consent.
3. Education about the use of ECT and its potential risks and expected benefits should be conducted with the patient and family. If possible, having the patient or family meet with other adolescents and their parents who have been through the ECT process is useful.
4. An independent psychiatrist should be consulted regarding the suitability of ECT.
5. An appropriate medical evaluation and anesthesia consultation should be obtained.
6. Consultation with an ECT specialist (in addition to the independent psychiatric opinion suggested in no. 4) for case review, ECT treatment suggestions, and conduct of ECT treatment is necessary.

Electroconvulsive treatment should be undertaken following the same symptom measurement and evaluation guidelines used for mania, and the side effects discussed earlier for pharmacologic intervention should be assessed. An initial course of 10 bilateral treatments using brief-pulse ECT is suggested on the basis of clinical research with this treatment and the available literature. This should be carried out under appropriate anesthesia and monitoring over a period of 3 to 4 weeks. Seizure length should be monitored with every treatment. Clinical improvement is expected to occur at about the fourth to sixth ECT treatment, with some patients showing significant improvement at the second or third treatment and others later on in the treatment course. A full course of ECT should be completed even if the patient appears to have experienced substantial clinical improvement by eight or nine treatments. If clinical improvement has not been fully obtained after 10 treatments, it is reasonable to increase the course to include two more bilateral treatments, leading to a final total of 12. Although the use of combined lithium therapy with ECT is controversial, it may be used with proper consultation and seizure monitoring. Valproate is an anticonvulsant and thus its use should not be continued during ECT. Judicious use of chlorpromazine can be helpful in controlling manic symptoms during the early stages of ECT if lithium is not being used concurrently.

The use of ECT in acute adolescent mania can be summarized as follows:

1. Consider the use of ECT if the patient meets the criteria outlined earlier
2. Educate and conduct a fully informed discussion with patient and parents or legal guardian
3. Obtain consultation and follow procedural guidelines outlined earlier
4. Carefully monitor clinical parameters before, during, and after ECT
5. Complete a full course of 10 bilateral ECT treatments even if patient improvement begins to occur earlier in the course of treatment
6. Follow successful ECT treatment with prophylactic thymoleptic treatment

Long-Term Pharmacotherapy Issues

Bipolar disorder is a chronic psychiatric illness, and long-term treatment is necessary both to provide prophylaxis against future episodes and to intervene aggressively if either depressive or manic symptoms recur. Effective long-term pharmacotherapy takes place as part of a comprehensive treatment package that addresses the unique personal, social, and academic-vocational needs of the patient. The underlying concepts regarding long-term pharmacotherapy are discussed in Section Three.

Careful long-term monitoring of the child's or adolescent's condition is essential and should be the shared responsibility of the patient, family, and the physician. The use of a mania or depression signs and symptoms checklist is a useful monitoring guide (Fig. 12–3). When used as part of an ongoing education program (which may include group support for either the patient, such as self-help groups, or the parents, such as parent support groups), this signs and symptoms checklist may help the patient or parent identify potential depressive or manic symptoms when they first occur and thus help them seek physician assessment and early intervention, which may abort the development of a more malignant mood swing. Patients and their families should be instructed to seek the treating physician's advice at any time if concerns about mood stability arise and not wait until the next scheduled appointment.

Consistent outpatient follow-up is essential for monitoring a patient's clinical condition and medication side effects. Additionally, important issues often arise (such as academic problems) in which the physician has an important role to play as an advocate for the patient and as an educator of other professionals (such as teachers) as to the functional effects of the disorder and appropriate interventions for these effects (see Section Three).

The frequency of outpatient visits must be individualized to patient needs. If the teenager has been euthymic, has stable serum levels, and is doing well socially and academically, then visits on a once every 2 or 3 month schedule are reasonable. For the teen who is experiencing symptoms, side effects, or other problems, visits as often as one or two times weekly may be appropriate. The timing of routine monitoring visits should be determined in discussions between the physician and patient/parent and should be part of the educational process regarding the illness and its optimal treatment.

Routine visits do not take the place of immediate assessment should significant symptoms or side effects arise. The physician must be available to see the patient within a day if significant concerns arise. A combination of routine monitoring and emergency availability is the optimal outpatient follow-up schedule for pharmacologic treatment.

Routine Monitoring

Routine monitoring includes the use of baseline evaluation measures applied longitudinally. The careful and systematic application of these measures will provide a useful addition to the regular office visit and may identify medical problems, symptoms, or side effects that would otherwise be unreported or unexamined. In addition, medical or psychiatric evaluations may need to be made if specific physical or psychiatric problems occur.

The use of the following scales should be continued to monitor the patient's physical status in the outpatient treatment phase:

1. The chosen extrapyramidal side effects scale should be completed at every outpatient visit if neuroleptics are used.
2. The AIMS should be repeated at 6-monthly intervals if neuroleptics are used.
3. MSSES should be completed at every outpatient visit.

Routine outpatient monitoring of the following baseline laboratory measures is suggested. If lithium is being used,

1. TSH at 6 month intervals
2. Specific gravity and creatinine clearance at 6 month intervals
3. Serum calcium at yearly intervals

Bipolar illness has two phases, mania and depression. You have experienced both of these. The chances are quite high that either mania or depression (or both) may recur. One way that you can try to prevent this is to continue taking your medication in the manner it has been prescribed. Another way you can try to prevent this is to take good care of yourself—avoid excessive use of alcohol, avoid use of illicit drugs, and get a good night's sleep every night. Sometimes, in spite of all of our best efforts, an illness returns. If this happens, the severity and length of the manic or depressive episodes can often be decreased if changes to your treatment are implemented as soon as possible. Part of your responsibility in taking care of yourself and controlling your illness is to contact your doctor as soon as any symptoms arise so that the necessary changes can be made in your treatment. If you are not sure if the symptoms that you are experiencing are signs of the illness coming back, it is better to seek advice from your doctor than to wait and see. Remember, the sooner that we can work together to stop relapses, the better your chances are of stopping the recurrence.

Your Symptoms of Mania Could Be:

1. _____   5. _____
2. _____   6. _____
3. _____   7. _____
4. _____   8. _____

Your Symptoms of Depression Could Be:

1. _____   5. _____
2. _____   6. _____
3. _____   7. _____
4. _____   8. _____

If you are experiencing two or more of these symptoms and they have lasted for 3 days or more, notify your doctor immediately. Do not wait for your next appointment; call your doctor at this number:_____

FIGURE 12–3 Signs and Symptoms Checklist: Is the Illness Coming Back?

If valproate is being used,

1. Liver function tests monthly for 6 months and then once every 6 months thereafter
2. Complete blood count, including platelets and WBC with differential every 6 months

Routine outpatient monitoring of the following symptom rating scales is suggested as follows:

1. MMRS—at each outpatient visit until the patient has been relatively euthymic for 6 months and then monthly thereafter. Should symptoms begin to reappear, monitoring should increase in frequency as appropriate.
2. BPRS—at each outpatient visit until the patient has been relatively euthymic for 6 months and then monthly thereafter. Should symptoms begin to reappear, monitoring should increase in frequency as appropriate.
3. OCI—not necessary for long-term outpatient follow-up.
4. Beck Depression Inventory (BDI)—see Section Two for a description of this self-rated

depression rating scale. This is a useful follow-up instrument because depressive episodes are more common than manic episodes, are often more difficult for an observer such as a parent to detect (compared with the behavioral symptoms of mania), and are less responsive to the prophylactic effects of thymoleptics. A BDI should thus be completed at the time of hospital discharge to determine the baseline BDI score and then at each subsequent outpatient visit.

CASE EXAMPLE

"Sick again—and so soon."

Eight weeks following adequate resolution of his clinical state (MMRS = 12; BPRS = 9), G.A. was discharged to the care of his community physician on a total dose of 1200 mg lithium daily, given in two equal doses. His serum levels in the hospital had consistently been 1.0 to 1.2 mEq/L, and he was not experiencing any significant side effects. All laboratory indices were within normal limits.

G.A. was seen at the hospital outpatient clinic once every 6 weeks to monitor his progress. Three months later his manic symptoms returned, although they were not as severe as previously, but he was hospitalized at his own request. The serum lithium level obtained at the time of admission was 0.4 mEq/L. His total daily lithium dose was 900 mg once daily. G.A. admitted that he had occasionally forgotten to take his medication but noted that this occurred relatively infrequently. When his outpatient physician was contacted, it was learned that G.A.'s lithium had been decreased to 900 mg some 4 weeks after discharge and his serum lithium levels had consistently been maintained at 0.4 to 0.5 mEq/L to avoid the possibility of side effects.

CASE COMMENTARY

This scenario provides an all too common example of what may occur when long-term lithium treatment is guided by the use of serum levels that are potentially insufficient to provide prophylaxis against future episodes. Unfortunately, rigorously controlled long-term follow-up studies in lithium-treated teenagers are lacking, but available evidence from extensive clinical experience and a scattering of research reports suggests that lithium serum levels in the 0.8 to 1.2 mEq/L range are necessary to produce a maximal prophylactic effect. It is important to try to maintain lithium levels in this range, particularly when side effects are not an issue.

Furthermore, specialist monitoring occurring more frequently than once every 6 weeks following hospital discharge is necessary. The period immediately following hospital discharge is one in which the risk of relapse is high, and clinical experience suggests that close clinical monitoring (once weekly or even more frequently if indicated) is necessary. After a reasonable period of time of euthymia has passed (6 months or more), monitoring may be changed to once every 3 to 4 weeks, with the expectation that should any change in the child's or adolescent's clinical condition occur, he or she should be seen immediately. The general guidelines that underlie decision making for long-term monitoring of pharmacotherapy are found in Section Three.

CASE EXAMPLE

"I've been taking this medication but I'm feeling blue."

W.R., a 13-year-old boy, has been stable on his valproate for 14 months at serum levels ranging from 55 to 70 mg/mL. He has few if any side effects and has otherwise been doing well socially. His academics have also started to improve, and he is once again developing a "future." Although he has been following his prescribed treatment religiously, his mood begins to drop as the "dog days of February" approach. His BDI scores, which have consistently been below 8, have climbed to 17 over the course of 2 weeks. He does not, however, meet the diagnostic criteria for a major depression. He is concerned that he will become depressed and lose all his hard-earned gains.

CASE COMMENTARY

Lithium and valproate are more effective for preventing the relapse of manic episodes than for depressive episodes. In an ongoing study of long-term outcome in adolescent bipolar 1 disorder, repeat depressive episodes were almost twice as common as manic episodes over a mean follow-up period of 5 years. Thus, the problem of depressive relapse is relatively common and needs to be effectively treated. Because subsyndromal depressive symptoms often precede the development of a major depression, the treatment of breakthrough depressive symptoms should be immediate and aggressive.

Unfortunately, there is a paucity of data on the optimal treatment of bipolar depression in this age group. The first strategy regarding relapse would be to raise the thymoleptic to a higher tolerable dose. In this case, the patient was relatively free of side effects but had a serum thymoleptic level in the lower end of the therapeutic range. Sometimes, simply increasing the thymoleptic dose to push the serum levels into the top end of the therapeutic range is sufficient to improve breakthrough depressive symptoms and to prevent the onset of a major depressive episode. If the patient is taking lithium, checking the TSH level is of value to ensure that early or subclinical hypothyroidism is not responsible for the symptoms under evaluation.

In terms of other alternatives, tricyclic antidepressants have not demonstrated clinical efficacy in adolescent unipolar depression, but no literature is available specific to their use in bipolar depression. Their use is associated with many side effects. Serotonin-specific re-uptake inhibitors (SSRIs) may be helpful but they may induce manic or hypomanic epi-sodes. The atypical antidepressants, bupropion and buspirone, may be of benefit in this situa-tion. One report of the use of light therapy—10,000 lux delivered in the morning and in the evening for 1 to 2 weeks—showed promising results in the amelioration of depressive break-through symptoms in thymoleptic-treated ado-lescents with bipolar disorder.

Given the currently available treatment op-tions and the scientific knowledge about their relative value, it is suggested that the first choice of intervention is to raise the thymolep-tic dose to obtain a serum level at the high end of the putative therapeutic range. If this is not possible or is not tolerated by the patient, the use of light therapy is suggested. This is a rela-tively well-tolerated intervention, and clinical experience and research on this treatment sug-gest that using a minimum of 2500 lux deliv-ered over a period of 1 hour twice daily is rea-sonable. Each hour-long treatment should be given in the morning and again in the evening. The morning dose should be administered be-tween 0600 and 0800 hours. The evening dose should be administered between 1800 and 2000 hours. Symptomatic improvement should be seen in 7 to 10 days.

If antidepressants are used, the clinician must consider their potential in inducing mania. An-tidepressants should only be added to maximize ongoing thymoleptic treatment, following the standard procedures for their use (see Chapter 11). The first choice of an antidepressant, given the current information available, should be ei-ther an SSRI or buspirone, and after ensuring that thymoleptic serum levels are in the thera-peutic range, these should be appropriately titrated to potentially effective doses.

Similarly, if breakthrough manic symptoms occur, the first strategy is to ensure that thy-moleptic levels are at the upper end of the therapeutic range. If breakthrough symptoms continue, a short course of a midpotency neu-roleptic (e.g., perphenazine, 16 to 24 mg daily, or flupenthixol, 3 to 6 mg daily) along with an antiparkinsonian medication (e.g., procycli-dine, 5 mg twice daily) should be used. In ad-dition, risperidone is being used to treat break-through manic symptoms by clinicians familiar with its use. If risperidone is chosen, the clini-cian should consult Chapter 13 for clinical sug-gestions regarding its use. Often daily doses of 1 or 2 mg will be sufficient. As with the break-through depressive symptoms described earli-er, treatment of manic breakthrough should be immediate and aggressive.

If thymoleptic monotherapy does not pro-vide sufficient prophylaxis against recurrences of depression or mania, the following steps should be undertaken:

1. A careful review of potential causal fac-tors outside the natural rhythm of the dis-ease must be conducted. The most im-portant is the use of illicit drugs or alcohol, which can lead to episodes of mania or depression, even in the presence of adequate thymoleptic coverage. In old-er adolescents, lifestyle issues such as a job that demands late-night work, or travel across time zones should also be considered.

2. Careful review of the long-term medica-tion treatment record should be complet-ed, with particular attention paid to en-suring that optimal serum levels of the thymoleptic have been obtained and compliance is adequate.

If these reviews are negative, a second thy-moleptic could be added to the first. If adequate prophylaxis is not obtained with this combi-nation at optimal serum levels of both com-pounds, midpotency neuroleptics or risperi-done may be helpful. The use of long-lasting injectable neuroleptics (such as flupenthixol) or oral clozapine (an "atypical" neuroleptic) may be indicated. If, in spite of these measures, breakthrough episodes still occur with some frequency and severity, then prophylactic out-patient bilateral ECT could be considered.

CASE EXAMPLE

"I've been doing well for a while. What now?"

W.R. has been doing relatively well over the last 6 months. His mood has remained euthymic, and he is attending school and "hanging out with his friends." Although his grades are not what they were prior to his illness, they are be-ginning to improve. His valproate serum levels have been stable and range from 75 to 85 μg/mL. G.A. and his parents request a special appointment to discuss his future treatment.

CASE COMMENTARY

One question almost invariably asked by a pa-tient or parent is, "How long will I be taking the lithium or valproate?" The answer depends on the natural history of the illness and the demonstrated efficacy of pharmacologic treatment for that patient. Bipolar affective disorder is a chronic psychiatric illness, with repeat episodes of both mania and depression continuing through the life cycle. Within this broad general framework, however, different patients will exhibit different particular courses. For example, one may suffer from severe frequent episodes, another may experience a long period of relative euthymia only to be followed by an unexpected return of either mania or depression, and a third patient may show an entirely different course. Unfortunately, no clinical or biologic variables are available that, when used alone or in combination, will help predict a patient's clinical course.

Thus a reasonable response to this important question is to review what is known about the chronicity of the disorder and then to identify the variability in any one individual's course. The clinician may well respond, "We don't know for sure. It depends on how your illness and its treatment progress."

A reasonable guideline for long-term pharmacotherapy of early onset bipolar disorder is that after one manic episode, the patient should stay on a thymoleptic for a minimum of 1 year following full resolution of the first episode. After two manic episodes or after one manic episode followed by a major depression, the patient will need to consider life-long thymoleptic treatment. Furthermore, during long-term thymoleptic treatment, there may well be periods of time in which more than one pharmacologic intervention will be necessary. The goals of treatment are to alleviate the episode in the acute phase and to prolong remission and prevent relapse in the chronic phase.

The general guidelines that underlie decision making for long-term pharmacotherapy are found in Section Three. They should be applied for this disorder as follows:

1. Educate the patient and family about the chronic nature of the illness and its expected treatment.

2. Develop an individually tailored medication monitoring program that includes routine evaluation of symptoms, side effects, medication serum levels, and pertinent laboratory measures.

3. Establish an emergency response procedure to allow for rapid and aggressive intervention if significant breakthrough symptoms of depression or mania appear.

4. Treat significant breakthrough symptoms immediately using the methods outlined earlier.

SUGGESTED READINGS

Alessi N, Naylor M, Ghaziuddin M, Zubieta J. Update on lithium carbonate therapy in children and adolescents. Journal of the American Academy of Child and Adolescent Psychiatry, 33:291–304, 1993.

American Academy of Child and Adolescent Psychiatry. Practice parameters for the assessment and treatment of children and adolescents with bipolar disorder. Draft, September 6, 1995.

Botteron K, Geller B. Pharmacologic treatment of childhood and adolescent mania. Child and Adolescent Psychiatric Clinics of North America, 4:283–304, 1995.

Chou JC-Y. Recent advances in treatment of acute mania. Journal of Clinical Psychopharmacology, 11:3–21, 1991.

Fetner HH, Geller B. Lithium and tricyclic antidepressants. Psychiatric Clinics of North America, 15:223–241, 1992.

Fristad M, Weller E, Weller R. Bipolar disorder in children and adolescents. Child and Adolescent Psychiatric Clinics of North America, 1:13–30, 1992.

Goodwin FK, Jamison KR. Manic-Depressive Illness. New York: Oxford University Press, 1990.

Jefferson JW, Greist JH, Ackerman DL. Lithium Encyclopedia for Clinical Practice. Washington, DC: American Psychiatric Association Press, 1987.

Kutcher S, Robertson H. Electroconvulsive treatment in acute adolescent mania. Journal of Child and Adolescent Psychopharmacology, 5:167–175, 1995.

Papatheodorou G, Kutcher S. Treatment of bipolar disorder in adolescents. In K Shulman, M Tohen, S Kutcher (eds): Mood Disorders Across the Life Span. New York: Wiley-Liss, Inc., 1996, pp 159–186.

Pollock JM. Carbamazepine side effects in children and adults. Epilepsia, 28:S64–S70, 1987.

Prien RF, Potter WZ. NIMH workshop report on treatment of bipolar disorder. Psychopharmacologic Bulletin, 26:409–427, 1990.

Vestergaard P. Clinically important side effects of long-term lithium treatment: A review. Acta Psychiatricia Scandinavia 67(Suppl):11–36, 1983.

CHAPTER 13

Psychopharmacologic Treatment of Acute Schizophrenia

Schizophrenia is a chronic mental illness that most often onsets during the later adolescent or early adult years, although it can occur in childhood. Current diagnostic practice applies similar syndromal diagnostic criteria for this disorder across the life cycle. Schizophrenia onsetting in early childhood must be carefully distinguished from a pervasive developmental disorder, particularly autism, whereas schizophrenia onsetting in adolescence must be differentiated from bipolar disorder or an Axis II diagnosis, particularly borderline or schizotypal personality disorder. The diagnosis of schizophrenia should follow from a thorough assessment of the patient, often best accomplished in an inpatient or day-treatment setting in which multiple parameters of functioning can be carefully measured. This assessment not only allows for more careful diagnostic ascertainment but also provides a baseline against which subsequent treatment interventions and developmental processes can be evaluated.

Because this diagnosis carries with it a host of psychological and social issues, it is not one to be offered lightly or without due assessment. Occasionally it may be difficult to be certain about the diagnosis, in which case a longitudinal evaluation that includes a comprehensive treatment trial is indicated. Cases with substance abuse or short-lived psychotic symptoms in the context of failure to achieve expected levels of social development often require such a longitudinal diagnostic-cum-treatment process. Nothing is to be gained and much may be lost in rushing into the diagnosis of schizophrenia. On the other hand, it is important not to try to "cushion the blow" by using euphemisms or alternative classifications if the child or adolescent clearly meets the diagnosis.

Schizophrenia onsets in a variety of forms. In some cases a lengthy prodrome is followed by an acute psychotic break. In other cases negative symptoms (such as social withdrawal and apathy) predominate and positive symptoms (such as delusions or hallucinations), while present, may be hidden or may occur only occasionally. In others the onset of the illness may appear to be sudden, possibly precipitated by the illicit use of psychoactive substances. Occasionally, the patient or family may present having already considered or even made a diagnosis of schizophrenia, especially if there is a family history of the disorder.

The use of a semistructured interview such as the Kiddie Schedule for Affective Disorders and Schizophrenia (K-SADS) (see Section Two) is of value in the diagnostic evaluation of a child or adolescent when a diagnosis of schizophrenia is being considered. Repeating this assessment some 4 to 6 months after the initial evaluation in cases in which the diagnosis is not certain can often provide useful information. It is helpful if this second interview is conducted by a clinician who was not involved in the initial diagnostic evaluation or subsequent patient management. An independent diagnostic evaluation is suggested for those cases in which the physician is relatively uncertain about the diagnosis.

The treatment of schizophrenia is multimodal. Medications are a necessary but not sufficient component of proper and comprehensive treatment. Education about the illness, individual and family counseling and support, academic or vocational assistance, social and life-skills enhancements, and occasional hospitalizations, all continued over the long term, are necessary for optimal outcome. The proper use of psychopharmacologic interventions in treating both the acute and long-term manifestations of this illness are necessary to allow for the optimal effects of needed psychosocial interventions.

CASE EXAMPLE

Childhood Schizophrenia: "She is quite unusual, could it be . . . "

P.O. was an 8-year-old girl who was referred for diagnostic assessment by her family doctor. Her parents had noticed increasingly withdrawn behavior and were aware that she seemed to be talking to "imaginary people" and "animals" for some time. More recently her family had observed her at times covering herself with a blanket, sometimes shouting aloud. She told her parents that "wolves" were chasing her. In addition, P.O. had begun to develop a variety of rituals that seemed to be in response to directions that she received from her conversations with various "animals." These rituals included putting milk out on the back doorstep in the evening, drawing the shades in her bedroom to a specific location every night, and insisting that her parents leave the living room lights on at all times.

P.O. had always been a withdrawn child who preferred solitary activities, although she did have some friends who would play with her occasionally. She was very interested in nature and would go on long walks through the countryside around her rural home. She had told her parents that she could communicate with animals by thoughts, and she sometimes reported seeing jungle creatures during her walks in the yard. Her parents had interpreted these stories as coming from an active imagination in a quiet and somewhat lonely child.

Academically, P.O. had demonstrated difficulties in spelling and other language-based activities. She enjoyed drawing, but a few months prior to her assessment, her teacher had contacted her parents and expressed concerns that P.O.'s pictures were becoming increasingly more unusual and "bizarre." She mentioned representations of wolves eating people and bleeding body pieces. When questioned about her art work, P.O. refused to discuss what she had produced.

When seen, P.O. presented as a withdrawn youngster with poor eye contact and a restricted or flat affect. She was initially hesitant about describing her "thoughts," but she gradually began to report on an elaborate delusional system of "animals" and "shadow people." She described auditory hallucinations that consisted of sentence fragments or single words that would either be directed toward her or spoken about her. She reported that the "shadow people" told her to provide food for "wolves" (hence the milk on the doorstep), and she described horrible visions of wolves eating people that frightened her.

A full diagnostic assessment was carried out. A positive family history of schizophrenia was found in the father's brother, and the father himself was noted to be "schizoid" and to spend much of his time writing to various government agencies about incidences of "toxic gas leaks" that he believed were occurring at a chemical plant near P.O.'s school. The mother was not forthcoming about her own family history but disclosed that her own mother had been hospitalized for "nerves," a hospitalization that had apparently lasted for many years.

Academic assessment identified multiple language difficulties and problems with attention and concentration. Social evaluations showed P.O. to have significant difficulties in age-appropriate social interactions. Psychological testing demonstrated an I.Q. within the low normal range but with an inconsistency across subtest scores. Projective testing that had been ordered by a psychologist with whom the family had previously consulted was reported as showing "cognitive slippage." Extensive staff observations confirmed the presence of withdrawn behavior and deficient social skills, auditory hallucinations, and delusional thinking. A diagnosis of schizophrenia was made, and a comprehensive treatment program developed.

CASE COMMENTARY

This case illustrates a relatively common presentation of gradually onsetting schizophrenia in a child. The pharmacologic management of this disorder is discussed here using this case for illustrative purposes. Although not discussed in detail, it is understood that proper psychopharmacologic treatment must occur within the context of optimal and comprehensive care, which includes those psychosocial, individual, and family features already identified. From the very beginning of treatment it must be kept in mind that the expected paradigm is that of chronic care with the goal of controlling acute symptoms, preventing relapse, and optimizing patient functioning across a variety of parameters.

CASE EXAMPLE

Adolescent Schizophrenia: "We are worried about our son. He's acting strangely."

A.J. was a 17-year-old boy who was brought to the emergency room after he had been found walking along a limited-access highway wearing no overcoat during a winter snowstorm. He was unkempt and agitated, and he told police officers that he was on his way to a neighboring city (40 miles away) because he had discovered a plot to poison the water supply. He had chosen not to take public transportation because "it is being watched" and had not taken the family car because he thought that his father may have been "in on the plot."

A medical assessment was essentially unremarkable, and a drug screen was negative. Psychiatric evaluation identified: paranoid delusions, auditory hallucinations (including hallucinations commanding him to do away with his parents), tangential thinking, loosening of associations, and ideas of reference in a clear sensorium. His affect was described as "flat" and "inappropriate," and there was no evidence of depressive or manic symptomatology. During the interview, A.J. became agitated and began to pace about the interview room. At one point he began to examine the ceiling and accused the physician of videotaping him. He then asserted that the doctor was part of the poisoning plot and attempted to "escape" from the hospital, but he was restrained by the police. A.J. refused admission to the hospital and was then certified under the terms of the mental health act and admitted to a safe and secure environment. When his parents arrived at the hospital they were relieved that he had finally obtained "help."

According to his parents, 12 months prior to hospitalization, A.J. had begun to do poorly at school. He blamed his performance on teachers who he felt were against him. At the same time, he began to distance himself from his friends and dropped off the basketball team, although he had worked hard to earn a place on the squad. He told his parents that the coach was "playing favorites" and that the other players on the team were "talking behind his back." As a result, A.J. decided to change schools, which he did. Soon after changing schools, however, he began to avoid going to school, complaining that his guidance counselor "had it in for him." Although his parents were unable to confirm this story, they agreed to let A.J. enroll in an alternative school program.

Here, however, similar complaints emerged, and soon A.J. decided to quit school altogether.

About this time A.J. became very interested in mysticism and philosophy. He would retire to his bedroom, pull the curtains, and read by candlelight. He began to sleep during much of the day and stay up during the night. When his parents tried to engage him in conversation he would avoid talking and soon stopped joining his family for meals. His older brother, who was quite close to A.J., found him increasingly difficult to relate to and told his parents that he felt that there was something "really wrong with A.J."

A.J.'s mother was concerned that her son might be depressed. She made a number of appointments with their family physician, all of which A.J. refused to attend. She contacted a counselor at a social service agency, who listened to her story and advised, "Leave the boy alone. He is just being a teenager."

Over time A.J.'s behavior became more unusual. He became convinced that the teachers and principal at his first high school had plotted to keep him from being successful. He told his parents that the neighbors across the street were spying on him but could not say why this might be happening. The day before A.J. left on his snowy mission, he was noted to have stayed awake for most of the night talking in a loud voice and arguing with someone, although no one else was present in the room with him. When his parents discovered that he had left the house, they contacted the police, who told them that A.J. had not been away long enough to be considered a missing person.

CASE COMMENTARY

This case illustrates an unfortunate although relatively common presentation of schizophrenia with an onset in adolescence. The acute nature of the presentation often follows a period of more gradual decline, as illustrated here. The pharmacologic management of this psychotic illness is discussed later using this case for illustrative purposes. Although not discussed in detail, it is understood that proper psychopharmacologic treatment must occur within the context of optimal and comprehensive care, which includes those features already identified. From the very beginning of treatment it must be kept in mind that the expected paradigm is that of acute symptom control and chronic care, with the goal of preventing relapse and optimizing patient functioning across a variety of domains.

Initial Pharmacologic Management

In the first case described, initial pharmacologic treatment can be planned and gradually instituted, perhaps over the course of a week or two. Issues such as patient and family education can be fully addressed before pharmacotherapy is begun. In the second case, the clinical presentation of the patient is a psychiatric emergency, and treatment needs to be initiated with that in mind. This does not mean that the principles of good psychopharmacologic treatment should be neglected; rather, they should be applied within the context of the individual presentation. The two somewhat different approaches that these cases require are described.

Baseline Considerations

In both scenarios, the following baseline considerations apply.

Medical Considerations

Medical considerations are outlined in Section Two. Of particular importance is the evaluation of those physical parameters that may be affected by pharmacologic treatment. Because the expected acute and long-term treatment will primarily be with antipsychotics, the following standardized baseline physical assessments are suggested:

1. Extrapyramidal Symptom Rating Scale (ESRS)—to assess extrapyramidal and dyskinetic symptoms
2. Abnormal Involuntary Movement Scale (AIMS)—to assess dyskinetic symptoms
3. Medication-specific side effect scales (MSSES)—(see Appendix IV for scales for typical antipsychotics, risperidone, and clozapine)

Patients who are beginning treatment with antipsychotics should be assessed on an ongoing basis for the presence of side effects. In the first case described as that of a psychotic yet relatively behaviorally stable youngster, once-a-day objective and subjective evaluations are probably sufficient during the medication initiation phase. In the second case, that of an aggressive and behaviorally uncontrolled psychotic teen, more frequent clinical monitoring including evaluation of side effects—at least two to four times daily—is suggested.

Laboratory Considerations

Laboratory investigations should assess those physiologic parameters that pharmacologic treat-

ment may affect in both the acute and long-term phases of treatment. Because treatment will be directed toward the use of neuroleptics, the following baseline laboratory measures are suggested:

Typical antipsychotics (e.g., chlorpromazine, perphenazine, flupenthixol): liver function tests

Atypical neuroleptics (including risperidone and clozapine): liver function tests and complete blood count (CBC), including white blood (cell) count (WBC) and absolute neutrophil levels

If typical antipsychotics are used, there is no good medical indication for routine weekly monitoring of the above-mentioned laboratory parameters during the treatment induction phase. However, if changes in the clinical condition of the patient occur (e.g., fever, vomiting, diarrhea) that may indicate an adverse reaction, then the appropriate laboratory tests should be obtained as clinically indicated. Otherwise, a repeat of baseline laboratory measures at the end of 2 weeks after the onset of pharmacotherapy and at discharge from the hospital (or 6 to 8 weeks later) should be sufficient.

If atypical neuroleptics are being used, then other monitoring protocols will have to be implemented, especially with clozapine. At this time clozapine is not considered a first-line medication for the treatment of schizophrenia in children and adolescents, although the available literature suggests that it may be potentially effective as such. Currently, it is recommended for those patients who have demonstrated treatment nonresponse to adequate trials of typical neuroleptics or experienced side effects of sufficient severity as to preclude an adequate medication trial with other more traditional compounds. Nevertheless, when treatment with clozapine is being initiated, a weekly CBC with WBC and total neutrophil count should be obtained. Continued treatment with clozapine is dependent on the maintenance of adequate WBC and neutrophil counts. A similar CBC monitoring strategy is recommended for continuation therapy as well. These are discussed more fully later.

Psychiatric Considerations

Baseline evaluation should include those symptoms that are the target of pharmacologic treatment. The following baseline symptom assessment measures are suggested:

1. Brief Psychiatric Rating Scale (BPRS): As described in Section Two, the BPRS provides a sensitive rating scale for the global assessment of severe psychiatric pathology, including cognitive, behavioral, and affective symptoms (see Appendix VI). The BPRS should be used weekly during the initiation of treatment as an

outcome measure. Once the patient is stabilized on medications, longer periods of time between assessments (once every 2 weeks if a day patient, or at each medication monitoring visit if an outpatient) is usually sufficient.

2. Positive and Negative Syndrome Scale (PANSS): As described in Section Two, the PANSS provides a useful measure of both positive (e.g., delusions and hallucinations) and negative (e.g., apathy and withdrawal) symptoms (see Appendix VI). When used consistently, this scale provides an excellent profile of symptom changes over time. Although the PANSS can be used to monitor weekly progress, it is perhaps best used with longer blocks of time, such as 6 to 8 weeks between evaluations. For patients undergoing long-term treatment, it is suggested that the PANSS be repeated at least two or three times per year (once every 4 to 6 months) to provide a robust symptom-monitoring measure.

In addition, various 10 cm Visual Analogue Scales (VAS) can be used to monitor symptoms that are especially problematic or underassessed in the above-mentioned scales. Some such target symptoms may be:

1. Concentration
2. Ability to tolerate ward milieu
3. Level of agitation
4. Number of hours of sleep at night
5. Ability to tolerate visits with family members

The symptom-directed VAS will most likely not be useful once acute symptom reconstitution has begun, but it can provide important information that can be used to direct pharmacologic treatment during the first few weeks of pharmacotherapy.

Antipsychotics

Typical antipsychotics are at this time considered to be the medications of choice in the management of child and adolescent schizophrenia. However, risperidone and clozapine, two relatively new atypical neuroleptics, represent potentially useful therapeutic compounds in this population and appear to be possibly better tolerated than many of the typical compounds. Other new antipsychotics such as olazapine are in clinical trials with adults and will not be reviewed here. This section addresses both the typical and atypical antipsychotics as they apply to use in children and adolescents, and their clinical use is illustrated.

The antipsychotics are often classified as outlined in Table 13–1. Although there are a large number of these compounds, data (both clinical and research) about their use in the psychotic

TABLE 13–1   Classification of Antipsychotics with Examples of Representative Compounds Potentially Useful in Treating Child and Adolescent Schizophrenia

Classification	Representative Compound
Phenothiazines	
Aliphatic	Chlorpromazine
Piperidine	Thioridazine
Piperazine	Perphenazine
Thioxanthenes	Flupenthixol
Butyrophenone	Haloperidol
Diphenylbutylpiperidines	Pimozide, fluspirilene
Dibenzodiazepine	Clozapine
Benzisoxazole	Risperidone

child or adolescent are often insufficient for endorsement of routine use for many of these compounds. Accordingly, Table 13–1 provides lists of classes and medications that may offer the clinician a sufficient armamentarium from the many classes and compounds that are available.

Phenothiazines and Other Typical Antipsychotics

As a group, the phenothiazines present a complex pharmacology and exhibit multiple actions in both the central and peripheral nervous systems. They possess dopaminergic, adrenergic, and muscarinic activity and may also affect the gamma-aminobutyric and peptide systems. Their mode of therapeutic action is thought to arise from their ability to antagonize dopamine-mediated neurotransmission at postsynaptic receptor sites.

As a result of this complex pharmacology, phenothiazines demonstrate a variety of important physiologic effects involving the central nervous system, the cardiovascular system, and the endocrine system. Their adverse effects are multiple and may appear in almost any system. Prescription of these compounds must accordingly follow a comprehensive understanding of their activity, which requires further study than is found in this chapter. Readers are referred to the reference texts listed in Section One.

Other typical antipsychotics from different categories exhibit similar efficacy and adverse effects profiles as those found with the phenothiazines, with some clinically important differences. The high-potency butyrophenone haloperidol, for example, is more likely to induce extrapyramidal side effects than the phenothiazines. This may be particularly problematic in adolescent males, who seem to be at greatest risk for these adverse events.

TABLE 13–2 **Expected Side Effects with Antipsychotic Treatment in Children and Adolescents**

Relatively Common	Relatively Uncommon	Rare
Sedation	Confusion	Gynecomastia
Sunburn	Impotence	Galactorrhea
Increased heart rate	Hypotension	Amenorrhea
Dystonic spectrum	Pruritus	Syncope
Akathisia or Akinesia	Skin rash	Ocular effects
Parkinsonism	Oral syndrome	Cholestatic jaundice
Withdrawal dyskinesia	Tardive dyskinesia	Hematologic disorders
Weight gain	Dizziness	Sudden death

The diphenylbutylpiperidine pimozide may be associated with electrocardiogram (ECG) abnormalities and with an increased risk of seizures and sudden death at higher doses (20 mg daily) and has an extremely long elimination half-life with oral dosing. Its use is usually limited in the psychotic disorders, but it is effectively prescribed at doses of 1 to 6 mg daily in children and adolescents with Tourette's syndrome (see Chapter 17).

Risperidone

Adverse events from the atypical antipsychotic risperidone may differ from those of the more typical neuroleptics already described. Reportedly, at therapeutic doses (2 to 8 mg daily) it exhibits significantly fewer extrapyramidal side effects and dyskinetic side effects, and thus seems to be better tolerated than the more typical antipsychotics. This may have important clinical implications, particularly with regard to patient compliance. Adolescents, who are at high risk for distressing and disabling extrapyramidal side effects, may particularly benefit in this respect. The data pertaining to this population, however, at this time are relatively limited, and while studies are underway, further detailed information on its efficacy and tolerability in children and adolescents is needed.

Pharmacologically, risperidone exhibits potent dopamine D2 receptor and serotonin 5HT2 receptor blocking effects. Its active metabolite, 9-OH-risperidol, exhibits a similar profile as the parent compound. Risperidone is rapidly absorbed following oral administration and is metabolized by the debrisoquine hydroxylation system. Most whites and Asians are rapid metabolizers of risperidone. The clinical significance of this phenomenon may be relatively minor (unlike most of the typical neuroleptics) because it is the combination of risperidone and its active metabolite that is thought to be related to its therapeutic efficacy and tolerability.

Peak plasma levels of the parent drug and its active moiety are reached in 1 to 3 hours. Using a multiple daily dosing strategy, steady-state drug levels are usually reached in 5 to 6 days. In adults, therapeutic efficacy and tolerability seem to be associated with a therapeutic window at a usual oral total daily dose of 6 to 8 mg given using a twice-daily dosing schedule. This amount may be lower in children and adolescents (1 to 4 mg total daily dose given twice daily). Medications that are known to affect the hepatic cytochrome P-450 II-D6 isoenzyme system (such as carbamazepine, phenobarbital, and cimetidine) may affect risperidone metabolism and its subsequent therapeutic and side effect profiles.

In children and adolescents, in addition to the known adverse effects of these compounds (see Tables 13–1 to 13–4), other considerations pertaining to growth and development are important. Questions such as the effect of antipsychotic medications on normal endocrine development during puberty are as yet largely unanswered and must be kept in mind. Nevertheless, these compounds have been successfully and safely used for many years in children and adolescents, and if the risk/benefit ratio supports their implementation, they should be prescribed by competent clinicians following careful monitoring procedures.

TABLE 13–3 **Dystonic-Type Side Effects in Children and Adolescents Treated with Antipsychotics**

Severe	Moderate to Mild*
Torticollis	Minor neck spasm
Opisthotonos	Minor back spasm
Carpopedal spasm	Mandibular or temporomandibular joint stiffness
Laryngospasm	Minor swallowing problems
Oculogyric crisis	Minor visual complaints
Perioral spasm	Minor chewing difficulties

*Moderate to mild side effects may be overlooked or dismissed as unnecessary complaints by the physician but are often experienced as quite debilitating by the patient. Because they usually respond well to minor dose decrements of the antipsychotic medication or antiparkinsonian agents, they should not be ignored but vigorously treated.

TABLE 13–4 Parkinsonian-Type Signs and Symptoms Induced with Antipsychotic Drug Use in Children and Adolescents

Occur at Any Dose (even low doses)	Usually at Higher Doses
Tremors	Pill rolling movements
Stiff walking	Shuffling gait
Less prosodic speech	Slow monotone speech
Difficulty swallowing	Dysphagia
Slowed body movements	Bradykinesia
Less facial expression	Masklike facies
Decreased body movements	Akinesia
Hypersalivation	Drooling
Restlessness	Akathisia

Possible Side Effects of Antipsychotics

As noted earlier, side effects are multiple and are briefly discussed within the framework of the physiologic system in which they occur. Although they are considered separately here, it is common to find patients with side effects across multiple systems occurring simultaneously. Thus, when patients who are being treated with antipsychotics are being monitored it is essential for the clinician to carefully assess each of the systems at risk.

Extrapyramidal Effects

These are thought to be dose related, although even small doses of antipsychotics may induce one or more extrapyramidal side effects. Adolescents may be particularly sensitive to dystonic reactions, and children and teens with mental retardation can show unexpected sensitivity to these compounds. Persons of Asian descent, regularly menstruating females, and first drug-exposure patients may also be more sensitive to extrapyramidal effects. Furthermore, recent re-evaluation of long-standing pharmacologic practice has suggested that the appearance of severe extrapyramidal side effects may signal the overshooting of the therapeutic dose range most associated with antipsychotic efficacy.

Dystonic Side Effects

Dystonic reactions typically occur early during treatment with neuroleptics. These are found on a spectrum from mild to severe and life threatening, and are listed in Table 13–3. Clinicians should be careful when examining their patients not to overlook mild manifestations of dystonias, such as back and neck stiffness, because these can be quite discomforting to the patient and may lead to treat-

TABLE 13–5 Useful Antiparkinsonian Medications for the Treatment of Antipsychotic-Induced Parkinsonian Side Effects*

Medication	Starting Dose	Usual Total Daily Dose Range
Amantadine	100 mg	100–400 mg
Benztropine	1 mg	2–6 mg
Diphenhydramine	25 mg	100–200 mg
Procyclidine	2.5 mg	5–20 mg

*Compounds other than those listed here are also available. Endorsement of their routine use in children and adolescents is limited by a lack of available data (clinical and research) on their efficacy and tolerability in this age group. Doses may be given on a bid or tid schedule.

ment noncompliance. These symptoms respond well to most antiparkinsonian medications and antihistamines, or low-dose benzodiazepines can also be helpful.

Parkinsonian Side Effects

The classic parkinsonian side effects are listed in Table 13–4. These also respond relatively well to antiparkinsonian medications (see Table 13–5).

Akathisia

Akathisia, subjective or objective motor restlessness, can be extremely distressing to the patient and might be confused with exacerbation of the psychosis. Some psychotic patients have been known to develop delusional elaborations to explain their sensations of akathisia ("There are radio waves in my stomach and legs." "Electricity is being shot through my body from my bed"). Thus, a high degree of suspicion of the possibility of akathisia is indicated on the part of the clinician. Unlike other parkinsonian side effects, akathisia does not respond well to traditional antiparkinsonian medication. It can be controlled by decreasing the dose of the neuroleptic or with the use of one of the medications listed in Table 13–6.

TABLE 13–6 Useful Medications in Treating Antipsychotic-Induced Akathisia in Children and Adolescents*

Medication	Suggested Starting Dose	Usual Daily Dose
Clonazepam	0.25 mg	0.25–2.0 mg
Propranolol	10 mg	10–30 mg
Diphenhydramine	25 mg	100–200 mg

*The suggested doses of medications are guidelines only; individual patients may require higher or lower amounts. Doses should be titrated to the individual patient's clinical needs.

Neuroleptic Malignant Syndrome

Neuroleptic malignant syndrome (NMS) is a relatively rare but potentially fatal antipsychotic side effect of uncertain etiology. Its appearance constitutes a true psychiatric emergency. Clinically, NMS presents with autonomic instability, severe extrapyramidal dysfunction, and hyperthermia. It may be more common in patients treated with neuroleptics combined with lithium. Left untreated, NMS can progress to loss of consciousness, rhabdomylysis, and death. Upon suspicion of NMS, the neuroleptic should be stopped immediately and appropriate symptomatic therapy instituted (e.g., fever control, electrolyte and fluid maintenance). Cardiac monitoring may be necessary. Medical consultation should be sought.

Although laboratory investigations often reveal elevated creatinine phosphokinase (CPK) and leukocytosis, these findings are not invariably present and indeed may occur after the initial onset of the clinical symptoms described earlier. The absence of an elevated CPK and leukocytosis does not mean that the patient does not have NMS or that immediate emergency treatment measures should not be initiated. Alternatively, the CPK can be elevated as a result of severe agitation or intramuscular (IM) injection. Laboratory indices are helpful in monitoring the clinical progression of NMS, but they should not be used as set in stone diagnostic indicators.

A number of pharmacologic interventions for NMS are available, but the value of their use in children and adolescents, beyond discontinuation of the neuroleptic and usual supportive treatment, has not been demonstrated. These are listed along with the suggested doses in Table 13–7.

Tardive Dyskinesia

The syndrome of dyskinetic involuntary movements can, unlike its name, occur at any time during neuroleptic treatment and may also occur spontaneously as part of the disease process of schizophrenia itself. Whereas it usually manifests itself in older females with a history of high-dose neuroleptic treatment over prolonged periods of time, its symptoms can be found in children and adolescents as well. Although it most commonly presents as rhythmic involuntary movements of the tongue, face, mouth, and jaw, it may also involve the extremities and the trunk as well. Fine vermicular movements of the tongue, best seen with the mouth open and the tongue lying flat on the floor of the mouth in a relaxed position, are considered to be among the earliest signs of tardive dyskinesia (TD).

TD can best be treated if detected early. The routine use of the AIMS (see Appendix III) at specified times during treatment is recommended as a method of detecting TD. However, assessment of possible buccolingual involuntary movements should be part of every medication-monitoring visit (see Antipsychotic Side Effects Scale—Objective Measurement in Appendix IV).

Treatment usually consists of decreasing the neuroleptic dose. Although this strategy may temporarily increase the amount of dyskinetic movements, in most cases it will lead to an eventual decrease in symptoms. No other medical intervention has been clearly established for ameliorating TD symptoms. Care must be taken to distinguish TD from the much more common withdrawal dyskinesias that can occur if a patient has not been fully compliant with medication use. Furthermore, clinical care of adolescent patients treated long term (5 years or more) with neuroleptics suggests that short-lived minor dyskinetic movements may occur and spontaneously remit, even without any changes in the medication regime. If neuroleptic treatment is effective and minor dyskinetic movements are noticed, it is prudent to observe the patient over 1 to 2 weeks before making changes in the medication regime to ensure that the signs noticed are indeed likely to be early manifestations of TD.

TABLE 13–7   **Medications of Possible Use in Treating Antipsychotic-Induced Neuroleptic Malignant Syndrome in Children and Adolescents***

Medication	Dose	Potential Adverse Effects
Dantrolene	1–5 mg per kg IV, or 25–100 mg PO, Q 4–6 h	Drowsiness, dizziness, fatigue, gastrointestinal distress (Seizures and hepatic injury reported in long-term use are rare.)
Bromocriptine	2.5–5 mg PO, Q 4–6 h to a maximum of 40–100 mg daily	Nausea, vomiting, postural hypotension, headache

*The value of these medications in this population above and beyond discontinuation of the neuroleptic and routine supportive medical treatment has not been clearly established at this time. Individual patients may requre doses different from those identified above. Treatment must be directed towards the clinical requirements of each individual patient.

The atypical antipsychotic clozapine may be significantly less likely to cause TD than the typical antipsychotics, possibly due to its lack of D2 blockade in nigrostriatal dopamine tracts. TD can occur with risperidone, and at this time it is unclear if its serotonin activity may offer some degree of protection against the development of TD in comparison with typical antipsychotics.

Anticholinergic Side Effects

Anticholinergic side effects are often identified by children and adolescents as a reason not to take their neuroleptic medication. Although they may seem relatively trivial in comparison with such potential problems as TD and NMS, they are quite uncomfortable and have a negative impact on the patient's quality of life. Accordingly, the clinician must pay careful attention to the monitoring and management of this class of side effects.

Anticholinergic side effects include such symptoms as dry mouth, xerostoma, blurry vision, mydriasis, nausea, constipation, urinary hesitancy and irritation, decreased sweating, and impotence. These can be exacerbated by some antiparkinsonian medications, particularly benztropine. Other medications with anticholinergic effects (such as some tricyclics, particularly clomipramine) will also increase the frequency and severity of these symptoms if given concurrently with neuroleptics.

These side effects can be best managed by first decreasing the neuroleptic dose and then, if necessary, decreasing or changing concomitant antiparkinsonian drugs, altering the use of other concurrent medications, such as antidepressants, or switching to another antipsychotic with a more modest anticholinergic profile.

Cardiovascular Side Effects

Cardiovascular side effects are most common with low-potency antipsychotics, such as chlorpromazine, and include othostatic hypotension, increased heart rate, syncope, dizziness, and ECG changes in children and adolescents. As a group these side effects are less common in children and adolescents than in adults or the elderly. Although the quinidine-like effect of phenothiazines can be manifested as longer QT and PR intervals or depressed ST segments on ECG, these changes are of little or no clinical significance, and if no baseline cardiovascular pathology has been identified, routine cardiac monitoring is not recommended.

Phenothiazine-induced hypotension is rare in children and adolescents, and should be treated symptomatically and by changing to a higher potency preparation, such as perphenazine or flu-

penthixol. Acute hypotensive episodes should be treated supportively. Epinephrine *should not be used* because it may further lower blood pressure. If pharmacologic intervention is required, phenylephrine may be considered. In children, a dose of 100 µg/kg (or 2 to 5 mg subcutaneously in adolescents) given subcutaneously or intravenously can be used. Continuous monitoring of heart rate and blood pressure is necessary to determine the effect of this treatment and to identify rebound hypertension or bradycardia, should they occur.

Hematologic Side Effects

Hematologic side effects occur rarely with the use of phenothiazines. A mild and clinically insignificant leukopenia may be noted in some patients; however, significant hematologic problems, such as agranulocytosis, pancytopenia, thrombocytopenia, aplastic anemia, and hemolytic anemia, are rare. Thus routine monitoring of the blood count is not indicated, although immediate appropriate laboratory investigation is necessary if symptoms consistent with a possible blood dyscrasia occur.

Dermatologic Side Effects

A variety of uncommon dermatologic side effects have been described with antipsychotic use, including pruritus, urticaria, erythema, eczema, and exfoliative dermatitis. The latter must be managed as a dermatologic emergency; the others may respond to a decrease in the neuroleptic dose or topical dermatologic preparations. In some cases, an alternative neuroleptic may be indicated.

The most common dermatologic side effect is sunburn, which results from an antipsychotic-induced increase in skin photosensitivity. It is not uncommon to see neuroleptic-treated children and adolescents with sunburns because they or their parents or staff members forgot, or didn't bother, to apply correct protective measures. Remember that even a short exposure to sunlight (1 to 2 hours) may lead to sunburn in this population. Neuroleptic-treated children and adolescents should use proper sunscreen (SPF-15 or higher for UVF and UVB light) on all sun-exposed skin areas and limit their exposure to direct sunlight. The wearing of a hat with a brim to shade the face and loose-covering clothing is recommended.

Gastrointestinal Side Effects

Common complaints include nausea, gastrointestinal (GI) distress, and constipation, as already discussed. An oral syndrome may occur, however, perhaps most commonly with patients receiving liquid antipsychotics. This consists of dry mouth, reddened mucous membranes, stomatitis, cracked lips, and occasionally, vesicles in the mouth. Some patients experience the "hairy tongue" phenomenon, and in rare cases a pseudomembrane formation may be found in the oral cavity. Treatment is symptomatic, and if liquid medications are being used tablets should be started instead.

Endocrine Side Effects

Various endocrine side effects have been reported. Serum prolactin will invariably be raised. Weight gain may be a serious problem, especially for adolescent girls. Water intoxication syndrome should be considered if significant rapid weight gain (2 kg or more in a day or two) is observed. Amenorrhea or other menstrual cycle disturbances may occur. Gynecomastia, although rare, often causes great concern for adolescent boys, who will quite often be too embarassed about it to bring it to their doctor's attention. Galactorrhea can occur but is also rare. Nevertheless, because teenagers, in particular, have strong feelings about their bodies and are often reluctuant or too embarassed to bring up such issues as milk expression, changes in menses, or swelling of breast tissue, it is necessary for the clinician to inquire about such side effects with dignity and sensitivity. The patient should be encouraged to report such problems spontaneously if they occur.

Sexual side effects have been described, but not in child or adolescent populations, possibly because the questions have not been adequately studied. Decreased libido, erectile difficulties including impotence, ejaculatory problems (inhibition or retrograde ejaculation), anorgasmia, and priapism have all been associated with neuroleptic use. These problems may be compliance-limiting factors, particularly in sexually active adolescents. Good clinical management includes careful explanation and monitoring of these side effects. Teenagers will rarely report such side effects spontaneously, and perhaps more than any other aspect of the medical monitoring of neuroleptic treatment, a supportive and nonjudgmental relationship with their clinician is often a necessary prerequisite to the proper identification and subsequent management of these adverse events.

Management of endocrine side effects begins with decreasing the neuroleptic dose. If the problem persists, an endocrine consultation is warranted. For weight gain, nutritional counseling, although theoretically appealing, is in actual clinical practice a waste of time and money. Even simple suggestions, such as increasing exercise, and substituting diet drinks for juice or sodas, while potentially beneficial, are often "forgotten" by the teen engaged in his or her pursuit of the ideal adolescent diet. For sexual side effects, changing the neuroleptic may sometimes be of benefit. In other cases, bethanechol, yohimbine, amantadine, cyproheptadine, or neostigmine may be of value, depending on the particular side effect experienced. If these compounds are to be used, it is advised that a urologic, gynecologic, or endocrine consultation be undertaken and that joint management of the patient be considered.

Sensitivity Syndromes

These rare phenomena can be life threatening. Usually, they tend to appear during the first few months of neuroleptic therapy, but they may occur when the medication is being discontinued. Cholestatic jaundice, agranulocytosis, eosinophilia, laryngeal and angioneurotic edema, and anaphylaxis can occur. If any of these are seen, the medications must be discontinued immediately and proper medical management initiated.

Clinically patients may exhibit hypersensitivity reactions to preparations that contain sodium bisulfite or the yellow dye tartrazine. Patients with well-established allergic reactions, particularly aspirin sensitivity, should undergo allergy-immunology consultation prior to treatment with tablets that may contain these compounds. Liquid preparations can be used until such testing is completed if there are significant concerns about this possibility.

Ocular Effects

At high doses and especially during long-term use of typical antipsychotics, ocular side effects have been reported. Lenticular pigmentation usually does not impair vision and is reversible if the medication is discontinued. If the patient exhibits neuroleptic-induced skin pigmentation, it is worthwhile to obtain an ophthalmologic consultation to determine if lenticular pigmentation is also present. Pigmentary retinopathy (retinitis pigmentosa) has been reported primarily with the chronic use of chlorpromazine and thioridazine. Thioridazine doses of 800 mg per day or higher are not recommended because of the increased risk of this condition at those dose levels. Visual acuity is impaired in patients with retinitis pigmentosa, and blindness can occur if the condition is not treated. Ophthalmologic consultation is indicated for those patients on long-term neuroleptic treatment who complain about decreased visual acuity.

The necessity for routine yearly ophthalmologic examination is not clear but may be considered for patients who are at high risk for this adverse effect.

Potential Drug Interactions

The clinical use of neuroleptic agents may be complicated by many potential drug interactions. Drugs that compete with various neuroleptics at the hepatic cytochrome P-450 system may all affect the metabolism of neuroleptics or have their own pharmacokinetics significantly altered. Table 13–8 lists potential drug interactions of common concern to child and adolescent psychiatrists.

General Issues in the Pharmacologic Treatment of Acute Schizophrenic Psychosis

The use of neuroleptic medications is clearly indicated for the presentation of acute schizophrenic psychosis and remains the foundation for all other types of necessary interventions. The goal of treatment in this phase of the illness is to obtain symptom resolution with a minimum of adverse events. The strategy used to attain this goal is optimal neuroleptic dosing.

Recent review of neuroleptic prescribing practice has identified little if any benefit of using high doses of these compounds. Generally, at high doses side effects increase in frequency and intensity without increased clinical improvement in symptoms. At very high doses, the patient's clinical presentation may become such that it is difficult to distinguish medication-induced symptoms (particularly negative symptoms) from those of the illness itself.

This suggests that adequate, that is, neither very

TABLE 13–8 Drugs with Potential Clinically Significant Interactions with Antipsychotics of Common Concern to Child and Adolescent Psychiatrists*

Antidepressants	Antihypertensives	Disulfiram
Antihistamines	Anxiolytics	Epinephrine
Carbamazepine	Buspirone	Lithium
Phenytoin	Cimetidine	Tobacco
Valproate	Alcohol	

*A prudent course of action when the clinician is uncertain about potential drug interactions with neuroleptics is to consult available pharmacologic listings or a pharmacologist. This list is condensed from Bezchlibnyk-Butler KZ, Jefferies JJ, Martin BA. Clinical Handbook of Psychotropic Drugs (6th rev ed). Seattle: Hoegrefe & Huber Publishers, 1996, with permission.

high nor very low, doses of neuroleptics are optimal for treatment. High doses of antipsychotics do not necessarily improve, and indeed can adversely affect, outcome. Low doses are likely to be ineffective. The art of pharmacologic management of children and adolescents who present with an acute psychosis is provision of optimal medication treatment, which in part relates to the manner in which the patient presents.

Pharmacologic Management of the Acute Phase: Gradual Initiation

The initiation of pharmacologic treatment in the acute phase varies according to the presentation of the patient. In the case of the young girl with schizophrenia described earlier, pharmacologic treatment can begin in a method quite different from that necessary for the adolescent male described earlier. Generally, patients who are relatively stable behaviorally and who are compliant with therapy can be treated as described here, using gradual initiation of neuroleptic treatment.

Gradual Initiation of Neuroleptic Treatment

Patients for whom this approach works best demonstrate the following criteria:
1. Relatively stable behavior (while they may be actively hallucinating and delusional, they are not a threat to others or to themselves)
2. Compliant with taking medications
3. Have a supportive family or other social system that agrees with and upholds the treatment prescribed
4. Are able to be monitored closely but do not require continuous observation
5. Have no concurrent medical or other psychiatric condition that significantly complicates their treatment
6. Understand the nature and purpose of their treatment, and provide either consent or assent to pharmacotherapy

Initial pharmacologic treatment is selected based on the following considerations:
1. Given what is known about the differential side effect profiles of the various available neuroleptic compounds in this particular population, what is the best medication to use?
2. Given that long-term treatment will most likely be necessary and may involve the use of long-acting preparations administered by IM injection, is there a compound that is

available in both oral and long-acting IM forms?

The following approaches are reasonable, based on these considerations:

1. If the patient is preadolescent, the clinician may decide to choose a low dose of a high-potency neuroleptic, such as the butyrophenone haloperidol, to start. Preadolescent patients are possibly less likely to experience the dystonic reactions, akathisia, and severe tremors associated with the initiation of neuroleptic treatment using high-potency compounds in teenagers. In addition, because haloperidol is available in many preparations including liquid, tablet, and long-term injectable, the clinician has a wide variety of options that can be used to deliver the medication in the most useful, effective, and tolerable manner. Alternatively, risperidone could be considered.

2. If the patient is an adolescent, choose a low to moderate dose of a medium-potency neuroleptic, such as the piperazine phenothiazine perphenazine or the thioxanthene flupenthixol, to start. Perphenazine may be slightly less sedating than flupenthixol, whereas flupenthixol may be slightly more likely to produce anticholinergic side effects than perphenazine. Flupenthixol is available in the depot form as flupenthixol decanoate, while perphenazine is not. Patients with a good response to perphenazine can be converted to depot treatment with either flupenthixol decanoate or another long-acting agent if this is later chosen as the optimal route for delivering the medication.

3. Although published studies are still limited, available clinical experience at a number of sites treating adolescents with first-onset schizophrenia suggests that the atypical benzisoxazole antipsychotic, risperidone, may be a useful agent, particularly in the patient who fits the gradual initiation profile described earlier. In this case (more fully described later), risperidone can be introduced at low doses. Risperidone at this time is only available in oral tablet form, and thus long-term pharmacotherapy with this agent is limited to those patients who are likely to be compliant with oral dosing.

Suggested treatment options are listed in Table 13–9.

In all cases in which neuroleptic treatment is initiated, except with the use of risperidone and clozapine, it is recommended that antiparkinsonian medications be concurrently prescribed. This practice should decrease the frequency or severity of acute dystonic reactions and distressing extrapyramidal side effects, thus making the medication more tolerable to the patient and improving long-term compliance with pharmacotherapy. When this strategy is employed, the physician must be careful to monitor the side effects specific to antiparkinsonian agents if they are used in excessive doses. Once the peak period for the onset of acute dystonic reactions and tremors has passed (6 to 8 weeks following the onset of neuroleptic treatment), the antiparkinsonian medication can be gradually withdrawn. Useful antiparkinsonian medications, along with suggested total daily doses, can be found in Table 13–10.

The choice of antiparkinsonian agent depends on the anticipated side effect profile of the medication, because each compound noted in Table

TABLE 13–9 **Suggested Initial Antipsychotic Medication Options for Child and Adolescent Schizophrenia Using the Gradual Medication Introduction Approach**[*]

Medication	Class	Starting Dose	Usual Daily Dose
Haloperidol	Butyrophenone	1 mg	5–15 mg[†,‡]
Perphenazine	Piperazine	4 mg	16–64 mg[†]
Flupenthixol	Thioxanthene	2 mg	6–12 mg[†,‡]
Trifluoperazine	Piperazine	5 mg	5–40 mg
Chlorpromazine	Aliphatic	25 mg	200–600 mg[†]
Thioridazine	Piperidine	10 mg	200–600 mg[†]
Risperidone	Benzisoxazole	0.5 mg	2–6 mg

[*]Dosing guidelines are suggested ranges only. Individual patients may react to similar doses differently, both in terms of the therapeutic effect and side effects. Acutely ill and agitated patients may require lower doses when stabilized than when in the agitated phase. Actual dosage must be carefully tailored to the patient's clinical condition. Once-a-day dosing is usually possible after the initial target dose has been reached. Some clinicians prefer to begin antipsychotic treatment in paranoid patients with a small test dose of medication that is less than the starting dose identified above.

[†]Liquid preparation available.

[‡]Long-term injectable preparation available.

TABLE 13–10   Anticipated Common Side Effects with Various Antiparkinsonian Agents

Medication	Common Possible Side Effects
Amantadine	Indigestion, nervousness, agitation, dizziness concentration difficulties, agitation; possible tolerance to drug effect may develop early (1 to 2 weeks) during use
Benztropine	Dry mouth, blurred vision, urinary retention, constipation, potential for abuse, possible negative effects on learning
Diphenhydramine	Sedation, daytime drowsiness
Procyclidine	Dry mouth, blurred vision, constipation, urinary retention, mild stimulant effect, giddiness, cognitive and perceptual disturbances, especially at high doses

13–10 provides relatively equal efficacy against tremors, rigidity, and akathisia. Amantadine may be slightly more effective in treating neuroleptic-induced akinesia, and benztropine may be more effective in treating dystonic reactions. Diphenhydramine may be most useful for akathisia and tremor, but less helpful with muscular rigidity. In cases where parkinsonian side effects prove troubling to the patient at neuroleptic doses that otherwise provide good clinical efficacy, combining agents (at least in the short term) is possible. For example, diphenhydramine may be effectively and safely combined with benztropine or procyclidine. However, the use of multiple antiparkinsonian medications should generally occur infrequently, if at all, during the process of gradual neuroleptic introduction, as described later. The clinician should also remember that these antidote medications may all have their own side effects (Table 13–10).

CASE EXAMPLE

Gradual Initiation of Antipsychotic Treatment in a Child with Schizophrenia: "Hopefully this will help."

Following a comprehensive assessment and education program on schizophrenia, P.O.'s parents agreed with the recommendation for a multimodal treatment program including antipsychotic medications. Following discussions with the physician, the decision was made to use haloperidol as the first-choice pharmacologic intervention. P.O. was included in this process

and was educated about the medication in an age-appropriate manner. She did not want to take "pills," so the mode of delivery chosen was liquid haloperidol added to her evening juice.

P.O. and her parents were informed about the details and method of the pharmacologic intervention. These included potential risks and benefits, method and timing of medication delivery, method of monitoring tolerability and efficacy, definition of an adequate therapeutic trial, expected length of the therapeutic trial, and possible outcomes at the completion of the therapeutic trial.

Treatment was begun using haloperidol 1 mg daily combined with 2.5 mg of procyclidine given twice daily. The procyclidine was crushed and given with jam in order to respect P.O.'s wishes not to take pills. She understood that the medicine was added to the jam. Once-daily objective and subjective assessment of possible side effects was conducted using the appropriate MSSES (see Appendix IV).

Following 3 days at the starting dose, the haloperidol was increased to 2 mg, given in a similar format. This was continued for another 3 days and again increased by 1 mg per day. This process was continued until the initial target of a total daily dose of 4 mg of haloperidol was reached. At this dose, P.O. showed minimal side effects and seemed to be tolerating the medication well. Accordingly, the haloperidol was maintained at this level for 6 weeks. Evaluation of symptoms was conducted weekly using the BPRS and Overall Clinical Impression (see Appendix V and VI).

A case review at the end of the 6 week therapeutic trial was conducted. At this time the AIMS was completed in addition to the usual tolerability and efficacy measures. P.O. showed improvement in psychotic symptoms, minimal side effects, and some gains in social functioning. It was decided to maintain her on her current medication regime and to re-evaluate it in 6 weeks. Accordingly, P.O. was discharged to outpatient care, which included weekly medication monitoring.

CASE COMMENTARY

This case example illustrates the essential features of gradual antipsychotic initiation, which are as follows:

1. Select an anticipated therapeutic target dose and determine the expected length of an adequate treatment trial (usually 6 to 8 weeks) at that dose.

2. Begin antipsychotic and antiparkinsonian medications simultaneously.
3. Increase the antipsychotic medication gradually (once every 3 days or twice weekly is suggested) to reach the anticipated target dose.
4. Monitor medication-specific side effects using appropriate rating scales (objective and subjective) frequently.
5. Increase or decrease antiparkinsonian medications as indicated given the results of the side effects monitoring.
6. Monitor therapeutic efficacy using appropriate rating scales weekly.
7. Attain the anticipated therapeutic dose and then maintain it for 6 to 8 weeks, continuing to monitor tolerability and efficacy as described earlier.
8. Comprehensively review the progress of the case and conduct additional medication tolerability measures such as the AIMS, following the completion of the initial therapeutic trial.
9. Make decisions about further neuroleptic dose requirements. If larger daily doses are indicated, set another target dose and proceed as described earlier, ensuring that an adequate treatment trial is obtained at the new target dose.

Pharmacologic Management of the Acute Phase: Rapid Initiation

The discussion of the use of antipsychotic medications in this section can be applied with some modifications to the treatment of acute psychotic states in manic or depressive disorders. For further information on these conditions, please refer to Chapter 12 for mania and Chapter 11 for depression.

In many cases, as in the example of the psychotic adolescent described earlier, gradual initiation of antipsychotic pharmacotherapy is not possible. In patients who present with the following clinical features, more rapid initiation of treatment is required to ensure their safety and that of others:

1. Aggression and violence
2. Uncontrolled behavior (including severe agitation)
3. Unpredictable behavior
4. Acute danger to themselves or others
5. Behavior in response to command hallucinations
6. Severe disruption of normal neurovegetative functioning

When rapid treatment is clinically necessary, the patient is best managed by an expert staff in a therapeutic hospital setting that can provide a safe, low-stimulation environment. At times, pharmacologic management of the patient with the above-mentioned profile will involve legal issues of committal, consent, and liability. It is important to follow the legal requirements of the jurisdiction in which the clinician practices, and it is essential to respect the patient's right to refuse or accept treatment. At the same time, it is also ethically and morally imperative that a patient who is in severe distress not be denied a potentially effective medical intervention. The issues pertaining to this common clinical scenario are discussed further in Section Three.

At all times during the pharmacologic management of this acute phase, the physician and treatment team must inform the patient of the medication treatment that he or she is receiving and treat the patient in a respectful and humane manner. The patient's disordered or aggressive behavior should not preclude him or her from being treated as an informed and respected individual.

The reasons for using particular medications, route of medication delivery, expected outcome (short term and long term, e.g., "This medicine will help you rest and sleep" and "This medicine will help take the voices away"), anticipated time to expected outcome (e.g., "You should begin to feel sleepy or tired in about a half hour" and "It may take up to 4 weeks or longer for the voices to go away, but you might notice that they are less demanding and bothersome after a few days of taking this medicine"), and potential side effects ("This medicine will make you feel drowsy and even sleepy. If you get up quickly, you may feel dizzy") should be carefully and consistently explained. Whenever possible, the child or adolescent's family should be involved in the treatment process. In some cases, responsible parents who have a good relationship with their child can assist in the pharmacologic management by offering explanations and providing needed reassurance. Further discussion, including useful patient care techniques for pharmacologic management of the acute psychotic state that can be applied to schizophrenia psychoses are found in Chapter 12 in the discussion of the treatment of acute mania:

Pharmacologic management of the acute psychotic state is governed by the following objectives:

1. Provide early and effective control of behavior.
2. Restore usual neurovegetative functioning.
3. Provide early and effective relief of psychotic symptoms.

These objectives are reached by applying antipsychotics in such a manner as to produce the desired therapeutic outcome with the minimal adverse effects possible.

Although a number of different pharmacologic strategies (described later) can be used to reach these objectives, the clinician must be aware of the expected time course and pattern of clinical improvement that will provide the framework for evaluation of the therapeutic efficacy of the chosen pharmacologic intervention. The patient and patient's family must also be informed of this expected time course for improvement. This information not only will help educate them about the treatment's usual clinical course but also in many cases will enable the patient and family to become active participants in monitoring the expected outcome. Table 13–11 illustrates the expected course during successful pharmacologic treatment of an acute schizophrenic episode.

Effective pharmacologic treatment of the acute schizophrenic episode is dependent in large part on achieving sufficient daily doses of a relatively well-tolerated neuroleptic. In general terms, a total daily dose of antipsychotic should reach at least 300 mg of chlorpromazine or its equivalent. Lower doses may not demonstrate the expected efficacy. A common problem among clinicians treating acutely psychotic children and adolescents is undertreatment, prescribing an insufficient dose of antipsychotic. Another common problem is overtreatment, prescribing an overly generous dose of neuroleptic. The first course of action often results in ineffective or unnecessarily prolonged treatment, whereas the second course of action often results in an increased rate of side effects without an increased therapeutic effect.

The proper choice of neuroleptic medication takes into account the nature and type of the patient's presenting symptomatology and attempts to fit the neuroleptic to the patient. For example, the patient who is severely aggressive and agitated, and who requires sedation for optimal clinical management, may best benefit from a neuroleptic that is high in sedative properties, such as, chlorpromazine. In this case, doses of chlorpromazine in the range of 300 to 600 mg daily (for an adolescent; lower in a child) will usually be sufficient to provide behavioral control without overdosing. The use of a less sedating neuroleptic, such as haloperidol, if applied without concomitant sedating or anxiolytic compounds, often results in extremely high daily doses for behavioral control, with the attendant increased

---

TABLE 13–11   Expected Course for Clinical Improvement in the Acutely Psychotic Schizophrenic Child or Adolescent Treated with Antipsychotics*

Clinical Indicator	Time of Expected Improvement from Initiation of Effective Neuroleptic Treatment[†]
Behavior during the day is relatively settled. The patient is not severely aggressive or hostile. He or she does not require continuous sedation to control behavior.	Significant improvements to reach these indicators should occur within 1–3 days.
The patient is able to fall asleep and maintain relatively continuous sleep for most of the night.	Sleep function should be restored or else show major improvements within 2–3 days.
The patient is able to engage in relatively normal eating and basic self-care routines.	These indicators should be generally present within 5–7 days.
The patient is able to tolerate minor stresses, such as short periods of time in a common room or appropriate family visits without a significant increase in behavioral disturbance.	These indicators should be generally present within 5–7 days.
The patient should be able to tolerate longer periods of time in situations that are more stimulating or demanding (such as ward milieu, longer family visits).	These indicators should be generally reached between 10 and 14 days.
The patient should begin to show a significant decrease in hallucinations and delusions.	These indicators should generally be reached between 2 and 3 weeks.
More normative social functioning should be significantly present (such as eating in a group, participating in group activities)	These indicators should generally be reached between 2 and 3 weeks.

*The suggested time course for reaching each clinical indicator will vary among patients depending on the severity of their illness and other factors. Therefore, they are to be used only as a guide.

[†]Effective antipsychotic treatment in the acute psychotic phase of schizophrenia is expected to be about 300 mg of chlorpromazine (or its equivalent) daily.

rate of side effects without increased antipsychotic efficacy.

In treating an acute schizophrenic episode with neuroleptics, more does not mean better. Physiologically optimal dopamine receptor binding in the central nervous system occurs at doses of 300 to 600 mg of chlorpromazine or equivalent. Higher doses are not likely to speed clinical improvement but may actually worsen it by inducing a variety of side effects (such as akathisia), which can be confused with the psychosis itself. This effect may possibly explain the occasional clinical observation in which the patient's psychosis improved when his or her neuroleptic dose was decreased.

The physician choosing a neuroleptic medication to treat the acutely psychotic schizophrenic child or adolescent must consider the following:

1. Given what is known about the differential side effect profiles of the various available antipsychotic compounds in this particular population and the nature of the particular patient's clinical presentation, what is the best medication to use?

2. Given that treatment will most likely be necessary in the long term and may involve the use of long-acting preparations given by IM injection, is there a compound that is available in both oral and long-acting IM forms?

Based on these questions, the following approaches are reasonable for acute management:

1. A sedating low-potency neuroleptic, such as chlorpromazine or thioridazine, can be used. These medications can be given in various forms—tablet, liquid, or injectable, as clinically indicated. When appropriate clinical improvement has been achieved (usually within the first 2 to 3 weeks), they can be substituted with either a medium-potency neuroleptic, such as perphenazine or flupenthixol, or with a long-acting injectable such as flupenthixol or fluphenazine decanoate (see later for a discussion on the use of injectable neuroleptics).

   Ideally this changeover should be gradual to minimize the potential of withdrawal effects. If substituting a medium-potency neuroleptic, it is advisable to decrease the low-potency neuroleptic dose by one third while introducing the equivalent amount (in chlorpromazine units) of the medium-potency neuroleptic. This should be maintained for 3 to 5 days, at which time two thirds of the remaining low-potency neuroleptic dose can be discontinued in favor of the equivalent amount of medium-potency neuroleptic. The final fine-tuning of the dose can then be made 3 to 5 days later. Alternatively, the clinician may choose to substitute the low-potency neuroleptic with the atypical antipsychotic, risperidone. This is discussed later under point 3.

2. A less sedating medium-potency neuroleptic, such as perphenazine or flupenthixol, can be used. This may need to be combined with occasional doses of a more sedating neuroleptic, such as chlorpromazine, during the first few days to weeks of treatment if the less sedating medication alone does not provide adequate behavioral control. Alternatively, in some cases a benzodiazepine such as lorazepam (2 mg per oral dose or 1 mg per sublingual dose, up to a daily maximum of 4 to 6 mg) can be used as a combination compound for behavioral control.

   Clinical experience with the combined neuroleptic strategy (low potency, e.g., chlorpromazine, plus medium potency, e.g., perphenazine) has been positive, with good therapeutic effects and tolerable side effects. The initial combined dose of antipsychotics is titrated to the patient's clinical condition, with the combined daily dose of the medications aimed at between 300 and 600 mg of chlorpromazine equivalents. As the patient shows improved behavioral control and requires less sedation, the dose of the low-potency antipsychotic is gradually decreased and the dose of medium-potency neuroleptic is increased proportionally. This procedure often results in a relatively smooth medication initiation phase because the doses of the low-potency antipsychotic can be spread out during the day as needed and the medium-potency antipsychotic can be given as a single bedtime dose. The low-potency neuroleptic chlorpromazine also is available in liquid and injectable form for use when tablets are inappropriate or if very rapid behavioral control is required.

   Some textbooks and articles argue against the combination of two neuroleptic medications, often from no good rationale other than the firmly held but unsubstantiated dogma of "one medicine is always to be preferred to two." As long as the clinician understands the rationale behind the use of combining low-potency and medium-potency neuroleptics and provides careful monitoring of both compounds separately and in combination, this pharmacologic approach not only increases therapeutic flexibility but may actually decrease the incidence of extrapyramidal and parkinsonian-type side effects that would accompany the use of a single medium-potency compound titrated to produce the same beneficial effect on severely disordered behavioral symptoms.

The use of adjunctive benzodiazepines to provide behavioral control, while clearly an accepted common practice in treating adult schizophrenic patients with acute psychosis, is not universally supported in children and adolescents. As explained in previous chapters, the use of benzodiazepines in children and adolescents is associated with a higher incidence of behavioral side effects than in adults. In some series, this occurs in up to 30 percent or more of patients. Thus, the risk of introducing problematic behavioral adverse events, especially disinhibition, exists if benzodiazepines are used but can be avoided if low-potency antipsychotics are used.

Some experienced child and adolescent psychopharmacologists, however, have successfully combined benzodiazepines such as lorazepam (4 to 6 mg daily) and clonazepam (1 to 3 mg daily) with both medium-potency and high-potency neuroleptics (such as haloperidol) in this population. Others have been less impressed with the therapeutic effects of this combination and have found that the problems associated with this approach often outweigh the expected benefits. At this time, no clear direction can be given regarding this issue. The clinician choosing to use a benzodiazepine-antipsychotic combination should carefully monitor patients so treated for the occurrence of benzodiazepine-induced behavioral side effects, taking care to differentiate these from psychotic symptoms. One benefit of the benzodiazepine-antipsychotic combination should be a lower incidence and decreased severity of akathisia. If clozapine is being used in acute treatment, however, the use of concomitant benzodiazepines is strongly discouraged because of the potential for respiratory difficulties, including respiratory arrest, with this pharmacologic combination.

In options 1 and 2, and indeed whenever neuroleptic therapy is instituted with "typical" antipsychotics, the concomitant use of antiparkinsonian medications is recommended in the short term. These have already been discussed.

3. The atypical antipsychotic risperidone can be used, either alone or combined with low-potency neuroleptics or benzodiazepines, as clinically indicated (see earlier discussion). Because risperidone at low doses is relatively nonsedating, it may need to be combined with an adjunctive agent during the early phases of treatment if the patient's behavior is not controlled by risperidone alone. Either low-potency neuroleptics (e.g., 25 to 50 mg chlorpromazine per dose) or benzodiazepines can be safely combined with risperidone if necessary.

If used alone, risperidone in adolescents should be started at a dose of 1 mg twice daily and increased to 2 mg twice daily after 3 to 5 days at the first dose level. The potential therapeutic window for risperidone in children and adolescents is 2 to 6 mg daily. Doses lower than 2 mg daily may not produce a significant therapeutic effect, and doses greater than 6 mg daily may be unlikely to show greater efficacy. Some studies in adults suggest that daily doses of 16 mg risperidone may provide a therapeutic effect for patients who have failed to respond at doses within the expected window. However, at the higher dose risperidone use is associated with significant extrapyramidal and parkinsonian side effects, and it seems to act more like a "typical" antipsychotic. Clinical experience and some early experimental evidence suggest that an initial target dose of 4 mg daily, given in two divided doses, is appropriate for the adolescent experiencing an acute schizophrenic psychosis. If expected clinical improvement does not occur as anticipated on this dose, it can be increased to 6 mg, given as 3 mg twice daily. Although the use of risperidone with children is limited, prepubertal patients may often respond at a total daily dose of 2 mg or less. Thus, the initial target dose and initiation strategy will need to be modified accordingly for this age group.

In some cases, patients who are not compliant with tablets (but show improved compliance with liquid medications) may be started with more typical antipsychotics and then switched to risperidone. Alternatively, the clinician may elect to use strategy 1 and switch the patient to risperidone rather than to a medium-potency typical neuroleptic. In this scenario, a withdrawal of the low-potency medication should proceed gradually, as already described, to minimize the risk of a withdrawal syndrome. In adolescents, one third of the total low-potency neuroleptic can be discontinued and 1 mg of risperidone, given twice daily, begun concurrently. Three to 5 days later, two thirds of the remaining typical neuroleptic dose can be discontinued and the risperidol dose increased to 4 mg daily (2 mg twice daily). Three to 5 days later, the rest of the low-potency neuroleptic dose can be discontinued.

Patients treated with typical neuroleptics, as in the above-mentioned scenarios, should also be concomitantly treated with antiparkinsonian medications. When they are switched over to risperidone, they will probably require significantly less antiparkinsonian medication and may indeed be able to forgo it altogether. These compounds should not be abruptly terminated. It is suggested that the patient be maintained on his or her antiparkinsonian medication at the same dose for 2 to 3 weeks following the discontinuation of the typical neuroleptic. At this time, the antiparkinsonian medication can be gradually tapered. A reasonable antiparkinsonian discontinuation schedule is given in Table 13–12.

Prior to the discontinuation of antiparkinsonian medications and during every discontinuation day, a careful evaluation of the patient's signs and symptoms of parkinsonian-type side effects should be completed using an appropriate side effects monitoring instrument, as described earlier. Should significant side effects occur with the withdrawal of antiparkinsonian medications, these may need to be re-established, even though risperidone in general is less likely to cause them. Another attempt at discontinuation could be made at a later date.

TABLE 13–12 **Suggested Discontinuation Protocol for Antiparkinsonian Medications***

Day 1	Decrease the daily dose by one quarter to one third
Days 4–6	Decrease the daily dose by one quarter to one third
Days 8–10	Decrease the daily dose by one quarter to one half
Days 12–14	Discontinue

*The discontinuation protocol is to be used as a guideline only. Individual patients will vary in their experience of withdrawal symptoms and return of parkinsonian symptoms. Careful clinical titration is necessary.

CASE EXAMPLE

Use of Neuroleptic Medication in the Acute Treatment of an Adolescent with a Severe Schizophrenic Psychosis

A.J. was admitted to an observation unit on an adolescent inpatient psychiatric service. His behavior was agitated and hostile. He threatened to kill the staff because they were "evil" and "plotting against" him. He reported that he was hearing "voices" that were telling him to escape by jumping out of the window. A supportive male nurse was assigned to provide him with constant care.

A.J. initially refused any medications despite reassurances from hospital staff and his parents. He kept demanding to leave and believed that he was being held in a "jail so that experiments could be made on his brain." He was convinced that his school principal had orchestrated the entire scenario, and a few hours after admission he attacked a nurse who had entered his room.

At that time, A.J.'s behavior become totally uncontrolled. Accordingly, he was physically restrained and given chlorpromazine, 50 mg intramuscularly (two separate injections at 25 mg per injection site). During this procedure, the reasons for the injection and verbal calming were continuously provided, and he was kept in a face-down prone position on his bed. Blood pressure and heart rate monitoring were provided. He was encouraged to rest and relax. One-half hour later, A.J. was much more subdued. At this time, he was again engaged in a discussion about what was happening to him and was encouraged to take the medications offered to him. This time he agreed and was given procyclidine 5 mg orally. A half-hour later he was asleep.

At this time, the attending physician and a nurse met with A.J.'s parents and discussed the tentative diagnosis and treatment options. After a wide-ranging conversation, A.J.'s parents agreed with the use of neuroleptic medications. Regular meetings were scheduled between parents and staff, and A.J.'s parents were given the name and number of a staff contact person who they could reach at any time.

Four hours later, the attending nurse reported that A.J.'s behavior was once again escalating. He was seen immediately by the physician and the behavioral escalation was confirmed. A review of his blood pressure and heart rate data showed no significant problems, and 100 mg of liquid chlorpromazine in 50 cc of orange juice was given. Cardiovascular monitoring and continuous nursing care were maintained. The patient's progress was reviewed by the physician at 2-hourly interviews by direct observation, and the physician was available to attend to the patient at any time judged necessary by the nurse monitor. Liquid chlorpromazine at oral doses of 100 mg were given as dictated by the patient's symptomatology.

Following this protocol, A.J.'s status was reviewed at 2000 hours, and he was examined for evidence of neuroleptic side effects. The presence of some mild parkinsonian side effects was noted, and an additional 5 mg of procyclidine was prescribed. A bedtime dose of oral liquid chlorpromazine of 150 mg was given at 2200 hours.

In the morning (0700 hours), A.J.'s progress and treatment were reviewed. He had been given a total of 550 mg of chlorpromazine over the previous 24 hours, and on this dose he had still exhibited episodes of agitated and hostile behavior, although he could be "talked down" by staff. He had not slept very well and although he had not demonstrated any aggressive episodes during the night, he was noted to be awake and talking in response to his voices for long periods of time. It was estimated that he had slept 4 hours.

A physical examination showed A.J. to have mild tremor and stiffness; otherwise, his neurologic condition was unremarkable. His cardiovascular parameters were reasonable and showed minor sinus tachycardia. Mental status examination showed continuing hallucinations and delusions but less agitation. The purpose of hospitalization and medical treatment was again discussed with A.J. by the attending physician and a staff nurse, and the risks and benefits of pharmacologic treatment were reviewed. A.J. consented to take chlorpromazine, and his consent was recorded in the medical and nursing records.

Because A.J.'s behavior was believed to be still unpredictable, and he was found to be easily agitated and combative, it was decided that multiple daily dosing with the sedating low-potency neuroleptic chlorpromazine (to optimize behavioral control) was the preferred method of medication delivery. The following outline of medication delivery was developed, using a total 1 day target of 700 mg of chlorpromazine because this was the approximate amount that the patient had required over the previous 24 hours to provide behavioral control and to assist in sleep:

Chlorpromazine 100 mg liquid PO at 0800, 1200, 1600, and 2000

Chlorpromazine 300 mg liquid PO at 2200
Procyclidine 5 mg tablet PO at 0800
Procyclidine 5 mg tablet PO at 2000

Blood pressure and heart rate were to be recorded prior to each chlorpromazine dose and one half hour following each chlorpromazine dose. Attending physician examination of the patient was scheduled for 0800, 1200, 1600, and 1800 hours. On-call physician examination of the patient was scheduled for 2000 and 2200 hours. Nursing staff were directed that no antipsychotic medication was to be given without the patient first being assessed by the treating physician.

As needed medication use was identified as chlorpromazine 100 mg liquid or 50 mg IM and benztropine 2 mg IM. As needed medication was not to be given without the physician being notified and agreeing to the use of the medication.

A standardized Medication Delivery Record, as outlined in Figure 13–1, was used to monitor and record A.J.'s acute pharmacologic management.

CASE COMMENTARY

This case illustrates a common clinical presentation and pharmacologic intervention for an acutely psychotic schizophrenic teenager. The patient was treated in a specialized adolescent psychiatric facility with expert staff. Every attempt was made to provide a safe and secure environment for him, to educate him about his clinical condition, to discuss treatment options with him, and to respect his rights and dignity. Within this framework, however, active pharmacologic intervention was necessary, and although IM medications were used because of behavior that could not be safely controlled otherwise, every attempt was made to continue reassurance and education about treatment throughout this process.

IM injections of chlorpromazine may provide good behavioral control in similar clinical situations. Although 50 mg may be needed for an adolescent (25 mg is usually sufficient for a prepubertal patient), only 25 mg should be given per injection site. Emergency IM injections are best given in the gluteus muscle with the patient in a face-down position. In those rare cases in which mechanical restraints are necessary, the patient should always be made as comfortable as possible while

Medication Delivery Record*

Patient: _____ Date: _____

Physician: _____

Morning review (issues arising from night monitoring that need to be addressed): _____

_____

_____

Total neuroleptic dose used over past 24 hours (in chlorpromazine equivalents): _____

Total estimated neuroleptic dose for today (in chlorpromazine equivalents): _____

Time: 0800

Blood pressure: _____ Heart rate: _____

Physical examination findings: _____

Summary of clinical condition: _____

Neuroleptic and dose given: _____

Other medications given: _____

Time: 0830

Blood pressure: _____ Heart rate: _____

Medication effect: _____

Observations and interventions: _____

_____

Time: 1200

Blood pressure: _____ Heart rate: _____

Physical examination findings: _____

Summary of clinical condition: _____

Neuroleptic and dose given: _____

Other medications given: _____

Time: 1230

Blood pressure: _____ Heart rate: _____

Medication effect: _____

Observations and interventions: _____

_____

Time: 1600

Blood pressure: _____ Heart rate: _____

Physical examination findings: _____

Summary of clinical condition: _____

FIGURE 13–1 Acute Pharmacologic Management for Child and Adolescent Psychosis: Physician Log

Neuroleptic and dose given: _____

Other medications given: _____

Time: 1630

Blood pressure: _____   Heart rate: _____

Medication effect: _____

Observations and interventions: _____

_____

Time: 2000

Blood pressure: _____   Heart rate: _____

Physical examination findings: _____

Summary of clinical condition: _____

Neuroleptic and dose given: _____

Other medications given: _____

Time: 2030

Blood pressure: _____   Heart rate: _____

Medication effect: _____

Observations and interventions: _____

_____

Time: 2200

Blood pressure: _____   Heart rate: _____

Physical examination findings: _____

Summary of clinical condition: _____

Neuroleptic and dose given: _____

Other medications given: _____

Time: 2230

Blood pressure: _____   Heart rate: _____

Medication effect: _____

Observations and interventions: _____

_____

*This record is provided as a template on which the unique medication management strategy for each patient can be placed. Although the outline should remain generally the same for most patients, the time of medication delivery is expected to vary. The use of this template helps ensure that all the required expected medical and nursing management of the patient, with regard to the provision of acute pharmacologic intervention, occurs. A new medication management strategy should be developed for each consecutive day in which acute pharmacologic treatment is necessary, and each day's medication management record should be altered appropriately.

FIGURE 13–1 *Continued*

in a face-down position and constant observation should be provided. The continued need for mechanical restraints should be formally reassessed at least at 10 minute intervals and blood circulation to extremities should be checked more often.

In most cases, if oral medications can be given the use of IM injection can be avoided. Liquid medicines and not tablets should be used during the acute phase. They are more easily swallowed and the patient is less likely to tongue liquid medication (see Chapter 12 for further practical hints regarding medication use during this phase).

As illustrated earlier, the attending physician must be very involved in the patient's immediate care and should frequently monitor the patient's physical condition and mental state. Antipsychotic medications should be given only after this monitoring has occurred. Expert nursing staff providing constant care not only ensures a safe and supportive environment for the patient but also allows for the early identification of behavioral escalation and other symptomatic changes. This awareness of behavioral changes further allows for early pharmacologic intervention, which has the goal of decreasing the frequency and severity of behavioral outbursts. Using this strategy, the treatment of the patient becomes proactive instead of reactive. Thus, the patient's symptoms can be controlled without overmedicating or undermedicating. This type of careful monitoring is necessary for the provision of optimal pharmacologic treatment to a child or adolescent suffering from an acute psychotic episode.

It is not good pharmacologic practice to leave standing medication orders for an acutely ill patient without frequent physician monitoring. Good clinical care demands constant nursing and frequent physician monitoring of the patient's condition. If prn orders are left, as in this case, a reasonable instruction to the nursing staff is that the physician must be called and the patient's clinical condition discussed before any prn order is given. The only exception to this rule is if the nurse (who has been trained in the recognition of acute dystonic reactions) suspects an acute dystonic reaction, in which case the proper treatment (benztropine 2 mg IM) can be given immediately and the physician then notified. In the opinion of many child and adolescent psychiatrists who treat large numbers of acutely ill psychotic patients, standing prn orders for an-

tipsychotic medications are a mixed blessing. They may provide a false sense of security for staff and be overused; for example, one nurse's assessment of agitated and dangerous behavior may be significantly different from another's. A better strategy is to involve either the attending or on-call physician at any time that the nursing staff believes that further neuroleptic dosing may be required. In this case, the prn medication orders will be less likely to be overused and will serve as a treatment guideline and management plan, having the effect of ensuring that sufficient amounts of the proper medications are easily available should they be needed.

Initial pharmacologic treatment in the above-mentioned case was based on obtaining behavioral control and normalizing vegetative functioning. A multiple daily dose strategy using a low-potency neuroleptic was chosen as a reasonable approach to achieve this goal and to provide sufficient sedation to allow for increased efficacy of verbal calming. The patient's clinical condition dictated the amount and frequency of medication use over the first 24 hours. This approach not only allowed for optimal titration of the neuroleptic dose but also provided an important learning curve for the physician and nursing staff, because they were able to carefully observe the clinical effect of each individual medication dose. This approach is an extremely useful strategy because there may be great individual variation in response to any single dose of an antipsychotic.

The second 24 hours were guided by a best estimate of the predicted medication effect. The total daily medication dose expected to be used that day was derived by taking the amount of medication used during the previous day, (because this seemed to provide reasonable clinical efficacy and was close to the expected therapeutic range for chlorpromazine, 300 to 600 mg daily) and spreading it out during the day using the information about the usual effect of a single dose on the patient's clinical status as observed on the previous day. More of the total daily dose was given at night to help with sleeping.

Side effects were carefully monitored. Physical examination by the physician was structured to occur at predetermined times. Blood pressure and heart rate were measured just prior to every medication dose and repeated one-half hour later to ensure that adverse events are identified early, should they occur. Instructions to nursing staff should identify minimal blood pressure and heart rate parameters that require immediate attention by the physician.

The attending physician and staff met with the patient's parents soon after the patient's hospitalization. This is essential to provide support and education for the child or adolescent's family and to obtain their informed consent or agreement for medical treatment. Failure to do this may lead to misunderstandings and difficulties that need not occur if this procedure is followed. Parents of a child or adolescent who is experiencing an acute psychotic break are likely to be frightened, concerned, worried, and distressed. Often this type of stressful situation can create or exacerbate family dysfunction. Because successful pharmacologic treatment will to a great degree depend on the relationship that not only the patient but also the family has with the physician and the clinical team, it is essential to take the time to meet with and support the family during the crisis.

A useful strategy at this time is to identify a member of the nursing staff who can provide an immediate liaison with the family. Parents or other family members will often have many questions that will arise from the initial meeting and will want someone to talk with about them. They will often be quite worried about how their child is doing and will want to have frequent updates on the child's condition. Giving the parents the name of a staff contact person and a telephone number where that person can be reached will usually be very helpful. In addition, regular meetings with family and staff should be scheduled. In some units a social worker may be involved in these: in other units, a nurse. These meetings can be used for multiple purposes: to provide support, to educate, to discuss treatment, and so forth.

The physician should be available to meet with parents or other family members as necessary. Usually these meetings need to be held more frequently during the early course of treatment and tend to decrease somewhat in number as the child or adolescent improves. When the child or adolescent is sufficiently well, he or she should be invited to join these meetings in whole or in part as indicated. These sessions can be used to provide a forum for the discussion of many issues and will provide continuity of care over the course of hospitalization that ideally could be carried out as needed during outpatient treatment as well.

Other Important Considerations for Pharmacologic Management of the Acute Phase of a Schizophrenic Psychosis

The appropriate use of neuroleptics in acute treatment of a schizophrenic psychosis is still the subject of discussion among seasoned clinicians. Two issues that are important to address within the context of that discussion may have immediate impact on patient care. These are the use of high-potency neuroleptics and the use of injectable neuroleptics.

High-potency neuroleptics such as haloperidol are an effective treatment for psychotic symptoms in adult schizophrenics. Many clinicians also use these compounds in the treatment of acute psychotic states in children and adolescents. There are concerns about the use of high-potency neuroleptics in this population. Clinical experience and some research suggest that adolescents in particular are at greater risk of developing dystonic reactions and severe parkinsonian symptoms when high-potency antipsychotics, as opposed to low- or medium-potency antipsychotics, are used. Further, the danger of overdosing with high-potency antipsychotics (e.g., rapid neuroleptization) to obtain behavioral control during the first phase of pharmacologic treatment in the acute psychotic state is well known. Given the availability of a number of equally effective compounds with less potential for these problems, the routine prescription of high-potency neuroleptics should not, in the opinion of some, be routinely used as a first-line pharmacotherapy in acutely ill psychotic adolescents. There may be a role for their use in that portion of the population who are prepubescent and/or who present with a clinical profile suitable for gradual induction of antipsychotic treatment, as described earlier. In these cases, small doses of high-potency antipsychotics using gradual upward titration, coupled with careful monitoring of side effects, may be preferred over the use of low-potency medications with their sedating potential.

Long-acting injectable neuroleptics are very useful in the long-term treatment of schizophrenia, and their use in this condition is described in Chapter 14. They should not be used to treat the child or adolescent who presents with an acute psychotic picture, even if the clinician is certain that the disorder is a schizophrenic psychosis and that the use of long-acting injectable neuroleptics will be indicated in its treatment. The use of long-term injectable neuroleptics in the acute phase simply does not provide the pharmacologic flexibility that is necessary to optimize symptom control. Furthermore, should the patient experience a severe adverse reaction to the medication that demands the discontinuation of treatment (such as NMS), the necessary clearance of the neuroleptic will be severely prolonged, with potentially unpleasant or even fatal consequences. This should not be confused with the use of short-term, injectable low-potency neuroleptics, such as chlorpromazine, which are useful in treating the acute state. Once the patient's clinical condition has been stabilized using oral neuroleptics, consideration can be given to the use of long-term injectable medications.

Common Clinical Problems Regarding Pharmacologic Treatment of Acute Schizophrenic Psychosis

Compliance

Difficulties with patient compliance are often encountered in this population, particularly with teenagers. This is discussed generally in Section Three, but some issues specific to neuroleptic use bear repeating here. First, many patients do not understand or appreciate the nature of their illness or its treatment. Thus, one of the essential factors for improving compliance is the effective education of patients and their caregivers about their illness, an ongoing process that begins at the time of diagnosis and treatment initiation and continues over the patient's lifetime. A second issue is that *all* the medications used to treat psychotic symptoms have unpleasant side effects. Some side effects (particularly the dystonias and severe extrapyramidal reactions) are more unpleasant and frightening than others, but the patient's mild subjective discomforts should not be ignored by the clinician. Optimal pharmacologic treatment includes not only obtaining symptomatic control but also minimizing side effects. Various strategies for this are outlined in Section Three. Of great value are the explanation of potential adverse effects to the patient and family and the assurance that many of these may be transient or dose related and will improve as the clinical condition improves and the total daily dose can be decreased.

Negative Symptoms

As is well appreciated, many schizophrenic patients will suffer from debilitating negative symp-

toms. In some cases, these symptoms may actually be the predominant clinical picture or may precede the development of a positive phenomenology by months or even years. There is some suggestion that patients with significant degrees of negative symptoms may show a poorer long-term outcome across a variety of social and vocational domains. Thus identification of and appropriate intervention for negative symptoms are important clinical issues. Common negative symptoms of schizophrenia are alogia, asociality, affect flattening, apathy, avolition, and attentional impairment.

First, the clinician must ensure that the medication itself is not responsible for the negative symptoms. The use of typical antipsychotics, especially at high doses, is known to possibly induce negative-type symptoms that may be difficult to distinguish from the illness itself. In many cases these can be treated by lowering the antipsychotic dose, or if that is not possible, by increasing antiparkinsonian medications. In addition, negative symptoms must be carefully differentiated from depressive symptoms, which are well recognized to occur in schizophrenic patients. If severe depressive symptoms are present, or if a depressive syndrome is found, the clinician is well advised to review the diagnosis of schizophrenia and possibly institute treatments appropriate for psychotic depression (see Chapter 11).

Second, patients with predominantly negative schizophrenic symptoms may benefit more from the use of an atypical antipsychotic, such as risperidone or clozapine. If this is the case, it is reasonable to begin pharmacologic treatment with one of the atypical antipsychotics, even if the patient is currently experiencing many positive symptoms, such as hallucinations and delusions.

Relapse or Plateau During Active Treatment

In some cases, patients may appear to relapse (symptoms increase) or plateau (symptoms do not continue to improve at the same rate as previously noted), even during active treatment. When this occurs, it often has one of the following causes:

1. The antipsychotic total daily dose prescribed is insufficient to produce an optimal clinical response—an under-medication problem.
2. A changeover from one antipsychotic to another is occurring, such as from oral to long-acting injectable, or from a typical to an atypical antipsychotic, and the dose titration

during the switch process has not been optimal—an undermedication problem.

3. The antipsychotic total daily dose prescribed is sufficient for optimal clinical response but another medication has been added (or the patient is ingesting another substance) that has either directly or indirectly decreased the efficacy of the neuroleptic—a pseudo-under medication problem.

4. The neuroleptic total daily dose prescribed is sufficient for optimal clinical response but is producing side effects that confuse or exacerbate the clinical picture—an overmedication problem.

5. The neuroleptic total daily dose prescribed is sufficient for optimal clinical response but the patient is no longer taking the same amount as previously—a compliance problem.

6. The clinical picture represents a blossoming of the psychosis because the symptoms that may have gone unrecognized previously are identified—not a medication problem but a clinical possibility.

Relapse is most often associated with possibility 5, and clinically this often occurs when the patient has been switched from liquid to tablet medication. A reasonable approach is to discuss this possibility with the patient while concurrently returning to the use of liquid medications until the issue can be clarified. The plateau is most often associated with possibilities 1 to 4, and the correct clinical intervention follows from determining which of these potential phenomena is occurring. Any degree of clinical suspicion about a medical problem or substance abuse should be followed up with the appropriate necessary investigations.

Treatment Resistance

A poor clinical response to any one neuroleptic may be expected in 20 to 30 percent of the child and adolescent schizophrenic population. There is some suggestion that the response to neuroleptic treatment in schizophrenia may improve somewhat with age, with older adolescents showing response rates similar to adult populations. The clinical approach to neuroleptic nonresponse should follow the guidelines offered in Section Three. However, a number of issues that apply to this population will be discussed here. First, it is essential to determine if the patient is indeed nonresponsive. To that end, the following questions should be asked.

Review of Potential Neuroleptic Nonresponse in Acutely Psychotic Children and Adolescents

1. Exactly what symptoms show nonresponse to treatment?

   In many cases, it may be found that the patient is actually responding to treatment if the correct assessment of expected symptom response is made. A potential mistake in this case is when the hallucinations and delusions are unrealistically expected to be completely controlled within a week of beginning pharmacologic treatment. Because it is highly unlikely that this will happen, even with the most optimal of available pharmacologic treatment, considering the patient to be nonresponding is incorrect. The pattern and degree of response must be compared with the expected pattern and degree of response outlined in Table 13–11.

2. Are the symptoms that are considered to illustrate nonresponse of the patient actually symptoms of the disorder, or have they been iatrogenically induced?

   The most common confusion between symptoms of the illness and symptoms of the treatment arises in the area of akathisia. In many cases, if the patient is experiencing akathisia he or she may demonstrate behavioral or cognitive symptoms that are difficult to distinguish from the schizophrenic psychosis. For example, the patient may be restless, pacing, or agitated. In some cases, the patient will provide a psychotic elaboration as an attempt to understand the physical sensations that he or she is experiencing: "Ants are crawling under my skin." "My legs are jazz, rock and roll, and rhythm and blues." In other cases, the patient will not or cannot describe the sensations and may express distress by suicidal ideation or behaviors. Thus, it is essential that a careful assessment of potentially iatrogenic symptoms be made prior to declaring a patient as treatment nonresponsive. In cases in which the clinician is uncertain, a reasonable strategy is to decrease the neuroleptic dose and observe the response over 1 to 2 weeks.

3. Has the medication been given in the proper dose for a sufficient length of time?

   One of the most common explanations for treatment nonresponse is inadequate pharmacologic treatment. This can be either underdosing (a total daily dose that is below the amount needed for symptom resolution), undertiming (a potentially effective dose continued for an insufficient length of time), or overdosing. Inadequate pharmacologic treatment is a problem not only found in rapid-initiation treatment but also in gradual-initiation treatment. Indeed, in the latter it may be more difficult to identify because in many cases the patient will obtain some symptomatic improvement but will plateau or even relapse. In such cases, increasing or decreasing the total daily dose to fall within the expected amount necessary for clinical improvement and continuing this over an appropriate length of time (6 to 8 weeks) is a reasonable strategy.

If this review demonstrates that treatment nonresponse is indeed present, the following strategies are reasonable to consider:

1. Change the total daily dose of the neuroleptic (optimize initial treatment)

    If the patient is a rapid metabolizer of the neuroleptic, the expected serum levels for the usual daily dose may not be realized and higher total daily doses will be required. Because neuroleptic serum levels are not easily available and their relationship to clinical outcome is not well understood, there is little if any indication to use these as a treatment guideline. A more reasonable approach is to titrate the antipsychotic dose to a new target dose and then hold at this level for a sufficient time to observe the potential efficacy of this strategy. The ceiling for this approach when dosing is increased is the onset of distressing or intolerable side effects that cannot be controlled other than by decreasing the total daily amount of neuroleptic used.

2. Combine the neuroleptic with another medication (augmentation)

    This strategy is sometimes useful, although controlled research trials are lacking. Clinical experience suggests that in some patients (particularly if there is a family history of affective disorder) the addition of lithium might be of benefit. If this strategy is chosen, the lithium should be added gradually and monitored carefully, following the approach outlined in Chapter 12. It is reasonable to consider this augmentation approach if maximization of the initial medication, as described earlier, is unsuccessful.

3. Switch to another neuroleptic (substitution)

    This strategy should be considered if maximization of initial treatment is not successful. In this case, although clinical lore suggests that substituting one class of typical neuroleptics for another (such as perphenazine, a piperazine phenothiazine, for flupenthixol, a thioxanthene) is reasonable, this strategy evolved in a time where alternative or atypical antipsychotics were not available. Currently, although this changing of one typical antipsychotic for another typical antipsychotic is not unreasonable, greater consideration should be given for changing from a typical to an atypical antipsychotic. In this case, risperidone (described earlier) or clozapine (see later) may be used. The choice of which compound should be used will depend on the preference of the patient and family. One of the choice-limiting factors in the experience of many clinicians has been the cost and weekly blood monitoring associated with clozapine use. This may lead many patients or their families to choose risperidone first, with clozapine kept as a future possibility. Nothing is inherently unreasonable with this strategy. However, it should be kept in mind that an expanding literature is showing the potential efficacy of clozapine as a first-line medication in the treatment of children and adolescents with schizophrenia. Educating and informing the patient and family about the relative known efficacies, risks, and benefits of these compounds are the responsibility of the physician.

Clozapine

Clozapine is a dibenzodiazepine that has been found to be useful in treatment-resistant adult schizophrenic patients and that has shown promise in the control of psychotic symptoms in child and adolescent schizophrenia. It may be of particular benefit in cases in which aggression or violence complicates the clinical picture. Unlike typical neuroleptics, clozapine is thought to interact primarily with dopamine D4 and serotonin 5HT2 receptors, primarily in the mesolimbic and mesocortical pathways. It seems to have less affinity for dopamine receptors in the nigrostriatal pathway and exhibits a different timing in its GABA interactions, which may explain its lower potential for inducing parkinsonian-type side effects, including tardive dyskinesia.

Clozapine is relatively poorly absorbed from the GI tract and shows an elimination half-life of 5 to 15 hours, which necessitates a multiple daily dosing regime. Adverse effects of clozapine in children and adolescents are listed in Table 13–13.

Medically serious side effects include seizures

TABLE 13–13 Potential Clozapine Side Effects in Children and Adolescents

Relatively Common	Relatively Uncommon
Sedation	Seizures
Transient low-grade fever	Neutropenia
Tachycardia	Eosinophilia
Postural hypotension	Agranulocytosis
Hypersalivation	Obsessions
Nausea	Compulsions
Constipation	
Weight gain	
Nocturnal enuresis	

TABLE 13–14 Suggested Dosage Titration for Initiation of Clozapine Use in Children*

Day	Dose	Total Daily Dose
1	12.5 mg AM	12.5 mg
2–3	12.5 mg AM and 12.5 mg HS	25 mg
4–5	12.5 mg AM and 25 mg HS	37.5 mg
6–7	25 mg AM and 25 mg HS	50 mg
8–9	25 mg AM and 37.5 mg HS	62.5 mg
10–11	37.5 mg AM and 37.5 mg HS	75 mg
12–13	37.5 mg AM and 50 mg HS	87.5 mg
14–15	50 mg AM and 50 mg HS	100 mg
16–17	50 mg AM and 75 mg HS	125 mg
18–19	75 mg AM and 75 mg HS	150 mg[†]
20–21	75 mg AM and 100 mg HS	175 mg
22–23	100 mg AM and 100 mg HS	200 mg
24–25	100 mg AM and 125 mg HS	225 mg[†]
26–27	125 mg AM and 125 mg HS	250 mg
28–29	125 mg AM and 150 mg HS	275 mg
30	150 mg AM and 150 mg HS	300 mg[†]

*These doses are suggestions only. Individual patients will vary with regard to therapeutic and adverse effects. Some patients may require and tolerate total daily doses of clozapine greater than those identified in this schedule.

[†]Potential therapeutic point—a reasonable course of action is to hold titration at this point and observe the therapeutic effects if the clinical condition suggests this is possible.

TABLE 13–15 Suggested Dosage Titration for Initiation of Clozapine Use in Adolescents*

Day	Dose	Total Daily Dose
1	12.5 mg AM	12.5 mg
2	12.5 mg AM and 12.5 mg HS	25 mg
3	12.5 mg AM and 25 mg HS	37.5 mg
4–5	25 mg AM and 25 mg HS	50 mg
6–7	25 mg AM and 50 mg HS	75 mg
8–9	50 mg AM and 50 mg HS	100 mg
10	75 mg AM and 75 mg HS	125 mg
11	75 mg AM and 75 mg HS	150 mg
12	75 mg AM and 100 mg HS	175 mg
13–14	100 mg AM and 100 mg HS	200 mg
15	100 mg AM and 125 mg HS	225 mg
16	125 mg AM and 125 mg HS	250 mg
17	125 mg AM and 150 mg HS	275 mg
18–19	150 mg AM and 150 mg HS	300 mg[†]
20	150 mg AM and 175 mg HS	325 mg
21	175 mg AM and 175 mg HS	350 mg
22	175 mg AM and 200 mg HS	375 mg
23	200 mg AM and 200 mg HS	400 mg[†]

*These doses are suggestions only. Individual patients will vary with regard to therapeutic and adverse effects. Some patients may require and tolerate total daily doses of clozapine greater than those identified in this schedule.

[†]Potential therapeutic point—a reasonable course of action is to hold titration at this point and observe for therapeutic effects if the clinical condition suggests this is possible.

and agranulocytosis. Seizures are rare (1.0 to 4.0 percent in adults) and may be dose related but have been reported in children and adolescents. If patients have a history of a seizure disorder (not including febrile seizures) and are currently not being treated with an antiepileptic medication, it is not unreasonable to introduce concurrent valproate therapy. Phenytoin is to be avoided. Neurologic consultation may be indicated in such cases.

An agranulocytosis rate of less than 1 percent for adults has been reported with clozapine use, and some evidence indicates that this may be increased by a factor of two in children and adolescents. This serious side effect tends to occur most frequently during the first 6 months of treatment and may preferentially affect females and persons of Finnish or Jewish descent. Thus, careful weekly monitoring of total WBC and absolute neutrophil counts is essential for clozapine treatment. Sudden drops in WBC or absolute neutrophil count should increase the possibility of a clozapine hematologic effect and appropriate interventions should be taken accordingly, as described later.

In children and adolescents, clinical experience suggests that the dosage schedule typically used in adults may be too aggressive, because the younger population seems to demonstrate increased sensitivity to clozapine's cardiovascular and sedative properties. Thus, treatment should be instituted with a dose of 12.5 mg daily taken as a target dose and increased for children as illustrated in Table 13–14 and for adolescents as illustrated in Table 13–15.

Clozapine dosage must be individualized for each patient. Should significant adverse effects occur, a reasonable course of action is to decrease the total daily dose to a point at which the side effects are not apparent and maintain the patient at that level for an additional 2 to 3 days. Following this, the dosage escalation can again be attempted as scheduled if sufficient clinical improvement has not occurred. As noted in each of these dosing schedules, some patients will require and tolerate doses of clozapine above 300 or 400 mg daily. Dose increments above these daily levels should be carefully titrated and physical parameters such as heart rate, blood pressure, and mental status should be monitored.

A target dose range of 150 to 600 mg daily is reasonable, but total daily doses of 300 to 450 daily are usually sufficient in most cases. Because clozapine's full therapeutic effect may take 6 months or more to optimize, when this medication is used in long-term care (see Chapter 14) dose titrations should be followed by sufficient time to monitor potential changes in symptoms or functioning.

One interesting clinical phenomenon that may occur with clozapine use is the attenuation but not dissipation of auditory hallucinations and delusions. In many cases, patients will describe that while they still hear the same voices and think the same thoughts, these seem much less compelling and important than previously. In many cases, they are able to ignore them or identify them as their "brain playing tricks" and are able to function much better, although their positive symptoms are not completely alleviated.

As has been suggested in studies of adults, reports of clozapine use in children and adolescents suggest a much lower frequency and severity of dyskinesias, extrapyramidal effects, and parkinsonian side effects than found in treatment with "typical" antipsychotics. Negative symptoms also seem to improve with this medication.

Children and adolescents who have been previously treated with typical antipsychotics can be switched to clozapine relatively easily. After baseline symptom and side effect evaluation the patient can have the original antipsychotic gradually withdrawn using a neuroleptic discontinuation schedule, as outlined earlier. When the original antipsychotic dose has been decreased by at least one half, clozapine can be started using the dosing schedules found earlier. Withdrawal of the original antipsychotic should continue until it is no longer being taken. However, as described earlier, antiparkinsonian medications should continue to be used for 1 to 2 weeks following discontinuation of the original neuroleptic and then should be gradually withdrawn.

The clinical use of clozapine is complicated by the risk of agranulocytosis. Thus, as described earlier, weekly monitoring of both WBC and absolute neutrophil count is essential. The next week's clozapine medication should not be prescribed until the physician confirms that *both* the WBC and absolute neutrophil count are within accepted limits (Table 13–16).

Clinical experience with long-term clozapine use in treatment-resistant adolescent schizophrenics has shown that WBC counts can vary substantially from one week to another. If the WBC or the absolute neutrophil counts show a value below the accepted lower limit, the physician should hold the clozapine for the next week. A WBC and absolute neutrophil count should then be repeated. In many cases, both the WBC and absolute neutrophil counts will be found to have climbed back into the acceptable ranges again. Thus, the clozapine can be restarted at the previous dose, and hematologic monitoring should occur as before. If the physician is concerned that although the WBC or absolute neutrophil counts have returned to within acceptable norms but the values lie in the lower range of these norms, taking an additional blood test midweek (3 to 4 days following restarting the medication) is a reasonable procedure.

For patients in whom the WBC and absolute neutrophil count remain below the acceptable level for 2 consecutive weeks, the clozapine should continue to be held. There is no clinical consensus at this time about reintroducing the medication. A reasonable approach is that in the face of an excellent clinical response in a previously treatment-unresponsive patient, the clozapine can be carefully reintroduced once the blood picture has stabilized. However, if this is the case clozapine treatment should be started de novo and gradually titrated upwards with careful monitoring of the hematologic parameters (twice weekly). If the blood picture yet again shows a decrease of total WBC or absolute neutrophil counts fall below accepted levels, clozapine treatment should not be attempted again.

The successful pharmacologic treatment of the acute phase of the schizophrenic onset as described here now moves into the chronic or long-

TABLE 13–16 Generally Acceptable Lower Limits for Total WBC and Absolute Neutrophil Counts in Monitoring Clozapine Treatment in Children and Adolescents

Index	Generally Accepted Limit*
Total WBC	4000
Absolute neutrophil count	2000

*If WBC drops below 3000 or the absolute neutrophil count drops below 1500, discontinue clozapine immediately and consult a hematologist.

term pharmacologic treatment phase. This is described in Chapter 14.

SUGGESTED READINGS

Frazer J, Gordon, CT, McKenna K, Lenane M, Jib D, Rapoport J. An open trial of clozapine in 11 adolescents with childhood-onset schizophrenia. Journal of the American Academy of Child and Adolescent Psychiatry, 33:658–663, 1994.

Goff DC, Baldessarini RS. Drug interactions with antipsychotic agents. Journal of Clinical Psychopharmacology, 13:59–67, 1993.

Kane J (ed). Risperidone: New horizons for the schizophrenic patient. Journal of Clinical Psychiatry, 55(Suppl):3–35, 1994.

Lieberman J, Kane J, Johns C. Clozapine: Guidelines for clinical management. Journal of Clinical Psychiatry, 50:329–338, 1989.

McClellan JM, Werry J. Practice parameters for the assessment and treatment of children and adolescents with schizophrenia. Journal of the American Academy of Child and Adolescent Psychiatry, 33:616–635, 1994.

Remington, G (ed). Novel neuroleptics in schizophrenia: Theory and clinical revelance. Canadian Journal of Psychiatry, 39(Suppl 2):S43–S80, 1994.

Richardson M, Haughland G (eds). Use of Neuroleptics in Children. Washington, DC: American Psychiatric Press, Inc., 1996.

Royal College of Psychiatrists. Clozapine—the atypical antipsychotic. British Journal of Psychiatry, 160(Suppl 17), 1992.

Steingard R, Khan A, Gonzalez A, Herzog D. Neuroleptic malignant syndrome: Review of experience in children. Journal of Child and Adolescent Psychopharmacology, 2:183–198, 1992.

Teicher MH, Gold CA. Neuroleptic drugs: Indications and guidelines for their rational use in children and adolescents. Journal of Child and Adolescent Psychopharmacology, 1:33–56, 1990.

Thompson C. The use of high-dose antipsychotic medications. British Journal of Psychiatry, 164:448–458, 1994.

CHAPTER 14

Long-Term Psychopharmacologic Treatment of Children and Adolescents with Schizophrenia

Schizophrenia is a chronic and debilitating mental illness that may have a variety of courses characterized by varying degrees of cognitive, social, vocational, and personal impairments. Recent evidence suggests that early onset of this disorder may be predictive of poorer global outcome over the long term. The very nature of schizophrenia demands that optimal treatment address multiple domains of disturbance and take into account the unique characteristics of the individual with the disease and the natural course of the disorder. Thus, treatment of schizophrenia is truly biopsychosocial in nature.

Effective pharmacotherapy, however, remains the cornerstone of successful long-term treatment for the child or adolescent with schizophrenia. Effective control of positive and negative symptoms provides the base on which successful psychosocial interventions can be built. Successful social and cognitive rehabilitation, family intervention programs, social skills training, community support, and economic advocacy depend on optimal pharmacologic interventions that control symptoms and prevent psychotic relapse. On the other hand, although pharmacotherapy remains necessary, by itself it is not a sufficient treatment for patients with schizophrenia. There is no place in good clinical practice for the prescription of pharmacotherapy without the envelope of psychosocial interventions.

Schizophrenia is an expensive disease. Although the suffering to individuals and their families cannot be economically measured, those studies that are available show that this illness comes with high direct and indirect costs. Patients with the most severe forms of the illness may account for the greatest proportion of those costs. Treatments that can decrease the disability of this group can thus be expected to provide an accrued economic benefit as well as the more obvious humanitarian one. Given that children and adolescents (the early onset group) with schizophrenia face a longer time course with this illness and that the onset of the disorder early in development may be expected to result in more severe and global dysfunction (see Fig. 14–1), early and optimal interventions in this age group are especially necessary to decrease the economic liability of this illness. Effective pharmacotherapy has demonstrated its cost effectiveness in this disorder, and thus its optimal provision by child and adolescent psychiatrists experienced in its use is necessary.

Diagnosis

The long-term pharmacologic treatment of children and adolescents with schizophrenia is, as is all pharmacologic treatment, premised on valid diagnosis and symptom evaluation. Although in most cases diagnostic uncertainty at this stage of treatment may be less of an issue than in the acute psychotic phase, the clinician must not approach chronic pharmacologic treatment with a closed mind about diagnostic issues. The necessity for and process of diagnostic re-evaluation during long-term pharmacologic treatment are discussed below, but the period in which long-term treatment is initiated provides an ideal opportunity for a diagnostic reassessment.

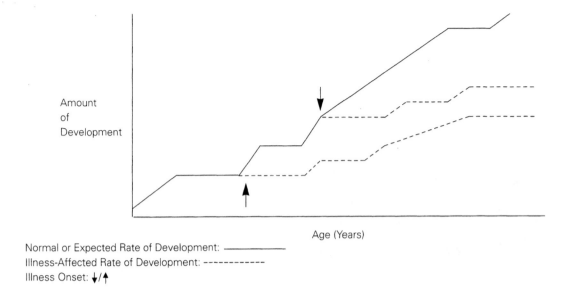

Normal or Expected Rate of Development: ————————
Illness-Affected Rate of Development: - - - - - - - - - -
Illness Onset: ↓/↑

FIGURE 14–1 Hypothetical Influence of Age of Onset on the Long-Term Outcome of Schizophrenia Demonstrating Potentially Greater Negative Endpoint Effect with Earlier Onset of the Illness: A Schematic Presentation

Although intense and detailed diagnostic reviews are perhaps not necessary at this time, it is useful to conduct a diagnostic minichallenge. This is best approached by identifying those psychiatric and medical disorders that are most likely to be confused with schizophrenia (Table 14–1) and then proving from the information on hand that the particular child or adolescent does not suffer from that particular disorder. This in effect challenges the clinician to act as a scientist and prove the null hypothesis. If this cannot be done from available information, the clinician should seek out those pieces of data that will allow him or her to do so. If this can be done, the degree of diagnostic certainty does increase.

Fortunately, the pharmacotherapy of schizophrenia is a rapidly evolving field. The development of new antipsychotic medications, many with improved tolerability and safety over those previously available, promises better and more effective control of symptoms and improved long-term outcome for those children and adolescents who develop this disorder. This chapter outlines the use of both the traditional and some of the newer antipsychotic medications in the long-term treatment of children and adolescents with schizophrenia. As might be expected, the availability of rigorously instituted research into many aspects of the long-term pharmacologic treatment of schizophrenic children and adolescents is as yet unavailable, although clinical experience with

many neuroleptic medications is extensive. As elsewhere in this book, the pragmatics of pharmacologic practice with this population are described from a combination of available research and extensive clinical experience.

The long-term pharmacologic treatment of schizophrenia has as its goals to provide symptomatic control (both positive and negative symptoms), to prevent relapse, and to improve quality of life.

Pharmacologic treatment is directed toward the attainment of all the above goals simultaneously, and in clinical practice they are usually found to be closely related. For example, medications can help provide symptomatic control only when they are titrated to the correct dose. Doses that are too low will not allow for this, and not only will the patient's ongoing symptoms interfere with his or

TABLE 14–1 Psychiatric and Medical Conditions Requiring Null Hypothesis Testing for a Diagnostic Mini-Review at the Onset of Long-Term Pharmacotherapy for Children and Adolescents with Schizophrenia

Psychiatric	Medical
Mania	Partial complex seizures
Psychotic depression	Genetic or developmental
Schizoaffective disorder	disorders
Drug-induced psychosis	

her quality of life, but the risk of relapse, with its attendant hospitalizations and further developmental delays, will be increased. Medications that are poorly tolerated by the patient, even if they provide reasonable symptom control, will lead to a decreased quality of life. Furthermore, patients who suffer side effects may well become noncompliant with treatment; as a result, symptoms may increase and relapse may occur. Thus, careful and optimal medication management is necessary for all the treatment goals described earlier.

Long-term pharmacologic treatment may be conveniently divided into two different but related strategies that identify different modes of medication delivery: oral medications and long-acting injectables. The pros and cons of each of these options are listed in Table 14–2.

The question that the physician faces with these choices is, What to recommend and at what time during the course of the illness should one route be chosen over another? In some cases, this will be clear. The adolescent who demonstrates poor compliance with oral medications leading to poor symptom control and relapse is clearly a candidate for depot neuroleptic treatment. The young child with well-controlled symptoms who is compliant with oral medications may be a candidate for depot neuroleptics when a chaotic family environment cannot be counted on to provide appropriate oral medication delivery and alternative methods for medication delivery (such as through a day treatment program) cannot be arranged. An adolescent with a first onset psychosis and a diagnosis of schizophrenia who is compliant with oral medication treatment may not be a candidate for depot treatment. An adolescent with a first onset schizophrenic paranoid psychosis who presents with homicidal delusions may conversely be a good candidate for depot treatment, even if seemingly compliant with oral medications.

Choosing Depot Pharmacotherapy

A depot neuroleptic is usually an esterized form of an oral agent dissolved in an oil vehicle, usually vegetable or sesame seed oil, that demonstrates a multicompartmental model of pharmacokinetics on clinical use. This compound is injected deep into a large muscle, where over a period of a few days the antipsychotic is taken up into fat stores. The medication is then gradually released from these fat stores into the blood stream. The ester form of the neuroleptic is hydrolyzed in plasma to produce free fatty acids and unbound antipsychotic. Release of the medication from fat stores can be prolonged for a long period of time. This pharmacokinetic feature may be important in the pharmacodynamic profile of these drugs in terms of their effect on relapse and side effects.

The clinical decision as to when and for whom to recommend depot neuroleptic treatment is not always clear; yet this decision may have profound consequences for the outcome of treatment, as illustrated in the following cases.

TABLE 14–2   **Long-Term Treatment with Neuroleptics**

Pro	Con
Oral Neuroleptics	
Provides patient with increased sense of control over treatment	Easily liable to compliance difficulties
Allows for greater ease in dose titration as clinically indicated	Must be administered daily
The oral forms have been shown to be the only effective medication for the patient, e.g., clozapine	Patient needs weekly hematologic monitoring with clozapine
Adverse effects usually quickly apparent	
Depot Neuroleptics	
Compliance increases with medication treatment	Compliance comes from the structure and not necessarily from the patient
Provides an ideal structure for regular patient monitoring	Forces the patient and caregiver to suspend other activities for medication maintenance
Demonstrates an extended interval between treatments	May create a psychological distance between the experience of treatment and illness
Requires injection	Requires injection
	Onset of adverse events may be delayed for a few days following an injection

CASE EXAMPLE

Let's Go for Injectable Treatment: Accepted

H.D., a 17-year-old boy with a diagnosis of paranoid schizophrenia, lived at home with his father who was not often present. H.D. was admitted in a paranoid psychotic state; he was suffering from persecutory delusions and he had on him written plans to shoot a number of his classmates. He accepted pharmacologic treatment only after all his legal appeals failed to lead to his release from the hospital. He was noted to be noncompliant with oral medications even when closely supervised. Eventually H.D. developed enough trust in his treatment team to accept its recommendation of depot neuroleptic treatment. His father supported this, as did the community follow-up services. He was discharged from the hospital taking flupenthixol 95 mg every 2 weeks, and he continued to show relatively good symptom control with minimal side effects. Follow-up included dose medical supervision and clinical case management with a day treatment and vocational component. Three years after his initial admission, he was stable and maintained his improvement.

CASE EXAMPLE

Let's Go for Injectable Treatment: Refused

G.S. was an 18-year-old boy with a diagnosis of paranoid schizophrenia. He had been admitted to two different hospitals in the past but had not complied with follow-up treatment. All his hospital admissions had been characterized by violent outbursts and paranoid delusions, often involving members of his family. He showed a relatively good response to acute neuroleptic treatment and seemed to accept the need for continued medication use. He was compliant with oral medications in the hospital setting. Although depot neuroleptics were strongly advised by the treatment team, neither G.S. nor his family would agree to their use, and he was discharged on oral medications with intensive community supports. Six months after discharge, G.S. discontinued his oral medications against the advice of his physician and then was lost to follow-up. About 1 year after his discharge, apparently while acutely psychotic, he murdered a family member.

CASE COMMENTARY

These two cases illustrate success and failure of chronic psychopharmacologic treatment in adolescents with schizophrenia as it relates to the use of depot medications. Although it may be overly simplistic to ascribe the differential outcome in these cases to the use of depot over oral compounds, the importance of depot neuroleptics in promoting compliance with medications is well recognized. Just when and with what type of patient should the physician strongly recommend their use is not always clear, however, and the use of depot medications in and of themselves certainly does not ensure a positive treatment outcome. Nevertheless, research and clinical experience have clearly defined that the optimal use of antipsychotic medication is necessary in the treatment of this disorder, and some guidelines as to which patients should be strongly advised to use the depot as opposed to the oral route of delivery are available.

The following decision scale (Fig. 14–2) re-

Clinical Feature	Consideration	
Compliant with oral medications	Yes	No**
Good therapeutic relationship	Yes	No
Reliable historian regarding symptoms	Yes	No
Educated about medication use	Yes	No
Reasonable supervision of oral dosing	Yes	No
Reasonable home environment	Yes	No
Reliable for follow-up monitoring	Yes	No
Good community support system	Yes	No
First episode	Yes	No
Paranoid homicidal or suicidal symptoms	Yes**	No
Violent history or potential	Yes**	No

Score 0 for each "Yes" response, 1 for each "No" response, and 2 for each "No**" or "Yes**" response. A total score or 0 is consistent with a recommendation of oral dosing. A total score of 2 or more is consistent with a recommendation for depot dosing.

This decision scale is meant to be used as a clinical guide only. It is intended to assist the clinician in the process of deciding whether to recommend depot neuroleptic treatment for the child or adolescent with schizophrenia. It is not a predictive or outcome scale. Clinical judgment on a case-by-case basis is necessary.

FIGURE 14–2 Choosing to Recommend Depot Neuroleptic Treatment: Decision Scale for a Child or Adolescent with a Schizophrenic Psychosis Showing a Good Response to Acute Neuroleptic Treatment

garding the use of depot neuroleptics is provided to assist in the decision-making process.

Choosing a Depot Neuroleptic

Once the decision has been made to choose a depot neuroleptic, the issue then becomes "which one." A number of possible choices that are available have similar efficacy and tolerability. However, as with all other psychotropic medications, there are subtle differences among them. As it is highly unlikely that the child and adolescent psychiatrist will need to use all the available depot neuroleptics, he should choose two or three compounds from those available and learn their particular pharmacokinetic and pharmacodynamic features well. This strategy is preferred to that of trying out all available depot neuroleptics. Table 14–3 provides a list of suggested depot neuroleptics that might provide sufficient clinical flexibility for use by a child and adolescent psychiatrist.

Given the choices of compounds above, what criteria can the clinician use to determine which medication will be most appropriate. Unfortunately, there is no exact science available to provide a useful guide, and a period of controlled trial and error may be necessary. Clinical experience, however, suggests that flupenthixol decanoate is generally well tolerated by the younger schizophrenic population and compared with haloperidol decanoate may be less likely to induce severe extrapyramidal side effects in adolescent boys. Fluphenazine decanoate and flupenthixol decanoate may be mildly more sedating than haloperidol decanoate, which may be a consideration for those patients in whom this may interfere with daily activities. Haloperidol decanoate may be less frequently associated with weight gain than either fluphenazine decanoate or flupenthixol decanoate and thus may be considered if body image issues are a major concern. In any case, as discussed in Chapter 13, the choice of a particular neuroleptic depends on a weighing of patient and chemical criteria to try to estimate the best potential "fit."

One useful factor that may assist in this process is that of the oral neuroleptic used to treat acute episode. If the patient has, for example, shown a good response to oral flupenthixol, he or she may be conveniently switched to injectable flupenthixol decanoate. Similarly, if the patient has demonstrated a good response to a piperazine phenothiazine (such as perphenazine), it is reasonable to consider the use of a depot version of the same chemical class (such as fluphenazine decanoate). Patients who respond to the butyrophenone haloperidol may respond similarly to haloperidol decanoate. This being said, however, many patients who show a good acute treatment response to one oral compound from a particular class (such as perphenazine) may do quite well on a depot compound from another class (such as flupenthixol). In the "art" of depot neuroleptic psychopharmacology there is no substitute for extensive clinical experience.

Beginning Treatment with a Depot Neuroleptic

Once a decision has been made to proceed with a specific depot neuroleptic treatment, the physician must convert the patient from the oral to the depot preparation. This conversion process is not without its difficulties and may be complicated by all or some of the following:

1. increase in symptoms because of insufficient neuroleptic dose during the crossover period
2. increase in side effects because of excessive neuroleptic dose during the crossover period
3. emergence of new side effects, withdrawal phenomena such as nausea and vomiting, because of excessively rapid discontinuation of oral antipsychotics

Accordingly, the conversion from oral to depot preparations must be carefully titrated to ensure as much as possible that neither of the above difficulties occur.

A number of conversion tables are available to assist the physician in this process, but the clini-

TABLE 14–3 Suggested Depot Neuroleptics for Use in Children or Adolescents*

Neuroleptic	Class	Usual Dose Range (mg)	Usual Duration of Action in Weeks
Flupenthixol decanoate	Thioxanthene	20–100	3
Fluphenazine decanoate	Piperazine phenothiazine	12.5–100	4
Haloperidol decanoate	Butyrophenone	25–150	4

*Medication doses and duration of action are guidelines only. Individual responses will vary, and dosing and time of delivery will need to be individually tailored depending on clinical presentation.

cal consensus is that although they may be useful guidelines they do not necessarily offer any real advantage over individualized strategies that are based on the clinician's understanding of the general pharmacokinetic issues involved and the unique pharmacodynamic responses of the patient. Some conversion tables were developed during the period when higher neuroleptic doses were routinely prescribed and are not necessarily applicable to current lower-dose practice. No conversion tables that are commonly available have been developed specifically for children and adolescents. In addition, available conversion tables cannot take into account the wide interindividual variations that occur with depot preparations. A potential danger with rigid adherence to such tables is that the clinician may inadvertently begin to treat the table instead of the patient. Thus, it is necessary to tailor make the oral to depot conversion for each patient.

Essentially, two different approaches can be taken in converting from oral to depot medication. The first approach uses a comparison of approximate oral to depot doses based on chlorpromazine equivalents. This, however, is not necessarily ideal because of the great individual variations in plasma levels at any one given dose of antipsychotic and the known interindividual variability in plasma levels of oral compared with equivalent injectable antipsychotic doses. The second and simpler method is beginning the depot neuroleptic at its lowest dose and then gradually increasing it as clinically indicated. Both these approaches are described later and only extensive clinical practice will provide the clinician with a useful conversion strategy. One important clinical point, however, should be kept in mind. Extensive experience with conversion from oral to depot preparations in adolescents with schizophrenia has identified that the use of the first conversion strategy is often associated with greater-than-necessary initial depot antipsychotic doses, perhaps because dosage amounts needed for maintenance are less than those needed to establish clinical remission in the acute phase.

In both methods described, it is reasonable to attempt a test dose of depot medication before going on the calculated dosing schedule. If the clinician chooses to give a test dose first, the following amounts are suggested:

flupenthixol: 10 mg
fluphenazine: 12.5 mg
haloperidol: 25 mg

In some cases (see Table 14–4), the initial dose can be considered as the test dose. In other cases, the test dose could reasonably precede the initial dose by 5 to 7 days.

TABLE 14–4 Approximate Chlorpromazine (CPZ) Dosage Equivalents for Selected Antipsychotics*

Medication	Delivery Method	CPZ Equivalent (mg)
Chlorpromazine (CPZ)	Oral	100
Perphenazine	Oral	10
Trifluoperazine	Oral	5
Flupenthixol	Oral	5
Haloperidol	Oral	2
Flupenthixol decanoate	Depot	50[†]
Fluphenazine decanoate	Depot	13[†]
Haloperidol decanoate	Depot	30[†]

*This table is provided as an approximate guideline only. Patient responses will vary greatly, particularly with depot medications. Clinical parameters should guide dosing, and each patient will need individualized medication management. The approximate conversions above also been established for adult and not for child and adolescent patients and thus may vary when applied to the younger age group.
[†]These doses are provided for the expected duration of the injectable dose; *these are not daily dose guidelines.* See text discussion of this important point.

First Method of Conversion from Oral to Depot Neuroleptics

One useful way to accomplish this conversion is to first express the total daily oral neuroleptic dose in chlorpromazine equivalents (see Table 14–4). Once this has been calculated, convert the chlorpromazine equivalents into the appropriate depot compound comparison. This will provide the clinician with an *approximate* target dose. Remember that this target dose is the total medication amount for the entire expected duration of the injectable dose; for example, if the calculation is for flupenthixol decanoate, the amount of the medication in milligrams (usual range is between 20–120) is for the entire 3-week period that follows a single injection. Unlike oral neuroleptics, the target dose is not expressed as a total daily dose.

Once this target dose has been identified, the patient should enter the conversion process. Again, clinical considerations will be the ultimate guide, but in principle, the practitioner must take care not to decrease the oral medication too quickly and not to increase the injectable too quickly.

During this process, it is important to keep two different pharmacokinetic parameters of the chosen depot medication in mind: the peak plasma level and the elimination half life (Table 14–5). These two pharmacokinetic factors play an important part in the optimal introduction of depot medication. The peak plasma level may identify a

TABLE 14–5 **Clinically Important Pharmacokinetics of Depot Antipsychotics***

Medication	Peak Plasma Level	Elimination Half-Life
Flupenthixol decanoate	4–7 days	8 days—single dose; 17 days—multiple doses
Fluphenazine decanoate	Two peaks occur, one at about 24 hrs; second at about 8–10 days	12–16 days—single dose; 100 plus days with multiple dosing
Haloperidol decanoate	3–9 days	18–21 days

*The pharmacokinetics described above have been developed primarily from studies in adults and may be expected to vary in children and adolescents. Individual patients may show different kinetic profiles, and clinical parameters must be used to guide dosing requirements.
Modified from Bezchlinyk-Butler KZ, Jeffries JJ, Martin BA. Clinical Handbook of Psychotropic Drugs (6th rev ed). Seattle: Hogrefe & Huber Publishers, 1996, with permission.

time in which the patient might be at highest risk for side effects. The elimination half-life can be used as a guide to determine dosing intervals, as steady state levels will be expected to take about 4 to 6 half-lives to reach.

Thus, as is evident from Table 14–5, the method of introducing different depot preparations may be slightly different depending on the medication chosen.

Once this information has been considered, it is reasonable to taper the oral medication in preparation of beginning the depot compound. Although some authors have suggested stopping the oral compound altogether, this is not necessary, and if done abruptly, may create withdrawal symptoms. A more practical approach is illustrated in Table 14–6.

On days 8 to 14, the injectable neuroleptic can be started at about 25 percent of the estimated total dosage per injection period (Table 14–7). For example, if it is estimated that an adolescent will require 100 mg of flupenthixol over each 3-week injection period, then the patient may be started on 25 mg IM at this time.

The timing of the second and subsequent injections is suggested by its estimated peak plasma level and elimination half-life. Table 14–7 provides suggested doses and timing for the introduction of depot neuroleptics. However, as individual patients may vary considerably in terms of their response to these compounds, clinical con-

siderations will need to be used to direct actual doses given. If a dose of injectable neuroleptic is considered slightly high, the next dose should not necessarily be decreased because the oral neuroleptic will be "washing out" during the time between depot doses.

Side effects should be used to help monitor dose requirements. If these suggest that the patient has sufficient neuroleptic in his system, one of two strategies is possible. The first is to decrease by 25 to 50 percent the total of the next injection dose; the other is to wait an additional 3 to 7 days prior to the next dose delivery. Although no hard and fast rules can be offered, clinical experience suggests that for flupenthixol and haloperidol, the preferred strategy may be waiting an additional few days but keeping the dose the same, whereas for fluphenazine, decreasing the dose but keeping to the timing of the schedule may be preferred.

The Second Depot Introduction Technique

The second depot introduction approach may be somewhat simpler than the first, but its use is not necessarily associated with either greater efficacy or fewer complications. This approach involves discontinuing the oral medication as suggested earlier in Table 14–6 and beginning depot treatment with the lowest possible dose, gradually increasing it over weekly increments to the estimated amount needed. This is summarized in Table 14–8.

Regardless of the method employed to effect the oral to depot conversion, concurrent antiparkinsonian medications should be continued throughout. After the patient has been stabilized on the depot neuroleptic for 3 to 4 months, the antiparkinsonian medication may be gradually discontinued.

Prolonged use of neuroleptic agents may be as-

TABLE 14–6 **Suggested Tapering Schedule for Oral to Depot Neuroleptic Conversion**

Day	Amount of Oral Neuroleptic to Be Discontinued
1	30–35 percent of the original total daily dosage
4	50 percent of the remaining total daily dosage
7	100 percent of the remaining total daily dosage
8–10	Begin first doses of depot (see Table 14–3)

TABLE 14–7 Suggested Doses and Timing of Depot Injections During the Oral to Depot Conversion Process*

Medication	Day	Dose
Flupenthixol decanoate	1	25 percent of estimated total dose per injection period
	7–10	50 percent of estimated total dose per injection period
	21	100 percent of estimated total dose per injection period
Fluphenazine decanoate	1	25 percent of estimated total dose per injection period
	7	25 percent of estimated total dose per injection period
	14	50 percent of estimated total dose per injection period
	28	100 percent of estimated total dose per injection period
Haloperidol decanoate	1	25 percent of estimated total dose per injection period
	10–12	50 percent of estimated total dose per injection period
	28	100 percent of estimated total dose per injection period

*These dosing schedules are suggestions only. Individual differences to depot neuroleptics vary, and doses will need to be titrated to each patient's clinical condition.

sociated with a decreased need for antiparkinsonian prophylaxis. Thus, once sufficient stability of depot dose has occurred, attempts can be made to gradually discontinue the patient's antiparkinsonian treatment. The optimal strategy to follow depends on the timing of expected peak plasma level for the compound that the patient is receiving. The antiparkinsonian drug can be gradually decreased by about 30 to 40 percent from total daily dose beginning 3 to 5 days following the expected peak plasma level of the depot injection. For example, if the patient is taking benztropine at a total daily dose of 4 mg, and is receiving flupenthixol every 3 weeks (expected peak plasma

TABLE 14–8 Suggested Doses and Timing of Depot Injections During the Oral to Depot Conversion Process*

Medication	Day	Dose (mg)
Flupenthixol decanoate	1	20
	7	40
	14	60
	28	Total estimated dose or as clinically indicated
Fluphenazine decanoate	1	12.5
	7	12.5
	14	25
	21	25
	28	Total estimated dose or as clinically indicated
Haloperidol decanoate	1	25
	7	50
	14	100
	21	100 or 150
	38	Total estimated dose or as clinically indicated

*These dosing schedules are suggestions only. Individual differences to depot neuroleptics vary, and doses will need to be titrated to each patient's clinical condition.

level of flupenthixol is 4 to 7 days), then the total daily benztropine dose can be decreased to 3 mg on or about days 10 to 12 following the injection. This dose should be maintained during the next injection as well. If there is no significant increase in side effects, a similar decrease at a similar time is reasonable.

This strategy continues until either the patient stops the antiparkinsonian medication altogether or a threshold of emergent side effects is reached. Even if the latter occurs, many patients can be managed by providing them with an antiparkinsonian agent (or increasing the dose of the antiparkinsonian agent) for the period of time beginning with each injection and ending some 3 to 5 days after the expected peak plasma level occurs. A similar strategy can be followed with medications used to treat akathisia.

CASE EXAMPLE

Adolescent Schizophrenia: Too Much, Too Soon

D.S. was a 14-year-old girl with a diagnosis of paranoid schizophrenia who had stabilized on perphenazine at a dose of 40 mg daily. She and her parents elected depot maintenance primarily for convenience of medication monitoring because she lived a great distance from the nearest mental health facility, and her family physician expressed a reluctance to monitor her medication. It was believed that the use of depot medication would allow for greater ease of medication monitoring and the family did not mind driving into the city to see the physician so long as this was only necessary once every 3 to 4 weeks. Accordingly, fluphenazine decanoate was chosen as the depot to be used.

D.S.'s perphenazine was decreased by 25 percent over 3 days, and she was then given 12.5 mg of fluphenazine decanoate. Side effect and symptom monitoring was provided every 2 days. On day 7, her perphenazine was once again decreased, to a level of 50 percent from the original total daily dose, and she was given 50 mg of fluphenazine decanoate on that day. Two days later she had significantly increased tremors, complained of stiffness, and on physical examination showed rigidity and cogwheeling, which had not previously been present. Her oral perphenazine was discontinued, and she gradually improved over the next 3 to 5 days.

CASE COMMENTARY

In the case of D.S., the clinician provided her with more neuroleptic medication than she needed, eliciting some unpleasant treatment-emergent adverse events in the process. First, her oral neuroleptic was not sufficiently decreased before depot treatment was initiated. Second, her first injection, although a reasonable first dose, showed its second plasma level peak just at the time that her second injection was given. The combined effect of these poorly timed injections and the insufficient oral taper led to the adverse events she experienced.

As a clinical guideline, it is better to err on the side of initial underdosing than overdosing during the conversion procedure because the risk of relapse over the month or so that this process occurs is quite low. Furthermore, if "topping up" is necessary, occasional oral doses can be used, although it is not recommended as a routine practice. Finally, although the concept of "loading doses" or depot neuroleptics has recently been raised, this strategy generally has little or no place to play in the treatment of children and adolescents.

Management Issues in Long-Term Neuroleptic Treatment

Regardless of the route of administration chosen for long-term neuroleptic treatment, a number of important management issues about the use of these medications occur. These can be identified as follows:

1. Overall pharmacotherapeutic strategies
2. Psychiatric and medical monitoring
3. Community and associated caregivers
4. Diagnostic reassessment
5. Drug abuse–misuse

Overall Pharmacotherapeutic Strategies

The optimal pharmacologic long-term treatment of schizophrenia is to provide the best possible symptomatic (both positive and negative) control with the minimum of adverse effects. This is done to optimize outcome, improve overall functioning, and provide prophylaxis against relapse. In addition, it is recognized that relapse may at times occur, even in the context of good long-term pharmacologic management. Thus, the early identification and treatment of relapse also becomes an important goal in long-term pharmacotherapy.

Generally, most clinicians try to obtain adequate symptom control on the lowest dose of neuroleptic possible whether delivered orally or by depot. This strategy attempts both to control positive symptoms and to improve negative symptoms. In many cases the total daily neuroleptic dose in long-term treatment will be lower than that used to treat the acute phase of the illness.

The lowest possible effective neuroleptic dose for long-term treatment cannot be calculated a priori, and individual differences are great. Therefore, no hard and fast rule nor indeed dosage guidelines can be given, and each patient's medication dose will need to be adjusted on the basis of clinical response.

Generally, however, the following procedural guidelines can be useful in assisting the physician in locating the potentially lowest effective neuroleptic dose range:

1. Titrate medications downward only after the patient has shown a prolonged period of stability to prevent early relapse. Remember that the critical period for relapse occurs within the first year following the resolution of the acute phase. Keep the patient on or close to the dose of antipsychotic medications originally begun (provided that side effects are tolerable) for about 12 months after beginning long-term pharmacotherapy.
2. Once step 1 has been successfully achieved, gradual dosage reductions, in the order of 10 to 15 percent, can be instituted, allowing for sufficient time to pass to evaluate the effect of this dosage reduction before again proceeding to another dosage reduction. This assessment of effect period should be at least 4 to 6 months in duration.
3. Modify antiparkinsonian and other treatments accordingly as the neuroleptic dose is gradually decreased.
4. Monitor for symptom relapse carefully, especially nearer the end of each assessment of

effect period, as this is the time when "break-through" symptoms are most likely to occur.

5. Do not accept unidimensional psychological or social "reasons" for relapse in the patient who is showing "breakthrough" symptoms during a period of neuroleptic dose reduction as an explanation for the patient's symptoms. As a general rule, the return of symptoms herald a relapse.

6. Treat all signs of relapse immediately and vigorously by increasing the neuroleptic dose to the level at which it was 6 to 8 months prior to the onset of "breakthrough" symptoms. Do not undertreat relapse. It may be necessary during these intervention periods to once again begin or else raise the dose of any other necessary medications such as antiparkinsonian compounds.

7. If "breakthrough" symptoms have been successfully treated, wait at least 4 to 6 months before beginning the next attempt at medication reduction and then reinstitute a reduction strategy at half the original reduction dosage amount.

8. If, while decreasing the antipsychotic dose, "breakthrough" symptoms occur on three separate occasions at or near a similar total oral daily (or depot monthly) dose, consider that the patient will need the dose currently being taken and hold off with further attempted decrements.

Patients and their families will often ask how long medication treatment will be indicated. It is essential to be clear and honest in response to this question. The answer will likely include the following information:

1. Medications are necessary but not sufficient in treating schizophrenia. They will help control symptoms, prevent relapse, and optimize outcome.

2. Although individuals differ, most patients with schizophrenia will need to take medications for the rest of their lives.

3. It is impossible to tell at the outset how long any particular patient will need to take a particular medicine and at what specific dose. Therefore, a method of medication monitoring must be put into place to help guide long-term treatment.

4. Taking medications for treating schizophrenia depends, like any other treatment, on weighing the risks against the benefits. These risks and benefits should be reviewed formally with patient and family ideally every 6 months and minimally once a year.

5. Time will help decide the length and type of long-term treatment. The patient, family,

and the physician will work together on this decision.

In some cases, if these guidelines are followed, patients may actually come off their medications entirely. Clinical experience suggests that this can occur in a small number of schizophrenic patients; however, such patients should still be followed up on a regular basis with intensive and vigorous pharmacologic interventions applied at the first signs of relapse. In exceptional cases, this type of intermittent neuroleptic treatment can provide sufficient pharmacologic control of symptoms.

The danger of this course of action, however, is how to ensure that effective interventions can occur if they are needed; patients are not likely to attend regular follow-up sessions if they are not undergoing active pharmacotherapy. Thus, the possibility of losing these vulnerable patients to follow-up occurs. Children or adolescents for whom there is careful and reliable monitoring (family or community treatment) may be less likely to face this problem.

On the other side of the coin (and unfortunately more commonly) are those patients who demonstrate relapse while undergoing pharmacotherapy and can be considered to show a kind of treatment resistance to prophylactic interventions. In these individuals, if all possible psychosocial interventions including social skills training and family counseling along with reasonable doses of "typical" antipsychotics, prove to be ineffective, the patient may require higher maintenance doses of medications or will need to be switched to another medication. Long-term clozapine treatment may be an alternative to "typical" oral or depot antipsychotics. The potential use of clozapine in this kind of treatment resistance should be considered following two relapses at expected prophylactic doses of "typical" antipsychotics. A potentially useful approach to decision making in schizophrenic children and adolescents who demonstrate treatment resistance to prophylactic neuroleptics follows:

1. Was the patient using "drugs" or were there psychosocial issues occurring that need to be addressed in treatment but to date have not been adequately dealt with (e.g., high expressed emotion family)? If the answer is *yes,* deal with the problem therapeutically. If *no,* go on to number two.

2. Was the dose of the maintenance medication too low? If the answer is *yes,* raise dose. If dose cannot be raised because of intolerable side effects or for other reasons, or if *no,* proceed to number three.

3. Is patient taking oral medications? If the an-

swer is *yes*, consider depot neuroleptics. If patient is already on depot neuroleptics and numbers one or two do not apply, proceed to number four.

4. Has patient had a previous relapse in which numbers one, two, and three did not apply? If the answer is *yes*, consider clozapine. If *no*, review patient management to ensure that adequate treatment monitoring and early intervention at the first signs of symptom breakthrough are occurring.

Psychiatric and Medical Monitoring

The purpose of psychiatric monitoring during chronic psychopharmacologic treatment is to evaluate the efficacy and tolerability of pharmacotherapy. This is perhaps best conducted in the following manner.

Symptom, functioning, side effects and other necessary assessments should be conducted at baseline, at the time that long-term pharmacologic treatment begins. A number of standardized assessment instruments (see Section Two) should be chosen to provide the necessary evaluations. These should then be applied as necessary over the entire course of treatment. A suggested selection of such instruments, useful in monitoring the long-term treatment of an adolescent with schizophrenia, is as follows, and the clinician should choose those that best meet the monitoring needs of any individual patient:

1. Symptom evaluation: the Brief Psychiatric Rating Scale (BPRS)
2. Symptom evaluation: the Positive and Negative Syndrome Scale (PANSS)
3. Side effects: a medication specific side effects scale (MSSES)
4. Side effects: the Abnormal Involuntary Movements Scale (AIMS)
5. Social functioning: the Adolescent Functioning Inventory (AFI)
6. Treatment-related issues: the Adolescent Illness Impact Scale (AIIS)
7. Quality of life: the Duke Quality of Life Inventory (DQOLI)
8. Global assessment: the Children's Global Assessment Scale (C-GAS)

The application of these various instruments depends on the issues under review. They should not all be used at every assessment point, because that would not only be extremely burdensome to the patient but also the information collected would be of little, if any, value. Some scales should be used frequently, others less so, and others only

occasionally. Scales that evaluate symptoms globally and scales that assess common and expected side effects should be applied at every patient visit. In this manner, they provide immediate important information that should be used in the decision-making process of pharmacologic management. This type of schedule is sensitive to the patient's clinical condition. A patient who is doing well may be monitored once every 3 to 4 weeks (monitoring occurring over periods of time longer than four weeks is not encouraged because it is unlikely to be effective in detecting symptom or side effect changes in sufficient time to introduce needed therapeutic interventions). A patient who is not doing well may be monitored once a week or even more frequently.

Table 14–9 provides suggested monitoring time frames for the assessment instruments described earlier.

The results of these structured assessments are of little or no value if they are not used to provide direction for ongoing pharmacologic treatment or if they cannot be readily reviewed to discern trends in patient functioning that may give subtle clues necessary for alterations in pharmacotherapy. Thus, their results should be displayed clearly, and the use of a yearly monitoring chart is suggested (Fig. 14–3). This monitoring chart has been filled in with a patient's BPRS scores as they were scored over the first 39 weeks of treatment. The entire chart should, however, be made up so as to allow for the scores of all 52 weeks to be entered on one page. A case description and commentary regarding the clinical use of this charting technique follow. Similar charts can be created for medication side effects monitoring, or these can be added to the symptoms monitoring chart simply by adding another scale running horizontally at the bottom of the page that measures MSSES scores. Side effects can then be easily evaluated concurrently with the symptom scores as measured by the BPRS, and the doses of neuroleptic medications (as seen later) should be written in whenever changes are made. This concise yet detailed graph is useful in long-term treatment monitoring.

TABLE 14–9 **Suggested Monitoring Guidelines for Chronic Pharmacologic Treatment of Schizophrenic Children and Adolescents**

Time Frame	Instrument
Every clinic visit	BPRS; MSSES
Every 3–4 months	AIMS; PANSS
Every 6 months	AFI; AIIS; DQOLI; C-GAS

Patient _____ , Attending Physician _____ .

BPRS SCORE

0 1 2 3 4 5 6 7 8 9 10 11 12 13 14 15 16 17 18 19 20 21 22 23 24 25 26 27

Week

Week	BPRS Score	Medication
1	10	perphenazine 32 mg daily
2	12	
3	10	
4	7	
5	10	
6	11	
7	10	
8	10	
9	11	
10	10	perphenazine 24 mg daily
11	10	
12	10	
13	10	
14	10	
15		
16	10	perphenazine 16 mg daily
17		
18	10	perphenazine 8 mg daily
19		
20	10	
21		
22	10	
23		
24	14	
25		
26	14	
27	13	
28	14	
29	14	
30	14	
31	16	
32	16	perphenazine 24 mg daily
33	16	
34	16	
35	16	
36	16	
37	13	
38	13	
39	13	

(continued to week 52)

FIGURE 14–3 Yearly Monitoring Chart: Symptoms as Rated by the BPRS

CASE EXAMPLE

Adolescent Schizophrenia: "I've been doing fine. Now what and what if."

E.D. was a 17-year-old boy who was diagnosed with schizophrenia and admitted to a long-term outpatient treatment program. His medication choice was perphenazine, and his total daily dose at the time of his admission to the program was 32 mg. Weekly medication monitoring visits were begun, and the BPRS was used as the symptom assessment tool. The pattern of E.D.'s BPRS scores is illustrated in Figure 14–3. At the tenth follow-up week, E.D. was still experiencing some mild extrapyramidal side effects and as he was doing relatively well symptomatically, the total daily dose of his perphenazine was decreased to 24 mg. On this dose he continued to do well from a symptomatic perspective and his side effects also improved. At the 16th treatment week his total daily perphenazine was decreased to 16 mg, and the frequency of his medication monitoring was changed to once every 2 weeks. At his next visit, his perphenazine was decreased to 8 mg. E.D. continued to do relatively well but on the 28th treatment week, the physician noticed that E.D.'s BPRS scores had started to creep upwards and were now averaging somewhere around 15 whereas previously they had been around 10.

Uncertain as to the meaning of this apparent but subtle change, the physician elected not to alter the medications but to increase the frequency of the symptom monitoring. Accordingly, E.D. was now assessed weekly. E.D.'s BPRS scores continued to rise gradually and by week 33, they were clearly into the high teens. No external factor could be identified that accounted for this change in symptoms, and compliance was judged to be good. The physician chose to increase E.D.'s perphenazine at this time to a total daily dose of 24 mg because E.D. has previously demonstrated a good therapeutic response and reasonable tolerability to the medication at this level. The weekly monitoring continued and 5 weeks later, E.D.'s BPRS scores had begun to return to more acceptable levels.

CASE COMMENTARY

This case shows the value of the use of a systematic rating scale measure of symptom severity and its charting over time to identify trends in the pattern of illness. In E.D.'s case, it could be argued that the physician decreased the perphenazine too quickly, but that may or may not have been the reason to explain the increase in E.D.'s symptoms. The physician's recognition of a pattern that suggested increased and persistent symptoms resulted in a reasonable first course of action—more careful monitoring. This confirmed the physician's concerns because the symptoms continued to subtly increase. This pattern suggested an impending relapse which was proactively dealt with by increasing E.D.'s medications back to a level that had previously provided adequate symptom control with reasonable tolerability.

The reaction of E.D.'s symptoms to this intervention was also similar to that usually seen in terms of the expected time line of response. The first expected feature is that the symptoms do not continue to worsen. That is, the clinical picture stabilizes. The second feature is that the symptom severity score begins to improve gradually and this improvement occurs over 2 to 3 weeks. An important clinical point about this expected pattern is that overaggressive pharmacologic interventions may not improve the rate of response but will most certainly increase the frequency and severity of adverse events. Thus, as illustrated in E.D.'s case, the most reasonable approach is to increase the medication to a tolerable dose that should lead to critical improvement and then to wait the necessary length of time to allow for proper evaluation of this intervention. Should symptomatic improvement not follow the pattern and time line described above, slightly higher doses of neuroleptic medication may be considered. In this case, depending on the severity of symptoms, short-term hospitalization (1 or 2 weeks) may be useful.

It is reasonable to argue that the type of pharmacologic intervention based on the early recognition of increased and persistent symptom exacerbation may have prevented a relapse of E.D.'s illness with its attendant hospitalization, loss of expected developmental trajectory, and increased economic costs.

If a patient taking depot neuroleptics develops a pattern similar to that noted in this case example, the physician has two choices in terms of pharmacologic management. The first involves increasing the dose of the next injection. Although this is a reasonable and useful strategy, in some cases it may not prove to be optimal. This approach may be particularly unsuitable in situations in which the next scheduled dose is 2 to 3 weeks away. The second choice involves adding an oral neuroleptic to the ongoing depot treatment. The amount of the oral medication can be more easily titrated to the patient's clinical condition, and the appropriate alteration in depot dose made at a later time. This strategy combines maximum flexibility with optimal symptom control. The concurrent administration of oral and depot neuroleptics for long periods of time is, apart from the rare case, not to be encouraged.

Medical Monitoring

The purpose of medical monitoring is to identify medication-induced adverse events as they occur. Although a plethora of potential adverse events are possible, in the chronic pharmacologic treatment of a child or adolescent with schizophrenia, these are unlikely to appear "out of the blue," particularly if the patient has been stabilized on a medication dose for a reasonable length of time. The most common periods of greatest risk for adverse events are associated with changes in the total daily dose or timing of neuroleptic medications. Both dose reduction and dose increments can lead to previously unexperienced or exacerbation of previously well-controlled side effects. Dose reduction is commonly associated with dyskinetic events, and dose increments with increased extrapyramidal or parkinsonian-type side effects.

The "gold standard" of medical monitoring is careful evaluation of subjective and objective side effects. At every medication monitoring visit, the appropriate MSSES should be completed, and the scores checked against previous records much as has been described for symptoms and illustrated in Figure 14–3. In addition, every patient treated with neuroleptic medications should undergo a standardized physical examination at each medication monitoring visit as outlined in Section Two. This information should be summarized and tabulated similar to that of the patient's subjective assessment. Careful documentation of medical issues during long-term treatment using these instruments should not only assist in optimal medication monitoring but also provide necessary information for use in medical and legal issues should they occur.

Interventions as to the treatment of side effects that emerge during chronic neuroleptic treatment vary depending on the cause of the side effects. Withdrawal dyskinesias are best left alone as they will tend to decrease over time. Increased extrapyramidal or parkinsonian-type side effects will need to be treated with the appropriate medications. It is important to remember here, as always, that patient complaints about side effects should be taken seriously, no matter how mild or insignificant they seem to be to the treating physician. Children and adolescents are no more likely than adults to put with physical discomforts arising from neuroleptic treatment, and if their legitimate complaints are not heard and dealt with, noncompliance with pharmacologic treatment may often be the outcome.

Laboratory monitoring depends on the neuroleptic compound being used. Good clinical guidelines are really only available for clozapine where weekly hematologic monitoring is necessary. Otherwise, there is little, if any, consensus on what constitutes appropriate laboratory monitoring in long-term neuroleptic therapy. A reasonable approach is to assess liver function tests once every 4 to 6 months, but many clinicians feel that even that is not necessary. No other routine monitoring laboratory tests need be performed. Obviously, if the patient develops clinical symptoms that are consistent with a potential side effect of the medication, the appropriate laboratory investigations should be undertaken.

If the patient is being treated by depot neuroleptics, the physician must be aware of the potential site injection issues arising with their use. Leakage of medication can occur at the injection site, thus decreasing the amount of medication delivered. A "Z-track" injection technique can decrease the likelihood of this problem. Indurations or inflammation although relatively rare, can occur at the medication site, particularly with prolonged use or with high doses. Patients should be instructed to apply ice to the site if they experience this problem and to contact the physician immediately. Alternating injection sites (e.g., right and left buttocks on alternate months) is a useful prophylactic strategy.

Given the amount of psychiatric and medical monitoring necessary for these patients, they are perhaps best treated in a clinic setting in which trained nursing staff and other caregivers are available to them. Using a medication clinic model (see Section Three) instead of the private practitioner or single-office practice model can provide the type of pharmacologic management that best meets the patient's needs. If this is not available in the community in which the patient resides, a competent and properly trained family physician may be an appropriate person to provide long-term medication monitoring. What is necessary in this scenario, is that the general practitioner have immediate access to the specialist if this is needed and that the patient be reviewed by the specialist on a regular basis (4–6 monthly intervals are reasonable).

Community and Associated Caregivers

The clinical choice as to the route of medication delivery must ultimately be made by the patient and family, and must follow from a process of education about the various options of treatment and fully informed consent as outlined in Section Three. In most cases, the child or adolescent being treated for schizophrenia will be provided with community or other outpatient services that may include all or some of the following: case management, day treatment, social and recreational interventions, individual or family counseling, group support networks, and medical follow-up.

Clinical experience suggests that whenever possible, discussion about issues regarding long-term medication strategy should include those individuals who will be most closely involved in the patient's community care. If community caregivers understand the rationale for medication monitoring (such as clinic visits once every month for those patients taking long-term injectable medications), they may be more likely to provide the child or adolescent patient with the needed support that chronic pharmacologic treatment requires. Failure to adequately involve community caregivers may lead to unnecessary and unhelpful complications.

CASE EXAMPLE

The Young Girl with Schizophrenia and Her "Helpful" Teacher

M.F. was an 11-year-old girl who had been diagnosed with schizophrenia. She had experienced a relatively good symptomatic response to a low dose of haloperidol (5 mg daily). When she was discharged from the hospital, she and her parents chose to continue medication treatment using oral haloperidol and concurrent benztropine (1 mg daily) treatment. As part of her community care, M.F. was placed in a day treatment program, where she attended a school classroom.

As part of her medication monitoring, additional benztropine tablets were made available to the school in case of an untoward reaction to haloperidol. Unfortunately, insufficient education about the potential use of this medication was given by the physician to the school staff.

Ten days after discharge, the attending physician received a telephone call from M.F.'s teacher. The teacher was beside herself with worry because M.F. was complaining of a stiff hand, and all the benztropine medication that had been provided to the school had already been used up. After further telephone discussion and reassurance, a meeting was held with the day treatment program staff and the teacher. M.F. had complained of feeling stiff one to two days after entering the school program. This complaint had elicited an immediate, caring and concerned response in her teacher that eventually resulted in one tablet (2 mg of benztropine) being given to M.F. It seemed that M.F. then quickly discovered that these type of complaints led to relatively rapid and positive responses. The teacher, in her desire to be helpful, had provided M.F. with much more benztropine medications than she required. Fortunately, this had not resulted in any toxic events, and once the teacher better understood some of the clinical issues involved in using prn benztropine properly she could pay more attention to the type of help-seeking behavior pattern that M.F. was developing.

CASE EXAMPLE

The Schizophrenic Adolescent with Erratic Clinic Attendance

P.M. was a 17-year-old boy diagnosed with schizophrenia. He had demonstrated a good response to his acute treatment and had chosen to take long-acting intramuscular flupenthixol, given at a dose of 80 mg every 2 weeks. As part of his community treatment program, he was provided with a case manager affiliated with a youth agency and a schedule of clinic appointments was set up for him.

Initially, P.M. followed his clinic schedule and he was occasionally accompanied to his appointments by his caseworker. After a few months, however, he began to miss appointments. When contacted by the clinic nurse, he would give the excuse that he and his "worker" were "doing rehabilitation."

An emergency meeting with P.M.'s caseworker and his youth agency supervisor identified that the caseworker was unaware of the necessity for regular clinic visits for proper medication management. Once this had been properly explained, P.M.'s clinic attendance record improved dramatically.

CASE COMMENTARY

In both of these cases the importance of involving community caregivers and educating them on the rationale and strategy of long-term medication use is clearly demonstrated. The onus is on the treating physician to ensure that effective communication about these and related pharmacologic issues takes place. Ideally, this should occur prior to the patient's discharge from the hospital and may require "booster" sessions during the course of the child or adolescent's treatment. These "booster" sessions should be held at regular intervals (once every 4 months is suggested) or when significant staff changes in community caregivers occur.

Of practical importance is the role of the physician in ensuring that the patient receive adequate counseling regarding the potential teratogenic effects of antipsychotic medications and appropriate information about birth control and sexually transmitted diseases. Female adolescents with schizophrenia may be more vulnerable for sexual abuse or misuse, and issues regarding sexuality, including gender identity, may be important for both females and males.

Diagnostic Reassessment

A psychiatric diagnosis is perhaps best understood as a hypothesis that identifies a characteristic syndrome, provides a relatively expectable prognosis, and suggests a particular course of treatment. Diagnostic nosology has not yet advanced to the point at which diagnostic certainty is 100 percent. In addition, in many psychiatric conditions (and in particular those of childhood and adolescents) cross-sectional evaluation must be combined with longitudinal assessment in order to make the most accurate diagnosis. Because both cross-sectional and longitudinal phenomenon may exhibit change, diagnoses are not "written in stone" and thus need to be critically evaluated as more information about the patient or the disorder is obtained over time.

Good psychopharmacologic treatment involves appreciation of this feature of psychiatric diagnosis and recognizes both the strengths and limitations of current diagnostic practice. This is particularly relevant as applied to the diagnosis of schizophrenia, which in its first onset may not be clear or which may be difficult to distinguish from an affective psychosis.

Diagnostic reassessment then should be a part of the long-term psychopharmacologic treatment plan for any child or adolescent with a diagnosis of schizophrenia. Ideally, this should be done at least annually (sooner if an event occurs that calls

into question the initial diagnosis, such as a clear-cut manic episode). This should include a review of initial presentation; a review of course of illness; a review of response to treatment (including symptoms, functioning, and so forth); and an application of a semi-structured diagnostic interview (Kiddie Schedule for Affective Disorders and Schizophrenia [K-SADS]).

After a diagnostic case reassessment, alterations or changes in the patient's course of treatment can be considered. Although this diagnostic reassessment should be undertaken by the treating physician, it should also involve other professional caregivers as well. Ideally, this diagnostic reassessment should be made explicit to the patient and the family, and they should be active participants in this process.

This type of approach has a number of distinct benefits. These are:

1. The reality of diagnostic uncertainty is acknowledged but at the same time a structured and careful process is identified as a strategy for decreasing this uncertainty.
2. It gives the patient and family a supportive forum in which to voice concerns about diagnosis, treatment, and outcome that might otherwise not become explicit but may implicitly affect their behaviors.
3. It gives a clear message to the patient and family that the physician is not closed-minded and is not only willing but also interested in critically evaluating the diagnosis.
4. It provides a supportive forum for the patient and family to further their education about the illness or its treatment.
5. It provides the physician with a built-in check on assumptions about any particular case.
6. It provides the physician and associated caregivers with a structure in which to update their knowledge about the disorder.

CASE EXAMPLE

"It is routine but it does have its purpose."

T.M. was a 14-year-old boy with a diagnosis of schizophrenia and a 1-year history of multimodal treatment for this disorder. He had been stabilized on depot flupenthixol at a dose of 30 mg every 3 weeks, was attending a day treatment program, and was receiving 4 to 6 hours a week of community caseworker services.

A diagnostic review using the methods described earlier was conducted about 1 year following his discharge from the hospital. During this review, information that had not been present at the time of hospital discharge was reconsidered. Specifically, a portion of the family history, concerning a paternal uncle who had been "sick in the old country" had been obtained following a lengthy and concerted effort by T.M.'s parents to track the story down. This information was strongly suggestive of a severe and chronic psychotic illness. In addition, clarification of family history on his mother's side revealed that a maternal uncle had not suffered from late onset depression, as had been suspected, but from Alzheimer's disease.

The psychiatric and semi-structured interviews, the review of T.M.'s course and response to treatment, and the new family information all pointed to a confirmation of the diagnosis of schizophrenia. The patient, family, and treatment team all believed that they were "on the right track" from a diagnostic perspective and were able to use this re-evaluation in further planning.

CASE COMMENTARY

The above scenario is not spectacularly exciting nor is it likely to incite riots in the street. Indeed, the reader could be forgiven for finding it just a little "humdrum." That, however, is exactly the point of the illustration. The diagnostic review process is not a circus. It is a careful and systematic re-evaluation of the patient. In most cases, it serves a confirmatory role. In some cases it serves as an agent of change. Both outcomes are to be expected and either outcome is satisfactory.

Drug Abuse or Misuse

Special attention must be paid to the issue of drug abuse or misuse in adolescent patients undergoing long-term treatment for schizophrenia. Available evidence from studies in this population suggests that drug abuse is significantly related to more frequent symptom relapse, increased use of medical facilities, and poorer overall outcome. Patients with a premorbid history of drug abuse or those who come from an environment in which recreational drug use is common may be at increased risk for drug abuse following the onset of their illness.

Adolescents are well known to engage in experimental use of illicit substances yet most do not go on to become drug abusers. The rates of drug abuse in schizophrenic teenagers expressed as a percentage of those who have experimented with drugs simply are not known, but it is unlikely to expect them to be significantly less than in the "well" population. On the other hand, chronically mentally ill teenagers may be at higher risk for drug abuse or misuse than their "well" counterparts. This may be due to one or more of the following reasons:

1. The adolescent may no longer "fit" into a peer group in which drug abuse or misuse is not condoned. Thus, a lack of peer antipathy to drug use is unavailable to provide a peer supportive structure against drug abuse-misuse.

2. Treatment programs for chronically mentally ill patients may often be located in urban neighborhoods in which drug abuse is endemic. Thus, illicit substances may be easily available.

3. The schizophrenic adolescent may be exposed (either in the hospital if treated on an "adult" unit or in outpatient settings) to adult patients who abuse or misuse drugs. This provides a potential "culture of acceptance" which the teenager may find hard to resist.

4. The adolescent schizophrenic may be suffering from symptoms that are either unrecognized (side effects, depressive feelings) or untreated. In this case, the teenager may turn to drugs in an attempt to self medicate.

5. The adolescent patient may be exposed to adult caregivers who themselves abuse or misuse drugs or who otherwise condone the recreational use of some illicit substances, thus providing negative role models.

6. The outpatient or inpatient treatment settings which the teenager encounters may not offer education about drug abuse or misuse and its attendant problems or may not directly address the issue of drug abuse at all. This type of laissez-faire attitude may actually serve to condone the use of illicit drugs by a kind of endorsement by neglect.

Drug abuse or misuse in adolescent schizophrenic patients may occur with illicit compounds that are obtained "on the street," by "trading medicines," or by misuse of prescribed medications. The following cases provide illustrations of each.

CASE EXAMPLE

"It's there and everyone does it."

R.C. was a 17-year-old boy with a 2-year history of schizophrenia. Premorbidly he had been known to be a multiple drug abuser, and his father was a known heavy "recreational" user of marijuana. Although his illness was relatively well controlled with depot neuroleptics, and he was engaged in an intensive community treatment program, he began to once again use various "street drugs," which led to increased symptoms, frequent emergency room visits, and multiple short-term hospitalizations. Community treatment staff were not willing to deal with R.C.'s drug abuse, and his caseworker "turned a blind eye" to the problem citing R.C.'s denial of illicit drug use as the reason. This caused a degree of conflict between the hospital and community program staff. Eventually, however, R.C. admitted to heavy illicit drug use, particularly crack cocaine, and identified multiple sources of supply in the area in which the outpatient treatment program was located. He agreed to enter a special drug treatment program to deal with this problem.

CASE EXAMPLE

"I'll trade you a blue one for two white ones."

E.W. was a 13-year-old girl who had a diagnosis of childhood onset schizophrenia and who was receiving oral neuroleptics and day treatment. Although she had been doing well and her symptoms had been relatively well controlled for some time, she began to exhibit "breakthrough" problems. These consisted of periods of irritability and short lived–psychotic-type symptoms. They were not consistent, however, and they would sometimes be present for a few days and then disappear, only to recur again. A case conference was held to discuss this issue, and a variety of hypotheses were entertained and followed-up, all to no avail in terms of identifying the pathoetiology of these symptoms. Some time later, the classroom teacher observed that E.W. was trading her medication with another patient. She was exchanging trifluoperazine for methylphenidate. After this entrepreneurial bartering was stopped, her "breakthrough" symptoms remitted.

CASE EXAMPLE

"The medicine you give me makes me feel good, if I take lots of it."

V.F. was a 15-year-old boy with a history of childhood schizophrenia treated with depot neuroleptics. He was quite sensitive to the parkinsonian side effects of these compounds and was being prescribed trihexyphenidyl 30 mg daily for their control by his outpatient psychiatrist. Concurrently, he was enrolled in a day treatment program and was seen weekly by a different psychiatrist who was the consultant to that program. V.F. was a difficult patient with restless and intrusive behavior. His psychotic symptoms seemed to be under relatively good control but his other problems made him difficult to manage in a classroom environment. The possibility of a comorbid attention-deficit disorder with hyperactivity (ADDH) was raised and his case was reviewed by the entire treatment team. During the course of this review, it became apparent that V.F. was receiving prescriptions for trihexyphenidyl from both psychiatrists. When this practice was identified and the antiparkinsonian agent was gradually discontinued, V.F.'s behavior improved. When this issue was discussed with him, V.F. responded that the trihexyphenidyl "gives me a buzz. I like that."

CASE COMMENTARY

These cases identify three potential patterns of drug abuse or misuse in the long-term treatment of schizophrenia. All three are adolescents, but these type of problems may occur in preadolescents as well, although teenagers may be more vulnerable to them.

In the first case, the patient was clearly known to be a substance abuser prior to the illness onset and had additional environmental risk factors. However, in spite of these facts and the clinical picture that he presented, some members of the treatment team were unwilling to consider or deal with the issue of drug abuse. This type of approach is not helpful to the patient. Treatment staff must understand the issues involved in drug abuse or misuse and support a therapeutic stance that no illicit drug use will be condoned. In addition, treatment programs for children and adolescents with schizophrenia should have a drug abuse or misuse component so that preventive and early identification strategies can be implemented. If this component is not available, it is necessary for the treating psychiatrist to advocate for its development. Such advocacy is necessary to help improve the pharmacologic management of this illness.

The second case illustrates a medication barter system that may be well recognized as occurring in adults with chronic mental disorders, but may be less well appreciated in children or adolescents. The treatment team considered a variety of hypotheses to account for the patient's symptoms. To their credit, they did not jump to conclusions about potentially explanatory models but tested out each possibility. They had not, however, considered the possibility of medicine trading as a reason for the symptoms they were observing. This should be counted as a possibility in children and adolescents as it does occur.

The third case demonstrates that drug misuse may arise from medications used in the treatment of the illness itself. In this case, the patient did experience distressing side effects which were improved by antiparkinsonian medications. He also discovered that his antidote medicine had other effects—decidedly not therapeutic but for him, pleasurable. Physicians must be aware that antiparkinsonian medications may be abused by some patients and conduct their long-term medication monitoring accordingly.

Parenthetically, the third case also illustrates the necessity for clarity in role as it applies to medication prescription and monitoring. This becomes very important when more than one physician is involved in a case. Most psychiatrists are aware of the dynamics that can arise when multiple caregivers are providing treatment. These same dynamics can be expected to be expressed around issues of medication management. Ideally, medication monitoring in the long-term treatment of the child or adolescent with schizophrenia should be the responsibility of one physician only. This will avoid "double doctoring" and the risks that this entails. Should emergencies or other issues regarding medication use arise, these are best dealt with by urgent discussions between the physicians involved.

Conclusion

The long-term pharmacologic management of the child or adolescent with schizophrenia entails the delivery of neuroleptic medications within the context of a comprehensive psychosocial treatment program. Antipsychotic medications are the cornerstone of the long-term management of this disorder. Their optimal use will help substantially to improve the long-term outcome of these patients.

SUGGESTED READINGS

Belanger M-C, Chouinard G. Technique for injecting long acting neuroleptics. British Journal of Psychiatry, 141:316, 1988.

Chamberlain R, Rapp CA. A decade of case management: a methodological review of outcome research. Community Health Journal, 27:171–188, 1992.

Deberdt R, Elens P, et al. Intramuscular haloperidol decanoate for neuroleptic therapy, efficacy, dosage schedule and plasma levels. Acta Psychiatra Scandinavica, 62:356–363, 1980.

Groves JE. Prescribing long acting neuroleptics. Drug Therapy, 9:89–93, 1979.

Hogarty GE. Prevention of relapse in chronic schizophrenic patients. Journal of Clinical Psychiatry, 54 (suppl 3):18–23, 1993.

Jann MW, Ereshefsky L, et al. Clinical Pharmacokinetics of the depot antipsychotics. Clinical Pharmacokinetics, 10:315–333, 1985.

Kane JM. Treatment of Schizophrenia. Schizophrenia Bulletin, 13:133–156, 1987.

Kane JM, Woerner M, et al. Depot neuroleptics: a comparative review of standard, intermediate and low dose regimes. Journal of Clinical Psychiatry, 47 (suppl 5):30–33, 1986.

King RA. Childhood onset schizophrenia: Development and Pathogenesis. Child and Adolescent Psychiatric Clinics of North America, 3:1–13, 1994.

Lohr D, Birmaher B. Psychotic Disorders. In M. Riddle (ed). Child and Adolescent Clinics of North America—Pediatric Psychopharmacology I. Philadelphia: W. B. Saunders Company, 1995, pp 237–254.

McClellan JM, Werry J. Practice parameters for the assessment and treatment of children and adolescents with schizophrenia. Journal of the American Academy of Child and Adolescent Psychiatry, 33:616–635, 1994.

McLellan, JM, Werry J. Schizophrenia. Psychiatric Clinics of North America, 15:131–148, 1992.

Meltzer HY, Cola P, et al. Cost Effectiveness of clozapine in neuroleptic-resistant schizophrenia. American Journal of Psychiatry, 150:1630–1638, 1993.

Middlemiss MA, Beeber LS. Issues in the use of depot antipsychotics. Journal of Psychosocial Nursing and Mental Health Services, 27:36–37, 1989.

Remington G, Adams M. Depot neuroleptics. In RJ Ancil, S Holliday, et al. (eds). Schizophrenia: Exploring the Spectrum of Psychosis. Chichester: John Wiley and Sons, 1994.

Teicher MH, Gold CA. Neuroleptic drugs: indications and guidelines for their rational use in children and adolescents. Journal of Child and Adolescent Psychopharmacology, 1:33–56, 1990.

Yadalam DG, Simpson GM. Changing from oral to depot fluphenazine. Journal of Clinical Psychiatry, 49:346–358, 1988.

CHAPTER 15

Psychopharmacologic Treatment of Attention-Deficit Hyperactivity Disorder

The pharmacologic treatment of attention-deficit hyperactivity disorder (ADHD) in children and adolescents is clearly the most studied and best understood of all the psychopharmacologic treatments in this age group. Nevertheless, important research into many aspects of the pharmacologic treatment for ADHD continues because many questions remain unanswered. Furthermore, the extent of available information on the pharmacologic treatments for ADHD does not necessarily correlate well with optimal clinical psychopharmacologic practice. From the vantage point of a child and adolescent psychopharmacologist, it is not uncommon to find children and adolescents who are receiving less than adequate pharmacotherapy for this disorder. On the other hand, some children and adolescents without clear-cut ADHD may be exposed to pharmacologic treatments that are not necessarily indicated in their cases.

Psychostimulant medication is clearly the current treatment of choice for ADHD in the practice of child and adolescent psychiatry. This category of medications includes dextroamphetamine, methylphenidate, and pemoline. Methylphenidate is the most commonly prescribed. Although rates vary across geographic regions, in the United States, 0.04 to 7.0 percent of primary school children, mostly boys, are treated with methylphenidate. These data compare with an estimated population prevalence rate of ADHD of about 5.0 percent. Thus evidence for gross overuse of this medication (as sensationalized in media reports and agitated by small but vocal special interest groups) is lacking. The core symptoms of ADHD, easy distractibility, difficulty in sustaining attention, problems with on-task functioning, excessive nonpurposeful motor activity, disorganization, and its associated functional impairments in classroom, peer, and family functioning, have been shown to respond to adequate treatment with stimulant medications in those children and adolescents who can tolerate them.

Recently, more studies of nonstimulant pharmacotherapies for ADHD have appeared. In part these investigations were instituted because not all children and adolescents with ADHD respond well to stimulant treatment. The effect of comorbid anxiety as a potential factor in choosing antidepressant rather than stimulant treatment was suggested in early reports, but later investigations proposed that many ADHD children, with or without comorbid anxiety, might respond to one or more of the following antidepressant medications: fluoxetine, desipramine, bupropion, monoamine oxidase inhibitors, venlafaxine, and others. Other compounds, including the alpha-2 noradrenergic agonists clonidine and guanfacine, also show promise (Table 15–1).

TABLE 15–1 **Potential Pharmacologic Treatments for Children and Adolescents with ADHD***

Well Established	Reasonably Established	Looking for a Home
Methylphenidate	Desipramine	Fluoxetine
Dextroamphetamine	Bupropion	Nortriptyline
Pemoline	Clonidine	Venlafaxine
		Moclobomide
		Buspirone

*The information used to compile this table was obtained from clinical experience and currently available literature regarding the pharmacologic treatment of children and adolescents with ADHD. Monoamine oxidase inhibitors (MAOIs) (including moclobomide) and guanfacine should be considered experimental therapies at this time.

Given the current state of knowledge about the pharmacologic treatment of ADHD and the variety of potential choices for treatment, the clinician may experience some difficulties in making the "best" first choice. General issues to consider when choosing a medication for first initiating pharmacotherapy are discussed in Section Three. These should be applied to the decision making process regarding the first choice of medicine in treating the child or adolescent with ADHD. In addition, the following issues should be reviewed as they apply to each particular patient:

1. Comorbid disorders
2. Previous or current medical concerns
3. Family history

Comorbid Disorders

ADHD often presents with comorbid disorders that might influence the choice of medication used to initiate treatment. Patients with "pure" ADHD or with comorbid conduct or oppositional disorders may do relatively well with stimulant treatment. Other patients may not be ideal candidates for stimulant treatment, and in those cases medication treatment can be initiated with an alternative medication such as a tricyclic antidepressant, buspirone, or a serotonin-specific reuptake inhibitor. Children and adolescents with ADHD who may be less likely candidates for initial treatment with a stimulant are identified as having (1) a comorbid psychiatric diagnosis of Tourette's syndrome, anxiety disorder, major depression, bipolar disorder, schizophrenia, or schizoaffective disorder. Note that recent opinion suggests that treatment with stimulants does not necessarily "unmask" or worsen tics in children or adolescents with Tourette's syndrome. In many cases, the ADHD symptoms contribute much more to the patient's impairments than do the tics. In this case it is not unreasonable to begin treatment with stimulants after careful evaluation of tic frequency and severity, and to monitor the effect

of this treatment on the tics. If stimulants are used and do increase tics, there is little evidence that this will be a permanent effect. In such a case, the stimulants could be withdrawn and an alternative medication (such as clonidine, desipramine, or fluoxetine) should be used. (2) The presence of severe or profound mental retardation (IQ less than 45 or a mental age of less than 4.5 years) may predict a poor response to methylphenidate in some cases.

Previous or Current Medical Concerns

A premorbid history of tics or current symptoms of tics may be a relative contraindication to stimulant treatment. The same considerations apply to this concern as for Tourette's syndrome. Height and weight that are significantly below age-expected norms may be a relative contraindication to stimulant treatment. However, the most important issue in this regard is the monitoring of growth velocity. Stimulant treatment should not be withheld simply because a child is smaller-than-average for age.

Family History

A family history of Tourette's syndrome may be a relative contraindication for stimulant treatment. The same considerations apply to this concern as for Tourette's syndrome. A history of a good response to stimulant treatment in a first-degree relative may suggest a similar response in the child.

Given the available literature on the pharmacologic treatment of ADHD, and a child or adolescent without one of these contraindications, most clinicians would argue that initial treatment should be instituted with one of the stimulant medications. Table 15–2 provides suggested first choices for the pharmacologic treatment of ADHD.

TABLE 15–2 **Suggested First-Choice Medications in the Pharmacotherapy of Children and Adolescents with ADHD***

Age Category	First Choice	Alternate	Alternate
Preschooler	Methylphenidate	Dextroamphetamine	Pemoline
School age	Methylphenidate	Pemoline or dextroamphetamine	Bupropion
Adolescent	Methylphenidate	Desipramine	Bupropion

*The suggestions regarding first-choice medications are based on clinical experience and the currently available literature regarding the pharmacologic treatment of children and adolescents with ADHD. The general principles identified in Section Three have been applied to this first-choice determination. Other writers may suggest other first choices.

CASE EXAMPLE

The Little Boy Who Couldn't Stop Moving: Treatment of ADHD

M.F. was a 7-year-old boy who was referred for possible medication treatment for his hyperactivity at his parents' request because, although his primary care physician had suggested methylphenidate, Mr. and Mrs. F. were concerned about giving their son this medicine and wanted another opinion. A psychiatric assessment confirmed a diagnosis of ADHD and no comorbid Axis I disorder was identified, although M.F. did have a number of oppositional symptoms. His parents were particularly concerned about his motor overactivity, his difficulty following directions and complying with their requests, his intrusive and persistent annoying of his older brother and younger sister, his inability to organize his living space, his time and activities, and his school performance. Although his parents and siblings were warm and generally supportive toward him, they noted that when he was "particularly hyper" he could bring chaos to the entire family.

M.F.'s teachers had always described him as having problems with paying attention in class. He was rarely able to get his class work completed on time and had developed a reputation as a disruptive influence on children who sat near him. Various behavioral methods had been attempted by his teachers, all to no avail. His workbooks were messy, he often misplaced his homework, and he had difficulty working in groups because he could not focus on the task at hand. His grades were low to average, and he had most difficulty with mathematics and reading. He was beginning to develop a self-image as a "rotten student," although his IQ test score was 120. Teachers at his school had begun to see him as a "difficult student" and had suggested that he be placed in a special behavioral class, but this was not available at his local school.

M.F. did have a number of good friends and was considered to be an excellent athlete, but he always seemed to underachieve on the playing field. He was a top-level soccer player and enjoyed all sports. His coaches, who applauded his natural athletic ability, described him as having trouble staying focused, and he was known sometimes to play as if he were partly asleep. A very good baseball player, he suddenly quit playing, complaining that the game was "too boring."

A family psychiatric history was unremarkable, except for M.F.'s father's self-description: "We are a lot alike. I have the same problems with organizing things, but I've learned to cope over the years." When this remark followed up with structured questioning, a possible diagnosis of adult ADHD was made.

After a full and detailed discussion about the diagnosis of ADHD and its pharmacologic treatment, M.F. and his parents agreed to a trial of methylphenidate concurrent with family counseling. Both M.F. and his parents were given educational materials about the disorder and its treatment and were encouraged to contact the local ADHD support group. In addition, they agreed to allow for detailed educational testing to determine if a learning disorder or speech and language problem might be contributing to his academic difficulties. Finally, they agreed to involve M.F.'s school in the baseline assessment and treatment process.

CASE COMMENTARY

This case illustrates a not uncommon presentation of a youngster with ADHD. In this case, the lack of a comorbid psychiatric disorder and the presence of a positive family environment suggest that M.F. may well show a positive response to methylphenidate treatment. The determination of a possible specific learning disorder is a useful baseline assessment, given the high prevalence of learning difficulties found in children with ADHD, some of which may not be able to be identified from intelligence testing alone. Family support, even for well-functioning families, combined with education about the disorder is a necessary component in providing comprehensive treatment for the child with ADHD.

Initiating Treatment

Baseline medical and laboratory investigations for stimulant treatment, in addition to a detailed medical history and physical examination (with particular attention paid to identification of tics), are as follows:

1. Medication-specific side effects scale (MSSES; see Appendix IV)
2. Complete blood count (CBC)
3. Height, weight, heart rate, and blood pressure

If pemoline is chosen, in addition to the above

tests the following baseline investigations should be completed:

1. Liver function tests
2. Careful assessment of any possible adventitious movements (the Abnormal Involuntary Movement Scale [AIMS] scale can be used for this; see Appendix III)

Baseline psychiatric assessment should include the following:

1. Evaluation of ADHD symptoms. Select one of the following, all of which may be found in Appendix VI: ADHD Symptoms Rating Scale, ADHD Rating Scale (ADHDRS), or Conners Parent–Teacher Rating Scale (CPTS). Teachers can use any of these instruments. If possible, using a common rating scale for parents and teachers is preferred for comparative purposes (see later).
2. Evaluation of attention and concentration. The Continuous Performance Task (CPT) or Cancellation Task (CT) can be used for this purpose. In many cases a clinician may not be inclined to conduct this part of the baseline evaluation as part of routine clinical care. However, the use of these assessments may be considered in some cases because these tasks capture a dimension of ADHD symptomatology that is not necessarily well obtained on parent or teacher rating scales.
3. Evaluation of social and family functioning, using a Visual Analogue Scale (VAS) defined by a specific symptom that is expected to be modified by stimulant treatment (Fig. 15–1).

   Alternatively, the Social Adjustment Inventory for Children and Adolescents (SAICA, see Appendix VII) can be used. However, outside of a research-driven investigation, it is not clear that the routine use of the SAICA will provide any more useful information for monitoring symptom change across a variety of domains than can be obtained by using various VASs.

It is therapeutically helpful to have all parties involved in the child's treatment complete these rating scales separately, allowing the child or adolescent, each parent, and the teacher to have input into the evaluation process. In addition, involving the child in systematically evaluating and recording his or her behaviors can become a blame-free learning process for all parties.

What often occurs (as seen in Fig. 15–2) is that the child rates his or her symptoms as being much less disturbing than either the parents or teachers rate them. This is not a manipulative act but difficulty in understanding how his or her behavior affects others. In most cases, children with ADHD do not feel ill, sick, or disturbed in the same way as when they have the flu or a sore throat. They tend to understand a sickness model that arises out of their own experience of other illnesses. Thus, it is to be expected that most ADHD children will not understand that in the absence of a physical experience of sickness their behaviors or difficulties with family, friends, or school could be identified as a problem requiring medical attention.

Parenthetically, in the absence of their awareness of how their behavior affects others, ADHD children and adolescents often experience their parents' and teachers' attempts to modify their activities as unnecessary and degrading. When this occurs, their self-esteem may suffer significantly and their behavior may become increasingly oppositional as a reaction to what they perceive as unfair and punitive criticism (which in many cases it may be!). In adolescents, this may in some cases lead to strenuous and overt rebellion against parental wishes. In some, these feelings may develop into significant dysphoria, which might be difficult to distinguish from a depressive disorder. Visually plotting the child's or adolescent's view of his or her behavior and comparing it with the views of parents and teachers are often the first steps in helping the child or adolescent understand the difficulties that have brought him or her to medical attention.

This process is often also helpful to parents and teachers as well. Visual plotting of symptoms and the different perceptions of them will assist parents and teachers in understanding that the child is not necessarily "bad" or lacking in a willingness to "do things right," but rather the child does not

Fighting with sister		
	Never	Constant
Family mealtimes		
	Not stressful	Very stressful
Playground activity		
	No fighting	Constant fights

FIGURE 15–1 Social and Family Functioning Scale Using a VAS in ADHD

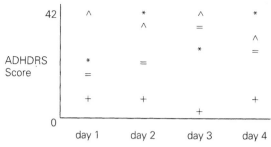

+, child (M.F.); =, mother; ^, father; *, teacher.

FIGURE 15–2 ADHD Symptom Severity Ratings Obtained by Different Observers Using the ADHDRS

experience his or her behaviors as a problem. These behaviors are, to borrow a psychotherapeutic phrase, ego syntonic. This new understanding can then become the beginning of therapeutic work with the child and family, and can provide a new foundation for judging the child's school-based difficulties.

In addition, when all parties are involved in the assessment of baseline symptoms and in monitoring outcome, they have a greater commitment to a common goal. Everyone's input is valued, and everyone's assessment of the situation becomes an important component in the measure of treatment efficacy. Thus, medication treatment is seen as one means to help everyone attain a similar goal. The treatment paradigm thus becomes one of cooperation rather than control.

A number of other issues in monitoring the outcome with methylphenidate treatment must also be considered. First, because standard preparations of methylphenidate have a short duration of therapeutic activity, treatment monitoring must reflect this. For example, asking a parent to complete a symptom assessment scale at 2200 hours, when the last dose of standard preparation methylphenidate was given at noon, will not identify any medication effect, even if it has been clearly present, because it will most likely have worn off before or soon after the child arrived home from school.

Second, the target location for methylphenidate treatment must also be clearly established. Is the medication to be taken only when the child is at school, or will the child take the medications in the evening and during the weekend as well? In many cases, physicians and parents may have strong opinions about this matter, well before they subject their views to any empirical evaluation. Whereas some believe that medicine should be taken only in the classroom setting to allow for

better classroom functioning, others think this may be too narrow a treatment goal. These physicians and parents note that the child spends much of his time with the family and point to studies that indicate that methylphenidate treatment improves parent–child interactions.

What is often useful in addressing this issue is to take a pragmatic, evaluative approach and have the child and parents assess medication effects on nonschool functioning to determine if the use of methylphenidate is reasonable outside the classroom. This can easily be done by ratings performed on the weekends; on some days the child takes methylphenidate and on other days does not. A similar strategy can be applied to evening assessments as well. With the information obtained using this approach, a more informed decision can be made as to the location and duration of methylphenidate treatment.

Methylphenidate

Methylphenidate is a stimulant piperidine derivative useful in the treatment of ADHD and narcolepsy. Although it has been postulated that its therapeutic effect in ADHD is via its ability to affect dopamine neurotransmission, a simple dopamine deficit model in the pathoetiology of ADHD is no longer considered to be a viable explanation of this disorder. Methylphenidate is available in both standard and sustained-release forms.

Methylphenidate is well absorbed following oral ingestion, and its absorption is enhanced if it is taken with food. It undergoes a large first-pass effect, exhibits relatively low plasma binding, and demonstrates a variable bioavailability of 30 to 80 percent. Peak plasma levels following oral dosing using the standard methylphenidate preparation are found at about 2 hours, and a half-life of 2 to 3 hours is usual. A single dose is completely eliminated in 12 to 15 hours, and its pharmacologic duration, which shows an onset of 30 to 60 minutes and a duration of 3 to 5 hours, parallels these kinetics. Recent findings suggest that methylphenidate efficacy may be related to its absorption phase, the so-called ramp effect. Thus multiple daily dosing is necessary.

The sustained-release preparation of methylphenidate demonstrates a relatively slower onset of action than is found with the standard methylphenidate tablet but a longer therapeutic action of 7 to 9 hours. Although some anecdotal reports suggest that the slow-release preparation may show less therapeutic efficacy compared with standard-form tablets, insufficient scientifically valid evidence exists to support this view. What is apparent in clinical practice, however, is that significant individual variability in therapeutic response is seen with all preparations of methylphenidate; thus treatment must be carefully tailored to the needs of the individual child or adolescent, whichever preparation is used.

Monitoring of methylphenidate treatment is clinical. Plasma and salivary levels are available in some locations but are unlikely to be useful. The side effects of methylphenidate are the same as found with stimulants in general. Reported severe adverse effects include toxic psychosis, alopecia, thrombocytopenia, Stevens-Johnson syndrome, and various hypersensitivity reactions and cardiovascular complications but these are rare. Common side events are dizziness, insomnia, irritability, headache, suppressed appetite, and dysphoria-crying. These have been identified from clinical experience and from the available current literature regarding methylphenidate treatment of children and adolescents with ADHD.

Most common side effects can be managed by altering methylphenidate dose amounts or the timing of doses. For example, if suppressed appetite is a problem, it (and consequent weight loss) can be avoided by providing a meal before bedtime, ensuring that the child eats a big breakfast, and encouraging the intake of healthy high-calorie drinks and snacks. In addition, the medication can usually be administered with or immediately following meals.

Although short-term treatment is unlikely to result in decreased height and weight, questions remain regarding the issue of potentially reduced growth velocity in children chronically treated with methylphenidate. Most long-term studies suggest that these effects, when they do occur, are minimal. Decreased weight velocity may be related to the anorexic effects of methylphenidate, and if this is the case giving the medication with meals (which has the added effect of improving its absorption) may be of benefit.

Behavioral side effects may arise with methylphenidate treatment. Although toxic psychoses are very rare and are usually associated with very high doses, methylphenidate treatment may exacerbate the cognitive, affective, and behavioral symptoms found in childhood mania and schizophrenia. If psychotic symptomatology is present, methylphenidate should generally not be prescribed. In special cases, it may be possible to administer methylphenidate to children or adolescents with mania or schizophrenic psychoses, provided that they are adequately covered by antipsychotic or thymoleptic medications, the patient is carefully monitored, and a rational clinical indication exists.

A behavioral rebound phenomenon has been described, and clinical experience suggests this may be more common than is often reported. Usually occurring near the end of the day, 5 to 15 hours following the last methylphenidate dose, it is characterized by irritability, oppositionality, motor or verbal hyperactivity, excitability, restlessness, and insomnia. This phenomenon is best managed by adding a small amount of standard-preparation methylphenidate, 5 to 10 mg, just prior to the time of usual onset. In some cases, the insomnia that occurs with methylphenidate treatment is a reflection of drug withdrawal occurring in the later evening and can likewise be treated with a small dose of 5 mg given 1 to 2 hours prior to bedtime.

Tics can occur with methylphenidate treatment, as they can with any stimulant. Some authorities argue that methylphenidate can unmask latent Tourette's syndrome. Although the tautology of this argument suggests caution in its adoption, nevertheless, the development of complex tics during methylphenidate treatment is a sufficient reason for switching to another medication. In these cases other stimulants should not be considered. The alpha$_2$-agonist clonidine or one of the antidepressant medications may be useful.

Methylphenidate is an effective treatment for the core symptoms of ADHD. In addition, it has been shown to improve classroom behaviors, general academic functioning, performance on arithmetic tasks, child–maternal interactions, and peer relationships. Of interest is that methylphenidate in therapeutic amounts can also improve the ability to play both video games and physical sports, such as baseball and soccer.

The therapeutic effects of methylphenidate are complex. For example, some but not all investigators suggest that lower doses may be primarily associated with improvement in cognitive tasks in general, and higher doses may primarily be associated with improvements in motor behavior. Some research suggests that particular cognitive tasks, such as the paired-associate learning task, may show errors at doses of methylphenidate approaching 1 mg/kg; hence lower doses, such as 0.3 or 0.5 mg/kg, are suggested to optimize this effect. These findings have not been demonstrated in all studies that have addressed this issue. Other cognitive tasks that measure vigilance or reaction time (such as the CPT) have not been shown to demonstrate cognitive difficulties at higher doses and may actually demonstrate a linear dose/response relationship. Thus, if clinically possible, behavioral, social, and cognitive functioning should be evaluated with regard to treatment outcome with methylphenidate.

Current dosing approaches suggest a daily target dose of about 0.5 to 1.0 mg/kg/day. This usually results in total daily doses of between 15 and 40 mg, although a maximal total daily dose may reach 60 mg or higher as long as side effects are minimal and increased doses are providing increased therapeutic efficacy (Table 15–3). Increasingly, clinicians and researchers are questioning the value of the milligram per kilogram dosing for methylphenidate and are using standardized dose approaches, titrating medications as per clinical response.

Initiating and Optimizing Methylphenidate Treatment

The dose of methylphenidate (if the standard preparation is used) is divided over the day to optimize therapeutic outcome across the various domains for which treatment is being sought. Two different initiation strategies that the clinician may wish to consider when beginning treatment with methylphenidate follow.

Strategy One: Single-Dose Approach for Children, Including Preschoolers

One useful approach is to start the child at a dose of 5 mg (2.5 mg if a preschooler) given in the morning and at noon and maintain that dose for a period of 3 days. At this time, clinical improvement and side effects should be assessed using standardized measures. This may then be increased by an additional 5 mg (2.5 mg for preschoolers) and again maintained for a period of 3 days. If late day or early evening dosing is being evaluated, similar amounts should be given at this time, as described earlier. This is then continued for a week, with further titration up or down being determined by clinical improvement and ad-

TABLE 15–3 **Suggested Initial Target Daily Dose Ranges of Methylphenidate in Treating Children and Adolescents with ADHD***

Target Daily Dose (mg/kg/day)	Target Daily Dose (mg/day)
0.5–1.0, in three divided doses	15–60, in three divided doses

*These target dose ranges are suggested on the basis of clinical experience and the currently available literature regarding the use of methylphenidate in children and adolescents with ADHD. Individual patient responses (therapeutic and adverse) may vary. These dose suggestions are guidelines only; actual doses must be tailored to the patient's clinical response. The therapeutically maximized daily dose may be higher or lower than the initial daily dose target. See Section Three for general principles regarding dose initiation and response optimization strategies.

verse events, as assessed using standardized outcome measures at the end of a week of treatment.

Strategy Two: Single-Dose Approach for Adolescents

If an adolescent is being treated for the first time with methylphenidate, a slightly different strategy is possible. An initial 5 mg test dose, if well tolerated, can be then followed by 10 mg, given in the morning and at noon. If a late day or early evening dosing is being evaluated, an additional 10 mg should be given at this time. This dose schedule can be continued for 3 to 5 days and then adjusted as suggested by outcome evaluation of therapeutic and adverse effects conducted at that time.

CASE EXAMPLE

M.F. Starts Methylphenidate

After discussions with M.F. and his family, and a week of baseline measurements (at home and at school), the physician instituted strategy three to begin methylphenidate treatment. A test dose of 5 mg was well tolerated, and both of M.F.'s parents reported that he showed a decrease in his motor activity and an improved ability to focus. Accordingly, the methylphenidate was begun at a dose of 5 mg, given at 0745 to 0800 in the morning (school began at 0900), and the school health officer dispensed an additional 5 mg to M.F. just before lunch (1200 hours). M.F.'s mother administered an evening dose (5 mg at 1800 hours). This was continued for 7 days, because it had been decided that M.F. would take his medication at home on the weekends as well. Following this, the results of the daily evaluations were compiled and compared with baseline scores. These are shown in summary form in Figure 15–3.

M.F.'s methylphenidate dose was then increased to 10 mg, given at the same times, and was continued for an additional 7 days. At this time the results of the daily evaluations were compiled and compared with baseline and treatment week 1 scores (see Fig. 15–3).

The results of this treatment evaluation reinforced the clinical impression of improvement in M.F.'s symptoms with methylphenidate treatment. The assessment also identified one other important issue; namely, that increasing the methylphenidate dose did not substantially alter the scores on the ADHDRS. Thus a clear clinical need for higher medication doses was not indicated.

As a result of this evaluation, M.F. was placed

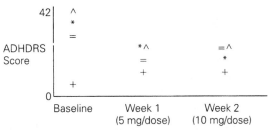

+, child (M.F.); =, mother; ^, father; *, teacher.

FIGURE 15–3 Evaluation of Outcome Using the ADHDRS in Initiating M.F.'s Methylphenidate Treatment

on methylphenidate, which he took at a dose of 5 mg in the morning, at noon, and with his evening meal. This regimen was continued during the weekend as well. Monitoring of side effects did not identify any significant treatment-emergent effects, and it was decided to continue M.F.'s medications using a once-every-4-weeks re-evaluation schedule until school ended for the summer holidays.

CASE COMMENTARY

The medication initiation strategies identified earlier (and described in the case of M.F.), although useful guides with which to begin treatment for many children and adolescents with ADHD, may need to be altered depending on the therapeutic effect and treatment-emergent side effects that occur. It must be kept in mind that, in addition to total daily dose *amounts*, the daily dose *timing* for an optimal therapeutic effect should also be individualized as much as possible. In some cases, standard-preparation doses of methylphenidate should be given three times daily. In some cases, a mix of slow-release and standard preparations may be necessary to provide optimal behavioral and cognitive effects.

The Insulin Model of Methylphenidate Treatment

Contrary to the study designs in much of the research literature regarding the use of methylphenidate, in which studies generally use fixed doses of one methylphenidate preparation and then measure the therapeutic effect across a number of different domains, the clinical use of methylphenidate attempts to maximize therapeutic outcome in as many identified domains as is reasonable. The

single-medication, fixed-dose model is a useful construct for application in many research strategies. In contrast, the art of clinical practice suggests that an insulin model of using medication may be of value in approaching methylphenidate treatment. In this model, long-acting and short-acting medications are used together to provide symptom control that is not attainable when only one preparation is used.

This model has three components (Table 15–4) and uses the titration of dose amount, type of preparation, and dose timing to target specific symptoms to maximize patient response.

Using these components, clinicians may modify methylphenidate treatment to reflect the various cognitive and behavioral treatment needs of each individual, including choosing which particular symptoms might need treatment at different times of the day. Similar to insulin treatment, both slow-release and standard preparations of methylphenidate may be used. This is demonstrated in the following cases.

CASE EXAMPLE

Young Boy Treated with Methylphenidate for ADHD

O.M. was a 9-year-old boy with ADHD comorbid with a diagnosis of oppositional disorder and a number of symptoms of conduct disorder. He was receiving special educational interventions and recently had been started on methylphenidate treatment. A dose of 10 mg, given in the morning between 0700 and 0730 hours, and 10 mg, given by a school counselor at lunch (between 1200 and 1230 hours), resulted in a marked improvement in O.M.'s behavior and classroom participation. His playground fighting, which had been a problem, had also decreased. Side effects were minimal, and treatment continued over a 1 month period showed O.M. to be functioning better academically.

TABLE 15–4   The Insulin Model of Methylphenidate Treatment

Treatment Component	Treatment Targets
Type of preparation (slow-release or standard tablet)	Core symptoms Academic success Classroom behavior
Titration of dose for each type of preparation	Family functioning Peer relationships
Timing of dose for each type of preparation	Extracurricular success

However, because O.M.'s mother worked outside of the home and could not get home by the time school ended, O.M. attended an after-school recreation program that began at 1600 hours. His behavior there continued to be problematic, and when his mother picked him up (usually around 1800 hours) he was "flying." The recreation program staff were unwilling to give O.M. any medications, because the program director had refused to allow them to do so (citing insurance reasons). He simultaneously threatened to discharge O.M. from the program because of behavior problems and continued to maintain this position, even after the physician and school counselor spoke to him about O.M. and his treatment. O.M.'s mother, a single parent, had no other reasonable alternative for child care and was very concerned about losing the recreation program placement. She was also hesitant to change the methylphenidate to another medication because it was working so well, and she was concerned about some of the potential side effects that could occur with alternative drugs.

After discussion with O.M., his mother, and the school counselor, it was decided to change O.M.'s methylphenidate regimen. He was given 10 mg in the morning, but the noon dose was changed to one slow-release tablet (20 mg). This combination resulted in a continued medication effect that persisted well beyond the time that O.M. participated in the after-school recreation program. Indeed, the therapeutic effect persisted into the late evening, and there was no evidence of a behavioral rebound effect. O.M.'s mother was exceedingly pleased with this change and felt that "finally, I can talk to him." O.M. was also pleased with the result because he was "not getting into trouble so much."

CASE COMMENTARY

This case example illustrates the successful use of the insulin model of methylphenidate treatment in which short-term and long-term preparations are used together to target time-of-day symptoms.

CASE EXAMPLE

Adolescent Treated with Methylphenidate for ADHD

K.J. was a 15-year-old boy with ADHD. In the past few years he had received sporadic methyl-phenidate treatment. When he had been taking the medication, he had shown a positive behavioral and academic response. However, his parents were not committed to his taking the medicine and often neglected to dispense it to him. K.J. did experience occasional nausea and decreased appetite, side effects that, although mild, nevertheless provided a rationale for non-compliance. Academically, he had been fortunate to attend a small local school with a low pupil to teacher ratio and a structured learning environment. Given this situation, he did relatively well academically, although below his potential. His peer relationships were good.

When he graduated to high school, K.J. chose to attend a large urban secondary school with class sizes that were two to three times greater than he had previously experienced. There was minimal structure in the learning environment. Soon after beginning high school, K.J.'s grades dropped drastically. Attempts to help him structure his work were unsuccessful. Homework became a family battleground because K.J.'s short attention span and poor on-task behaviors resulted in sloppy, unfinished assignments. Although he maintained good peer relationships, K.J.'s parents noticed that he was spending more and more time with teens whose own academic records were marginal and that his attitude toward school was becoming increasingly more negative.

Furthermore, although he had always been "hyper," his behavior at home was becoming more disruptive to the family. Conflicts between K.J. and his siblings escalated because he continued to intrude on them at times scheduled for schoolwork completion. A number of attempts were made to provide home tutors and school-based structure for K.J., all to no lasting avail. He designed plans to help him control his behavior, which he understood was a problem, but with no success.

Finally, his parents decided that they would provide a united front to encourage the continuous use of methylphenidate in an attempt to help K.J. "turn things around." K.J. agreed with this plan. Methylphenidate treatment was begun with a test dose of 10 mg, which showed an immediate effect on the core symptoms, and treatment was started at 10 mg, given in the morning and at noon. Although this showed a good therapeutic effect with no significant side effects, K.J. did not want to take a tablet at school (a common occurrence in children and adolescents). Accordingly, he chose to take a slow-release tablet of methylphenidate at about 0730 in the morning. This was also effective during school hours but had worn off by evening, making it difficult for K.J. to do his homework. A dose of 10 mg, of standard-preparation methylphenidate was added, which K.J. took with his evening meal. He began his study time an hour later.

With this regimen, his on-task effort and concentration showed considerable improvement, and he was able to successfully complete his homework with good results. His at-home behavior also improved significantly, and his grades showed a gradual but consistent improvement on this treatment regimen. K.J. reported a mild degree of insomnia as the evening dose wore off around 2300 hours but felt that he would put up with it because "the stuff works for me."

CASE COMMENTARY

These cases illustrate how the insulin model can be effectively used in treating children and adolescents with ADHD. The use of this model allows for improved titration of the medication dose and effect. The "right" amount of medication can be delivered at the "right" time of day. Because the right amount and right time can vary among individuals, a flexible, empirically driven dosing strategy is preferred. In many children and teenagers, the unwillingness to take medications at school, as in K.J.'s case, will lead to consideration of long-acting agents, and targeting of ADHD symptoms in the after-school home environment may best respond to the regular, shorter-acting preparation.

Applying an "N of 1" Model to Assist in Evaluating the Response to Methylphenidate

Methylphenidate is also uniquely suited to a more sophisticated evaluation of treatment efficacy, the single-case design or "n of 1" trial. Methylphenidate's rapid onset and offset of action make a repeated-measures design, in which active medication is compared with placebo over sufficient alternating conditions to provide enough power for statistical analysis, very useful. In addition, because of the potentially differential dose-related effects on cognition and behavior, a variable baseline using two or more dosage choices can be built into the basic structure of the n of 1 trial.

In a sophisticated use of this strategy, doses of 5 mg of methylphenidate may be randomly alternated with doses of 10 mg and placebo. As long as each treatment condition is similar in duration (1 day to 1 week), and each condition is experienced for a minimum of 10 or more times (days) over the course of the evaluation, statistical analysis of the results of the assessment should be possible. For example, using measures of core symptoms (such as the ADHDRS, a cancellation task, and a side effects scale) on a daily basis carried out over 1 month, the clinician can demonstrate not only global efficacy of methylphenidate treatment but also (if present) a differential cognitive and side effect profile of various doses. Usual clinical practice, however, may not need to be that complicated, and a modification of this approach can be useful.

In this modification, following a 3-day baseline assessment, a standard dose of methylphenidate is given alternatively with placebo, each over an alternating 3-day period for a total of 12 days. Thus, placebo is given on days 1 to 3 and 7 to 9. Active medication (e.g., 10 mg of methylphenidate) is given on days 4 to 6 and days 10 to 12. Global outcome scores and side effect scale scores are obtained daily, and the means of each treatment block are compared.

If the results suggest a medication effect (Fig. 15–4), the dose of the active drug may be decreased and then increased slightly to determine if less or more medication provides equivalent or better efficacy, and the process is continued. For example, days 1 to 3 (methylphenidate 5 mg dose), days 4 to 6 (methylphenidate 15 mg dose), days 7 to 9 (same as days 1 to 3), and days 10 to 12 (same as days 4 to 6) could be used (see Fig. 15–4). This type of protocol is especially useful in those cases in which the patient or parent has serious concerns about the value of expected dose ranges of methylphenidate treatment. This design also allows the clinician to better assess the optimal possible effect of different doses on a variety of measures, because there is no need to limit oneself to evaluating core symptoms, or side effects and various VAS measures of peer and family functioning can be easily added.

When used to assist in clinical evaluation, the data shown in Figure 15–4 provide reasonable evidence for a positive medication effect. The strength of this association is further supported by repeating the A and B blocks of the initial placebo/10 mg dose evaluation at the end of the entire trial and obtaining a result very similar to that found during the initial 12 days. Furthermore, it also seems from Figure 15–4 that the 5 mg dose of methylphenidate provides less therapeutic effect as measured by the ADHDRS than the 10 mg dose, but the 15 mg dose provides little if any additional therapeutic benefit to the 10 mg dose. This evaluation method can be further strengthened if the clinician determines an a priori target range for an expected therapeutic effect. If the on-active medication blocks fall into that

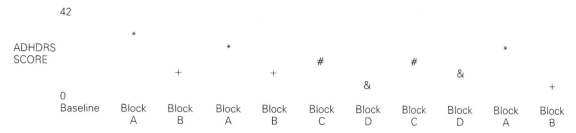

The baseline and each block are of 3 days' duration. The total length of this trial is just over 1 month (33 days).

The ratings shown are both parents' rating averaged for each block using the ADHDRS. In usual clinical practice, evidence of repeated effect over two blocks (ABAB) is often sufficient.

*, placebo; +, methylphenidate, 10 mg doses; #, methylphenidate, 5 mg doses; &, methylphenidate, 15 mg doses.

FIGURE 15–4   A Sophisticated "N of 1" Methylphenidate Trial in a 13-Year-Old Boy

range, this provides more certainty for considering the result as a positive response.

Long-Term Treatment

Once treatment response is established and the optimal dose for that response is identified, the issue of long-term use of methylphenidate arises. ADHD does not just disappear, nor do most children with ADHD "grow out of it." Thus, a significant number of children and adolescents may face long-term pharmacotherapy as part of an optimal multimodal treatment approach to this chronic disorder. As with other psychotropic agents used in the treatment of children and adolescents, scientifically valid studies regarding long-term treatment with methylphenidate are fewer than necessary. Of those studies that do exist, most suffer from significant design flaws that make their interpretation difficult. Furthermore, most long-term outcome (5 years or more) studies were not constructed in such a way as to provide information about the *optimal* long-term use of methylphenidate. Yet, recent critical reviews of this topic suggest that when the quality of the long-term study is taken into account, a demonstrable benefit of long-term methylphenidate treatment may be seen in specific domains. Thus, as in other psychiatric conditions, long-term pharmacotherapy with methylphenidate is an empirically determined process in which the risks are weighed against the benefits and periodic re-evaluations must be conducted regarding the necessity of continued methylphenidate treatment.

To this end, periodic evaluations of the continued efficacy of methylphenidate should be part of any long-term treatment strategy. The view that tolerance to the effect of methylphenidate on core ADHD symptoms, peer functioning, and family functioning develops over time, although part of clinical lore, has not been established. On the contrary, most available evidence suggests that whereas tolerance to some of the side effects (such as suppression of appetite or increased heart rate) of methylphenidate does occur, the therapeutic effects are unlikely to show a similar pattern. Clinical experience suggests that in many cases of reported "tolerance" to the therapeutic effects of methylphenidate, other explanations—usually a lack of proper compliance (either inadequate frequency or amount of dose taken)—more reasonably account for the decrease in therapeutic effect. Thus, in cases in which the clinician identifies an apparent diminution in methylphenidate's therapeutic efficacy, the first step is to carefully review the multiple aspects of child, teen, and family activities that might have an impact on compliance. Common factors negatively affecting compliance with methylphenidate treatment are as follows:

1. Inadequate child and parent education regarding the ADHD disorder and methylphenidate treatment
2. Misunderstanding of the clinician's instructions about dose amounts or dose frequency
3. Parental experimentation with dose amount or dose frequency
4. Parental fears about the possible harm to their child arising from the use of medications
5. External influences on parent or child, such as negative, unsubstantiated, and sensationalized media reports about methylphenidate or pressures from uninformed friends or family members
6. Child or adolescent opposition to taking medication
7. Teasing or other negative input from friends or peers

8. Life stresses that provoke a behavioral and emotional response that mimics some symptoms of the initial disorder

9. Behavioral side effects that arise from the use of concurrent and unreported drugs, including illicit substances and over-the-counter or health food store/natural remedy preparations

A common issue arising in long-term methylphenidate treatment is that of discontinuing the medication for specific periods of time. This practice is the so-called drug holiday. Although the use of drug holidays is popular among many clinicians, no scientifically valid research exists that suggests such a strategy is either optimal or desirable. In everyday clinical practice, drug holidays could be an opportunity to evaluate the continued efficacy or need for methylphenidate treatment, but they are not so designed. Usually, drug holidays are scheduled to occur when the child or adolescent is not attending school, often over a vacation period. The medication is discontinued over this time to decrease the child's or adolescent's exposure to the medication. Such a practice, based on no valid rationale, may actually have deleterious effects on long-term outcome if the return of previously controlled symptoms has a negative impact on a child's peer and family relationships.

The drug holiday pattern of pharmacotherapy suggests that methylphenidate treatment is basically a pharmacologic intervention targeted toward improving school functioning. Although this is one goal of methylphenidate pharmacotherapy, it must be recognized that other important aspects of a child's and adolescent's functioning are equally valid treatment targets. These include peer relationships, family relationships, aggressive behaviors, and recreational activities (such as reading, dyadic quiet games, sports, etc.). Success in these areas is essential to the development of a child's or adolescent's positive self-image and improved psychosocial functioning in both the short and long term. If methylphenidate treatment clearly improves a child's or adolescent's functioning in these other vital areas and then is withdrawn for a drug "holiday" of dubious if any medical benefit, the net effect of this procedure may well be a negative long-term outcome if psychosocial gains already made are lost or expected psychosocial development is derailed.

The relative risks and benefits of periods off methylphenidate do need to be carefully considered, and there is no reason to globally prescribe continuous treatment if good clinical reasoning suggests that a holiday may be of benefit. Such a case could be a child who exhibits significant anorexia and either weight loss or delayed weight gain with methylphenidate treatment that cannot be modified by dose manipulation strategies. This patient may benefit more from stopping the methylphenidate for a period of 4 to 6 weeks, especially over the summer, if he or she is in a situation in which the core symptoms of ADHD are less likely to interfere with usual functioning, for example, a holiday at the family cottage as opposed to a demanding camp experience. Full and open discussion of these issues with the patient and parent are necessary to allow for appropriate decision making about drug holidays to occur.

Another issue in long-term methylphenidate treatment still too often found in clinical practice is the belief that loss of therapeutic effect of methylphenidate occurs postpubertally. There is essentially no reasonable evidence for this clinical myth, and many adolescents (or adults) with ADHD show a positive therapeutic response to methylphenidate treatment. Furthermore, there is no evidence that adolescents will demonstrate significant euphoric responses to therapeutic amounts of methylphenidate or that the use of methylphenidate to treat ADHD in teenagers will in and of itself lead them to abuse this medication. Thus, the onset of puberty per se is not a reason to either discontinue successful and needed methylphenidate treatment or to not consider instituting it if indicated.

The approach to periodic re-evaluation of the continued necessity of methylphenidate treatment can take a number of courses that can be tailored to patient needs and clinician preference. In all cases the following guidelines should be applied:

1. Select a time of year in which the disruption to a child's functioning that may occur if an effective treatment is withdrawn will be minimal yet target symptoms can be properly evaluated. For example, withdrawing methylphenidate during the first month of a school year when a teacher is beginning to assess and categorize the students in a class is not a good idea. Neither is withdrawing methylphenidate during or just prior to school examinations, or when the child's family decides to take a 1 week car-touring holiday a good idea.

2. Identify the target symptoms and the duration of the medication withdrawal period.

3. Assess the target symptoms using the same instruments that were used previously during past evaluations of symptoms.

4. Use the same assessors (patient, parents, teachers) as were used in previous evaluations.

Once these evaluations have been completed, one of the following three methods of evaluating the continued efficacy-necessity for methylphenidate treatment may be used:

Method 1

1. Daily measurement of target symptoms over a reasonable period of time (1 week suggested).
2. Discontinue methylphenidate treatment (no gradual withdrawal is necessary).
3. Complete measures of target symptoms daily over a reasonable period of time (the same length of time as in point 1).
4. Begin methylphenidate treatment as previously taken prior to medication withdrawal.
5. Complete measures of target symptoms daily over a reasonable period of time (the same length of time as in point 1).
6. Review all rating scales for evidence of an on/off/on effect.

Using this method, a positive trial is suggested by a return of symptom scores to the approximate levels identified at the initial baseline (before treatment with ·methylphenidate was ever begun) when methylphenidate is withdrawn and a return in symptom scores to the approximate levels identified prior to beginning the current withdrawal paradigm (when the patient was taking methylphenidate) when methylphenidate is again added.

Although this method is somewhat limited in terms of its statistical validity and predictive power, the strength of this method is that it is simple and can provide more useful clinically relevant information than the usual clinical practice of stopping the medication to "see how it goes without it." Furthermore, although clinically useful designs that can be evaluated using statistical methods are preferred, it is important to remember that statistical and clinical validity are not necessarily congruent. For example, a study may identify a statistically significant phenomenon that may be an artifact of the study design or analysis and may not be of clinical value. Similarly, a clinically valid phenomenon may occur but not achieve statistical significance because of analytic power variables. The physician, in the final analysis must make *clinical* sense of the data.

Method 2

1. Daily measurement of target symptoms over a shorter period of time (usually daily).
2. Withdrawal of methylphenidate and reinstitution of methylphenidate using an on/off/on design that is alternated daily for 8 to 10 continuous days. This gives a measure of at least six periods (days) on medication (including baseline and endpoint) and similarly equal periods (days) off medication. Measure target symptoms daily.
3. Compare the mean results generated by the "on" periods to the mean results generated by the "off" periods.

Using this method, a positive medication effect is suggested by four features. First, the mean scores of the "on" days should be substantially and clinically different than the mean scores of the "off" days. Second, a sawtooth pattern of scores should be evident over the course of the assessment period, with "on" day scores on most days being similar to each other and usually different from "off" day scores. Third, "on" day scores should be similar to scores obtained when the patient was on medication prior to beginning the assessment protocol. Finally, the "off" day scores should be similar to those obtained at baseline (if these are available), prior to the initiation of any methylphenidate treatment.

This method may be a more powerful validator of a true clinical response to methylphenidate than method 1. Because it does not take any more time or effort than method 1, it is preferred. It does, however, take more careful involvement by the parents and patient in the entire process, because if the on days are confused with the "off" days, the entire sequence will be invalid. Thus, there may be cases in which patient or parent reliability or ability to follow through with this more complicated protocol may be so problematic that the simpler design of method 1 will be more clinically useful, even though it is less powerful than method 2.

Method 3

1. Daily measurement of target symptoms over a long period of time (3 to 4 weeks).
2. Make identical placebo-methylphenidate capsules (either the physician, a clinic nurse, or pharmacist should place methylphenidate tablets in larger capsules) or obtain placebo methylphenidate tablets.
3. Obtain a randomized number list to direct dispensing of active (methylphenidate tablet inside a capsule) and placebo (nothing inside an identical capsule) capsules.
4. Place the capsules or tablets into two different and clearly labeled (e.g., bottles A and B) bottles, with one bottle containing the active and one bottle containing the placebo preparations.
5. Give a responsible parent (or other adult) clear written instructions about which days to dispense from which bottle; for example, on days 1, 2, 5, 7, 8, 9, 13, 14, 17, and 19 dispense one capsule at 0800 hours, one capsule at 1200 hours, and one capsule at 1700 hours

from bottle A. On all other days, dispense one capsule at 0800 hours, one capsule at 1200 hours, and one capsule at 1700 hours from bottle B. Measure symptoms daily.

6. Continue the medication trial as directed by the random numbers assignment until both conditions (placebo and active) have reached a minimum of 10 conditions (days) each.

7. Collect the scores for all days and use a computer statistical program (either a t test or a Mann Whitney U test) to evaluate statistical significance between drug on and drug off conditions.

8. Make sure that the statistical significance and observed clinical effect are similar.

9. Compare the on values to scores obtained during methylphenidate treatment and the off values to scores obtained at baseline, before any methylphenidate treatment was initiated (if these are available).

This method provides the strongest validation of treatment effect because it combines a statistically sound approach with a clinically sound approach. However, it takes much longer to apply, is much more complicated—both for the clinician, who must ensure that the placebo capsules are properly made up and dispensed, and for the parent, who must follow a complicated dispensing procedure. Therefore, the use of this method creates the most risk for implementation problems, and there may be many cases in which it is just not clinically feasible. Furthermore, it is not clear that in most cases it will provide information that will be clinically more useful than that provided by other methods described earlier. The clinician may choose to use this evaluation method in cases in which method 1 or 2 provide equivocal results or in cases in which the resources are available (e.g., very dedicated and meticulous parents or a therapeutic setting such as a day treatment center) to manage the complexities of its implementation.

In any case, systematic use of one of these methods described will provide a clinically useful strategy to determine if methylphenidate treatment is still indicated over time, or if the necessary therapeutic dose needs to be adjusted. For example, one common clinical issue that arises is the need for increasing doses of methylphenidate as a child grows in order to maintain the therapeutic effect. This is not necessarily a sign of tolerance to methylphenidate but more likely is a result of needing a higher total daily dose because of increased growth. In these cases, the total daily dose will increase but the dose per kilogram will remain essentially the same. Each of the evaluation strategies described here can be easily modified to evaluate the need for a higher dose of methylphenidate as well.

As part of a multimodal treatment program for ADHD, careful assessments of methylphenidate efficacy should be conducted at regular intervals, 9 to 12 months apart. Decisions to continue, alter, or stop methylphenidate treatment can then be made in part by using the information obtained from these withdrawal trials. Dealing with ADHD children and adolescents who are treatment refractory to methylphenidate is now discussed.

Other Stimulants Useful in Treating ADHD

In addition to methylphenidate, two other stimulant medications can be used to treat the core symptoms of ADHD. Although significantly fewer studies of various effects of treatment with either dextroamphetamine or pemoline are available compared with methylphenidate, both of these compounds have been shown to effectively ameliorate the core symptoms of ADHD. They may be useful in the following cases:

1. The patient has side effects that limit methylphenidate treatment.

2. The patient or parents prefer a nonmethylphenidate stimulant treatment.

3. The patient has not shown an adequate response to methylphenidate but the use of another stimulant is reasonably indicated.

In cases in which other stimulant medications are chosen, the clinician must inform the patient and parent that these medicines are from a similar class as methylphenidate. This is necessary because patients and their parents may often not be aware of this, and they might refuse methylphenidate treatment because it is a stimulant and not simply because it is methylphenidate. Furthermore, the relative risks and benefits, including the knowledge base used to guide rational treatment of dextroamphetamine and pemoline compared with methylphenidate, should be discussed.

Dextroamphetamine in its extended-release forms has a slightly longer period of efficacy than standard methylphenidate, but it may not be quite as effective in some cases. In addition, it may cause more anorexia and weight loss than methylphenidate. Otherwise, its side effects are quite similar to those found with methylphenidate. Pemoline has a delayed onset of action, up to 3 weeks from the onset of treatment, although this can be decreased somewhat by a more aggressive dose initiation (described later). Pemoline may be associated with a higher incidence of insomnia than methylphenidate, and unlike methylphenidate and dextroamphetamine, pemoline treatment can cause hepatic damage in some cases. Thus, if treatment with pemoline is chosen, liver function tests must be obtained at baseline and at regular intervals (suggested once every 2 months) during treatment.

Dextroamphetamine

Dextroamphetamine is indicated for the treatment of children with ADHD. It is also used in the treatment of narcolepsy. Commercially available preparations of dextroamphetamine (both Spansules and tablets) contain tartrazine, which may cause allergic reactions in some individuals. Although the plasma half-life of the longer acting form is about 10 hours, individual variations in the duration of therapeutic effect can be quite pronounced.

Dosing of dextroamphetamine is generally half that of methylphenidate. Thus if 5 mg of methylphenidate would be used, 2.5 mg of dextroamphetamine should be used. A reasonable target daily dose range for initiating treatment is 10 to 30 mg, given in three divided doses. General guidelines for initiating and optimizing pharmacotherapy are found in Section Three.

Treatment can be initiated using 5 mg of dexedrine or dextroamphetamine sulphate tablets (in younger children, a dose of 2.5 mg should be used), given in divided doses twice or three times daily. Doses may be increased by 5 mg increments (2.5 mg in younger children) every 3 to 5 days until a total daily dose of 30 mg (15 mg in younger children) is reached. The dose can then be stabilized at this level for a week and its effects evaluated using the methodology described earlier for methylphenidate. Once an initial response has been established, the dose can be increased or decreased by 5 mg increments (2.5 mg in younger children) to determine if additional improvements are possible at higher doses or if similar improvements are sustainable at lower doses.

Once an effective total daily dose of dexedrine is established (Table 15–5), the longer-acting dextroamphetamine (as a resin complex) or the extended-release preparation of dextroamphetamine sulfate (also known as Spansules) can be used. Side effects and dosing management techniques are similar to those described for methylphenidate.

Long-term treatment studies using dextroamphetamine are not available, and a decision to use dextroamphetamine or dextroamphetamine sulfate must weigh the expected risks against the benefits. If this medication is used in long-term treatment, regular evaluations of its continued therapeutic utility need to be carried out, usually in 9 to 12 month periods. This is best realized by gradual withdrawal of the medication using standardized symptom rating scales to measure the effect of this procedure on the core symptoms of

TABLE 15–5 Suggested Initial Target Daily Dose Ranges with Dextroamphetamine Treatment for ADHD in Children*

Usual Target Daily Dose Range (mg/kg/day)	Usual Target Daily Dose Range (mg/day)
0.15–1.0, in two or three divided doses	10–30, in divided doses

*These target dose ranges are suggested on the basis of clinical experience and the currently available literature regarding the use of dextroamphetamine in children with ADHD. Individual patient responses (therapeutic and adverse) may vary. These dose suggestions are guidelines only; actual doses must be tailored to the patient's clinical response. The therapeutically maximized daily dose may be higher or lower than the initial daily dose target. See Section Three for general principles regarding dose initiation and response maximization strategies.

ADHD. This process is described under method 1 of the earlier section on methods of medication withdrawal evaluation. The optimal length of time for dextroamphetamine treatment has not been established, and studies of its use in the adolescent population are insufficient to provide adequate guidelines for this population.

Pemoline

Pemoline is an oxazolidinone derivative stimulant that produces a similar pharmacologic effect as seen with methylphenidate. It is well absorbed orally and peak plasma concentrations occur at 2 to 6 hours. Pemoline has a plasma half-life of up to 13 hours. Children may show an increased elimination half-life following multiple dosing. Once-a-day dosing is thus usually sufficient. Plasma levels have not been correlated with therapeutic effect, and a marked individual variation in response to specific doses is known to occur. Unlike methylphenidate and dextroamphetamine, the therapeutic response to pemoline may take up to 3 weeks to manifest.

In addition to the side effects found with methylphenidate, pemoline use is reported to be associated with the following: increased incidence of insomnia, hepatic damage (usually a hypersensitivity reaction, although deaths related to hepatic damage with pemoline use have been reported), seizures, and dyskinetic movements. Pemoline treatment is usually started with a dose of 18.75 mg given once daily in the morning and increased by 18.75 mg weekly until a total single daily dose of 75 mg is reached (Table 15–6). Using this initiation scale, the therapeutic effect of pemoline usu-

TABLE 15–6 **Suggested Initial Pemoline Target Daily Dose Ranges in Treating Children and Adolescents with ADHD***

Target Daily Dose (mg/kg/day)	Usual Target Daily Dose (mg/day)
0.6–4.0, in once-daily dose	37.5–112.5 (or higher), in once-daily dose

*These target dose ranges are suggested on the basis of clinical experience and the currently available literature regarding the use of pemoline in children and adolescents with ADHD. Individual patient responses (therapeutic and adverse) may vary. These dose suggestions are guidelines only; actual doses must be tailored to the patient's clinical response. The therapeutically maximized daily dose may be higher or lower than the initial daily dose target. See Section Three for general principles of dose initiation and response maximization strategies. Pemoline use may be associated with hepatic damage so liver function testing is necessary.

ally does not become evident until 3 to 4 weeks of treatment, although side effects can of course be manifested earlier. Reasonable clinical practice suggests that during this dose escalation phase, weekly monitoring of side effects and bimonthly monitoring of the potential therapeutic effect using standardized instruments are sufficient.

More recently, some authors have advocated a jump-start approach to pemoline treatment. This strategy initiates treatment with a dose of 18.75 mg given in one daily morning dose, increased by 18.75 mg every 3 to 4 days to a dose of 75 mg given once daily in the morning. Apparently not associated with an increased frequency of side effects, this more aggressive dosing technique is reported to be associated with a somewhat earlier onset of action, 2 to 3 weeks. If this dosing strategy is used, side effects evaluation should take place more frequently (every 3 to 4 days), and therapeutic assessment should occur weekly.

Long-term studies of pemoline treatment are not available, and the decision to use pemoline in the long term must weigh the potential risks against the benefits of this approach. If this medication is to be used over a prolonged period of time, regular evaluations of its continued therapeutic utility need to be conducted. These should occur at every 9 to 12 months and are best conducted following method 1 described earlier in the section on medication withdrawal methods for methylphenidate. Unlike methylphenidate, pemoline withdrawal should be more gradual, with a drug discontinuation schedule of 18.75 mg every 3 to 5 days. The drug-free period should continue for a minimum of 3 weeks, with ratings conducted on a weekly basis. Pemoline therapy should then be restarted and sufficient time al-

lowed (4 weeks) before completing standardized evaluations. Use of this method should allow for an adequate clinical assessment of the continued value of pemoline therapy as follows:

1. Obtain a prewithdrawal evaluation of all target symptoms and side effects.
2. Gradually withdraw pemoline (18.75 mg every 4 to 5 days).
3. Repeat evaluation of target symptoms and side effects weekly beginning 1 week after withdrawal is complete and continuing for 4 weeks.
4. Reintroduce pemoline using the jump-start technique described earlier, using the prewithdrawal level as the target for the total daily dose.
5. Repeat evaluation of target symptoms and side effects weekly beginning 1 week after the initial pemoline dose has been reached and continue weekly measures for 4 weeks.
6. Compare the weekly mean scores from the medication-free phase with the scores obtained from the pre- and postmedication withdrawal ratings.

Using this strategy, a positive effect of pemoline is suggested if a clinically meaningful increase in target symptoms occurs during the medication-free phase compared with the prewithdrawal phase and if these symptoms show clinically meaningful improvement when the medication is again restarted.

Specific Issues Regarding the Clinical Use of Stimulant Medications

A number of issues commonly arise that physicians may encounter regarding the clinical use of stimulants. These include potential for abuse, drug-drug interactions, rare side effects, tics and stimulants, other (non-ADHD) possibilities for stimulant use, and medical emergency—overdose.

Potential for Abuse

Stimulant drugs (particularly amphetamine, which is not indicated for ADHD treatment) may have abuse potential in some individuals. Euphoric effects of dextroamphetamine, methylphenidate, and pemoline can be seen. The strength of the effect is relatively mild and is found more commonly with dextroamphetamine, less so with methylphenidate, and little if at all with pemoline. However, although much has been made of the abuse potential of the stimulants used in the treatment of ADHD, there is no compelling evidence that when prescribed properly, stimulants become drugs of abuse or increase the propensity of children or adolescents to abuse other drugs. Stimulant abuse can occur but is usually found in the context of adolescent multiple drug abuse or in long-term intravenous drug users, particularly when usual street supplies of heroin and cocaine dry up. These chronic drug abusers tend to attempt and solubilize stimulant preparations for intravenous use, resulting in talc granulomatosis and other severe medical problems.

Methylphenidate, pemoline, and dextroamphetamine treatment of children and adolescents with ADHD will in and of itself not create future drug abusers. Some clinicians have indeed argued the exact opposite, that successful treatment of childhood ADHD with stimulants may decrease later substance abuse in this population. However, prudent clinical practice suggests that in the child or adolescent who is a known drug abuser, if medication treatment for ADHD is deemed necessary, the use of nonstimulant compounds such as desipramine should be considered.

Drug-Drug Interactions

Drug interactions are relatively uncommon with the stimulants and thus quite easy to remember. Although some differences in drug-drug interaction among the stimulants do occur (see later), as a class they should not be prescribed concurrently with MAOIs and narcotics. Both methylphenidate and dextroamphetamine can decrease the hypotensive effects of guanethidine, although this is unlikely to be a major issue with most children. These and other common potential drug-drug interactions are listed in Table 15–7.

Rare Side Effects with Stimulant Use

Common side effects of stimulant use have already been identified. Given the high frequency of

TABLE 15–7 **Drug-Drug Interactions with Stimulants***

Methylphenidate and Dextroamphetamine	
MAOIs	Guanethidine
Phenobarbital	Tricyclic antidepressants
Phenytoin	Primidone
Methylphenidate	Dextroamphetamine
Sympathomimetics	Beta-blockers
Theophylline	
Warfarin	
Phenylbutazone	
Fluoxetine	

*Potential drug-drug reactions with pemoline have not been well studied.

their use, the clinician should also be aware of rare events. These include depression, leukocytosis, alopecia, hypersensitivity reactions, and psychosis (both mood and nonmood types), the latter being dose dependent and usually only seen with high doses. Although lowering of the seizure threshold can be accomplished by toxic doses of stimulants, there is no evidence that stimulants actually produce a clinically significant lowered seizure threshold at the usual therapeutic ranges. On the contrary, with careful monitoring of anticonvulsant levels, they can be safely combined to treat children and adolescents with comorbid ADHD and seizure disorders.

Tics and Tourette's Syndrome

As discussed under methylphenidate treatment, stimulant medications have been described as inducing or exacerbating tics. There is insufficient evidence, however, that their use is of pathoetiologic significance in Tourette's syndrome. Furthermore, the concept of stimulant medications unmasking a tic disorder is a tautology, adding little to our understanding of the complex relationship between stimulant use and tics.

Many children and adolescents exhibit transient minor motor tics of many varieties. These by themselves should not contraindicate the use of stimulant medications. Of prime importance is the careful clinical examination for and documentation of tics prior to the implementation of stimulant treatment. If minor simple tics appear for the first time or previously present simple tics are mildly exacerbated with successful stimulant treatment, a reasonable clinical strategy is to continue the medication and carefully monitor the frequency and severity of the tics. If complex tics occur, simple tics become severe, or vocal tics develop, prudent clinical care suggests that stimulant treatment be discontinued and alternatives, such as clonidine, bupropion, or desipramine, be used instead.

Patients with Tourette's syndrome and ADHD have often not been considered to be candidates for stimulant treatment. More recent opinion however, suggests that in those children or adolescents with Tourette's syndrome in whom ADHD symptoms contribute in a significant way to the patient's morbidity, their use should be considered. Many children and adolescents will not experience an increase in tic severity or frequency when treated with stimulants. Those who do will usually see these increases remit on discontinuation of the stimulant. Thus, it is not unreasonable to treat with stimulants while carefully monitoring the frequency and severity of tics. In cases in which stimulant treatment is found to exacerbate tics, alternatives, such as clonidine bupropion, desipramine, or other medications (see later), can be used.

An alternative approach is also reasonable. The clinician, in discussion with the patient and family, may elect to initiate treatment with a nonstimulant medication in a child or adolescent with ADHD. In this case, the choice of compound should follow the suggestions discussed later.

Other Potential Psychiatric Indications for Stimulant Treatment

In addition to the treatment of ADHD, stimulants have been reported to be helpful in treating a variety of conditions, most often for ameliorating symptoms of impulsivity, motor restlessness, aggressivity, and attention difficulties. Information about stimulant use to treat the disorders in which these symptoms are manifest is minimal and often unreplicated. The following list identifies the potential use of stimulants in treating other psychiatric disorders, where they may be considered for a therapeutic trial as part of a comprehensive treatment plan. Their use in these disorders should proceed as in all pharmacologic trials, using clear assessment techniques following from a careful evaluation of potential risks and benefits and with the appropriate decision-making procedures and informed consent:

Narcolepsy*
Pervasive development disorders
Mental retardation
Fragile X syndrome
Preschool-aged children (under 6 years of age) with ADHD symptoms

Medical Emergencies with Stimulant Use

Stimulants are often used for the treatment of young children, a population that may be at increased risk for accidental poisoning. Education about the need to take preventive measures as well as the proper storage of medications is imperative. Inadvertent overdoses, however, can and do occur. Symptoms of stimulant overdose are those arising from autonomic hyperactivity. These include elevated blood pressure, seizures, tachycardia, organic brain syndrome, hyperthermia, and psychosis.

Children or adolescents who overdose on stimulants should be admitted to the hospital for monitoring and treatment. Chlorpromazine, orally as the liquid or intramuscularly, may be used to treat the psychotic symptoms. It has the added effect of decreasing elevated blood pressure as well. Cooling and the use of antipyretics are indicated for the fever, and seizures are usually self-limiting but

*The use of methylphenidate has been well established in narcolepsy.

will respond to intravenous diazepam if they are prolonged.

Nonstimulant Treatments for ADHD

Although stimulants are generally considered to be first-line pharmacologic interventions for children and adolescents with ADHD, not all patients will tolerate or respond to adequate trials of a stimulant medication. Although the exact number of true stimulant nonresponders is unclear, recent estimates put this at about 20 to 25 percent of ADHD patients. Thus, a substantial number of children and adolescents may be expected to require pharmacotherapeutic alternatives to stimulants.

At this time it is not clearly possible to predict on an individual basis which child or adolescent will or will not respond adequately to stimulant treatment. A number of clinical features have been identified that may be associated with a greater likelihood of stimulant nonresponse. These can be best classified under the categories of treatment history and clinical psychiatric presentation.

Factors of Potential Use in Identifying Stimulant Nonresponse in ADHD

Treatment History

1. The patient has demonstrated treatment resistance to stimulant pharmacotherapy.
2. Side effects experienced with stimulants are intolerable and either affect compliance at a dose in which significant clinical improvement has occurred or else limit the application of an adequate treatment trial.

Clinical Psychiatric Presentation

A comorbid anxiety disorder may result in stimulant nonresponse. In addition, there may be instances in which the clinician believes that initiating treatment with stimulant medications may not be in the patient's overall best interests. Such factors may include one or more of the following:

1. Psychosocial issues—an unstable environment in which the proper drug administration or medication monitoring does not take place or in which the risk potential for abuse of stimulants by the patient, family members, or others is high
2. Unstable or brittle psychosis
3. Significant medical difficulties, such as delayed growth or mental retardation (IQ $\leq$ 45)

In deciding whether to use nonstimulant medications in the treatment of ADHD, the clinician must clearly identify if he or she is choosing a nonstimulant medication as a first choice or because a previous trial of a stimulant medication has resulted in true treatment resistance or intolerable adverse effects. This is a crucial difference. The choice of a nonstimulant medication in the first-choice strategy may be reasonable for a particular case if the method for determining among various potential medications outlined in Section Three is followed. If that is the case, then it is reasonable for the physician, on the basis of best clinical judgment, to choose a nonstimulant medication as a first-line treatment for a child or adolescent with ADHD.

Alternatively, the patient or parent may have strong opinions about the use of stimulants and will not agree to stimulant treatment, regardless of clinical advice to the contrary. Sometimes, however, patients and parents who oppose stimulant treatment will agree to nonstimulant treatment over no pharmacologic treatment at all. This scenario is not all that uncommon and should be identified and resolved as part of the collaborative model of treatment planning discussed in Section Three. Given the available and rapidly increasing evidence on the efficacy of a variety of nonstimulant medications in treating child and adolescent ADHD, it is not unreasonable for a clinician to agree to use one or more of these compounds should this be the outcome of discussions with the patient and parents.

If a previous trial of stimulant medication has failed (despite attempts at optimization) or if adverse effects were of a frequency or severity that might limit the use of a stimulant medication, then the physician should consider the use of nonstimulants in the context of a patient who is treatment refractory to stimulants. The general issues regarding this determination and how to address this pharmacotherapeutically are outlined in Section Three. Following from this, the clinician can use nonstimulant medications as either (1) substitution therapy, to replace one medication with another, or (2) augmentation therapy, to add another medication while continuing with the first compound. Thinking about the issue of nonstimulant treatment for ADHD in this manner will help clarify the often confusing suggestions for treatment found in the current literature and will assist the physician in clinical problem solving.

The nonstimulant pharmacologic treatments for ADHD that are available can be classified as follows: antidepressants, alpha-adrenergic agents, and neuroleptics. All have their risks and benefits. None have been optimally investigated in this disorder, although a number of research reports and case studies are available in the psychiatric literature regarding their use in ADHD. Table 15–8 lists some potential nonstimulant medications for treating ADHD and provides the author's impressions regarding their use.

TABLE 15–8   Nonstimulant Pharmacologic Treatments to Consider for Use in Treating Children or Adolescents with ADHD*

Class	Medication	Impressions
Antidepressant	Amitriptyline	Many anticholinergic side effects, sedation a problem, not recommended because of potential side effects
	Imipramine	Many side effects, tolerance to therapeutic effects reported
	Nortriptyline	Reasonably tolerated, no evidence for increased efficacy in ADHD comorbid with depression
	Desipramine	Reasonably tolerated, caution because of potential cardiotoxicity, may be useful in adolescents
	Bupropion	Reasonably tolerated, potential to induce seizures at high doses, may exacerbate tics, may be useful in patients with comorbid anxiety, not for patients with bulimia
	Fluoxetine	Reasonably tolerated, must begin treatment with low doses
	Moclobemide	Monoamine oxidase A inhibitor, reasonably tolerated, minimal data, other MAOIs not recommended.
	Venlafaxine	Serotonin norepinephrine reuptake inhibitor, early studies appear promising
Alpha-adrenergic agents	Clonidine	Cardiovascular side effects, may be more useful in "hyperaroused" cases, slow clinical improvement—1 month or more—means patience needed, may be useful in patients with tics
	Guanfacine	Investigational, use not recommended
Neuroleptics	Thioridazine or Haloperidol or Risperidone	Low doses of these neuroleptics show potential efficacy, side effects and concerns about tardive dyskinesia limit use, may be of value in patients with low IQ or in comorbid conduct disorder, careful monitoring for dyskinesia necessary
Other	Buspirone	Some evidence for efficacy, generally well tolerated

*If using these compounds, remember that symptom response may not be immediate. Four to 8 weeks may be necessary for determining the response to many of these agents.

If one of the medications mentioned in Table 15–9 is used for the treatment of ADHD, the same baseline and evaluative procedures should be followed as explained elsewhere in this book for compounds of their class. Generally, doses needed for ADHD symptom improvement are lower than those used in treating other disorders in which these compounds are indicated (i.e., depression or psychosis). This is particularly true if antidepressants or antipsychotics are being used because higher doses are unlikely to produce significantly more benefit and will be associated with increased frequency and severity of side effects. Suggested initial target dose ranges for antidepressants and neuroleptics in treating ADHD are found in Table 15–9).

Combining Pharmacologic Treatments for ADHD

Medications useful in treating ADHD may be combined in two different cases: (1) when ADHD is co-morbid with another psychiatric disorder and (2) when the treatment response to monotherapy is suboptimal (full or partially treatment refractory).

CASE EXAMPLE

ADHD and Bipolar: What a Combination

R.L. was an 18-year-old boy with a long history of ADHD and learning problems for which he had never received pharmacologic treatment. He experienced a major depression in early adolescence, and his first manic psychosis occurred at age 17. He responded to pharmacologic treatment and was maintained, with good symptom control, on carbamazepine. His ADHD symptoms, however, did not improve, and he remained quite functionally impaired by them. Desipramine at a total daily dose of 100 mg was found to improve his concentration and to decrease impulsivity, with noted functional improvements in vocational and social pursuits. When the desipramine dose was decreased to 75 mg daily, his ADHD symptoms worsened significantly but again lessened at a total daily dose of 100 mg. R.L. still continues on this successful pharmacologic combination.

CASE COMMENTARY

In this case, a good outcome was obtained for a difficult pharmacologic management case. Prescription of a stimulant medication may or may not have resulted in an exacerbation of psychosis or "flipping of mood." An antidepressant medication may also have precipitated a mood switch. In such a case the clinician will need to consider the relative risks and benefits of each potential pharmacologic intervention and choose that which seems most reasonable. Unfortunately, there are no clear scientifically derived guidelines available to help the clinician in weighing the relative risks and benefits. Thus, careful monitoring of the patient's clinical status is necessary when using such combinations.

Totally or Partially Refractory to Stimulant Treatment

CASE EXAMPLE

"Well, it helps a lot but not quite enough. If I raise the dose, he gets nausea."

K.I. was a 10-year-old boy with ADHD and comorbid dysthymia who was initially treated with

TABLE 15–9 Suggested Dose Ranges for Antidepressants and Neuroleptics in Treating Children and Adolescents with ADHD*

Medications	Initial Target Dose Range	Suggested Starting Dose
Antidepressants		
Imipramine	50–150 mg/day	Child, 10 mg
		Teen, 25 mg
Desipramine	50–150 mg/day	Child, 10 mg
		Teen, 25 mg
Nortriptyline[†]	50–150 mg/day	Child, 10 mg
		Teen, 25 mg
Fluoxetine	5–20 mg/day	Child, 5 mg
		Teen, 5 mg
Bupropion	50–150 mg/day	Child, 50 mg
		Teen, 50 mg
Neuroleptics		
Thioridazine	50–100 mg/day	Child, 10 mg
		Teen, 25 mg
Haloperidol	0.5–2 mg	Child, 0.5 mg
		Teen, 1.0 mg
Risperidone	0.5–1.0 mg	Child, 0.5 mg
		Teen, 0.5 mg
Other		
Buspione	20–60 mg/day	Child, 5 mg bid
		Teen, 10 mg bid

*The compounds selected for this table are those that in the opinion of the author show the best risk/benefit ratio for nonstimulant ADHD treatment. Other options are available. Medication doses are given as guidelines only; some patients may need higher or lower doses, as the clinical picture indicates. The use of clonidine is described in Chapter 16. Neuroleptic use must be clearly clinically indicated.

†There is some evidence that there is a possible therapeutic window for the efficacy of nortriptyline in ADHD. This has been reported as serum levels of 50–150 mg/mL. If this medication is used, monitoring of serum levels is reasonable.

methylphenidate. At a total daily dose of 30 mg, he showed an improvement in symptoms of 40 percent from baseline. His mood, however, remained low, and when attempts were made to increase his methylphenidate he developed nausea and "crying jags." His mother had been successfully treated for a depressive disorder with fluoxetine, and at the time of K.I.'s treatment review it was decided to attempt an augmentation strategy instead of trying another stimulant medication. Accordingly, fluoxetine was added at a starting dose of 5 mg daily. It was maintained at this level for 8 weeks. At this time, reassessment showed an additional improvement in the ADHD symptoms and a mild brightening of mood. The fluoxetine was increased to 10 mg for another 8 weeks, with no increased effect on ADHD symptoms but with a good effect on the low mood. The next pharmacologic issue that arose was the mother's question, "Does he need to be on two medicines at the same time?"

CASE COMMENTARY

The issue raised earlier is what is the best strategy to pursue if the child or adolescent is not showing an adequate response to initial stimulant treatment. Three potential strategies are available: optimization, substitution, or augmentation. If optimization has failed (as in this case), general clinical lore suggests the use of a substitution strategy, and this entails a change to another medication, often another stimulant. However, in some cases (such as described here) an augmentation strategy may be preferred. The general issues regarding this common clinical problem are discussed in Section Three.

When a successful augmentation strategy is used, the clinician often cannot be certain if the observed therapeutic effect was caused by the combination treatment or if it would have occurred with substitution alone. In this case it may be reasonable to consider discontinuing the first medication at some later point to help differentiate this issue. Appropriate symptom monitoring should accompany this procedure.

In an augmentation strategy, the same baseline and monitoring procedures as apply to the monopharmacologic use of the augmenting agent apply during the augmentation as well. Thus, if the clinician chooses to use fluoxetine, as in this case, the baseline medical procedures are carried out and the expected duration of treatment parameters are followed. Evaluation of treatment effect is then similarly carried out.

Although there is only a rudimentary litera-ture concerning augmentation strategies in children and adolescents with ADHD, clinical experience suggests that a substantial number of these patients may be helped with augmentation approaches. At this time, however, clear and scientifically valid guidelines for choosing substitution over augmentation strategies are not available.

Adult ADHD Treatment

Although the treatment of adults with ADHD is not usual in the routine therapeutic practice of the child or adolescent psychiatrist, colleagues in adult psychiatry often ask for second opinions regarding the use of stimulant treatment in adults with a presumptive diagnosis of ADHD. If such a case is assessed, great care must be taken in determining the diagnosis of ADHD from retrospective information about childhood histories provided by adult patients who may be coincidentally comorbid with a variety of psychiatric conditions (particularly antisocial personality disorder or substance abuse). Whenever possible, corroborative information should be sought. Furthermore, the available evidence for the efficacy of stimulant treatment in adult ADHD is at this time inconclusive, with wide efficacy outcomes reported (23 to 75 percent).

An especially difficult group to sort out are adults with concurrent drug abuse who present with some of the core symptoms of ADHD. Because many of these symptoms can directly result from drug abuse alone, prudent clinical practice would be to avoid pharmacologic treatment of this population until it is clear that the patient is no longer using drugs and sufficient time has passed to allow for a clear evaluation of a symptom baseline that is relatively free from residual drug abuse effects (6 months is suggested). When pharmacologic treatment is believed to be indicated, the use of nonstimulant medications, such as venlafaxine, fluoxetine, or desipramine, should be considered first.

If stimulant treatment of adults is being contemplated, it is essential that the following conditions be met:

1. No substance abuse currently or within the last 6 months
2. Clear history of child-onset ADHD, with child functional impairment arising from the disorder
3. Patient meets current criteria for ADHD

Whenever possible, the following should be obtained:

1. Corroborative history from a parent or sibling of childhood ADHD
2. Copy of the child and adolescent school record

In all cases, if stimulant treatment is selected, it should incorporate the following:

1. As part of the baseline psychiatric assessment, a complete drug and alcohol history
2. As part of the baseline laboratory assessment, a drug and alcohol screen, including serum and urine, liver function tests, and CBC
3. A placebo-controlled evaluation of therapeutic efficacy
4. The input of responsible adults in the rating of symptom response during the placebo trial

Given the recent evidence for the efficacy of desipramine in treating adult ADHD, the prudent clinician may make this medication their first-line choice with this population.

SUGGESTED READINGS

Barkley R. Attention Deficit Hyperactivity Disorder: A Handbook for Diagnosis and Treatment. New York: Guilford Press, 1990.

Green WH. Child and Adolescent Clinical Psychopharmacology. Baltimore: Williams & Wilkins, 1995.

Green WH. The treatment of attention-deficit hyperactivity disorder with non-stimulant medications. Child and Adolescent Psychiatric Clinics of North America, 4:169–195, 1995.

Greenhill LL. Attention-deficit hyperactivity disorder: The stimulants. Child and Adolescent Psychiatric Clinics of North America, 4:123–168, 1995.

Hallowell EM, Ratey JJ. Driven to Distraction. New York: Simon & Schuster, 1994.

Hunt RD, Capper L, O'Connell P. Clonidine in child and adolescent psychiatry. Journal of Child and Adolescent Psychopharmacology, 1:87–102, 1990.

Osman B, Greenhill LL (eds). Ritalin: Theory and Patient Management. New York: Mary Ann Liebert, 1991.

Patrick KS, Mueller RA, Gualtier CT, Breese GR. Pharmacokinetics and actions of methyphenidate. In Meltzer HY (ed): Psychopharmacology: The Third Generation of Progress. New York: Raven Press, 1987, pp. 1387–1395.

Rapport MD, Denney C, DuPaul GJ, Gardner MJ. Atention deficit disorder and methylphenidate: Normalization rates, clinical effectiveness and response prediction in 76 children. Journal of the American Academy of Child and Adolescent Psychiatry, 33:882–893, 1994.

Safer DJ, Krager JM. A survey of medication treatment for hyperactive/inattentive students. JAMA, 260:2256–2258, 1988.

Sallee F, Stiller R, Perel JM. Pharmacodynamics of pemoline in attention deficit disorder with hyperactivity. Journal of the American Academy of Child and Adlescent Psychiatry, 31:244–251, 1992.

Wender P. The Hyperactive Child, Adolescent and Adult. New York: Oxford University Press, 1987.

CHAPTER 16

Psychopharmacologic Treatment of Autism and Mental Retardation

The pharmacologic treatment of autism and mental retardation is discussed together in this chapter. The two often coexist and may manifest similar associated symptoms. Self-injurious behavior (SIB), for example, is common in both conditions and is often a treatment target regardless of the specific diagnosis. They are not the same, however, and their pharmacologic treatment is not identical. Nevertheless, it is reasonable to approach the pharmacologic treatment of these disorders from both categorical and dimensional perspectives, that is, to consider pharmacologic interventions based on (1) the ability to globally improve the core symptoms of a specific disorder (more important for autism, in which a syndrome comprised of these core symptoms is clearly identifiable) and (2) the ability to improve associated symptoms that are not necessarily part of the defining characteristics of any one disorder (important for both autism and mental retardation).

Thus, pharmacologic treatments directed at the core symptoms of each disorder are outlined as well as particular pharmacologic interventions directed at target symptoms of behavior and cognition that often coexist with but are not defining characteristics of each disorder. In neither autism nor mental retardation should any pharmacotherapy be prescribed outside of a comprehensive psychosocial treatment program that includes behavioral interventions for symptoms (such as self-injury) often targeted for pharmacologic treatment.

Medications that are commonly used in these disorders include high-potency neuroleptics, methylphenidate, lithium, carbamazepine, opiate antagonists, clomipramine, clonidine, propranolol, and the serotonin-specific reuptake inhibitors (SSRIs) (Table 16–1). Low-potency neuroleptics should be avoided because of their sedative side effects, and although a number of other drugs have been suggested, evidence for their efficacy and tolerability is lacking. Thus, in this chapter the use of the following will be described: haloperidol (a high-potency neuroleptic), fluvoxamine (an SSRI), carbamazepine, propranolol, and naltrexone. Lithium use is described in Chapter 12, other SSRIs in Chapter 11, and clonidine in Chapter 17.

Although the potential medication treatments for autism and mental retardation overlap considerably and are so presented in Table 16–1, they are not identical and need to be approached differently.

As suggested by Table 16–1, no one medication or group of medications has clearly demonstrated superiority in treatment of these disorders. Thus, in most cases treatment will proceed on the basis of careful identification of target symptoms, careful selection of the medication that might be most

TABLE 16–1 Medications Commonly Considered in the Treatment of Children and Adolescents with Autism*

Haloperidol[†]	Propranolol[†]	Imipramine
Clomipramine	Clonidine	Lithium[†]
Fluvoxamine	Naltrexone[†]	Fenfluramine
Methylphenidate[†]	Buspirone	Sedating agents
Carbamazepine[†]	Valproate	
Pimozide	Trifluoperazine[†]	

*Suggestions regarding these medications are made from clinical experience and currently available literature regarding the pharmacologic treatment of autism in children and adolescents.
[†]May be suitable for specific indications in children or adolescents with mental retardation.

helpful for the specific child (risks and benefits determination), optimization of pharmacologic effect, and careful monitoring. The general principles that underlie this process are found in Sections Two and Three.

Autism

Autism is perhaps best understood as a complex neuropsychiatric syndrome of early developmental onset. It is characterized by profound and chronic disturbances in social interaction, severe problems with language, the presence of perseverative and compulsive-like behaviors, an intense need for environmental "sameness," and a markedly restricted range of functional activities. Associated phenomena commonly found with this disorder include mental retardation, aggressive behaviors directed toward other people and inanimate objects, and self-injury. Although its pathoetiology is unknown, recent studies have identified abnormalities in central nervous system (CNS) neurochemistry, specifically within the serotonin, dopamine, and opiate neurotransmitter networks. Medications that have been shown to have positive effects in ameliorating some of the core symptoms of the disorder are those that are known to effect CNS changes in these same neurotransmitter systems. In current diagnostic classification (DSM-IV and ICD-10), autism is included among the various pervasive developmental disorders in Table 16–2.

Psychopharmacologic studies that have evaluated one or more of the compounds identified in Table 16–1 across most of the diagnostic categories within the class of pervasive developmental disorders (whichever diagnostic system is used) are not available. Clinical experience, however, suggests that, except for Rett's disorder (Rett's syndrome), the information obtained from pharmacologic studies in autistic children and adolescents can be applied generally to other pervasive developmental disorders as well. Higher functioning individuals who may meet criteria for Asperger's syndrome may also be an exception and will require a careful evaluation of appropriate target symptoms for pharmacologic treatment. Keep in mind that there may be unknown differences in pharmacokinetics or pharmacodynamic responses to specific medications across different diagnostic categories. The following discussion is based on what is currently known.

As with other mental illnesses, there is no known "cure," pharmacologic or otherwise, for autism. Psychotropic agents, however, can be a useful part of an overall treatment plan, which includes psychosocial, behavioral, and language interventions. As such, in treating autism medications may be used to

1. Decrease the severity of many of the core symptoms of the disorder
2. Help control harmful or dangerous associated behaviors (such as self-injury)
3. Improve the patient's accessibility to psychosocial and language interventions
4. Improve the overall quality of life for the patient and his or her caregivers

CASE EXAMPLE

"She is just different."

F.S. was a 6-year-old girl who was referred for an inpatient psychiatric assessment because of "delays in development." She had received a number of previous psychiatric and psychological outpatient assessments, none of which had been completed because of parental decisions to withdraw F.S. from every assessment attempt. Finally, authorities from the therapeutic school program that she was attending demanded a full inpatient review of her case as a prerequisite to her continuing in the program. Because no other program would consider her application for admission, her parents reluctantly agreed to the school's demands.

Initial diagnostic consultation revealed a severely disturbed young girl who exhibited minimal interaction with the interviewer and spent most of her time playing with colored strings brought by her mother. F.S. demonstrated no understandable verbal language, and receptive language was very limited. The psychiatric his-

---

TABLE 16–2 Diagnostic Classification of Pervasive Developmental Disorders

DSM-IV Pervasive Developmental Disorders	ICD-10 Pervasive Developmental Disorders
Autistic disorder	Childhood autism
Retts's disorder	Atypical autism
Childhood disintegrative disorder	Rett's syndrome
Asperger's disorder	Other childhood disintegrative disorders
Pervasive development disorder NOS	Overactive disorder associated with mental retardation and stereotyped movements
	Asperger's syndrome
	Other pervasive developmental disorders
	Pervasive developmental disorder unspecified

tory revealed that these severe social, behavioral, and language difficulties had been present for many years, and although her mother tended to deny their severity, ancillary reports from the child's pediatrician and the early-age day care program identified that F.S. had never been able to function in an age-appropriate manner. When a preliminary diagnosis of autism was raised, F.S.'s mother became extremely distraught and withdrew F.S. from the hospital. As it turned out, when other reports were made available, this diagnosis had first been made at least 3 years previously and subsequently had been raised a number of times as well. Every time this had occurred, the parents had refused further evaluation or assistance.

Five months later, F.S.'s mother returned and requested readmission. In the interim, she had been to see a number of orthomolecular practitioners who had refused a psychiatric label but had instead suggested F.S. might have a "learning problem" and provided dietary manipulation, including megadoses of various vitamins and folic acid. Unfortunately, F.S.'s condition had not changed, and indeed she had developed a number of aggressive behaviors, including hitting and screaming, repetitive banging of her head to the point of bruising, and throwing her food. Furthermore, the school had discharged her, stating that they could not work with the family. In addition, F.S.'s mother could not obtain any consistent child care because no single caregiver could control the child's behavior. This led to a family crisis because the mother was faced with the prospect of losing her job, and the father, who was often out of town on business, could not take over his daughter's daily care.

F.S. was readmitted for a full diagnostic evaluation, which resulted in a diagnosis of pervasive developmental disorder—autism. Extensive educational and therapeutic work was conducted with the family, and a full psychosocial intervention program was instituted.

After 2 months, however, a variety of milieu interventions and behavioral techniques had not provided improvement in core symptoms or adequate control of the aggressive and disruptive behaviors. F.S.'s difficulties continued to place great stress on her parents, and they often found that they could not provide the consistent structure she needed during the times that she spent at home with them (usually weekends). After some time of resisting suggested pharmacologic intervention, F.S.'s parents finally agreed to a trial of low-dose haloperidol.

CASE COMMENTARY

This case illustrates a number of important features in the pharmacologic treatment of autism. In some cases the parents have resisted the diagnosis and thus potentially effective interventions have been delayed. In other cases, ineffective or inappropriate treatments may have been used, including megadoses of various vitamins and minerals, which may actually cause harm if not properly taken. Vitamin B_6 may in some cases be prescribed for the child by an "alternative healer" or even a shop owner. Although there may be some anecdotal evidence that this treatment might benefit selected children, its indiscriminant and unmonitored use can lead to peripheral neuropathy.

The therapeutic and educational aspects of care for the child's family and psychosocial-behavioral-language treatments are essential. Psychopharmacologic interventions are only part of a comprehensive treatment program. Medication use may often be resisted by family members who have concerns about side effects or who feel that drugs will cause more harm than good. In many cases, medications are used as a last resort to try to modify behaviors after other treatment modalities have failed, either because the family has resisted their use or staff does not consider the option of combining pharmacologic with psychosocial interventions from the onset of treatment. Ideally, pharmacologic interventions should be applied from the onset of treatment and should be part and parcel of the entire treatment package.

Also of importance, the child with autism may receive medications across a range of settings, including the home, institution, day treatment program, or a combination of these. Psychosocial interventions can vary significantly across these settings, and symptom expression may also be somewhat setting specific. Thus it is important to evaluate symptom response to pharmacotherapy across all treatment settings simultaneously. This often necessitates more extensive planning than would be expected if all treatment were setting specific. Parents, educators, and other mental health professionals all need to understand and participate in the assessment, measurement, and monitoring of pharmacologic treatment, and hence good communication across settings and careful attention to rater reliability in symptom measurement are essential to a proper evaluation of the therapeutic efficacy and tolerability of psychopharmacologic treatment.

Initial Pharmacologic Management

As also might be expected from Table 16–1, there is no clear-cut consensus on what the preferred first-choice medication for treating the autistic child or adolescent might be. In most cases, this choice is determined by the target symptoms that are the focus of pharmacologic intervention. Thus, if hyperactivity is a target, methylphenidate or clonidine may be chosen. If rituals are a target, an SSRI such as fluvoxamine may be a reasonable choice. If aggression is the target, naltrexone or haloperidol could be used. This symptom-directed approach to treatment may be misleading, however, because many autistic children exhibit more than one of the above symptoms. In addition, more than one of these target symptoms may be improved by more than one medication. Thus, in thinking about selecting a first choice medication for initiating pharmacologic treatment in autism, it is reasonable that, in addition to using the guiding principles to select a first-choice medication (see Section Three) the physician also consider the following question: Which medication(s) are most likely to positively affect not only the chosen target symptom but also the other problematic disturbances demonstrated by this particular patient?

Some experienced clinicians suggest classifying the autistic child's difficulties in the manner indicated in Table 16–3 as a guide to selecting initial psychopharmacologic treatments. Combination pharmacotherapies may be needed to optimize the clinical response in autistic children. These should be implemented using the augmentation approach described in Section Three. Planning for this possibility should precede the initiation of pharmacotherapy.

An alternative approach is to select a broad-spectrum medication as a first-choice treatment and augment using a symptom-specific agent if symptom improvement is inadequate. Using this approach, the physician treating the autistic child may reasonably elect to choose a broad-spectrum medication such as haloperidol or fluvoxamine for initial pharmacologic treatment (Table 16–4) Other compounds can then be added as necessary to target those symptoms that have not shown an adequate response to optimization of monotherapy.

High-potency neuroleptics used in low to moderate doses (haloperidol 1 to 4 mg daily) are a reasonable first-line approach to treating children and adolescents with autism. Various symptoms of the disorder may improve with this treatment, making the child more amenable to psychosocial interventions. More recently, SSRIs have been described as possibly useful in improving many of the core symptoms of autism. Other compounds have also been studied, some of which may target specific symptom clusters (such as methylphenidate or clonidine for the hyperactive cluster of symptoms) or specific symptoms (such as naltrexone or propranolol for aggressive behaviors). Initial pharmacologic management should be directed at the core symptoms of the disorder be-

TABLE 16–3 Clinically Heuristic Subtypes of Autistic Symptoms and Selected First-Line Medication Treatments*

Suggested Subtype	Medication	Alternate
Rage, impulsivity, aggression	Clonidine	Methylphenidate or haloperidol
Obsessions, tantrums, sleep disturbance	Clomipramine	Fluoxetine or sertraline
Panic type	Propranolol	Clonazepam
Self-injury type	Naltrexone	Clonidine or haloperidol

*Although there is little, if any, substantial research that clearly supports this classification, many experienced clinicians use this thinking to assist them in their considerations regarding first-line medications.

TABLE 16–4 Suggested Medications for Initiating and Fine Tuning Pharmacotherapy with Autistic Children*

Initiate with	Fine tune with	Fine tune for
Haloperidol	Methylphenidate	Hyperactivity, aggression
	Clonidine	Hyperactivity, aggression
Fluvoxamine	Naltrexone	Self-injury, hyperactivity
Risperidone‡	Propranolol	Aggression, panic
	Carbamazepine	Aggression
	Fluvoxamine†	Rituals, aggressions
	Sertraline‡	Rituals
	Clomipramine	Rituals

*These suggested medications are derived from clinical experience and the currently available literature on the treatment of autism in children. Other clinicians may approach the issue differently. The physician is advised to consider the guidelines for selecting initial pharmacologic treatments (found in Section Three) in choosing the pharmacologic strategy.

†Use these compounds if haloperidol is chosen as the initiation medication.

‡Early open trials with this compound are encouraging, but systematic large-scale scientifically valid studies are yet unavailable. See Chapter 13 for a discussion regarding risperidone.

cause some of the related symptoms may also show significant improvement with core-directed pharmacologic treatment. If significantly disruptive behaviors, such as aggression, that are associated with but are not core symptoms continue after optimal treatment of core symptoms has been achieved, these can be additionally targeted at that time.

Baseline Evaluation

Medical Considerations

Medical considerations are those outlined in Section Two. Of particular importance is the evaluation of those physical parameters that may be affected by pharmacologic treatment. Because the expected initial treatment will often include the use of high-potency neuroleptics or SSRIs, the following standardized baseline physical assessments are suggested. If neuroleptics are chosen,

1. Extrapyramidal Symptoms Rating Scale (ESRS)—to assess extrapyramidal symptoms and involuntary movements (see Appendix III)
2. Abnormal Involuntary Movement Scale (AIMS)—to assess dyskinetic symptoms (see Appendix III)
3. Medication-specific side effect scales (MSSES) for each medication chosen (see Appendix IV)

If SSRIs are chosen, use the medication-specific side effect scale for antidepressants (see Appendix IV).

In addition to baseline assessment with these instruments, the child should be formally assessed weekly using the same scales as at baseline. Because the ESRS includes a section on involuntary movements (as does the MSSES for neuroleptics), the AIMS needs only to be completed once every 6 months. If a positive response to treatment is identified (see later) and side effects are well tolerated, the following schedule for the use of these scales is suggested. If neuroleptics are used, (1) the ESRS should be completed at every outpatient visit or medication monitoring point thereafter. (2) The AIMS should be repeated at 6-monthly intervals. If either neuroleptics or SSRIs are used, MSSES should be completed at every outpatient visit.

Laboratory Considerations

Laboratory investigations should assess those physiologic parameters that pharmacologic treatment may affect both in the short term and, because chronic treatment may be indicated, in the

long term as well. Because expected treatment will include either high-potency neuroleptics or SSRIs, the following baseline laboratory measures are suggested.

High-Potency Neuroleptics   Routine baseline laboratory tests are not necessary unless clozapine is being used. At this time, routine use of clozapine is not recommended for autism. For information about the use of clozapine, see Chapter 14.

SSRIs   Routine baseline laboratory tests are not necessary if treatment with an SSRI is chosen. There is no value in conducting expensive laboratory evaluations of serotonin, dopamine, or opiate metabolism because these are usually only available in specialized research centers and have not demonstrated any diagnostic or treatment predictive validity.

Psychiatric Considerations

Baseline evaluation should include those clinical features that are the target of pharmacologic treatment. The following baseline measures for the overall symptoms of autism are suggested: the Aberrant Behavior Checklist (ABC), the Childhood Autism Rating Scale (CARS), or the Real Life Rating Scale for Autism (RLRSA) (see Appendix VI). Similarly, specific behaviors or aspects of cognitive functioning may be the target of pharmacologic interventions. In these cases, those measures that best reflect these specific treatment targets should be used at baseline and in evaluation. Some useful measures include the following:

1. For stereotypies—the Timed Stereotypies Rating Scale or a clinician-constructed scale providing a rating of the frequency, duration, and severity of those particular stereotypies that are specific to a particular patient.
2. For symptoms of hyperactivity, attention, and impulsivity—the Attention Deficit Hyperactivity Disorder (ADHD) Rating Scale or the Conners Teacher Rating Scales can be adapted to the patient's clinical presentation and are easily completed by trained mental health workers or educators. The Conners Parent Rating Scale or the ADHD Rating Scale can be used by parents to evaluate their child's symptoms in the home environment.
3. For SIB—perhaps the best method of evaluation is to use a 10 cm Visual Analogue Scale (VAS) for each specific behavior that is a target of intervention.

These rating scales (both overall and specific) should be repeated once every 2 weeks during the acute phase of treatment. Symptom changes may occur slowly in this condition, and pharmacologic treatment often takes 2 to 3 months to produce any significant changes. Once the optimal treatment response has been obtained, less frequent standardized symptom monitoring is necessary. For long-term treatment, the following schedule is suggested. For overall symptoms, the use of one of the three overall syndrome scales (ABC, CARS, or RLRSA) at intervals of 3 months is recommended. For specific symptoms, they should be administered monthly, or at every medical assessment, whichever is the more frequent. For SIB ratings, they should be used weekly.

Initiating Treatment

Pharmacologic treatment may begin after baseline measures have been completed and informed consent obtained from the parents or legal guardians who have been educated about medication treatment alternatives and their risks and benefits. In the initial pharmacologic treatment of the overall symptoms of autism, the clinician has one of two choices. The first choice is to use high-potency neuroleptics and the second is to select one of the SSRIs.

The available research literature is relatively scanty regarding both of these possibilities, but more studies have been reported on the use of high-potency neuroleptics (particularly haloperidol) than on SSRIs. A theoretically intriguing possibility, the use of medications with combined dopaminergic and serotonergic effects (risperidone or low-dose flupenthixol), awaits proper evaluation, although case reports of risperidone use (at doses ranging between 1.0 and 4.0 mg daily) are encouraging. Methodologically reasonable studies of haloperidol, when taken as a whole, have shown improvements in stereotypies, attention, social withdrawal, and maladaptive behaviors. These findings seem to be independent of the sedative effects of haloperidol (which are minimal at the recommended doses), and there is suggestive evidence that haloperidol may have positive yet independent effects on improving maladaptive behaviors and attention.

With respect to side effects, however, dyskinesias are relatively common. According to some estimations, this can reach 30 to 40 percent of cases. However, it is important to keep in mind that these types of movements often occur in autistic children who have never been treated with antipsychotic medications. Thus, baseline assessment of potential atypical movements must be exceedingly thorough to allow for more reasonable determination of the possible pathoetiology (treatment emergent or not) should they be seen following the initiation of pharmacotherapy. If properly assessed prior to treatment and carefully monitored, in the

hands of an experienced psychopharmacologist these may be less of a clinical concern than the persistence of the prolonged and severe symptoms of the disorder itself. The great majority of reported dyskinesias are also associated with neuroleptic withdrawal and can be managed with slower and prolonged medication withdrawal schedules.

Interest in the potential clinical utility of SSRIs has arisen from the findings of serotonin system dysregulation in autism. Although early enthusiasm for the therapeutic efficacy of fenfluramine has waned because of subsequent negative reports of its value in treating the symptoms of autism, a number of studies, albeit mostly open and uncontrolled trials, when taken as a whole, suggest that SSRIs, or a tricyclic antidepressant with a demonstrated serotonin effect (clomipramine), may be useful in decreasing repetitive behaviors, aggression, restlessness, and agitation and in increasing social relatedness. The more classic noradrenergic antidepressants, such as imipramine and desipramine, do not seem to demonstrate these effects.

Given the state of current knowledge about the pharmacologic treatment of the symptoms of autism, the choice of pharmacologic agent depends in part on the differential expected frequency and severity of side effects among the two classes of medications. The short- and long-term side effects of neuroleptics are generally well known, although no studies evaluating their continuous use from early childhood into middle adulthood are available. Furthermore, the research literature may not be the most useful guide to the prediction of short-term side effects because those studies in which the dose of haloperidol was increased or decreased rapidly tend to report the highest incidence of sedation and extrapyramidal events. Both these side effects can be clinically modified by using slower dosage increments or decrements.

The short- and long-term side effects of the SSRIs in children are not known, and although the available data suggest that in the short term the side effects are relatively benign and approximate those found in studies of adult depressives, no evaluations of their long-term effects in this population are available. In this situation, a frank discussion of these issues with parents is essential, and the decision as to which compound should be tried first should be made mutually following informed consent.

Neuroleptic Treatment

If a neuroleptic is selected, haloperidol is the medication of choice given the weight of available information to date, although some clinicians prefer to use risperidone, and some evidence supports the use of pimozide. Haloperidol, however, has undergone the most extensive investigation of any neuroleptic in this population. The efficacy of this medication in improving the core symptoms of this disorder may be related to the reported disturbances of dopamine functioning in autism.

Haloperidol

The elimination half-life of haloperidol is 12 to 36 hours, and steady-state levels are reached within the first week of treatment. Doses can be given once daily and if taken at bedtime may assist in the onset of sleep and will decrease the experience of daytime side effects because peak plasma levels are reached 1 to 4 hours after administration. The usefulness of haloperidol serum level monitoring in autism has not been established and is not recommended. Some evidence from studies in psychotic adult populations indicate that haloperidol may have a pharmacodynamic profile consistent with a therapeutic window and that high doses (greater than 10 mg daily) are unlikely to provide any additional clinical benefit but do increase the incidence and severity of side effects. Although this information is not available for autistic children, it is prudent to keep this possibility in mind (see Chapter 13 for a detailed discussion).

Haloperidol is highly bound to plasma proteins and is metabolized in the liver. Concomitant administration with some SSRIs is likely to significantly increase serum haloperidol concentrations. Other potentially problematic drug interactions include: potentiation of atropine-like side effects when used with antiparkinsonian agents, significantly decreased oral absorption when given with antacids, potential cardiac conduction problems with some antihistamines, significantly decreased haloperidol serum levels with carbamazepine, and increased neurologic and sedative side effects if used concurrently with valproate. Other drug interactions may occur, and good clinical practice includes conducting a literature search for potential interactions prior to prescribing concurrent medications. It is also important to educate the family about potential drug interactions and to advise them to check with the prescribing physician prior to administering any other pharmacologic agent to the child.

Acute extrapyramidal reactions to high-potency neuroleptics are possibly less common in children than in adolescents. Contrary to the recommended prophylactic use of antiparkinsonian agents when treating psychotic adolescents with neuroleptics, these medications (Cogentin, benztropine, procyclidine, and others) are not necessarily indicated when low doses of haloperidol (0.5 to 2.0 mg daily) are used to treat autistic children. If these reactions do occur, low doses of nonsedating antiparkinsonian medications (procyclidine at a total daily dose of 5 mg) should be used.

Given the limited verbal communication of autistic children, it is imperative that frequent medical monitoring of side effects occurs. At the onset of treatment, it is suggested that this be undertaken daily, with less frequent (once every 2 to 5 days) clinical monitoring occurring after the dose has been stabilized (see later). The routine use of standardized side effect scales should be included, as described earlier.

Particular care needs to be taken to avoid exposure to extremes of heat and humidity, and sunscreens and UV-protective sunglasses should be worn as appropriate to avoid photosensitive reactions. Fluid intake should be carefully monitored. The possibility of akathisia should be considered if the child shows behavioral deterioration, especially increased motor restlessness, which may be incorrectly labeled as increased hyperactivity or increased irritability. Should this occur in the presence of an otherwise positive clinical outcome, clonazepam, given in a dose of 0.125 to 0.25 mg twice daily, can be used. A test trial of clonazepam continued over 2 to 3 days may help clarify the diagnosis of akathisia and provide symptomatic relief.

If any serious untoward reactions occur, such as fever, rigidity, pruritus, or polydipsia, the medication should be held and appropriate laboratory investigations undertaken (e.g., white blood cell count [WBC], CPK, liver function tests, electrolytes). If laboratory tests and careful clinical observation do not support a drug reaction, the medication can be safely restarted at the same daily dose.

The dose of haloperidol found to be clinically useful in a number of studies has been between 0.5 and 2.0 mg/day, with maximal daily doses of 4 mg reported. A useful clinical guideline in initiating haloperidol treatment is to give a test dose of 0.5 mg in liquid form in the late morning or early afternoon of day 1. It is possible to add the liquid medication to lunch, snack foods, or drink. However, it is important that the entire amount of medication be taken. If this strategy is used, it may be prudent to provide a small amount of the child's favorite food or drink to which the haloperidol elixir has been added, and when that has been fully consumed, provide the rest of the snack or meal.

If this initial dose is well tolerated, it can then be given at bedtime or with dinner, once daily. A reasonable initial total daily target dose range is 0.5 to 2.0 mg of haloperidol per day. Because doses of 0.5 mg daily are potentially likely to be of significant clinical benefit, this amount should be continued for a reasonable length of time (6 to 8 weeks is suggested) prior to increasing the dose to 1.0 mg given once daily. Monitoring of therapeutic and adverse effects should be conducted in the manner described earlier. Another useful method that may decrease the incidence and severity of side effects is to amend the dosing schedule after 4 to 6 weeks on 0.5 mg daily to alternating 0.5 mg/day with 1.0 mg/day and continuing this alternating schedule for 2 weeks before increasing the dose to 1.0 mg given once daily.

Once a daily dose of 1.0 mg is reached, this should be maintained for a minimum of 6 to 8 weeks before further dosage increases are implemented. Monitoring of side effects and treatment outcome should take place as described earlier. If, following 6 to 8 weeks of treatment at 1.0 mg daily, side effects are well tolerated, the dose should be increased to 1.5 mg daily and maintained for an additional 6 to 8 weeks. Further dosage increments designed to optimize pharmacotherapy (see Section Three) should follow the same pattern as described earlier and should be increased until the side effects become problematic or therapeutic effects are lost. If the latter occurs, the dose of haloperidol must be decreased, not increased, because the clinician may have dosed the patient through a possible therapeutic window.

Some clinicians suggest that younger children may be slower to demonstrate a treatment response to haloperidol than older children. Thus, if haloperidol is used in autistic children under the age of 3, it may be prudent to extend the treatment assessment time from 8 to 10 or 12 weeks to allow more time for possible medication effects to occur prior to proceeding to the next dosage level.

Although the above-mentioned dosage schedule is more conservative than that reported in the clinical trials of haloperidol, it has the advantage of minimizing the incidence and severity of side effects. Furthermore, it allows for optimal monitoring of potential symptom change at each dosage level of haloperidol. The entire protocol can take a number of months to complete. However, given the known clinical course of autism and the clinical advantages of "starting low and going slow," this is a situation in which haste might make waste, or at the very least, cause problems that would otherwise not occur.

Serotonin-Specific Reuptake Inhibitor Treatment

If SSRIs are chosen, a number of compounds are available for use. These include fluoxetine, sertra-line, fluvoxamine, and paroxetine (see Chapter 11 for more detailed information regarding SSRIs). The tricyclic clomipramine may also be considered, but given its side effect profile, potential cardiotoxicity in overdose, and the unlikelihood of showing increased efficacy when compared with the SSRIs, its first-line use in autism is not recommended by some clinicians. Others find it quite useful, particularly in children with sleep difficulties. Careful cardiac monitoring is necessary if it is used. Although not all the SSRIs have been evaluated in autism, there is little to suggest that any one will differ substantially from any other in terms of efficacy. Taken as a whole, published studies of SSRIs in autism show that when used in doses similar to those used in the treatment of adult depression, they may be effective in decreasing repetitive behaviors, aggression, restlessness, hyperactivity, and agitation, and in improving social relatedness. There may, however, also be a therapeutic response to low-dose SSRI treatment, and in the absence of dose-finding studies of various compounds, gradual and consistently evaluated dose increments are necessary.

Side effects may distinguish the various SSRI compounds, and pharmacokinetic profiles may play a role in deciding which medication to choose. For example, fluvoxamine may be slightly more likely to induce gastrointestinal distress, whereas fluoxetine has been reported to cause agitation and restlessness. In some cases, the long half-life of fluoxetine may be of value because medications may be taken once every 2 days after the steady state has been reached. On the other hand, this may delay the institution of other treatments if fluoxetine proves to be relatively ineffective, and a number of medication-free weeks are then necessary for drug washout to occur. These issues should be discussed with the child's parents, and a medication that best fits the particular needs of the patient should then be selected.

Currently, it is thought that all SSRIs produce their therapeutic effects through activity at various serotonin receptors, thereby influencing functional activity within serotonin neurotransmitter systems. SSRIs are structurally diverse, yet all are potent and selective inhibitors of serotonin uptake and have little or no effect on noradrenergic or dopaminergic systems at therapeutic doses. As a group of compounds, the SSRIs are extensively metabolized, primarily by the liver, and are highly bound to plasma proteins. All are long-acting drugs and can be given as a single daily dose. Apart from fluoxetine, steady-state concentrations are achieved in 7 to 14 days. Fluoxetine, which is metabolized to an active compound, norfluoxetine, has the longest half-life (up to 2 weeks).

All the SSRIs are relatively safe in overdose and have minimal cardiovascular effects. Headaches do occur and other neurologic side effects, such as tremor, dystonia, and myoclonus, have been reported. An akathisia-type syndrome, possibly secondary to initiating treatment at too high a dose, has been described, mostly with fluoxetine. Sedation may be experienced, possibly more with fluvoxamine or sertraline, and manic or hypomanic symptoms, although rare, have been reported to arise with all SSRIs. Gastrointestinal side effects are those that are expected with serotonin re-uptake inhibition and include nausea, bloating, and diarrhea. Allergic reactions do occur but are rare. Further information regarding this class of medications can be found in Chapter 11.

CASE EXAMPLE

Broad-Spectrum Approach to Treating Autism: Let's Go with Fluvoxamine

After extensive discussions with F.S.'s parents and the provision of various reading materials pertaining to the different medication possibilities, a joint decision was reached to implement a trial of fluvoxamine treatment. A consent form regarding the use of fluvoxamine was signed by both parents, target symptoms were selected, and appropriate baseline measures were completed. The parents' rationale for the choice of fluvoxamine was that it was less likely than haloperidol to cause neurologic side effects, especially tardive dyskinesia. Risperidone was considered to be "too experimental." In addition, it was thought to be more sedating than fluoxetine and because F.S. often experienced difficulty falling asleep, they felt that this would be of benefit to her.

Fluvoxamine

Fluvoxamine is well absorbed orally and can be given with food without affecting its absorption. This allows for increased ease of administration to an autistic child, to whom the medication can be given along with a food "treat." The half-life ranges from 12 to 24 hours, and once steady-state concentrations are reached (about 7 to 10 days) the drug can be administered in a once-daily dose. Some evidence from the adult literature suggests that fluvoxamine given in a once-daily bedtime dose is associated with fewer reported side effects than doses given once or twice during the daytime. This may be caused by a relationship between the experience of side effects and the timing of the peak plasma level of fluvoxamine,

which occurs about 2 to 8 hours following oral administration.

Cardiovascular effects of fluvoxamine are generally considered to be clinically insignificant, and its autonomic effects, as measured by its effect on salivation and pupil dilation, are not significantly different from placebo. Fluvoxamine has minimal proconvulsant activity, and when accompanied by careful clinical and laboratory (anticonvulsant plasma levels) monitoring, it may be safe to use in patients who have a concurrent seizure disorder.

Fluvoxamine may be the least plasma protein–bound of the SSRIs; nevertheless, its protein binding is about 70 to 80 percent, and thus it can displace other drugs and elevate their free plasma levels, potentially leading to problematic drug interactions. Similarly, fluvoxamine competes with other compounds for metabolism through the cytochrome P-450 system. This competition can affect the serum levels of many other drugs, especially anticonvulsants (carbamazepine and phenytoin). In addition, fluvoxamine should be used cautiously if administered with warfarin (the plasma level of warfarin can be significantly elevated) or with other medications that have serotonin activity because the combined use of serotonin-active compounds can lead to the development of a serotonin syndrome (see Chapter 11).

In treating autistic children with fluvoxamine the list of potential drug interactions is extensive. Two of the most commonly occurring clinical considerations follow. First, fluvoxamine has been reported to significantly increase the plasma level of propranolol, which may be considered for use (possibly in combination with fluvoxamine) to treat those aggressive or SIB symptoms that may not improve substantially, even if other autistic symptoms show significant change. Thus, this combination of medications has the potential to lead to propranolol toxicity, and if they are used concurrently cardiovascular function must be monitored carefully. Second, some autistic children may have concurrent asthma and may be treated with theophylline, the plasma levels of which can be substantially increased if fluvoxamine is added. In this clinical situation, care must be taken to monitor theophylline levels and to increase the fluvoxamine dose very slowly.

Fluvoxamine should be given as a test dose of 25 mg with a favorite food. If necessary it can be crushed into jelly or jam. If this dose is well tolerated, it can then be given as a once-a-day dose at bedtime. The dose should be increased in 3 to 4 days by 25 mg to a daily dose of 50 mg. At that time this dose should be maintained for a minimum of 6 to 8 weeks to determine its potential effect on the target symptoms. If significant improvement is not obtained, the dose should again be increased in 25 mg increments every 3 to 4 days until a total daily dose of 100 mg is reached. If side effects are minimal and significant improvement is not obtained following 6 to 8 weeks at this level, the dose should once again be increased using the same titration schedule and monitoring side effects. This pattern should be repeated until the pharmacologic use of fluvoxamine has been optimized. If side effects limit dose increments but the therapeutic effect has been good, the medication should be decreased to a daily dose just below that at which side effects limit its use. If higher doses seem to be associated with a loss of therapeutic efficacy, this suggests that a return to a lower dose is indicated.

CASE EXAMPLE

Trying Out the Fluvoxamine

Using the dosage schedule described earlier, fluvoxamine treatment was prescribed for F.S. in addition to all her other intervention modalities. By this time she had left the hospital for an institutional treatment setting because she was believed to be too disruptive for a day treatment program, and her parents were unable or unwilling to manage her at home on a daily basis. Staff at F.S.'s new setting were trained in the use of the treatment assessment instruments, and appropriate medical monitoring was put in place.

F.S. tolerated the medication well. At a total daily dose of 150 mg, there was substantial improvement in her symptoms as measured by the RLRSA. Her most marked improvement was noted in the subscales of sensory motor behavior, affectual reactions, and sensory responses. She continued to show SIB and although the frequency of her head banging had decreased by about 25 percent, she still required daily interventions to prevent her from harming herself.

Her fluvoxamine dose was gradually increased to 200 mg daily, with continued improvement in symptoms. Because F.S. was not experiencing any significant side effects at this dose, after assessment over 8 weeks the dose was increased once again, this time to 250 mg daily. At 250 mg F.S. experienced diarrhea and her appetite decreased substantially. In addition, she appeared to be more sluggish in the morning and somewhat sedated. Accordingly, her medication dose was decreased to 200 mg daily. Two weeks following this dose adjustment, her side effects had improved signifi-

cantly, and thus the dose of fluvoxamine was maintained at 200 mg per day over the next 8 weeks. Reassessment using the RLRSA (Appendix VI) and the OCI (Appendix V) showed an increased improvement in overall scores from the evaluation completed at a dose of 150 mg. Of particular interest was that the decrease in her SIB, which now occurred infrequently, was much less severe and was more easily redirected with minimal behavioral interventions.

CASE COMMENTARY

This illustrates a common issue in treatment, determining the optimal response to pharmacologic intervention (see Section Three for a discussion of the general principle underlying this topic). In F.S.'s case, fluvoxamine was being given at a total daily dose of 150 mg, and she was experiencing minimal side effects. It was thus quite reasonable to increase her dose to determine what the outcome at a higher dose would be. Once again, at this new target dose of 200 mg daily, although more improvement had occurred, she was still relatively side effect–free. In this case, with good physical health and positive symptom change, it was reasonable to carefully increase the dose of the medication. It must be remembered that the dosage range is a guideline for optimal dosage. Some patients will show a good clinical response with minimal side effects at doses below the lower limit; others will require doses above the upper limit for maximal therapeutic effect. The dosage must be determined clinically using rational dosing strategies that allow for proper identification of therapeutic efficacy.

Initial Pharmacologic Treatment of Autism—Practice Points

1. After careful diagnosis and baseline assessment, the clinician should identify target symptoms for pharmacotherapy.
2. For initiating pharmacotherapy, a broad-spectrum medication, such as haloperidol, risperidone, or an SSRI, can be chosen as first-line treatment.
3. Treatment effects may take up to 8 weeks or longer to become apparent at each dose level, and thus medication dose changes should allow for sufficient time between each dose to determine the therapeutic efficacy at each dose level.
4. Combined pharmacotherapies may be

necessary if initial optimized broad-spectrum treatment does not provide sufficient control of target symptoms.

Specific Clinical Problems

Treatment nonresponse is all too common in treating autism. Unfortunately, few if any studies are available to guide the practitioner in this issue, and even case series are few and far between. A number of different strategies may be suggested. The guiding principles are addressed in Section Three. The first is to ensure that optimal treatment with monotherapy has indeed occurred. For each specific medication used, the most appropriate dose continued for a sufficient length of time is essential. If this has not occurred, dosage adjustment and treatment duration must occur to allow for optimal initial treatment.

The second option is medication substitution. This involves switching from one first-line medication to another, such as from an SSRI to a neuroleptic or from a neuroleptic to an SSRI. Although there is a theoretical rationale for this procedure in that some autistic children show peripheral markers consistent with serotonin dysregulation and others show peripheral markers consistent with dopamine regulation, there is no study that has shown these peripheral disturbances are predictive of the response to particular compounds. This approach is not unreasonable, however, and should be considered first. It has the advantage of using a single compound that makes monitoring of compliance and side effects easier.

A third approach is to augment the initial treatment. In such cases, an SSRI can be added to a neuroleptic. Careful monitoring of side effects is essential, and elevation of neuroleptic serum levels may occur. If this strategy is chosen, an SSRI other than fluvoxamine should be chosen. Alternatively, propranolol, clonidine, naltrexone, methylphenidate, or buspirone augmentation may be considered. In these cases, it is useful to choose an agent that will target the most troublesome symptoms that the child is exhibiting.

In other cases, the suggestion of a comorbid psychiatric condition, such as a bipolar disorder, or a medical problem, such as a seizure disorder, may direct the choice of the augmenting agent. Lithium can be considered if augmentation is directed by the clinical suggestion of mania. Carbamazepine or valproate can be considered if augmentation is directed by the clinical suggestion of seizures.

Whatever agent is chosen, it is important to make clear that augmentation is quasi-experi-mental, and the informed consent documentation should reflect this. If two medications are used, care must be taken to avoid drug interactions (e.g., lithium augmentation of SSRIs may result in a serotonin syndrome and lithium augmentation of haloperidol may result in increased rates of neurotoxicity), and side effect monitoring must reflect the expected side effects of each compound.

Self-Injurious Behavior

SIB may pose a particularly difficult treatment challenge in the autistic child. In some cases, SIB may improve substantially with broad-spectrum pharmacologic interventions, such as haloperidol, risperidone, or an SSRI alone. In other cases, SIB may continue to be a problem, even when optimized pharmacologic treatment using a broad-spectrum compound has been accomplished.

CASE EXAMPLE

"He hits and hits and hits."

R.E. was a 9-year-old boy who was undergoing multimodal treatment for autism. This included haloperidol at a dose of 1.5 mg, given once daily. On this pharmacologic regimen, he had demonstrated significant improvement in attention and social relatedness and decreased hyperactivity. However, he exhibited frequent and severe SIB, which had improved only minimally with neuroleptic treatment. Attempts to increase his haloperidol dose were associated with distressing side effects. Various behavioral strategies had been attempted, all without significant positive effects. A case conference was held to determine if any other pharmacologic interventions could be considered.

CASE COMMENTARY

There were a number of medication choices that could be considered in this case. Of the available agents, perhaps the two most likely to provide relatively rapid improvement in SIB are the beta-blocker propranolol and the opiate antagonist naltrexone. Although rigorous placebo-controlled studies of large populations with SIB are lacking, both agents have shown positive results in a variety of case reports and open trials. Taken as a whole, this literature suggests that in cases in which SIB complicates the clinical presentation in autism, one of these medications should be considered.

Given the available information, it is not

possible to determine which agent, propranolol or naltrexone, if either, is superior in the control of SIB. Thus, the specific characteristics of each individual case will need to be considered in the selection of a drug for an initial trial. In some cases, this will be readily apparent, as in a child with severe asthma or diabetes mellitus, in which the use of beta-blockers would be contraindicated. In other cases, parent or patient preference, based on expected side effect profiles, may be the determining factor. In every case, informed consent is necessary before treatment is instituted. Clinical experience suggests that combined behavioral and pharmacologic interventions in SIB may improve results over the use of either agent alone.

Propranolol

If propranolol is chosen, a medical evaluation to ensure that the child does not suffer from any conditions for which this drug is contraindicated is necessary, including asthma, diabetes mellitus, cardiovascular disease, and hypothyroidism. Laboratory tests should include a fasting blood glucose and possibly an ECG. Other serologic or physiologic tests are not needed. Peripheral indices of cardiovascular functioning need to be followed carefully, and heart rate and sitting and standing blood pressure should be monitored daily. Clinically significant changes in these parameters (heart rate less than 50 beats/min and sitting blood pressure less than 80/50 mmHg) should lead to downward adjustment of the dose.

In older children or adolescents, a reasonable initial starting dose of propranolol is 10 mg, given three times daily (total daily dose of 30 mg). The expected therapeutic range for propranolol is 100 to 640 mg per day, with a reasonable initial daily target dose range being 100 to 300 mg. A reasonable strategy for dose increments is to give the medication on a three-times daily schedule, increasing the total daily dose by 30 mg daily every 3 to 4 days until a total daily dose of 120 mg is reached or side effects (particularly bradycardia or orthostatic hypotension) limit further increases. At that time, the dose should be maintained for a minimum of 4 to 6 weeks in order to fully determine the potential therapeutic efficacy of this dose. Further dose changes, guided by side effects and therapeutic response, can then be made.

Younger children may require lower doses (30 to 160 mg daily) of propranolol. Thus in autistic patients under the age of 6 or 7, an initial daily target dose range of 40 to 80 mg may be set. In addition, the elimination half-life of propranolol may be decreased in younger children, so consideration of a four times daily dose (qid) should be given. If this is done, the following protocol is useful: 5 mg orally, qid for 7 days, then increase to 10 mg qid for 6 to 8 weeks. If substantial improvement does not occur, increase the dose to 15 mg qid for 4 to 6 weeks. If adequate symptom control is not obtained at this dose, use graduated increases by monitoring therapeutic effect and treatment-emergent adverse events to optimize pharmacotherapy.

Some clinicians report that the effective therapeutic use of propranolol is accompanied by effective "cardioblocking," usually associated with a resting pulse rate of about 60 beats/min. Others report reasonable results at doses that do not show similar cardiac effects. In many cases, patients may be able to tolerate high doses of propranolol without demonstrating significant adverse events. Total daily doses of over 600 mg have been reported, and total daily doses over 300 mg are not all that rare. The patient taking propranolol *must* wear a medic-alert bracelet that cannot be easily removed.

Propranolol may be safely added to haloperidol (it may, however, increase chlorpromazine or thioridazine levels), and when used in conjunction with high-potency neuroleptics may allow for improved control of SIB, along with a decrease in the neuroleptic dose without diminution of other symptom control. In addition, propranolol is known to demonstrate some antiparkinsonian effects and may be particularly helpful in cases in which neuroleptic-induced tremors or akathisia complicate the clinical picture. It is important to remember to discontinue propranolol gradually because rapid reduction in high-dose treatment may lead to rebound tachycardia. If propranolol is added to SSRIs, the potential for fluvoxamine to significantly elevate propranolol levels must be taken into account.

Asperger's syndrome may occasionally be considered for pharmacologic treatment. Unfortunately, few clear guidelines are available. Children and adolescents with Asperger's syndrome need to be differentiated from those with schizotypal personality disorder. They present with a flat affect, a need for sameness, and obsessive ideation. They are generally insensitive to social cues and demonstrate reasonable language skills in the presence of deficient language pragmatics. They may demonstrate extensive social anxieties and should not be confused with those individuals who suffer from avoidant personality disorder or social phobia. In the author's experience, they may benefit from low-dose SSRI (fluoxetine 10 to 20 mg daily) or buspirone (30 to 90 mg daily) treatment. These interventions often reduce anxiety symptoms, decrease withdrawal, and increase social relatedness, although it is not known if these outcomes occur independently of each other.

Naltrexone treatment is described later in this chapter in the treatment of aggression occurring in the context of mental retardation.

Pharmacologic Treatment of SIB in Autism—Practice Points

1. First, optimize the broad-spectrum pharmacologic treatment.
2. If SIB continues, consider propranolol or naltrexone augmentation of ongoing pharmacologic treatment.
3. Acknowledge and carefully monitor for potential drug interactions with augmented medication treatments.

Long-Term Psychopharmacologic Treatment for Autism

Although autism is a chronic disorder, little is known about the long-term psychopharmacologic treatment of this disturbance. As with any chronic psychiatric illness, the decision to undertake long-term pharmacologic treatment weighs the risks against the benefits of continued medication use. Thus, for each patient these factors must be independently assessed. At this time, a prudent guideline is to evaluate the entire treatment program annually. A review of psychopharmacologic treatments should be part and parcel of this review. A gradual decrease in medications may be indicated to determine if the medicines still contribute significantly to symptom control. If this strategy is chosen, gradual medication withdrawal is necessary, particularly with haloperidol, with which too rapid decreases may precipitate withdrawal dyskinesia. Alternatively, there may be a decision to attempt further pharmacologic treatments to optimize a treatment response, including augmentation strategies. If this course of action is considered, care must be taken to ensure that proper evaluative methods are followed to allow for proper evaluation of therapeutic efficacy with each change in pharmacotherapy.

Mental Retardation

Mental retardation by itself or mental retardation comorbidly with other psychiatric disorders may occur and be a target for pharmacologic intervention. The optimal treatment of children and teens with moderate to profound mental retardation includes a combination of psychosocial, behavioral, and pharmacologic strategies. Medications may be useful in treating symptoms of an Axis I disorder; facilitating, learning, and promoting social interactions; and suppressing behaviors that are harmful to the patient or to others. Medications most commonly used are low doses of high-potency neuroleptics. In some cases, lithium or carbamazepine is often prescribed for nonspecific behavioral problems. Opiate antagonists and beta-blockers may be useful in treating SIB or aggression.

The pharmacotherapy of mental retardation, although similar, may not be identical to that of autism. For example, there are few if any clear-cut core symptoms of mental retardation, such as those that can be defined within a syndromal context for autism. Second, a number of pharmacologic interventions developed on the basis of a presumed pathoetiology of autism (e.g., the SSRIs following the identification of possible disturbed serotonin metabolism in some autistic children) have not been so defined for mental retardation. Practically, physicians do not really treat the "symptoms" of mental retardation as they may do for autism. Instead, target symptoms that are causing distress or danger to the patient or caregivers are usually the focus of pharmacologic interventions.

Pharmacologic treatment in mental retardation may be exceedingly complex for a variety of reasons. Some of these, of course, also apply to children with a pervasive developmental disorder such as autism. These are as follows:

1. Concerns about the validity of applying diagnostic criteria as outlined in DSM-III-R or DSM-IV to the classification of psychiatric illness in the intellectually handicapped
2. Uncertainties regarding the diagnosis of Axis I disorders appearing in intellectually handicapped individuals caused by variability in phenotypic presentations
3. Difficulties in obtaining information about inner states from intellectually handicapped individuals
4. Lack of sufficient systematic studies of pharmacologic treatments in both Axis I disorders and nonspecific disturbances of behavior in this population
5. Lack of systematic studies regarding psychopharmacologic treatments in subtypes of mental retardation (i.e., fragile X, Prader-Willi, Down syndrome, etc.)
6. Insufficient knowledge about the pharmacokinetics and pharmacodynamics of psychotropic agents in individuals with particular

genetic or metabolic disorders associated with mental retardation (such as the effect of some psychotropic agents on the clinical progression of oligosaccharides, e.g., Tay-Sachs disease)

The major clinical issues in treating behavioral disturbances in intellectually handicapped individuals are as follows:

1. Differentiating symptoms of specific Axis I psychiatric disorders from nonspecific behavioral disturbances
2. Choosing a pharmacologic agent with proven therapeutic efficacy for the disorder or symptoms(s) identified
3. Monitoring carefully target symptoms and side effects using multiple informants and inferring possible side effects from observable behaviors (such as nausea manifesting itself as a loss of appetite)
4. Ensuring that, as much as possible, given the cognitive developmental level of each specific individual, informed consent (or assent) is given and the rights of the child or adolescent (including the right to treatment) are protected

Traditionally, the neuroleptic drugs are often used in the treatment of behavioral disturbances in intellectually handicapped individuals. Clinical reviews and systematic study of this practice are limited, and there is some concern that, in the absence of a psychotic disorder, these medications may exert their effects through nonspecific effects. A reasonable guideline is to carefully evaluate the patient for a possible Axis I psychiatric disorder first. If an Axis I disorder seems a likely possibility, then pharmacologic interventions directed at that disorder are a reasonable first step. If an Axis I disorder cannot be identified, then behavior-specific pharmacologic interventions are appropriate.

CASE EXAMPLE

Treating Aggression in a Mentally Retarded Teen

T.R. was a 15-year-old girl with moderate mental retardation (IQ, 55 to 65) of idiopathic origin. She had been treated in the same day treatment program for the previous 7 years and generally had an unremarkable course. Eight months prior to assessment her behavior had begun to deteriorate. Over the course of a few weeks she became increasingly aggressive, irritable, and argumentative. Her food intake increased, and she started to steal food from other children, causing numerous fights. Although in the past she had always responded well to "time outs," she now actively resisted them. At home, her mother found her to be restless and easily agitated. She resisted going to bed and would often play her radio loudly at odd hours of the night. If limits were set for her, she would threaten and occasionally strike out at her mother, although this had never occurred previously. This pattern of behavior continued for about 2 to 3 months, with periods of time during which she was much worse and periods of relative stability.

She was assessed by a physician, who treated her with perphenazine at a dose of 24 mg daily and with benztropine at a dose of 2 mg daily. This led to an improvement in her behavior, but she exhibited side effects of sedation and marked tremors. Increasing the benztropine led to constipation and increased fluid intake, presumably because of dry mouth. Attempts to decrease the neuroleptic dose led to a return of behavioral problems.

T.R.'s parents were very concerned about the long-term effects of neuroleptic medications and watched carefully for signs of tardive dyskinesia. According to her parents (although not observed by her treatment staff or physician), T.R. developed "lip smacking." At the parent's insistence, she was withdrawn from her neuroleptic, at which time her behavior quickly worsened. Now, however, she began to exhibit additional symptoms including aggressive sexual behaviors, such as attempting to forcefully disrobe some of the boys in the treatment program and frequent self-stimulation through masturbation. This was upsetting to the treatment program staff, other patients, and her parents.

A psychiatric assessment revealed a history of bipolar disorder in her maternal grandfather (treated with ECT) and major depression in her mother (three distinct episodes over her lifetime). Her paternal uncle had been treated for alcoholism, and her paternal grandfather "would have been an alcoholic if he had admitted it." A variety of nonspecific behavioral disturbances were described in other family members, but information about them was sketchy because they lived in rural regions of a southern European country where psychiatric diagnosis was uncommon and psychiatric treatment was only sporadically available.

Although clear-cut DSM-IV diagnostic criteria were not met in this patient, a tentative diagnosis of mania was made and, following extensive discussions with her parents, the child, and the day treatment staff, a trial of carbamazepine was agreed on. The parents felt that carbamazepine instead of lithium was indicated because their daughter already had "bad" acne and was overweight. In addition, they were worried that if lithium were used her tremors, which had been quite marked with perphenazine treatment, would return.

CASE COMMENTARY

Although there are no clear-cut guidelines on the optimal choice of medication in this case, carbamazepine is a reasonable medication to select. Although carbamazepine is an imino-stilbene anticonvulsant with structural similarity to the tricyclic antidepressant imipramine, it has antimanic and antiaggressive properties and in studies of adult mania has been reported to perform well in mixed affective states. It has also been found to decrease severe impulsive aggression, emotional lability, and irritability in non–affectively disordered populations, but it is not known to negatively affect cognitive functioning. Compared with neuroleptics, carbamazepine does not tend to induce extrapyramidal side effects nor tardive dyskinesia. There is an available, albeit small, psychiatric literature regarding its efficacy in a variety of behavioral disturbances, including its use in mentally retarded individuals. Finally, there is an extensive literature on the use of this compound in epileptic children, and its pharmacokinetics and side effects (at least in that population) are understood. Alternatively, valproate may have been considered; its use is described in Chapter 12.

Baseline Evaluation

Medical Considerations

Medical considerations are those outlined in Section Two. Of particular importance is the evaluation of those physical parameters that may be affected by pharmacologic treatment. Because the expected initial pharmacotherapy will often be directed toward the treatment of disruptive or aggressive behaviors, a low dose of a high-potency neuroleptic may be used. If this is the case, haloperidol is suggested at the doses described earlier for autism. If haloperidol is used, then the appropriate baseline monitoring should be instituted. In some cases, such as the case described earlier, thymoleptics such as carbamazepine may be chosen. In other cases in which specific behaviors, such as SIB, are a problem, naltrexone or propranolol may be used. The following baseline assessments are

suggested if the clinician chooses to institute carbamazepine or naltrexone treatment.

If either carbamazepine or naltrexone is used, potential side effects need to be evaluated using a MSSES, which can be found in Appendix IV for each medication. If carbamazepine is used, a screening neurologic examination should be conducted with particular attention paid to nystagmus, diploplia, and cerebellar signs. The presence and severity, or the absence, of these symptoms should be recorded.

Laboratory Considerations

1. Complete blood count, including WBC with differential and platelets
2. Serum electrolytes and serum iron
3. Liver function tests
4. TSH and free T4
5. ECG

Psychiatric Monitoring

Those scales that measure the identified target symptoms should be used. These are discussed in Section Two and many examples of these may be found in Appendix IV

Carbamazepine

Carbamazepine's exact mode of therapeutic action in decreasing aggressive behaviors and improving mood stability is unknown, although GABA-agonist activity and sodium channel stabilization of its antikindling effects may be involved. Carbamazepine is metabolized by the liver and has an active anticonvulsant and neurotoxic metabolite (10,11-epoxide carbamazepine) that complicates the interpretation of the parent compound serum levels, because it is not routinely measured in most laboratories. Carbamazepine's elimination half-life varies from 12 to 60 hours, and peak levels occur 2 to 6 hours following oral administration, with steady-state levels reached within 4 days. With repeated administration at therapeutic doses, the elimination half-life decreases to 5 to 20 hours because of autoinduction of hepatic enzyme systems. Thus, in pharmacotherapy with carbamazepine it is common for steady-state serum levels of this drug to fall significantly, anywhere between the second and fifth week of treatment. This can lead to a decrease in its therapeutic activity, and thus, when treatment is initiated, serum levels need to be carefully monitored and corrected by appropriate dosage increments.

Adverse effects of carbamazepine may be severe and include agranulocytosis, aplastic anemia, clinically significant thrombocytopenia, exfoliative skin eruptions, and acute idiosyncratic hepatitis. Although these are relatively rare, they must be kept in mind during the entire treatment course, and careful clinical and laboratory monitoring is necessary during the entire course of carbamazepine treatment. Carbamazepine is contraindicated in patients with known hypersensitivity to tricyclic compounds and a history of hepatic, cardiovascular, or hematologic disease.

The more common side effects are those related to total daily dose, the amount of individual doses given, the sensitivity of the individual, or the rapidity of dose increments. These are neurologic (ataxia, clumsiness, dysarthria, diploplia, dizziness, sedation, nystagmus); gastrointestinal (nausea, diarrhea); hematologic (transitory and reversible mild leukopenia, thrombocytopenia); hepatic (mild reversible increases in liver function tests); and metabolic (decreases of serum sodium concentration). Less common but important adverse effects are its cardiovascular (slowing of intracardiac conduction) and thyroid (decreases in T3 and free T4 with long-term treatment) effects.

Behavioral side effects also may occur with carbamazepine and need to be considered in any case in which worsening of the clinical condition occurs with carbamazepine treatment. The exact incidence of the following potential behavioral side effects is not known. However, clinicians should carefully evaluate them prior to beginning treatment, because behavioral side effects may be very difficult to distinguish from the symptom profiles of various Axis I disorders, or of behavioral disturbances that themselves may be targets of treatment. Some potential behavioral side effects to consider are irritability, agitation, delirious states with hallucinations, insomnia, and obsessive thinking. Manic and psychotic symptoms have also been reported. If these features complicate carbamazepine treatment and it is unclear whether they are secondary to the medication or are part of the evolution of the clinical syndrome, a prudent course to follow is to discontinue the carbamazepine and monitor the patient for 3 to 4 days. Ancillary medications, if any, should be maintained at the same dosage. If the symptoms are caused by carbamazepine, they should subside substantially over that time. If not, they will persist or worsen. Decisions can then be made regarding the further use of carbamazepine. If carbamazepine is to be restarted, a conservative dosing schedule, such as follows, should be instituted.

When carbamazepine treatment is initiated, the following schedule for routine medical and laboratory monitoring is suggested for the first 8 weeks of treatment:

1. Assessment of side effects, including specific neurologic evaluation before each dosage increase and 3 to 4 days following each dosage increase (when a new steady-state level has been reached)
2. Weekly standardized side effect evaluation using a carbamazepine-specific side effects scale
3. Weekly monitoring of CBC with WBC and differential and platelets, hepatic enzymes, and carbamazepine serum levels
4. Evaluation of serum electrolytes and serum iron once sustained therapeutic levels have been attained (about 6 weeks)
5. ECG once sustained steady-state therapeutic levels have been attained (about 6 weeks)

In long-term therapy, once stable therapeutic levels have been reached and after the dose has been properly adjusted to account for the autoinduction phenomenon described earlier, the following schedule for routine monitoring is suggested:

1. Assessment of side effects, including specific neurologic examination and side effects scale evaluations at each follow-up visit
2. Every 3 to 4 months, CBC with differential, liver function tests, serum electrolytes, and serum carbamazepine levels
3. Every year, TSH and serum iron levels

Whereas transient decreases in hematologic indices are common and will often improve without any intervention, minor dosage adjustments are sometimes necessary. It is suggested that if hematologic indices fall below the following values, the medication should be held and urgent hematologic consultation obtained. If low levels persist, therapy with carbamazepine may need to be discontinued.

1. WBC—levels drop to <4000 white cells/mm^3
2. Absolute neutrophil count—<1700 cells/mm^3
3. Erythrocytes—levels drop to <4 × 10^6 mm^3
4. Platelets—levels drop to <100,000 mm^3
5. Hemoglobin—levels drop to <11 g/dl
6. Reticulocytes—count drops to <3 percent
7. Serum iron—levels rise to >150 mg/dl

Furthermore, if any of the following physical symptoms appear, immediate laboratory testing of hematologic indices is necessary: rash, sore throat, fever, lethargy and malaise, vomiting, jaundice, easy bruising or bleeding, neurotoxic symptoms, or mouth ulcers. In the presence of these symptoms, the prudent course is to withhold the medication until the results of the tests are available (usually the next day). If the results are negative, the medication can be restarted using the same dosage. If more than 3 days elapse, it is prudent to restart the medication at half the original daily dose and gradually increase it to previous levels.

Because of its high degree of plasma binding and competitive hepatic metabolism, drug interactions with carbamazepine are common. These are numerous and the clinician should consult a detailed reference regarding these prior to prescribing carbamazepine and should educate the child and parent about other medications to avoid. A list of potential drug interactions that may be more commonly expected in children or adolescents follows:

Erythromycin	Alprazolam
Doxycycline	Lithium
Valproate	Many neuroleptics
Phenobarbital	Oral contraceptives
Amitriptyline	Theophylline
Imipramine	

This is not a comprehensive list of all possible drug-drug interactions with carbamazepine. The clinician should consult the appropriate sources if uncertain whether a particular medication combination may lead to a drug-drug interaction.

Whenever MR children are treated with carbamazepine, it is useful for their parents to be given a Medications Monitoring Record (see Section Three) to help them monitor their child's pharmacotherapy. A good guideline is to ask the parent not to begin any other medication for the child until first informing the clinician.

Carbamazepine treatment usually should be started with doses of 100 mg daily given with food in divided doses. In small children or in cases for which compliance is a problem, an elixir preparation or "sprinkles" are available. Although carbamazepine can be added to foods, the same caveats regarding this practice apply, as described earlier for autism. The dosage should be gradually increased by 100 mg per week to a target of about 800 to 1000 mg daily in adolescents and 300 to 800 mg daily in children. Because of a more rapid elimination half-life of carbamazepine in young children, the daily dose should be given in three parts; a twice-daily dosage is acceptable for adolescents. The use of a slow-release preparation may improve compliance while providing a smoother pharmacokinetic profile and thus lessening side effects. Diploplia is an early manifestation of neurotoxicity with carbamazepine and provides a simple and reliable method of clinical monitoring.

Once the target dose has been stable for 1 week, therapeutic serum levels should be used to direct further adjustments. Although there is no clearcut evidence for specific therapeutic serum levels in treating behavioral disturbances, most investigators have used the suggested therapeutic levels obtained from the pediatric literature to provide seizure control. Levels of 8 to 12 µg/mL (20 to 50 µmol/L) are usually recommended. Dose adjustments should take place in 100 mg increments, and serum levels should be drawn 1 week after the last dose adjustment to guide further increases. Serum levels should be drawn 12 to 14 hours following the last dose to ensure that the proper trough levels are measured.

Self-Injury Behavior in Mental Retardation

Opiate antagonists have been studied in SIB based on the hypothetical model of opiate function in SIB in which SIB is thought to be a self-addictive phenomenon resulting from increased amounts of endogenous opioids (and subsequent mild euphoria) that occur following injury. Naloxone, an opiate antagonist, is only available in injectable form and has a very short duration of action. Thus the orally administered opiate antagonist naltrexone is perhaps more clinically useful. Naltrexone may be best suited for use in those cases in which (1) the aggressive symptoms are not caused by an Axis I disorder and (2) specific SIB symptoms can be clearly identified and measured (e.g., hitting, cutting, head banging, etc.)

CASE EXAMPLE

Self-Injury in a Mentally Retarded Child

E.H. was an 11-year-old boy with severe mental retardation (IQ, 40 to 54). He had exhibited the SIBs of biting and scratching. He required periodic restraint and wearing of a football helmet for self-protection. A pharmacologic consultation was requested to determine if any medications could be useful in decreasing these SIBs. Following a comprehensive diagnostic evaluation, baseline assessment, and parental consent, naltrexone treatment was instituted. When a daily dose of 1.5 mg/kg was reached, his SIBs decreased significantly, and he was able to be cared for in a more dignified and supportive manner.

CASE COMMENTARY

The opiate agonist naltrexone may sometimes be useful in treating aggressive behavior or SIB in the context of mental retardation. In other cases, haloperidol, risperidone, or propranolol may be considered. In other cases, carbamazepine or lithium may be helpful. The use of these medications is discussed in this chapter, except for lithium, which is discussed in Chapter 12, and risperidone, which is covered in Chapter 13. Naltrexone, which is relatively expensive in comparison with the other medications, is now described.

Naltrexone

Naltrexone shows variable oral bioavailability and demonstrates a serum half-life of 1 to 3 hours, with a duration of action of 1 to 4 hours. The dosage must thus be relatively frequent and should be titrated to the putative duration of action following careful monitoring of symptoms. It has a weakly active metabolite, 6-naltrexol, and may exhibit an unusual flipped S dose/response curve in which its therapeutic action may appear, disappear, and then appear again as the dose is increased. It has a relatively benign side effect profile and, apart from mild sedation, is generally well tolerated. No laboratory measures are necessary for baseline evaluation or monitoring.

Naltrexone has demonstrated clinical utility in cases of SIB and has also been used in treating individuals with autism, in which it has been reported to decrease withdrawal, increase communicative speech, improve social relatedness, as well as decrease SIB. Its long-term side effects secondary to continuous use are not known, but it can lead to increased serum luteinizing hormone, adrenocorticotropic hormone, and cortisol levels because of its tonic inhibitory effects on the release of some hypothalamic hormones. The clinical effect of this is unclear, and the rationale for routine laboratory monitoring of these indices is unknown.

Naltrexone treatment in children should be initiated with a dose of 12.5 mg given two times daily. This dose should be maintained for at least 3 weeks. If significant symptomatic improvement is not obtained by that time, the dose should be increased to 25 mg given two times daily and once again maintained for 3 weeks to allow for proper evaluation of its effect. In adolescents, the dosage could start at 25 mg, given two times daily and be increased using the same schedule to 50 mg twice daily. If breakthrough behaviors occur, the dose should be given more frequently and titrated to tolerability. Giving naltrexone together with a small dose of a high-potency neuroleptic is not contraindicated. Some reports on mania in the adult literature suggest that opiate antagonists may potentiate neuroleptic activity; however, this remains to be studied properly. Nevertheless, this combination may be of benefit in the child who shows a partial response to neuroleptics but in whom SIB continues to be clinical problem.

An additional clinical problem often seen in patients with mental retardation is hyperactivity, although it is often difficult to characterize. If this symptom is of sufficient severity to merit pharmacologic intervention, then the clinician should use the same approach to treatment as described in Chapter 15. Generally speaking, methylphenidate is a reasonable first-choice compound in this case.

At the time of this writing, a number of experimental treatments for autism and mental retardation have been reported. They include buspirone, an adrenocorticotropic hormone analogue, amisulpride, bromocriptine, and various vitamin therapies. With the exception of buspirone, none of these are recommended for use until further properly conducted studies evaluating their efficacy and side effects are available. Buspirone demonstrates a relatively benign side effects profile and may be considered in augmentation strategies if first-line medications such as high-potency neuroleptics or fluvoxamine have proven only partly effective.

Long-Term Pharmacologic Treatment in Mental Retardation

The guidelines for long-term treatment of behavioral disturbance in mental retardation are not established. Prudent clinical practice suggests that the need for medications be re-evaluated at regular intervals. A reasonable guideline is to review all treatment procedures at least once a year. Pharmacologic treatment should be part of that review, and the medications may be gradually tapered and stopped to determine if they are still required to assist in behavioral control. Should they still be necessary, as determined by an increase in symptom ratings, the medication can be restarted.

Alternatively, it may be decided to attempt other pharmacologic interventions to attempt to provide even better symptomatic control. Should this be considered, careful evaluation of the best approach should be undertaken because combination and augmentation strategies in this situation have not been adequately assessed. In addition, sufficient time should be allowed at each dosage level to determine the potential therapeutic efficacy of this strategy.

SUGGESTED READINGS

Aman MG. Assessing Psychopathology and Behavior Problems in Persons with Mental Retardation: A Review of Available Instruments. Rockville, MD: U.S. Department of Health and Human Services, 1992.

Aman MG. Efficacy of psychotropic drugs for reducing self-injurious behavior in the developmental disabilities. Annals of Clinical Psychiatry, 5:171–188, 1993.

Aman MG, Singh NN (eds). Psychopharmacology of the Developmental Disabilities. Berlin: Springer-Verlag, 1988.

Arnold LE, Aman MG. Beta blockers in mental retardation and developmental disorders. Journal of Child and Adolescent Psychopharmacology, 1:367–373, 1991.

Cook EH, Leventhal BL. Autistic disorder and other pervasive developmental disorders. Child and Adolescent Psychiatric Clinics of North America, 4:381–399, 1995.

Evans RW, Clay TH, Gualtieri CT. Carbamazepine in pediatric psychiatry. Journal of the American Academy of Child and Adolescent Psychiatry, 26:2–8, 1987.

Farber JM. Psychopharmacology of self-injurious behavior in the mentally retarded. Journal of the American Academy of Child and Adolescent Psychiatry, 26:296–302, 1987.

Kleijinen J, Knipschild P. Niacin and vitamin B_6 in mental functioning: A review of controlled trials in humans. Biological Psychiatry, 29:931–941, 1991.

McDougle CJ, Price LH, Volkmar FR. Recent advances in the pharmacotherapy of autism and related conditions. Child and Adolescent Psychiatric Clinics of North America, 3:71–90, 1994.

Pinder RM, Brogden RN, Swayer R, et al. Pimozide: A review of its pharmacological properties and therapeutic uses in psychiatry. Drugs 12:1–40, 1978.

Ratey J, Mikkelsen E, Sorgi P, et al. Autism: The treatment of aggressive behaviors. Journal of Clinical Psychopharmacology, 7:35–41, 1989.

Sloman L. Use of medication in pervasive developmental disorders. Psychiatric Clinics of North America, 14:165–182, 1991.

CHAPTER 17

Other Conditions for Which Psychopharmacologic Treatment Is Indicated in Children and Adolescents

In addition to the syndromes and symptoms described in earlier chapters that are often the focus of psychopharmacologic treatment in child and adolescent psychiatry, a number of other conditions that may bring a child to psychiatric evaluation are amenable to pharmacologic interventions. This chapter discusses the most common of these conditions. These range from those that have psychiatric diagnoses, such as Tourette's syndrome or simple chronic tic disorder, to those that are not necessarily psychiatric in nature, such as enuresis, but which may be encountered during the psychotherapeutic treatment of a child, adolescent, or family. It is important that the clinician be familiar with the various treatment options available for these conditions as well. This chapter reviews the pharmacologic treatment for the following disorders: Tourette's syndrome, tic disorder, bulimia, anorexia nervosa, enuresis, personality disorders, insomnia, phase four sleep disorders, and disruptive behavior and aggression.

Tourette's Syndrome

Tourette's syndrome is an inherited hyperkinetic disorder of motor, vocal, and behavioral tics, the symptoms of which range from mild to quite severe. Of diagnostic and treatment importance is that Tourette's syndrome may often arise comorbidly with attention-deficit hyperactivity disorder (ADHD), obsessive compulsive disorder (OCD), major depression, and various anxiety disorders.

CASE EXAMPLE

A Young Adolescent with Tourette's Syndrome and Poor Tic Control

P.D. was a 14-year-old boy with Tourette's syndrome who was referred for reassessment of his pharmacologic treatment. A diagnosis of Tourette's syndrome had been made 7 years previously, and he had been treated initially with haloperidol, with some success in reducing his motor and vocal tics. However, he exhibited problems with compliance, although according to his referring physician, he had experienced no significant side effects from the medication. For about 2 years prior to this assessment, he was taking haloperidol about 2 mg daily on a prn basis, determined by his assessment of need.

P.D.'s parents had separated when he was about 8 years of age, and he lived with his mother and two younger siblings. His mother reported being overwhelmed with the responsibilities of child rearing and had herself been admitted to the hospital suffering from "nervous breakdowns" at least three times over the previous 5 years. At the time of P.D.'s assessment, the local child protective agency had become involved in monitoring his youngest brother at the request of a school teacher, who had been concerned about the level of care that he was receiving.

P.D.'s mother accompanied him to his appointment. She seemed unclear about the nature of his illness and the purpose of his medication treatment. She felt confident that she could, however, look after his medications. Nevertheless, she was very concerned about side effects from "drugs" and described some of her own experiences with "bad effects."

P.D. also seemed quite unclear about both the nature of his disorder and the medications. He voiced no concerns about taking medicines, but he admitted that he often forgot or could not be bothered to take them. He wanted his tics to "go away" because he felt uncomfortable with them, particularly in social situations.

The consulting physician completed a full physical examination of P.D. This included careful ratings of tic frequency and severity using the Yale Global Tic Severity Score (YGTSS) and the Hopkins Motor/Vocal Tic Scale. In addition, the physician completed a 10-minute videotaping of P.D. as an additional evaluation of tic severity. Following this, a discussion of useful medications for tics was held.

TABLE 17–1 Suggested Medications for Treating Children and Adolescents with Tourette's Syndrome

Medications for Tics*	Medications for Associated Disturbances
Haloperidol[†] Pimozide[†] Clonazepam	Methylphenidate—inattention, hyperactivity Clonidine—aggression, hyperactivity Buspirone—anxiety Fluoxetine—obsessions Clomipramine—obsessions

*In some cases, the use of haloperidol or pimozide may not only improve tics but may also improve some of the associated symptoms of the disorder. Similarly, some of the medications listed under Medications for Associated Disturbances may by themselves improve tics. In deciding on a first-line treatment for children and adolescents with Tourette's syndrome, the physician should review the guidelines for decision making regarding initial pharmacotherapy found in Section Three.

[†]Suggested as reasonable choices for first-line medications.

CASE COMMENTARY

This case describes a young adolescent with Tourette's syndrome. It also illustrates one of the common issues regarding the pharmacologic treatment of this disorder. What is conspicuous by its absence is information about the patient's school and social functioning. Difficulties regarding family functioning are hinted at but not pursued. Instead, the physician has chosen to focus on the tics. Indeed, in this example the clinician has overfocused! The use of multiple and relatively equally valid instruments in the measurement of one symptom (such as tics) is inappropriate and unnecessary.

Although tic symptoms of sufficient severity are of course a target for pharmacotherapy, they are not a sufficient target in patients with Tourette's syndrome. These children and adolescents will often have moderate to severe difficulties with attention, hyperactivity, social functioning, academics, and getting along with family members. In some cases, these difficulties may contribute as much or even more to the child's or adolescent's functional problems than the tics themselves. In many cases, the use of other medications directed at these symptoms will lead to as much or more functional improvement as the treatment of the tics themselves (Table 17–1). The take-home message in the pharmacotherapy of Tourette's syndrome is as follows: By all means treat the tics if these are a problem but do not ignore other pharmacologically treatable symptoms. Indeed, some ex-

perienced clinicians suggest that when presented with a Tourette's syndrome patient they assess for ADHD and OCD, treat the *most* disabling symptoms first, assess the outcome, and then decide on further pharmacologic interventions if necessary.

Optimized monotherapy using either haloperidol or pimozide in some cases may improve the tics and many aspects of functioning in this disorder. However, some cases may require a combination of medications to treat a wide range of disturbances. In such cases, treatment should be initiated first with haloperidol or pimozide, and the other medication should be added if necessary once optimal effects with the first are obtained.

Baseline Medical Assessment

Because initial treatment for the tic components of Tourette's syndrome is usually with a low dose of a high-potency neuroleptic—either haloperidol or pimozide—those medical assessments that pertain to treatment with those compounds need to be obtained at baseline. In addition to a comprehensive medical history and physical examination, the following are suggested:

1. The Extrapyramidal Symptom Rating Scale (ESRS; see Appendix III)
2. The Abnormal Involuntary Movements Scale (AIMS; see Appendix III)
3. The Medication-Specific Side Effect Scale (MSSES; see Appendix IV)

Baseline Laboratory Assessment

This should include evaluation of those physiologic parameters expected to be of importance in the monitoring of low-dose, high-potency neuroleptic treatment:

1. CBC
2. Liver function tests
3. ECG if pimozide will be used

Baseline Psychiatric Assessment

This evaluation should include:

1. A tic severity rating scale (see Appendix VI for suggestions) or a simple tic counting chart that uses a minimum of a 5-minute assessment window
2. Appropriate Visual Analogue Scales (VAS) for other treatment targets
3. Assessment of social functioning scale, such as the adolescent Autonomous Functioning Checklist or the Social Adjustment Inventory for Children and Adolescents (SAICA)—see Appendix VII

Initiation of Treatment

Medication treatment of Tourette's syndrome usually begins with low doses of a high-potency neuroleptic, either haloperidol or pimozide (Table 17–2). Although haloperidol is perhaps the most

TABLE 17–2 Suggested Medications for Use in Treating Tics in Tourette's Syndrome*

Medication	Initial Dose	Initial Target Daily Dose Range
Haloperidol	Children, 0.25 mg daily	Children, 1–2 mg
	Teens, 0.50 mg daily	Teens, 2–4 mg
Pimozide**	Children, 0.5 mg daily	Children, 4–6 mg
	Teens, 1.0 mg daily	Teens, 4–10 mg

*These suggestions have been determined on the basis of clinical experience and the available current literature regarding the pharmacotherapy of Tourette's syndrome in children and adolescents. Individual patients will vary in their therapeutic and adverse event responses; thus dosing must be individualized depending on the patient's clinical needs. Optimization of pharmacotherapy may require higher or lower daily doses than those identified above.

**Because of potential cardiotoxicity at higher doses, do not exceed doses of 10 mg daily in children or 20 mg daily in adolescents. Increase the dose beyond 8 mg daily in children and 14 mg daily in adolescents *only* if cardiac function is carefully monitored and no other reasonable strategies for pharmacotherapy are available.

commonly used, pimozide may have fewer extrapyramidal side effects. However, at higher doses pimozide may express greater cardiac effects and lower the seizure threshold more than haloperidol. In terms of efficacy in tic control, there is little reason to choose one medication over the other. However, many physicians prefer haloperidol, perhaps because of greater familiarity with this compound or because of concerns about potential cardiotoxicity with pimozide. Both are described later. Further information about haloperidol may be found in Chapter 16, and the antipsychotic medications as a group are discussed in Chapter 13.

Haloperidol

Haloperidol is a butyrophenone-derivative neuroleptic. It has strong dopaminergic activity and is less sedating and less likely to cause hypotension and hypothermia than chlorpromazine or other phenothiazines. It does, however, cause relatively more extrapyramidal side effects. This issue may be of importance, particularly in adolescents, who seem to be more sensitive than adults to the extrapyramidal effects of neuroleptics.

Haloperidol is well absorbed orally and exhibits a bioavailability of about 60 percent. It demonstrates a high degree of protein binding (about 92 percent), and peak plasma levels are obtained 2 to 6 hours following a single oral dose. It is available in intramuscular form as well, and when used in the treatment of agitated psychotic patients (not suggested for children or adolescents), maximum serum levels are found in 10 to 20 minutes, with its peak pharmacologic action noted at about 30 to 45 minutes. Also available in a long-term injectable form as haloperidol decanoate, it can be used for the long-term maintenance treatment of schizophrenia. An intramuscular injection of a single dose of haloperidol decanoate typically reaches a peak plasma level in 6 to 7 days and is usually repeated monthly (range, 3 to 5 weeks) to maintain steady-state plasma levels.

Haloperidol undergoes hepatic metabolism, and its potential side effects are described more fully in Chapters 13 and 16. Of particular importance to haloperidol, however, is its potent inhibition of P-450 2D6 and its potential effect on other drugs metabolized by this pathway. Poor metabolizers, which may include a higher proportion of African-Americans and Chinese, show higher plasma levels of haloperidol at specific daily dose levels. The clinical significance of P-450 2D6 inhibition in treating children and adolescents with Tourette's syndrome is unclear because this population would most likely receive low doses (1 to 4 mg daily).

In addition, care must be taken when combining haloperidol with other psychotropic medications not to cause inadvertent and potentially toxic increases in the plasma levels of other psychotropics metabolized by P-450 2D6 (Table 17–3). This may be of importance in treating children and adolescents with Tourette's syndrome because some of these medications may be used to target the associated symptoms of the disorder.

In addition, because many adolescents experience extrapyramidal side effects with haloperidol treatment, if this medication is initially given in doses over 4 mg daily, it is suggested that prophylactic antiparkinsonian medications also be considered. Although severe dystonic reactions are uncommon at this low dose, distressing extrapyramidal symptoms can occur. Because these may limit further medication compliance, it is not unreasonable to cover the teenager with an antiparkinsonian medication such as procyclidine (5 mg twice daily) and gradually discontinue this 6 to 8 weeks later after the high-risk window for the onset of these adverse events has decreased. See Chapter 13 for further information regarding this issue.

Finally, physicians should be aware that haloperidol preparations may contain the yellow dye, tartrazine, which may cause severe allergic reactions in sensitive individuals. Children and adolescents who are allergic to aspirin may be more likely to experience some sensitivity to tartrazine.

When used in the treatment of Tourette's syndrome, the initial daily target dose of haloperidol is 1 to 4 mg. In young children, treatment is often begun using doses of 0.25 or 0.5 mg daily, given in liquid form. In adolescents, the initial dosage can be 0.5 to 1.0 mg daily. Sufficient time should be allowed to elapse between dose increments in order to assess the therapeutic response; 2 to 3 weeks may be a reasonable time frame. Although some clinicians prefer to use twice-daily dosing, this is not really necessary given the long half-life of haloperidol. If the child or adolescent tolerates the dose well, it can be given later in the day or at bedtime as a single daily dose. Most children

and adolescents will demonstrate reasonable decreases in tics at doses of haloperidol of 1 to 4 mg daily. As discussed in Section Three, optimization strategies should be used to maximize treatment outcome.

Pimozide

Pimozide is a diphenylbutylpiperidine derivative neuroleptic. Unlike most traditional neuroleptics, it demonstrates predominantly D2 receptor antagonism and has little effect on catecholamines, apart from dopamine. The practical results of its central nervous system (CNS) acetycholine and GABA effects are unclear. Clinically, pimozide may lower the seizure threshold and, although it has comparatively weak anticholinergic effects, these may still occur, especially at higher doses. Its alpha-adrenergic blocking activity may be associated with its cardiovascular effects, and it is known to cause ECG changes, including ? prolonged QT interval, U waves, and T-wave inversions. Doses of more than 20 mg per day are not recommended because of concerns about sudden deaths reported at these levels. ECG monitoring is recommended during pimozide treatment. This should occur at baseline and 2 to 3 days following each dose increase.

Although it is less sedating and may be less likely to affect temperature control than phenothiazine neuroleptics, pimozide nevertheless shares many of the potential side effects of these compounds (see Chapter 13). In addition, pimozide use has been reported to be associated with facial edema, light sensitivity, visual disturbances, and nocturia, although these side effects are rare.

Pimozide is rapidly absorbed following oral dosage and undergoes extensive first-pass metabolism. Peak plasma levels are reached 4 to 12 hours following an oral dose, but there is no known correlation between plasma levels and clinical response. Pimozide has an elimination half-life that extends from 50 to 150 hours or more, and thus requires only once-a-day or even once-every-2-days dosing.

In Tourette's syndrome, pimozide has been reported to be as effective as haloperidol in short-term treatment and may be better tolerated. As with haloperidol, insufficient information is available regarding its long-term use in Tourette's syndrome. Initial treatment is usually begun with doses of 0.5 mg daily in prepubertal children or 1 to 2 mg daily in adolescents. A symptomatic improvement of about 70 percent is considered to be a reasonable target of treatment, and at steady state daily doses of pimozide in Tourette's syn-

TABLE 17–3 **Commonly Used Psychotropics That Also Inhibit P-450 2D6**

Fluoxetine	Moclobemide	Fluphenazine
Paroxetine	Desipramine	Perphenazine
Sertraline	Thioridazine	Chlorpromazine

Adapted from Pollock, B. Recent developments in drug metabolism of relevance to psychiatrists. Harvard Review of Psychiatry, 2:204–213, 1994, with permission.

drome generally range from 4 to 8 mg, although higher doses are reasonable if further efficacy and good tolerability are identified. As with haloperidol, dosage increments are best spaced 2 to 3 weeks apart to allow for adequate determination of therapeutic efficacy and side effects at any one given daily dose.

CASE EXAMPLE

P.D. Chooses Treatment and then Augmentation

Because an adequate trial of neuroleptic had not been applied in his case and P.D. had seemed to receive some benefit with minimal side effects from haloperidol in the past, it was suggested that P.D. try haloperidol again. P.D. and his mother agreed to this suggestion. Haloperidol was begun at a dose of 1 mg daily and was increased to a level of 2 mg in 2 weeks. On this dose, P.D. demonstrated about a 50 percent improvement in his tics. Although he was complaining of no physical symptoms and his ESRS and MSSES showed no changes over baseline, his mother refused to allow for further increases in the dose of his medication. Her reasoning was that 3 mg daily was much too high a dose, and no amount of discussion or education about the medication dosage and treatment could change her mind. P.D., however, complained that although his symptoms were much improved, he wanted further relief. But he also refused more haloperidol, and neither P.D. nor his mother would consider a switch to pimozide. They were not adverse to his taking another medication to "help the Haldol work."

After many hours of fruitless discussion regarding these matters and a prolonged assessment period for further evaluation of the haloperidol treatment, the physician agreed to add another medication to "help the Haldol." Because P.D. had reported a number of anxiety symptoms at baseline and over the course of treatment, the clinician suggested clonazepam. This was initiated at a dose of 0.25 mg daily, with an initial target dose range identified as 1 to 2 mg daily (see Chapter 9). Three days later it was increased to 0.5 mg daily, given in divided doses.

At a dose of 0.25 mg clonazepam given twice daily, the frequency of P.D.'s tics decreased and he reported feeling "much better inside." The physician had finally contacted the school to enlist their assistance in dispensing P.D.'s med-ication because P.D.'s mother complained about her inability to do so, and P.D. himself was not the most reliable in this matter. The school nurse, who was on site all day, was willing to take on this task, and the necessary legal and educational issues were addressed.

During the weekends, P.D. took responsibility for his own medications because his mother did not "want to be bothered." Although he still occasionally "forgot" to take his medications, follow-ups at 2 months and 6 months showed much improved compliance than at baseline, with continued good symptom control. P.D.'s mother was particularly pleased with the outcome, mostly because she had "told the doctor all along that P.D. needs a helper drug for the Haldol."

CASE COMMENTARY

This case describes an augmentation approach to maximizing pharmacotherapy. In this case, the rationale for choosing this strategy instead of the tried and true technique of optimization with monotherapy was patient and parent wishes not to pursue this course. In such a case, augmentation is a reasonable alternative, even if in the clinician's opinion it is not the first choice. The issues regarding this are discussed in Section Three.

At this time, a number of antipsychotic medications other than haloperidol or pimozide may be considered in the treatment of Tourette's syndrome. Trifluoperazine in doses of 2 to 15 mg daily may be of use, but it offers no benefit over haloperidol or pimozide. The atypical neuroleptic risperidone in doses of 1 to 3 mg daily may be of value, particularly if reports of fewer side effects than typical antipsychotics stand up to study in this population. A number of other medications may also be useful, either as a first-line alternative to a neuroleptic or as an augmentation strategy. These are listed in Table 17–4, along with suggestions for their consideration.

In addition, methylphenidate may be combined with either haloperidol or pimozide to treat attention, concentration, hyperactivity, and impulsivity problems in Tourette's syndrome patients. Although Tourette's syndrome and tics in general are considered by some to be a contraindication to stimulant treatment because stimulants may exacerbate tics, extensive clinical experience and some research suggest that this is not necessarily the case. If careful baseline assessment and continued

TABLE 17–4 **Potential Uses of Medications Other than Haloperidol or Pimozide in Treating Tourette's Syndrome**

Medication	Possible First Line	Possible Augmentation or Combination	Suggestions
Risperidone	×		Useful in patients who tolerate haloperidol or pimozide poorly
Clonidine	×	×	Useful in patients with comorbid ADHD/behavior problems
Desipramine		×	Same as for clonidine; watch cardiovascular effects
Fluoxetine		×	Same as for desipramine but without cardiac concerns; watch interaction with antipsychotics
Clonazepam		×	Useful in patients with comorbid panic/anxiety but may be helpful in those without
Clomipramine		×	Useful in patients with obsessive or compulsive features

monitoring of tics are done, methylphenidate can be used if clinically indicated. Should tic symptoms worsen with stimulant treatment, this can then be discontinued. If the physician chooses to use a stimulant in this situation, adding measures of tic severity to an n of 1 study on the effect of methylphenidate on hyperactive symptoms (see Chapter 15) is a useful assessment strategy.

Long-Term Treatment

Because the effects of long-term treatment with these medications are not well understood, it is reasonable to review their use on a yearly basis. The general issues involved in such a review are discussed in Section Three. If drug discontinuation is chosen, this should be done gradually. Careful evaluation of symptoms both prior to drug discontinuation and for a reasonable time thereafter is necessary. Because of the prolonged washout of antipsychotic medications, a drug-free period of 2 to 3 months may be necessary in order to allow for a proper evaluation of their effects.

Treatment of Tourette's Syndrome— Practice Points

1. Pharmacotherapy should target tics and associated symptoms that impair functioning. The most disabling symptoms should be addressed first.
2. Initial pharmacologic treatment may include either haloperidol or pimozide.
3. Combined medication treatments may be necessary to address the entire range of target symptoms.

4. Chronic treatment should be carefully monitored for efficacy and tolerability, including periodic attempts designed to determine the continued optimal efficacy of pharmacologic treatment.

Tic Disorder (Non-Tourette's Syndrome)

Tics are generally classified as simple or complex, and may have a lifetime prevalence of 5 to 20 percent in children and adolescents. The treatment of Tourette's syndrome was discussed earlier, and the medications of choice are haloperidol or pimozide, with alternatives such as clonidine or clonazepam. In some cases, however, patients with moderate to severe tics but without Tourette's syndrome may seek treatment. Often this is initiated either because of concerns about Tourette's syndrome or because the tics (particularly if facial) may be embarrassing to the individual or cause problems in social functioning.

In other cases, children or adolescents with behavioral, attention, or obsessive symptoms will present with chronic tics. Syndromal diagnosis in this population may not be positive because many will not meet threshold criteria for Tourette's syndrome, ADHD, conduct disorder, or OCD. In most cases it will not be clear if the problem is a chronic simple tic disorder with functional impairment or an early onset of a more malignant multiple tic disorder. Although many patients with this symptom complex can learn to manage with proper support and education, others may exhibit a functional disability that approaches moderate or greater severity. These children should not be denied pharmacological treatment because their disorder does not meet the diagnostic criteria for Tourette's syndrome, particularly if reasonably effective and well-tolerated interventions are available.

CASE EXAMPLE

A Young Boy with Chronic Simple Tic Disorder and Behavior Problems

W.A. was a 10-year-old boy who was referred for assessment of possible Tourette's syndrome. He had exhibited eye-blinking tics for 3 years prior to assessment. Although they seemed to be stress related, they were present constantly, in all situations—school, home, and play. There were no other motor tics, and no respiratory tics had ever been noted. These eye-blinking tics were socially embarrassing. W.A. was often the brunt of cruel jokes and seemed to be an easy target in the schoolyard for bullying, which he felt was the result of his being "different than the other kids."

In addition to the tics, W.A. had a number of other problems. He was not doing very well academically, and his teachers often complained to his parents about his disruptive classroom behavior and his difficulties in completing his assignments. He was not popular among his peers and often got himself into difficulties because of his "jokes" about them. As he put it, "I just get it into my head and out it comes." At home he was often felt to be irritable and would frequently instigate conflicts with one of his three siblings.

A family history in first-degree relatives was unremarkable. However, W.A.'s father became concerned that one of his uncles had suffered from Tourette's syndrome after seeing a television special on this topic. Although he had not been able to confirm this, W.A.'s parents, who had nevertheless been concerned about his tics and other problems, proceeded to a psychiatric assessment of his condition.

No clear-cut Axis I disorders could be identified at assessment, except for the chronic simple tics, although the physician did wonder about possible ADHD. W.A. was medically fit, and a review of his medical history with the family physician confirmed this. Following a detailed discussion of these findings with W.A. and his parents, it was decided to attempt pharmacologic treatment of the tics because of the severe social impairments that W.A. and his parents both felt were at least in part due to the eye-blinking tics he experienced. The presence of other symptoms of a behavioral and attentional nature were also identified as potentially amenable to pharmacologic intervention.

CASE COMMENTARY

This case illustrates the problem of subsyndromal symptoms and chronic tics identified earlier. It is not clear in this case (and indeed, in many cases) if the tics and behavioral problems relate in a causal or correlational fashion. In such a clinical situation, the physician may wish to consider a pharmacologic intervention that addresses both the tics and behavior problems. A number of possible pharmacologic interventions are available that do not include the antipsychotics discussed earlier. The suggested first-line medication in this situation is clonidine, because it may be of value in improving both tics and the behavioral symptoms.

In other cases, anxiety symptoms that may not meet the criteria for an anxiety disorder predominate. In the context of moderate to severe distress or functional impairments in a patient with tics and anxiety symptoms, clonazepam treatment may be considered (Table 17–5).

Initial Treatment

Baseline medical and laboratory evaluations include those that may be expected to change during treatment. For clonidine, the following are suggested, in addition to a complete history and physical examination.

1. Specific clonidine side-effects scale (see Appendix IV)
2. Heart rate and blood pressure
3. Liver function tests

Psychiatric baseline evaluations should include a measure of tic severity and frequency, and an ob-

TABLE 17–5 Suggested Medication Choices for Non-Tourette's Chronic Tic Disorder in Children and Adolescents

Medication	Suggested Clinical Indication
Clonidine	If the patient presents with concurrent symptoms of hyperarousal, such as short attention, impulsivity, hyperactivity, irritability
Clonazepam	If the patient presents with concurrent symptoms of anxiety, such as rumination, excessive worry, or multiple functional complaints

jective assessment of related disturbances that might also be a target for treatment. In the latter case, VASs are practical and useful.

Clonidine

Clonidine is an imidazoline derivative hypotensive agent that has received some study in the treatment of anxiety, mania, schizophrenia, and attention-deficit disorder, in addition to tics and other behavioral aspects of Tourette's syndrome. It is known to stimulate a variety of alpha-2-adrenergic receptors in the CNS. Clonidine is well absorbed orally and percutaneously following topical application to the chest or upper arm using a transdermal preparation. Peak plasma levels are obtained 3 to 5 hours following oral dosing and 2 to 3 days following transdermal application. Although its half-life varies from 6 to 20 hours, its pharmacodynamic effect is thought to last for 6 to 8 hours following oral ingestion, thus necessitating the use of multiple daily dosing. Common side effects in part reflect its alpha-2-agonist activity and are as follows:

Drowsiness	Nausea
Dizziness	Vomiting
Headache	Rash
Fatigue	Weakness
Nightmares	Orthostatic hypotension
Sedation	Vivid dreams
Dry mouth	Withdrawal syndrome

These common side effects have been identified from clinical experience and a review of the available current literature on clonidine treatment of children and adolescents. Abrupt withdrawal of clonidine should be avoided, even if the patient is taking a low dose of the medication, because it may be associated with a withdrawal syndrome that can range from mild to severe. Should this occur, treatment with small doses of clonidine followed by a more gradual withdrawal may be useful. Symptoms of the clonidine withdrawal syndrome include:

Hypertension	Headache
Nervousness	Sweating
Agitation	Tremor
Restlessness	Palpitations
Anxiety	Hiccups
Insomnia	Muscle pains
Increased salivation	Abdominal pain

In addition to its use in Tourette's syndrome, clonidine may be of value in ADHD and in treating some of the symptoms found in children or adolescents with autism. The suggested role for clonidine treatment in Tourette's syndrome, ADHD, and autism is found in those chapters that address those disorders. Currently no guidelines have been established to help the practitioner in selecting those patients who may benefit most from clonidine treatment. In general, children with symptoms of tics, inattention, hyperactivity, and poor frustration tolerance may be considered as possible candidates for clonidine treatment.

Unlike neuroleptic treatment for tics, in which the daily dose of medications used is usually substantially less than that chosen for treating psychosis, the dose of clonidine is quite similar for all its child and adolescent indications. Oral dosing is typically begun with a target dose of 0.05 mg. This is followed by an initiation strategy of 0.05 mg given once daily, increased by 0.05 mg every 4 to 7 days to an initial target dose. The initial target daily dose range is 0.15 to 0.20 mg daily, given in divided doses of 0.05 mg three or four times daily. Maximal doses are usually in the range of 0.15 to 0.30 mg daily, given in three or four divided doses, although in some cases, if the medication is well tolerated, a total daily dose of 0.50 mg may be achieved. Optimization strategies for clonidine treatment should follow the guidelines described in Section Three.

Clonidine may have a delayed rate of therapeutic onset; therefore, reasonable clinical practice suggests that once the initial target dose of 0.05 mg given three or four times daily (0.15 to 0.2 mg daily) is reached, it should be held for 2 to 6 weeks to establish its potential efficacy. In addition, clinical experience suggests that some children and adolescents may demonstrate mild daily withdrawal-type symptoms, particularly insomnia and restlessness late in the evening, if the last dose of the day is given 6 or more hours before bedtime. Furthermore, some evidence suggests that up to 20 percent of children treated with clonidine may require an upward adjustment of their total daily dose several months after treatment onset, because partial tolerance to the therapeutic effect of clonidine may occur over time.

If clonidine treatment is successful, some children and adolescents may be successfully switched from an oral to a transdermal preparation if they prefer. The skin patch form is best applied to the chest or upper arm; absorption from other parts of the body may differ. The optimal time frame for each patch is 5 to 7 days. Because the total amount of medication per patch is slightly more than is needed for the entire treatment period, care must be taken not to exchange the patch more quickly than indicated earlier to avoid overdosing. Three patch strengths are available: the 3.5 cm size (approximately equivalent to 0.1 mg/24 hr), the 7 cm size (approximately equivalent to 0.2 mg/24 hr), and the 10.5 cm size (approximately equivalent to 0.3 mg/24 hr). Once the optimal total daily dose is established, the closest patch equivalent can be applied.

Transient skin reactions are relatively common with the use of the transdermal patch. Often, however, they may occur as a result of the patient using an adhesive overlay to more securely fasten the skin patch. These mild reactions can be managed by alternating the location of the patch between the chest and upper arm locations. Occasionally, skin reactions can become so problematic that they require a return to oral dosing. In some cases, oral dosing following discontinuation of transdermal treatment may be associated with a return to localized or generalized rashes. Disposal of used skin patches must be done carefully to ensure that other individuals in the family, particularly infants or young children, do not have access to them. Fold the patch in half, with the sticky sides together, place it in a fastened bag or other container, and immediately dispose of it in a secured container.

CASE EXAMPLE

Young Boy Treated with Clonidine for Tics and Behavior Problems

W.A.'s parents chose clonidine treatment and, although he expressed some negative feelings about using a medicine, he was interested in determining if this would "get rid of the tics." Clonidine treatment was begun at a dose of 0.05 mg given in the morning. No significant side effects were reported at this dose, and 4 days later it was increased to 0.10 mg given in divided doses. This dose was maintained for a week, and his tics and side effects were again evaluated.

At this level, W.A.'s blood pressure showed no baseline diastolic changes and no significant orthostatic drop. Although he complained of headaches, there was no increase in their severity rating from baseline. His eye blinking was rated by his parents as 25 percent decreased. W.A.'s self-rating of his tics showed no improvement. The physician's use of a tic evaluation scale (Appendix VI) suggested mild improvements.

It was decided to increase the clonidine dose to 0.15 mg daily, given in three divided doses— morning, early evening, and before bed. A repeat assessment carried out 1 week later showed a parental tic rating of 80 percent improvement from baseline. The physician rating was consistent with a moderate to excellent response. W.A. self-rated his tics as decreased by 50 percent.

Target behavioral symptoms had also been evaluated using various specific VASs. There was global improvement across all the various behavioral targets, ranging from 60 percent in terms of classroom behavior (W.A.'s parents were in weekly contact with his teacher) to 40 percent in his home irritability. W.A. reported that he still was being picked on at school. W.A.'s diastolic blood pressure was not significantly different from baseline, and he had no orthostatic drop. He was complaining of headaches but, once again, there was no increase from baseline measures. No other side effects were identified.

Accordingly, a short-term program of social skills behavioral treatment was planned for W.A., focusing on his peer relationships. Because both W.A. and his parents felt encouraged about his improvement, it was decided that he would continue on his clonidine at least until his social skills treatment was completed. A follow-up appointment was made for 2 months in the future, and W.A. and his family were encouraged to call if any problems arose or if they wishes to discuss any changes in the clonidine treatment.

Six weeks later, W.A.'s mother called to report that W.A. was having difficulty falling asleep. A review of his course to date identified that his parents had changed his dose schedule to morning, noon, and 1500 hours, when he returned home from school. This change in dosage schedule had been followed by the sleeping difficulties that his mother now described. At the physician's request, the last dose of the day was once again moved to between 1900 and 2100 hours, with a resulting improvement in W.A.'s sleep disturbance.

When next seen, W.A. continued to maintain a good response to clonidine treatment. His social functioning had improved somewhat, but both he and his parents realized that this would be an ongoing issue, requiring further psychotherapeutic interventions. Discussion about continued clonidine treatment led to the decision to gradually withdraw the medication to determine if it was still of value, and W.A.'s clonidine was decreased to 0.05 mg, given in the morning and in the late afternoon. A review of his progress 3 weeks later indicated that the tics as well as his behavior problems had increased in frequency. Increasing the dose back to 0.15 mg daily was accompanied by improvement, but not to the level of symptom control achieved prior to the initiation of drug tapering. Subsequent increase of the clonidine to 0.05 mg given four times daily achieved the same symptom control as had been obtained previously on 0.15 mg daily. It was mutually decided that further decisions about possibly discontinuing the medication would be put on hold for 6 to 9 months.

CASE COMMENTARY

This case illustrates a number of issues commonly arising during clonidine treatment: the potential for interdose rebound symptoms and the possibility of tolerance or a need to increase the initially effective dose when tapering of medication leads to a return of symptoms. Using rational pharmacotherapy strategies, these can often be dealt with reasonably. If optimization strategies provide an insufficient therapeutic outcome, the clinician might consider augmentation of clonidine with clonazepam. Guidelines for long-term treatment with clonidine have not yet been clearly defined, and good clinical practice includes careful monitoring and periodic re-evaluation of medication efficacy and tolerability (see Section Three).

Treating Non-Tourette's Chronic Tic Disorder—Practice Points

1. Ensure that other treatment methods are unsuccessful and that patient distress or functional impairment is present.
2. If behavior problems, such as attention difficulties, impulsivity, or overactivity, are present, consider clonidine as an initial treatment.
3. If anxiety symptoms complicate the picture, consider clonazepam as an initial treatment.
4. Careful systematic monitoring of efficacy and tolerability is indicated, and chronic treatment should include regular periodic evaluation to determine optimal pharmacologic treatment.

Bulimia Nervosa

This eating disorder of unknown etiology is characterized by periods of secretive binging and, in many cases, purging accompanied by endocrine and metabolic abnormalities. Up to one third of patients may have a prior history of anorexia nervosa. Major depression, substance abuse, and Axis II disorders can often complicate the clinical picture. Epidemiologic studies suggest that the prevalence of bulimia nervosa is about 2 percent, with the disorder often first onsetting in adolescence.

At this time, although pharmacologic treatments for bulimia nervosa have been investigated in adult populations, few if any systematic and controlled studies have been conducted in adolescents. Thus, the clinician is left with the common problem in child and adolescent psychopharmacology—extrapolating from adult data into a younger and different population. Psychotherapeutic interventions can be useful in patients with bulimia nervosa, particularly cognitive behavioral or group therapies. Medications should thus be reserved for those patients with significant symptoms and functional impairment who have not been responsive to optimal psychotherapeutic interventions. Furthermore, when medications are used in bulimic patients, they should be part of a comprehensive treatment package and should be prescribed in conjunction with a psychotherapy known to have demonstrated efficacy in this disorder.

Patients whose primary disorder is a severe Axis II disturbance or substance abuse and who demonstrate bulimic symptoms as part of a mixed state of psychiatric disturbance are not good candidates for pharmacologic treatment of bulimia. In this population, if pharmacologic treatment is to be considered, low-dose neuroleptics that affect both dopamine and serotonin system functioning (see later under personality disorder) may be of value.

Given the information available to date, no one pharmacologic intervention clearly stands out as the optimal medication treatment for every case. Given the impulsivity and Axis II problems demonstrated by many bulimic patients, care must be taken in the prescribing of medications, even those that have demonstrated some possible clinical utility in this disorder. Thus, traditional monoamine oxidase inhibitors (MAOIs) with their rigorous dietary considerations, and lithium, with its potential for toxicity in the presence of sodium loss (through vomiting or diuretic/laxative abuse), would not be recommended as a medication of first choice in this population. Other medications should be avoided altogether because they may induce serious side effects more commonly found in bulimic patients than in other patient groups. An example of this is the antidepressant bupropion, which may be associated with a higher incidence of seizures when used in bulimic patients.

In addition, substantial long-term studies of

pharmacotherapy in bulimic patients are few, and the advantage of medications over long-term psychotherapies has not been demonstrated. Thus, the pharmacologic treatment of bulimia nervosa remains largely empirical and directed toward the short term (2 to 6 months). Patients who demonstrate a good response (a decrease in bulimic symptoms of >50 percent), however, may be considered as candidates for longer term treatment if continued efficacy and tolerability can be demonstrated.

Baseline Medical Assessment

Baseline medical assessment consists of a thorough history and physical examination. An MSSES (see Section Two) should be completed prior to beginning any drug treatment. Baseline laboratory investigations should include the following:

1. Serum electrolytes, CBC, and liver function tests
2. Serum and urine drug screen
3. ECG

If significant physiologic abnormalities are identified at baseline testing, then medication treatment should be delayed until further medical investigations have been conducted and it is deemed that the use of a specific pharmacologic intervention will be relatively safe. Periodic monitoring of all the laboratory measures listed earlier is necessary because bulimic patients are known to under-report the frequency and severity of their binges and purging behaviors. Excessive vomiting and laxative or diuretic abuse can lead to metabolic disturbances that will increase the likelihood of adverse effects from medical treatment, and thus frequent laboratory evaluations are needed.

Initial Pharmacologic Treatment

The suggested initial choice of medication for the pharmacologic treatment of an adolescent with bulimia is one of the serotonin-specific reuptake inhibitors (SSRIs) (Table 17–6). Although fluoxetine has been most extensively studied in both short- and long-term treatment, sertraline, with its minimal effect on weight gain and its relatively low rate of serious drug-drug interactions, may be a possible alternative. These medications may show potential efficacy with a much more attractive risk/benefit ratio than any of the other alternatives. The use of these compounds is detailed in other chapters (e.g., Chapter 11), and the reader is referred there for information regarding these medications. The daily dosage is similar to that

TABLE 17–6   Medications of Potential Use in the Pharmacologic Treatment of Bulimia in Children and Adolescents*

Medication	Probably Useful	Demonstrated as Probably Useful in Adults but Not Recommended in This Age Group
Fluoxetine	×	
Sertraline	×	
Monoamine oxidase inhibitors		×
Lithium		×
Tricyclic antidepressants		×
Anticonvulsants		×

*These suggestions are based on clinical experience and the currently available literature on the pharmacologic treatment of bulimia. Given the paucity of studies in children and adolescents, the clinician should carefully evaluate the risks and benefits of using pharmacotherapy for this disorder in this population. Guidelines for decision making regarding this issue may be found in Section Three.

used in the treatment of major depressive disorder, except that for fluoxetine daily dosages of 60 or 80 mg may be necessary.

CASE EXAMPLE

Bulimia, to Treat or Not to Treat, That Is the Question . . .

O.V., an 18-year-old girl, was referred by a local youth service agency for psychiatric assessment and pharmacologic consultation regarding treatment of her "bulimia." Psychiatric history elicited a 5-year duration of substance abuse that included alcohol, marijuana, hashish, cocaine, amphetamines, and LSD. In addition, O.V. reported two arrests for "trafficking" and one arrest for "breaking and entering." She had been convicted once and was currently on probation. She had been offered a treatment program for her substance abuse but had refused. O.V. was also engaged in prostitution, an activity that she relied on for her income. Her violent outbursts and assaults on a shelter volunteer staff member and another female resident had resulted in her being asked to leave the youth shelter where she had been staying.

O.V.'s bulimic symptoms consisted of occasional binges of "everything that I can get my hands on" and food cravings, "especially when I'm coming down off a high." She engaged in occasional purging behaviors, admitting to one or two episodes of self-induced vomiting over the past month, but denied any laxative or diuretic use. She described occasional episodes of self-mutilation, usually burning herself with a cigarette butt or cutting her wrists when, as she put it, "I needed a place to get my head together for awhile," which would often lead to a short-term inpatient admission. She had never followed up on any outpatient psychiatric treatments.

No history of psychosis, mood disorder, or other Axis I psychiatric illness could be clearly identified. She stated that she knew nothing about her family history and refused to let the physician contact them. She also refused to let the physician contact her primary care physician and would not name one (although she did state that she had at least three who she saw occasionally and who prescribed for her "medicines for my nerves"). O.V. refused any laboratory investigations, including a drug screen and an HIV test.

When the clinician voiced doubts about the value of using any medications to treat her bulimic symptoms and suggested that these should be addressed as part of a comprehensive treatment package that included a substance abuse program, she became quite angry and hostile, and left the office in a rather unpleasant manner. The referring source, when contacted, stated that she had not returned to the agency for further services.

CASE COMMENTARY

This case illustrates that there are patients who, while they may clearly require psychiatric services, have not made the pharmacologic treatment of their eating disturbance a priority. Prescribing a medication in such a situation will serve no useful purpose.

Pharmacologic Treatment of Bulimia Nervosa—Practice Points

1. Medications should be used to augment or enhance psychotherapeutic interventions.
2. Careful baseline and continued monitoring of serum electrolytes and ECG may be necessary in this population.
3. Only those medications with a clearly positive benefit/risk ratio should be considered, such as SSRI antidepressants.

4. The presence of bulimic symptoms in a complex of severe Axis II disturbance or substance abuse is a relative contraindication for pharmacotherapy directed primarily at the bulimic problem.

Anorexia Nervosa

At this time, although a plethora of medications have been evaluated in treating this disorder (largely in adults), no medication has clearly demonstrated efficacy. Furthermore, given the metabolic complications that can arise in patients with anorexia nervosa and the effects of these on increasing the potential for serious medication-induced side effects, the dangers of medication use clearly outweigh the benefits. Thus, it is recommended that no pharmacologic treatment directed primarily at anorexia disorder be attempted. If anorexia nervosa exists comorbidly with another psychiatric illness, such as a major depression or OCD, pharmacologic management appropriate to that disorder may be undertaken, but only if more conservative measures, such as cognitive or interpersonal psychotherapy, have been proven by themselves to be ineffective, and then only with very careful weekly medical monitoring (serum electrolytes, weight, blood pressure, heart rate, ECG) using medications that have a low level of cardiotoxicity, such as SSRIs for depression.

Pharmacologic Treatment of Anorexia Nervosa—Practice Points

1. Medication treatment directed primarily at symptoms of anorexia is not indicated.
2. Medications may be used to treat patients in whom anorexia nervosa exists comorbidly with another psychiatric disorder known to potentially respond to a particular pharmacotherapy. If this course of action is chosen, the least cardiotoxic compound should be used and weekly monitoring of weight, electrolytes, blood pressure, and ECG should be instituted.

Enuresis

The etiology of functional or primary enuresis, as it is sometimes called, is not fully understood but may be related to delayed maturation of CNS mechanisms that control the micturition reflex.

Enuresis may occur nocturnally or during the daytime as well. Children who exhibit both day and night wetting require further medical investigations other than the usual initial urinalysis recommended for those who exhibit nocturnal or daytime wetting alone. Enuresis should be differentiated from marked urinary frequency, which is usually self-limiting over a relatively short period of time, and incontinence. Children presenting to a clinician for treatment of enuresis may also have an underlying structural urinary tract abnormality. Those who present with the following associated clinical features should be referred for medical evaluation above and beyond a baseline urinalysis:

Abnormal urinalysis

Around-the-clock wetting

History of frequent urinary tract infections

Failed optimal pharmacologic treatment

The efficacy of pharmacologic treatment of functional enuresis has been relatively well established in the child and adolescent population. Nevertheless, some clinicians argue that medications may remain an option to be considered only when other forms of nonpharmacologic intervention have been unsuccessful or are not possible, such as when the child is staying away from home overnight, for example, summer camp. They recommend that behavioral techniques, such as bedtime voiding routines coupled with the bell-and-pad apparatus, should be given an adequate trial first. If significant enuresis continues to be a problem, medications should be used because prolonged enuresis can have a negative impact on a child's or adolescent's self-esteem and social activities.

Other clinicians note that in many cases parents or children cannot or do not wish to take part in behavioral treatment regimens for enuresis. A common complaint in family members of the nocturnal enuretic is that the bell-and-pad apparatus is often more useful in waking them than it is in waking the patient. As discussed in Section Three, the clinician should provide the patient and family with the necessary information about the various treatment modalities for this condition and allow for a collaborative decision-making process to occur regarding initial treatment. In some cases, patients and parents may wish to proceed directly to pharmacologic interventions.

According to some authors, nocturnal enuresis may respond to treatment directed toward constipation using diet, bulk fiber agents, and occasional lubricants. This may be effective in 30 percent or more of the population without any other interventions needed. If this is chosen as a prebehavioral therapy and prepharmacotherapy approach, the use of oral bulk fiber preparations and lubricants is suggested at a frequency of two to three times per week. Caution should be exercised with regard to the excessive use of lubricants on normal bowel function, and it is expected that such treatment would only need to last until the appropriate changes in diet take effect.

A number of options in medication use are available. They are listed and first-choice suggestions are made in Table 17–7. Most medicines used in treating enuresis are tricyclic antidepressants, although 1-deamino-8-arginine-vasopressin (DDAVP) is also quite useful, although perhaps less familiar to psychiatrists.

If a tricyclic is being considered as a first-choice pharmacotherapy for enuresis, potentially useful tricyclics and issues regarding their choice may be of value in the process of clinical decision making (Table 17–8).

TABLE 17–7   Suggested Medications for Treating Enuresis

First Choice	Alternate Choices
DDAVP or Imipramine	Desipramine Clomipramine Oxybutynin

TABLE 17–8   Tricyclic Medications of Value in Treating Enuresis

Medication	Treatment Issues to Be Considered
Desipramine	Rapid treatment onset Total daily dose usually 25–100 mg (1–2.5 mg/kg) Concerns regarding potential increased sudden death risk Careful cardiac (ECG) monitoring suggested Less studied than impramine
Imipramine	Rapid treatment onset Total daily dose usualy 25–100 mg daily Higher rates of anticholinergic side effects Possible therapeutic levels of 60 mg/ml or higher
Clomipramine	Rapid treatment onset Total daily dose usually 25–100 mg High rates of anticholinergic side effects Possible therapeutic window 20–60 mg/mL Less studied than imipramine

Baseline Evaluation

Baseline medical evaluation should include a detailed medical history and physical examination. If a medical or structural problem is suspected, the child should be referred to the appropriate medical specialist. Baseline laboratory evaluation should include the following:

1. CBC
2. Serum creatinine and blood urea nitrogen
3. Urinalysis, routine and microscopic (include specific gravity determination)
4. ECG (if a tricyclic is being used)
5. Blood and urine glucose determination

CASE EXAMPLE

Tricyclic Antidepressant Treatment of Enuresis in a Young Adolescent Boy

P.B. was a 13-year-old boy referred by his outpatient therapist for possible pharmacologic treatment of enuresis. P.B. gave a history of nocturnal enuresis that went back "as far as I can remember." Apart from the enuresis, no psychiatric diagnosis was identified. He had been receiving outpatient psychotherapy twice weekly for about 1 month to help him in dealing with the accidental death of his younger sister, who had been involved in a traffic accident as a passenger on a school bus. Although he reported that he was "doing OK," he described occasional "bad dreams" or nightmares, and difficulty falling asleep. His symptoms did not, however, meet diagnostic criteria for posttraumatic stress disorder. There had been no significant change in his enuretic symptoms associated with this severe life stress.

A meeting with P.B.'s parents confirmed the history and identified that enuresis averaged about three to five nights per week. Two previous attempts using "bell-and-pad" techniques had been unsuccessful. P.B. had refused to attend summer camp because of this problem and avoided overnight activities with his friends. He was becoming more concerned about this problem because he had recently begun to excel at skiing and had joined a competitive team, which necessitated his being away from home for races and training. He was very concerned about the enuresis and was quite keen to attempt medication treatment.

After full discussion of the options, imipramine treatment was selected. It was also believed that its sedative effects might lead to improved sleep, both in terms of falling asleep and decreasing the "nightmares."

CASE COMMENTARY

Imipramine is a reasonable first choice in selecting a pharmacotherapy for enuresis. In this case, its sedative effect was also of potential benefit for other, nonrelated symptoms suffered by the patient. DDAVP is also quite costly in comparison with imipramine, and this may be a factor for many families in choosing between the two compounds.

CASE EXAMPLE

P.B.'s Treatment

Following a test dose of 25 mg given at noon, imipramine treatment was initiated at a dose of 25 mg given in the evening. An initial target daily dose range of 50 to 100 mg was identified, and 75 mg chosen as the midpoint. The dose was raised by 25 mg every 5 days until 75 mg was reached. This was maintained for 2 consecutive weeks to allow for evaluation of outcome. An ECG was obtained 1 week following the attainment of the initial target dose.

At a daily dose of 75 mg, 25 mg taken when he returned home from school around 4 pm (1600 hours) and 50 mg taken about 1 hour before bedtime. P.B. experienced a good therapeutic response of about 80 percent improvement in the frequency of nocturnal enuretic episodes. He subsequently was also able to better control his evening fluid intake and, with this combined treatment paradigm, was able to attend training and racing sessions with his skiing teammates. A follow-up 2 months later showed him to be taking the medication without adverse effects. He was essentially asymptomatic with regard to the enuresis.

CASE COMMENTARY

This case illustrates a positive response to imipramine treatment in enuresis. The issue of how long treatment should continue remains to be resolved.

Imipramine

Imipramine is a dibenzapine derivative tricyclic antidepressant currently used in the treatment of major depression. It is also indicated for the treatment of enuresis in children ages 6 and older. The exact action in enuresis is not known but may involve inhibition of urination by either peripheral or central means.

Imipramine is well absorbed following oral administration and undergoes hepatic metabolism through the P-450 2D6 system. Thus it is expected that its metabolism will be affected by any compounds that inhibit the P-450 2D6 enzyme. In addition to its effect on norepinephrine uptake, imipramine interacts strongly with the serotonin, histamine, and acetylcholine systems. Many of its side effects are associated with its actions on these systems. Common side effects in children and adolescents treated with imipramine are those found with all medications of this class, but with more sedative, gastric, and anticholinergic symptoms than found with desipramine. These are listed in Table 17–9.

Although the doses of imipramine used in treating enuresis ($<$2.5 mg/kg, 10 to 100 mg daily) are rarely associated with clinically significant changes in cardiac function, prudent clinical practice suggests that in addition to baseline ECG determination, the ECG should be obtained 3 to 5 days following each increase in dosage. Suggested parameters for cardiac ECG monitoring in children and adolescents treated with tricyclic medications are found in Chapter 11.

Peak plasma levels of imipramine occur 1 to 2 hours following oral ingestion. Plasma half-life varies between 8 and 16 hours. Thus, oral dosing can be once daily when steady-state levels are reached. Some commercial preparations of imipramine may contain tartrazine, to which some children and adolescents may be allergic. In some individuals this may induce bronchial spasm, which may occur more frequently in patients who are sensitive to aspirin.

Dose indications for imipramine treatment of enuresis are in the range of 1.0 to 2.5 mg/kg/day. Clinically, this works out to between 25 and 100 mg daily, usually given in divided doses, with the majority of the daily dose given in the evening to assist in sleep induction and decrease daytime sedation. However, in most cases the entire dose can be given before bedtime. Because imipramine's onset of enuretic action is rapid (2 to 4 days), the length of time needed to evaluate its therapeutic efficacy is minimal, and the intervals between dose increases are primarily determined by how well the patient tolerates the medication. Some evidence suggests that combined imipramine-desipramine serum levels of more than 60 mg/mL are necessary for a therapeutic response. Thus, judicious use of serum levels, if they are available, may assist in dosage adjustments, although this is not usually necessary unless the lack of therapeutic response to a reasonable dose suggests a compliance or rapid metabolism concern.

A reasonable dosing schedule is as follows: Treatment may be initiated by taking a test dose of 10 mg. In older children and adolescents, 25 mg orally about 1 hour before bedtime is a reasonable starting dose. In younger children, 10 mg may be sufficient. If this dose is not effective but the medication is well tolerated, the dose can be increased to 50 mg daily (20 mg daily for younger children) within 1 week. Using this same schedule, the dose can be increased to a maximum of 100 mg daily. Because imipramine comes in 10, 25, and 50 mg strengths, this allows for flexibility in dosing. There is some evidence that those patients who experience nocturnal enuresis during the first third of the night may benefit from a dosing regimen in which half the dose is given in the mid-afternoon and the other half of the dose is given 1 hour before bedtime.

Long-Term Treatment

Imipramine treatment of enuresis should be continued for 6 to 8 weeks prior to consideration of medication withdrawal. Chronic imipramine treatment for enuresis may often be associated with relapse if the medication is withdrawn. Restarting the medication after relapse may not lead to a similar level of therapeutic response. These considerations must be kept in mind when long-term treatment possibilities are discussed. Prudent use of imipramine in enuresis includes periodic re-evaluations of continued need for treatment and side effects.

Desmopressin Acetate

An alternative medication is desmopressin acetate, an antidiuretic hormone analogue. Desmopressin acetate is a synthetic polypeptide structurally related to arginine vasopressin. Because

TABLE 17–9 Side Effects of Imipramine Treatment in Children and Adolescents

Neurotransmitter Involved	Side Effects
Norepinephrine	Tremors, insomnia, sexual dysfunction, tachycardia
Serotonin	Anxiety, gastric distress, headache, agitation, restlessness
Histamine	Sedation, drowsiness, weight gain, hypotension
Acetylcholine	Dry mouth, blurry vision, constipation, urinary retention, memory problems, sinus tachycardia
Alpha$_1$-blockade	Dizziness, orthostatic hypotension, tachycardia, sedation

many enuretic children show abnormal nocturnal secretion of the antidiuretic hormone, it was postulated that nocturnal use of desmopressin acetate would mimic the expected usual increase of nocturnal antidiuretic hormone secretion. It is delivered by nasal spray or solution, and acts to decrease the urinary flow rate by increasing renal absorption of water without affecting serum sodium, potassium, or creatinine concentrations.

Desmopressin acetate is given intranasally by spray. Its antidiuretic effect onsets in about 30 to 60 minutes and lasts from 5 to 20 hours, although individual variation in these times does occur. Clinically significant side effects are relatively rare, and most side effects, when they do occur, are mild. Of note, increased blood pressure can occur with intranasal doses greater than 40 μg, but doses of 20 μg generally show little or no effect on heart rate or blood pressure. Dose-dependent increases in plasma factor VIII and inducement of platelet aggregation can occur, and if patients with bleeding disorders or von Willebrand's disease are considered for treatment of enuresis, imipramine should be selected as the first-choice medication. If desmopressin is used in these patients, clinicians inexperienced in their care should seek the assistance of a pediatrician or hematologist for monitoring bleeding and platelet indices.

Potential side effects of desmopressin acetate treatment include the following:

Hypertension	Nostril pain
Gastrointestinal complaints	Epistaxis
Flushing	Rhinitis
Conjunctivitis	Nausea
Ocular edema	Cough
Lacrimation difficulties	Sore throat
Dizziness	Chills
Headache	Clotting
Nasal congestion	problems

These side effects may occur but are relatively rare and are usually associated with doses above the recommended therapeutic range.

Drug-drug interactions with DDAVP are also relatively uncommon but can occur with the following:

Lithium	Alcohol
Epinephrine	Carbamazepine
Heparin	

Desmopressin acetate is applied intranasally into the high nasal cavity. Children, adolescents, and their parents will need to be taught how to apply it properly. One spray dose of desmopressin nasal spray is equal to 10 μg and spray doses can only be given in multiples of 10. The usual starting dose is 20 μg, one spray per nostril given about one-half hour before bedtime. If after 1

week there is not a significant reduction in nocturnal enuresis, the dose can be increased to 40 μg (two sprays per nostril). Doses above 40 μg are not suggested. If successful amelioration of symptoms occurs at 20 μg, the dose can be decreased to 10 μg to determine if the lower amount will provide sufficient control.

The long-term effects of desmopressin treatment have not been well studied, although chronic treatment of up to 1 year's duration has been reported. Prudent clinical practice suggests that periodic evaluation of the continued need for desmopressin be undertaken, perhaps at 3-monthly intervals. There is some evidence that dosage requirements may change over time, with either increases or decreases in the initial dose being needed to provide control of enuresis.

Pharmacologic Treatment of Functional Enuresis—Practice Points

1. Conduct a proper evaluation of the wetting problem, considering the possibility of a medical condition.
2. Select either a tricyclic antidepressant (imipramine or desipramine) or desmopressin acetate.
3. Continue pharmacotherapy for 6 to 8 weeks and then evaluate to determine continued need for treatment.
4. Consider long-term treatment if relapse occurs following discontinuation of medication after the acute treatment stage.
5. Consider the possibility of prn pharmacotherapy, which could be directed toward specific conditions (such as sleepovers or camp) if the patient has mild symptoms with minimal functional impairment. If this route is chosen, evaluate the use of the medication well in advance of its expected use.

Personality Disorders

Pharmacotherapy of personality disorders is an area under active study in adults, yet few if any satisfactory reports are available for adolescents. The diagnosis of personality disorder is not usually applied to children. Of all the personality disorders, borderline personality disorder (BPD) has received the most detailed investigations. In this population, low-dose, high-potency neuroleptics, the MAOIs tranylcypromine and phenelzine, and the SSRI fluoxetine have shown some promise. Thymoleptics and anticonvulsants have not clearly demonstrated utility, and benzodiazepines are contraindicated.

The diagnosis of BPD in adolescents is complicated by the presence of mood disorders, and recently available evidence shows that this diagnosis should not be applied when an adolescent is experiencing a depressive or hypomanic episode. Adolescent substance abusers will often meet criteria for BPD because of the CNS effects of the substances they are abusing. Thus, although this diagnosis must be approached with caution in the adolescent population, it nevertheless can occur and cause considerable distress and functional morbidity. Current treatment of adolescents with BPD usually applies a variety of psychological treatments, none of which have been validated in this population. Self-regulatory strategies, including problem solving, coping skills, and cognitive behavior interventions in the context of an expected interpersonal relationship, may be helpful. Only a few studies of pharmacologic interventions are available, and controlled studies are lacking. However, some evidence for efficacy with pharmacologic treatments is available, and medications should be considered in those adolescents with BPD who are exhibiting severe disturbances that may lead to significant morbidity or mortality (Table 17–10).

Given the clinical characteristics of the borderline population, in particular the presence of mood instability, impulsivity, and the high rate of self-injurious behaviors, the use of medications

TABLE 17–11 Suggested First-Choice Medications in Treating Adolescent Borderline Personality Disorder

Medication	Initial Dose	Initial Target Daily Dose Range
Flupenthixol	1 mg daily	1–3 mg daily, single dose
Haloperidol	1 mg daily	1–5 mg daily, single dose
Risperidone*	1 mg daily	1–3 mg daily, single dose

*Should be considered experimental.

with significant potential for toxicity in overdose should not be considered. This includes the MAOIs tranylcypromine and phenelzine, and any tricyclic antidepressant. Low-dose neuroleptics prescribed concurrently with low doses of prophylactic antiparkinsonian medications may be the drugs of choice, given the information currently available and the risk/benefit ratio when compared with other available medications (Table 17–11). Of particular interest in this population are low-dose neuroleptics, which show both dopamine and serotonin effects because the behavioral and affective symptoms of BPD may be mediated by these neurotransmitter systems. These medications include flupenthixol and risperidone.

CASE EXAMPLE

Double, Double, Toil and Trouble: The Borderline Adolescent

K.L. was a 17-year-old girl referred for psychopharmacologic consultation by an adolescent outpatient mental health clinic, where she was receiving individual and group psychotherapy. She had been given a psychiatric diagnosis of BPD, and her case manager believed that medications might be of value to help her with her impulsivity, depression, and mood reactivity.

Diagnostic evaluation confirmed the presence of an Axis II disturbance of BPD. A past major depression of 10 months' duration that had spontaneously remitted 2 years previously was identified. In addition, substance abuse, including alcohol and "soft drugs," was present. A pregnancy had been terminated by therapeutic abortion 6 months previously, and a medical history was positive for a sexually transmitted disease. She was HIV negative as tested 1 month earlier but continued to engage in unprotected intercourse. She had been arrested twice for shoplifting but had received suspended sentences in both cases.

TABLE 17–10 Potentially Useful Pharmacologic Interventions for Adolescents with Borderline Personality Disorder: Clinical Suggestions

Medication	Consider Use	Avoid Use	Unclear
Haloperidol	×		
Flupenthixol	×		
Risperidone	×		
Tranylcypromine		×	
Phenelzine		×	
Tricyclics		×	
Benzodiazepines		×	
Lithium		×	
Antiepileptic thymoleptics			×
Serotonin-specific reuptake inhibitors			×

*The suggestions in this table have been determined by clinical and research experience and a review of currently available information regarding the pharmacologic treatment of this population. Decision making about the use of psychopharmacologic treatments should be made using the guidelines described in Section Three. No literature regarding optimal pharmacologic treatment of children with this disorder is available.

Recently, K.L. had moved into a therapeutic group home for adolescent girls. She had started attending a local secondary school with some success. She identified these changes as positive and attributed much of this to her psychotherapeutic involvement. A detailed family history was not available because K.L. had cut off all contact with her family a number of years previously. She denied a history of sexual abuse but reported a history of being "hit" by her father when he had been drinking.

A discussion of the medication options, their risk/benefit ratio, and a realistic appraisal of their potential efficacy led to her choice of flupenthixol as a pharmacologic intervention. Further, she agreed to allow the group home staff to dispense her medications, and they agreed to participate in symptom monitoring. Target symptoms of dysphoria (assessed using the Beck Depression Inventory), impulsivity (assessed using the Ward Scale of Impulsivity), and global self-rating (SCL-58) were identified at baseline.

Treatment of Borderline Personality Disorder

Baseline medical and laboratory investigations are the same as for high-potency neuroleptics and, in addition to a medical history and physical examination, include the following:
1. MSSES (see Appendix IV).
2. ESRS (see Appendix III).

Baseline psychiatric evaluations are tailored to the target symptoms. It is suggested that they include:
1. Self-assessment of dysphoria/distress (Beck Depression Inventory; see Appendix VI).
2. An impulsivity scale (Ward Scale of Impulsivity; see Appendix VI).
3. A global self-measure of general functioning (SCL-58).
4. An objective measure of global functioning (Global Assessment of Functioning; see Appendix V or Autonomous Functioning Checklist; see Appendix VII).

Flupenthixol

Flupenthixol is neuroleptic of the thioxanthene class that in higher doses (>9 mg daily) is indicated in the treatment of psychosis and in lower doses (3 to 6 mg daily) has demonstrated antidepressant effects of a magnitude similar to both tricyclics and SSRIs in adult populations. Flupenthixol exhibits dopamine (D1 and D2), serotonin (5-HT2), and alpha-1-adrenergic activity. Low doses (1 to 3 mg/day), but not high, (9 to 18 mg/day) doses of flupenthixol are associated with

maximal activation of its serotonergic effects, combined with a moderate dopaminergic effect.

Absorption following oral administration is good, and its long half-life allows for once-daily dosage. It is available in a long-acting injectable form, which allows for flexibility and good monitoring of compliance in chronic use. Its side effect profile is similar to that found with other neuroleptics of its class (see Chapter 13), and side effects are less severe at low doses (1 to 3 mg daily) than at typical antipsychotic doses. Nevertheless, prudent clinical practice suggests that prophylactic antiparkinsonian agents such as procyclidine (5 to 10 mg daily) should be prescribed concurrently with flupenthixol treatment.

Treatment should be initiated with 1 mg daily and continued for 8 weeks at this dose. Evaluation of the therapeutic effect should be made at that time. Potential adverse effects should be monitored weekly. If this dose is well tolerated and the therapeutic effect is not maximal, the dose should be increased to 3 mg daily taken at bedtime and maintained for a minimum of 8 continuous weeks. Outcome evaluation should occur every 2 weeks, with weekly monitoring for adverse events during this time. Because compliance can be a serious issue with the BPD population, whenever possible a responsible adult should be enlisted in the process of dispensing the medication on a daily basis.

CASE EXAMPLE

Fire Burn and Cauldron Bubble

K.L. experienced no significant side effects on 1 mg of flupenthixol, and this dose was raised to 3 mg following 4 weeks of treatment. Her initial dose of procyclidine was maintained at 5 mg daily throughout. Although her course of treatment was not uneventful, she persisted in taking her medication throughout and demonstrated a compliance rate of about 80 percent (took her flupenthixol at least 80 percent of the time it was given to her).

At the end of 8 weeks at 3 mg daily (16 weeks in total), her treatment course was reviewed with her and her counselor at the group home. K.L.'s self-report scales showed significant improvements. Her Beck Depression Inventory had decreased from a baseline score of 23 to 10, and her SCL-58 scale score had changed from 133 to 93. The Ward Scale of Impulsivity, which had been scored by her counselor, showed a decrease from a prepharmacology value of 13 to a value of 5. Reports from the group home staff were positive regarding her behavior, she seemed to be particularly better in controlling her angry outbursts, and she was getting along better with staff and other residents. Her psychotherapist reported that she was "working" in therapy.

K.L. was given the choice of continuing the medication. She stated that she wanted to do so because "I feel better and I'm getting my s--t together." She elected to continue with oral medication, although she realized that an injectable preparation was available. Her procyclidine was gradually tapered and discontinued, with no onset of extrapyramidal side effects, and she was seen once-monthly for medication and side effect monitoring for a period of 8 months, at which time she moved to another city to be with her boyfriend, who had taken a job there.

CASE COMMENTARY

This case illustrates, among other things, a very important aspect of the pharmacologic treatment of adolescents with BPD. As a rule, they "vote with their feet"; that is, if they feel that the medication is helpful to them, many will want to continue it, in spite of their histories of impulsivity and previous treatment noncompliance. Unfortunately, the long-term effects of low-dose flupenthixol are not well described, and the same precautions that are taken with chronic use of any neuroleptic medication should be followed here as well. Prudent clinical practice includes regular monitoring for treatment-emergent side effects (once a month), especially for early signs of tardive dyskinesia. Although no scientific guidelines are available, clinical experience suggests that medication treatment should continue for at least 6 months to 1 year, while optimal psychotherapeutic and social interventions are implemented. At that time, gradual dosage reduction, leading to medication discontinuation, may be carried out to determine if pharmacotherapy is still indicated.

Pharmacologic Treatment of Adolescent Borderline Personality Disorder—Practice Points

1. Careful diagnosis is necessary, and particular attention should be paid to a possible mood or substance abuse disorder presenting similar symptoms.
2. Benzodiazepines are contraindicated.
3. Low-dose, high-potency neuroleptics may be useful, particularly those with both D2 and 5-HT2 activity (such as flupenthixol).

4. Begin treatment with concurrent administration of an antiparkinsonian medication, such as procyclidine.
5. Assessment of tolerability should occur weekly, whereas assessment of efficacy should occur every 2 to 3 weeks.
6. An initial treatment trial of about 16 continuous weeks at target doses, with at least 8 continuous weeks at the maximal limit of the target dose, is necessary to determine potential efficacy.
7. Careful consideration of potential risks and benefits, close side effects monitoring, and periodic evaluation of the need for pharmacotherapy are essential in long-term treatment with low-dose neuroleptics.

Insomnia

Insomnia may occur frequently in children and adolescents, and in most cases pharmacologic treatment is not indicated. Insomnia may be classified as primary (transient or chronic) or secondary (transient or chronic). Primary transient insomnia most often occurs following an acute psychosocial or physiologic stressor, such as the death of a family member or a circadian phase shift secondary to transoceanic air travel. Secondary insomnia can result from medical disorders, psychiatric illness (such as depression), substance abuse (including alcohol and caffeine), or as a side effect of medical treatment, for example, with carbamazepine. Pharmacologic interventions are generally reserved for primary insomnia, because treatment of the underlying condition usually alleviates secondary insomnia.

In children and adolescents, behavioral techniques and good sleep hygiene procedures are the preferred initial interventions. Sleep hygiene concerns are very important in this population, particularly in teenagers. Specific approaches to ensure optimal sleep hygiene are found in Table 17–12.

TABLE 17–12 Sleep Hygiene Techniques of Use in Treating Primary Insomnia

Stop	Begin
Don't take the following after noon: Nicotine Caffeine (including cola drinks) Alcohol Over-the-counter medicine (such as appetite suppressants) Don't use the bedroom as a kitchen	Regular exercise Going to bed at same time Develop a bedtime routine

Young children who exhibit problems with insomnia may have developed behaviors that impinge on their ability to fall asleep. Such factors as parental presence in the bedroom and soothing activities (holding, feeding) may become linked to falling asleep, and in their absence the child may experience difficulties. Older children may have insomnia secondary to anxiety or worries or as part of an Axis I disorder, such as generalized anxiety disorder. Adolescents may exhibit difficulties in falling asleep because of worries or a psychiatric illness. In many cases, however, the disruptions in routine sleep-wake cycles caused by weekend behaviors of staying up very late and then sleeping in may be at issue. Identifying potential psychiatric or other conditions that might underlie sleep problems is necessary. A thorough diagnostic assessment will assist in this endeavor. In addition, the keeping of a sleep diary in which the child or adolescent (or parent) provides daily recordings is useful in characterizing the nature of the difficulty and providing a baseline for monitoring treatment outcome. Detailed polysomnographic studies are not initially indicated, but unsuccessful application of optimal behavioral and pharmacologic treatments should lead to a referral to a sleep specialist if this is available.

Primary insomnia can be further broken down into two categories: (1) transient (1 month or less in duration) and (2) chronic (more than 1 month in duration). Given the current state of knowledge of the pharmacologic treatment of child and adolescent insomnia, it is suggested that for primary transient insomnia, medications be used only when other methods have failed or when a clear-cut short-term solution is necessary. For primary chronic (defined as greater than 30 days) insomnia, medications may be useful either as a short-term (1 to 2 week) adjunct to behavioral and sleep hygiene treatments or as a possible solution to an otherwise treatment-unresponsive problem that is leading to functional impairments. Medications to consider in these situations are found in Table 17–13.

When choosing a medication to treat insomnia in this condition, all the caveats that pertain to the risks and benefits of that particular class of compounds apply. These can be reviewed in the various chapters in which they are discussed. The clinical use of the nonbenzodiazepine hypnotics, although not sufficiently investigated in this population, are reviewed later.

If a benzodiazepine is chosen for the treatment of primary transient insomnia, it should be remembered that all benzodiazepines will shorten sleep latency. However, not all show the same onset of hypnotic effect, with flurazepam, temazepam, and quazepam providing a relatively rapid onset of action. Triazolam (an ultra–short-acting benzodiazepine), also demonstrates a relative rapid onset of action, but it is not recommended for use in this population. It has a propensity to lose its effect after more than a few days of use and its withdrawal is associated with the risk of rebound sleep difficulties. Long half-life benzodiazepines may be more likely to produce sedation and reduced daytime performance than ultra-short half-life compounds, which, however, can lead to rebound insomnia and a cycle of self-

TABLE 17–13 **Potential Pharmacologic Treatments for Primary Insomnia in Children and Adolescents***

Type of Insomnia	Medication	Comments
Transient	Flurazepam[†] Temazepam Quazepam	Use for only 1–7 days, then gradually discontinue
Transient	Zopiclone[†] Zolpidem	Use for only 1–7 days, then gradually discontinue
Transient or chronic	Chloral hydrate[†]	Use for either 1 or 2 weeks, then gradually discontinue
Chronic	Flurazepam Temazepam Quazepam	Use for only 1–2 weeks in combination with other nonpharmacologic treatment, then gradually discontinue
Chronic	Doxepin[†] Trazodone[†]	Use only in low doses in combination with other nonpharmacologic treatment and attempt to periodically discontinue by gradual taper

*Pharmacologic treatment of sleep disorders should always occur in the presence of other interventions, such as relaxation training, a sleep hygiene program, and behavior treatments (graduated extinction). The use of sedative medications, such as antihistamines, is not recommended.

[†]Suggested as potential first-line choices.

medication to deal with what are essentially pharmacologically induced effects. Thus, both long-acting and ultra–short-acting benzodiazepines are not suggested for the treatment of insomnia.

Furthermore, there is no good evidence that the initial hypnotic efficacy of benzodiazepines persists beyond 12 weeks of continuous treatment, and findings from some adult studies suggest that beyond 2 to 3 weeks of continuous benzodiazepine treatment, hypnotic effects are not significantly greater than with placebo. Thus, treating insomnia with benzodiazepines is a short-term proposition.

The use of a low dose of the tricyclic antidepressants doxepin (10 to 25 mg 1 hour before bedtime) or trazadone (25 to 50 mg 1 hour before bedtime) is a potentially useful adjunct to nonpharmacologic treatment in primary chronic insomnia. Doxepin exhibits the strongest antihistamine effect of any tricyclic, and daily doses of 10 to 25 mg are unlikely to be associated with any cardiotoxicity. Alternatively, chloral hydrate at doses of 500 mg to 1 g is a safe and often helpful medication if used as recommended in Table 17–13. Its use, however, is associated with increased hepatic metabolism, and it is highly protein bound so as to displace other drugs from protein binding. Thus the potential for drug-drug interactions must be considered in its use. The use of L-tryptophan or barbiturates is not recommended.

CASE EXAMPLE

And So to Bed, Perchance to Dream . . . Primary Transient Insomnia in an 11-Year-Old Boy

D.N. was an 11-year-old boy referred for treatment of primary insomnia by his family doctor. Three weeks prior, D.N.'s best friend's mother, with whom he was quite close, had died of cancer. D.N. had accompanied his best friend to a special religious service that required him to fly to a city that was two time zones away. He returned home 2 days later and was unable to fall asleep at night. This problem persisted despite sleep hygiene behavior interventions.

D.N. had no premorbid history of psychiatric illness, and there was no history of significant sleep problems. A family history was similarly unremarkable. Although he was highly motivated to carry on with his behavioral sleep treatment, he was becoming discouraged because it was not proving to be effective. He was having some difficulty during the day paying attention in class and felt drowsy but did not nap. His parents were concerned about how he

was functioning. Following a discussion of available pharmacologic treatments for primary transient insomnia, D.N. and his family chose to try zopiclone.

Treatment of Primary Transient Insomnia with Zopiclone

Baseline medical and laboratory investigations can be limited to medical history and physical examination if zopiclone treatment is being considered. A specific medication side effect scale completed prior to the initiation of treatment is useful. A VAS used to rate the severity of insomnia as identified by both the child and parent is sufficient for monitoring therapeutic outcome. Alternatively, a sleep diary can be used.

Zopiclone is a cyclopyrrolone that is not chemically related to benzodiazepines but is thought to influence the GABA-A receptor complex. It is relatively well absorbed, and peak plasma concentrations are reached within about 2 hours following oral administration. Zopiclone undergoes extensive hepatic metabolism and has one partially active metabolite. Its elimination half-life varies with age but is approximately 6 to 8 hours in young adults. Treatment requires a once-daily dose given 1 to 1½ hours before bedtime.

Studies of zopiclone use in children and adolescents have not been reported. In adults, significant improvements in sleep latency, sleep quality, number of awakenings during sleep, and sleep duration have been reported across a number of different studies, with a dose of 7.5 mg (3.75 mg in the elderly) showing hypnotic efficacy. Higher doses have not led to increased therapeutic efficacy. Zopiclone may be particularly effective in increasing the amounts of stage four and stage two sleep.

Short-term zopiclone use at doses not exceeding 7.5 mg daily is not usually associated with rebound insomnia or other withdrawal phenomena, especially if the medication is gradually discontinued. If these do occur, they are usually less severe than those reported with benzodiazepines. Although some impairment of acute psychomotor functioning or memory with doses above 7.5 mg has been reported with zopiclone use, these effects are generally not evident within 8 to 10 hours following oral dosing, thus potentially showing fewer next-day effects than are found with some benzodiazepines. Afternoon effects on psychomotor functioning, including driving skill impairments and memory loss, have not been demonstrated with short-term zopiclone use. Combined use of zopiclone and alcohol can lead to additive effects on performance impairment.

Zopiclone is not known to cause euphoria, and

there is no solid evidence of a high abuse potential with this medication. Its abuse has been reported in patients who were known multidrug abusers, and, accordingly, it should not be prescribed to that population. Reported side effects are generally similar to placebo in frequency, apart from dry mouth and a bitter taste, which may affect up to 4 percent of those treated. Drug-drug interactions have not been extensively studied. Concurrent administration of zopiclone and carbamazepine may reduce the plasma concentration of both medications, necessitating more careful monitoring of carbamazepine therapy.

CASE EXAMPLE

Treating with Zopiclone

D.N. was started on zopiclone at a dose of 3.75 mg 1 hour before bedtime taken for three consecutive nights. A telephone conversation with D.N. and his mother revealed that he was not sleeping any better, but he did not report any side effects. The dose was then increased to 7.5 mg at the same time daily. When seen 2 days later, D.N. reported improved sleep and no side effects. This was corroborated by his mother. Zopiclone treatment was continued for 1 week, the daily dose was decreased to 3.75 mg for 3 days, and then it was withdrawn altogether. D.N. did not experience any side effects on this regimen, and his sleep returned to normal.

CASE COMMENTARY

This case illustrates the use of a novel sedative-hypnotic medication that has a number of advantages over the benzodiazepines. It shows equal efficacy to hypnotic benzodiazepines and may demonstrate fewer side effects. Its full potential for withdrawal symptoms has not been adequately evaluated, however, and although the manufacturer suggests that this medication be discontinued without tapering, prudent clinical practice is to taper this medication as described in D.N.'s case. As with all other medication treatments for transient insomnia, zopiclone should only be used in the short term (1 week or less) and then only as part of a comprehensive sleep hygiene program.

Night Terrors and Somnambulism

These disorders are relatively common (5 to 15 percent of children and adolescents), but disorders of stage four sleep occurring in children and adolescents only rarely continue into adulthood. Night terrors are characterized by recurrent episodes of abrupt awakening from sleep, associated with intense fear, excessive autonomic discharge, and confusion. Children with night terrors are severely agitated on awakening and generally are unresponsive to comforting. Morning amnesia regarding the event is common. Somnambulism or sleepwalking is well described by its name.

In general, pharmacologic interventions are used in the treatment of night terrors if the disorder is severe, is long lasting, or leads to significant disruptions in the home. Pharmacologic treatment of somnambulism is rarely, if ever, indicated and only needs to be considered if the sleepwalking is persistent and a threat to the patient's safety. Pharmacologic treatment of these disorders always occurs within the context of other psychotherapeutic interventions.

Night terrors can be treated by either a benzodiazepine or imipramine. Diazepam, given in doses beginning at 2 mg to a maximum of 5 mg 1 hour before bedtime, may be helpful. Clonazepam in doses ranging from 0.5 to 1.5 mg given 1 hour before bedtime can also be used. The possibility of morning hangover effects with diazepam suggests that clonazepam may be tried first. These treatments have usually only been applied for the short term (up to 1 week's duration), but this may be sufficient to alter the pattern of the disturbance. It is not recommended that either of these treatments be continued for more than 2 weeks, and care must be taken to provide gradual withdrawal of the medications to avoid rebound effects.

Another potentially useful medication that should be considered if longer term treatment is indicated is the tricyclic antidepressant imipramine. Doses of 10 to 50 mg given about 1 hour prior to bedtime may provide good symptom control. At such low doses, cardiotoxicity is not usually a concern, but the routine cardiac monitoring parameters in imipramine use identified earlier in this chapter should apply. The side effects of tricyclic antidepressants are further discussed in Chapter 11.

The optimal duration of successful pharmacologic treatment in these disorders is not known. By and large, because they are usually self-limited, long-term therapy is not necessary. If diazepam or clonazepam is used, 1 to 2 weeks of treatment followed by gradual discontinuation is suggested. If imipramine is used, 2 to 4 weeks of initial treatment are not unreasonable as long as the medication is well tolerated. Patients who experience symptom relapse following withdrawal of benzodiazepine treatment may be considered for longer term intervention using imipramine. Prudent clinical practice suggests that if longer term treatment is initiated because of a return of symptoms on discontinuation of medications, periodic evaluation (approximately every 2 to 3 months) using gradual medication taper can be used to determine if pharmacotherapy is still indicated.

Pharmacologic Treatment of Night Terrors and Somnambulism— Practice Points

1. These disorders typically require treatment only in severe and persistent cases, because they are usually self-limiting.
2. Short-term use of diazepam or clonazepam (1 to 2 weeks) may be useful.
3. Imipramine in doses of 10 to 50 mg daily may be useful and more suitable for longer term (2 to 4 weeks) use.
4. Periodic evaluation (every 2 to 3 months) for pharmacologic treatment is necessary if long-term (more than 2 months) treatment is indicated.
5. Don't treat nightmares with medications!

Disruptive Behavior and Aggression

Disruptive behavior may occur as a defining part of a particular psychiatric syndrome, such as ADHD or conduct disorder. Alternatively, it can occur as a phenomenon associated with another psychiatric disorder, such as schizophrenia or mania. In some cases, aggressive or violent actions may occur outside of a diagnosable psychiatric syndrome. In children or adolescents in whom severely disruptive or aggressive behaviors create significant disturbances in their environment and impair the child's or adolescent's social, interpersonal, family, or academic functioning, these behaviors may, in some cases, be the target of psychopharmacologic interventions.

In considering the use of pharmacologic agents for the treatment of disruptive or aggressive symptomatology, it is necessary to carefully determine the category of disruptive disturbance that the child or adolescent is exhibiting, because the pharmacologic interventions for similar symptoms may be different. For example, if the behavioral disturbances are secondary to a psychotic state or disordered mood (such as in schizophrenia or mania), the treatment approach is directed toward the underlying psychiatric disturbance, and the disordered or aggressive behaviors demonstrated by the patient are targeted as one of many symptoms that would be expected to improve with effective treatment of the primary condition. Aggressive or disruptive behaviors that occur as part of the syndrome of ADHD may also in many cases improve with successful pharmacologic treatment of that disorder. In other cases, disruptive or aggressive behaviors may be the primary considerations for treatment, such as in an adolescent with intermittent explosive disorder. A categorizing scheme for disruptive disturbances useful for pharmacologic interventions is suggested in Table 17–14.

In many cases, children or adolescents may fall into more than one of the categories in Table 17–14. This is perhaps most commonly observed with those individuals who meet diagnostic criteria for comorbid disorders involving one of the following: ADHD and conduct disorder, or ADHD and oppositional disorder. In these cases, primary pharmacologic intervention should be directed toward the treatment of the ADHD component of the comorbid state.

A number of medications are available for use in children or adolescents who exhibit severe disruptive or aggressive behaviors (Table 17–15). In gen-

TABLE 17–14 Suggested Conceptual Categorizations for the Pharmacologic Treatment of Disruptive Behaviors and Aggression in Children and Adolescents

Category	Description	Treatment
Syndromal disturbance	Disruptions and aggression occur as defining parts of a specific psychiatric syndrome, e.g., ADHD	Treat the specific syndrome
Associated disturbance	Disruptions and aggression occur secondary to a specific psychiatric syndrome, e.g., mania, schizophrenia, organic brain disorder	Treat the primary disorder
Primary disturbance	Disruptions and aggression occur as primary defining characteristics of a psychiatric syndrome, e.g., conduct disorder, intermittent explosive disorder, organic disorders	Treat with medications and other therapies
Unrelated disturbance	Disruptions and aggression occur sedonary to clear-cut environmental stimuli only, e.g., fighting with a sibling or parent, gang-related behavior	Use nonmedication treatments

TABLE 17–15 **First-Line Medications for the Treatment of Severe Behavioral Disturbances and Aggression in Children and Adolescents**

Medication	Suggested Indications
Stimulants	Aggression associated with ADHD or conduct disorder
Lithium	Intermittent, explosive aggression; episodic aggression associated with organic brain disorders; conduct disorder
Carbamazepine	Intermittent, explosive aggression; episodic aggression associated with organic brain disorders
High-potency neuroleptics	Severely aggressive conduct disorder; behaviors associated with organic brain disorders
Propranolol	Intermittent explosive aggression; episodic aggression

eral, those patients who exhibit episodic aggressive episodes with rapid-onsetting anger and rage seem to be more amenable to pharmacologic interventions than those with a relatively stable and high baseline level of aggression alone. In all cases in which pharmacologic interventions are used to treat aggressive behaviors, they should be yoked with behavioral or cognitive therapies as well.

In choosing a first-line medication for treating aggressive or severely disruptive behaviors, the clinician should follow the framework suggested in Table 17–14 and apply the questions regarding this choice found in Section Three. In all cases in which disruptive behaviors and aggressive acts are found in the context of a syndromal disturbance or an associated disturbance, the initial pharmacologic management should be that of the primary psychiatric disorder. If significant disruptive and aggressive behaviors remain following a good therapeutic response to the pharmacologic treatment of the primary disorder, the patient may be a candidate for combining pharmacologic treatments. In these cases, augmentation strategies (see Section Three) can be used.

Baseline Considerations

In any choice of treatment, the following baseline considerations apply.

Medical Considerations

Medical considerations are those outlined in Section Two. Of particular importance is the evaluation of those physical parameters that may be affected by pharmacologic treatment. In addition, a careful neurologic evaluation should be carried out for the presence of an underlying seizure disorder. The appropriate medication monitoring scales and laboratory considerations for baseline evaluation depend on the medication chosen and are found in those chapters of this book in which the medications listed in Table 17–15 are discussed.

Psychiatric Considerations

Psychiatric evaluation should include those symptoms that are the target of pharmacologic treatment. When aggressive behaviors are the major focus of treatment, the following baseline symptom assessment measures are suggested:

1. Overt Aggression Scale (OAS; see Appendix VI)
2. Ward Scale of Impulsivity—Inpatient or Outpatient Form (see Appendix VI)

In addition, for those children and adolescents who exhibit disruptive behaviors and aggression as a feature of ADHD (syndromal disruption), specific ADHD rating scales should be used (see Section Two). A relatively new rating scale—The New York Teacher Rating Scale—may be useful in evaluating the effects of pharmacotherapy on the aggressive and other antisocial behaviors often associated with ADHD (see suggested readings for scale reference).

CASE EXAMPLE

Nutin' but Trouble: A Young Boy with Aggression and Antisocial Behavior

U.Y. was an 11-year-old boy referred by his school following continued altercations with other children, which included behaviors such as swearing, fighting, rock throwing, and attempted extortion. He was accompanied by his ·mother, a single parent living on social assistance, to the assessment.

A review of U.Y.'s history revealed a long-standing problem with "overactivity," impulsivity, and aggression. He had been identified as a "problem child" when he first entered the public school system in kindergarten. Although he was referred for psychological assessment in first grade, this had never been carried out for reasons that were unclear. Teachers' reports identified learning problems, especially in language, short attention span, hyperactivity, impulsivity, and persistent aggressive behaviors directed at his classmates. U.Y. had been placed in a special education class for children with "emotional-behavioral needs" but had not been successful academically or socially.

U.Y.'s mother described similar at-home behaviors and found him "impossible." She had two other younger children, with whom she also felt unable to cope. She stated that she had not sought any "help" for U.Y. because "it doesn't matter what I do, he's gonna turn out like his dad." U.Y.'s biologic father was, at the time of U.Y.'s assessment, serving a jail sentence for armed robbery.

U.Y. met the diagnostic criteria for ADHD and conduct disorder. A formal education-learning assessment was initiated. Social supports for his mother (child case worker) and a structured after-school program for U.Y. were put into place. A behavioral modification program using a token economy was begun in the classroom, and lithium carbonate treatment was started for his aggression.

At a total lithium dose of 1200 mg daily, U.Y.'s serum level was 0.7 mEq/L. He was experiencing some urinary frequency and complained of "shakes." His medication was kept at this dose for 3 weeks. At the end of this time, there was little substantial change in his OAS scores. Teachers at school reported some improvement in classroom behaviors but no change in playground conflicts. A serum lithium level obtained at this time was 0.3 mEq/L, and U.Y.'s mother agreed that she may have "sometimes forgotten" to give him the medicine.

CASE COMMENTARY

This case illustrates an inappropriate approach to pharmacologically treating aggressive and antisocial behavior in children. U.Y. clearly suffered from comorbid ADHD and conduct disorder, in addition to a problematic social environment and inadequate parenting. In this case, psychosocial interventions directed toward his behavioral problems and family-social environment should have been coupled with proper pharmacologic treatment of his ADHD and conduct disorder (see Chapter 15). Ideally a stimulant medication, such as methylphenidate, would have been an appropriate first choice.

Practical Treatment Issues

Once the type of disruptive behavioral problem has been determined, an appropriate first-choice medication should be chosen. Medication treatment should be initiated as described in previous chapters for the particular compound selected. In most cases, the same target dose range as identified in previous chapters for each medication is suitable for the treatment of aggressive behaviors as well. Antipsychotic medications are the exception, and doses used to treat psychotic symptoms are, in general, too high for initial consideration in treating behavioral and aggressive disturbances. Total daily dose ranges for neuroleptics in this case are usually similar to those required to treat tic symptoms (haloperidol, or its equivalent, 2 to 4 mg daily).

With any compound chosen, treatment is initiated gradually following a reasonable baseline assessment period (2 to 3 weeks are suggested). When the initial target dose is reached, a 2 to 3 week period of continued therapeutic evaluation is necessary to establish therapeutic efficacy of the initial target dose prior to consideration of further dose changes or other optimization strategies.

A good response to treatment should be followed by a medication maintenance phase that should last from 4 to 6 months. During this time, optimization of nonpharmacologic interventions directed at controlling disruptive behaviors and aggression should take place. Following this maintenance phase, the medication can be gradually decreased with appropriate evaluation periods (2 to 3 weeks) of assessment following each dose reduction. Because antipsychotics may be quite slow to leave the body compared with other medications used for similar therapeutic purposes, if they are being withdrawn it is reasonable to extend this observation and evaluation period to 6 weeks following each dose modification. Significant increases in disruptive or aggressive behaviors occurring during the dose de-escalation process should be treated by returning the daily dose to the initial therapeutic level followed by another dose maintenance phase of 2 to 3 months. After this time, further dose-reduction strategies can again be employed if necessary.

No child or adolescent pharmacologically treated for disruptive or aggressive behaviors should have their medications continued for more than 6 consecutive months without a medications review. In many cases, this review might identify that the patient may benefit from further pharmacologic optimization strategies to improve symptomatic control. In other cases, it may be found that the patient may require less medication to provide similar levels of symptomatic control. Various withdrawal strategies useful for particular compounds are found in the appropriate chapters of this book.

SUGGESTED READINGS

Bilwise DL. Treating insomnia: Pharmacological and non-pharmacological approaches. Journal of Psychoactive Drugs, 23:335–341, 1991.

Campbell M, Gonzalez N, Silva R. The pharmacologic treatment of conduct disorders and rage outbursts. Psychiatric Clinics of North America, 15:69–85, 1992.

Corrigan P, Yudofsky S, Silver J. Pharmacological and behavioral treatments for aggressive psychiatric inpatients. Hospital and Community Psychiatry, 4:125–133, 1993.

Dahl R. Child and adolescent sleep disorders. Child and Adolescent Psychiatric Clinics of North America, 4:323–341, 1995.

Erenberg G. Pharmacologic therapy of tics in childhood. Pediatric Annals, 17:395–404, 1988.

Garfinkel PE, Garner DM. The Role of Drug Treatments for the Eating Disorders. New York: Brunner Mazel, 1987.

Hoehns JD, Perry PJ. Zolpidem: A nonbenzodiazepine hypnotic for treatment of insomnia. Clinical Pharmacy, 12:814–828, 1993.

Kutcher S, Papatheodorou G, Reiter S, Gardner D. The successful pharmacologic treatment of adolescents and young adults with borderline personality disorder: A preliminary open trial of flupenthixol. Journal of Psychiatry and Neuroscience, 20:113–118, 1995.

Leibowitz SF. The role of serotonin in eating disorders. Drugs, 39:335–485, 1990.

Mellinger GD, Balter MB, Uhlenhuth EH. Insomnia and its treatment. Archives of General Psychiatry, 42:225–332, 1985.

Miller LS, Klein RG, Piancentini J, Abikoff H, Shah MR, Samoilov A, Guardino M. The New York Teacher Rating Scale for disruptive and antisocial behavior. Journal of the American Academy of Child and Adolescent Psychiatry, 34:359–370, 1995.

Reiner WG. Enuresis in child psychiatric practice. Child and Adolescent Psychiatric Clinics of North America, 4:453–460, 1995.

Roy-Byrne PP, Cowley DS (eds). Benzodiazepines in Clinical Practice: Risks and Benefits. Washington DC: American Psychiatric Press, 1991.

Stein G. Drug treatment of the personality disorders. British Journal of Psychiatry, 161:167–184, 1992.

Stewart JT, Myers WC, Burket RC, Lyles WB. A review of the pharmacology of aggression in children and adolescents. Journal of the American Academy of Child and Adolescent Psychiatry, 29:269–277, 1990.

Trestman RL, de Vegvar M, Siever LJ. Treatment of personality disorders. In A Schatzberg, C Nemeroff (eds): Textbook of Psychopharmacology. Washington DC: American Psychiatric Press, 1995, 753–768.

Wachsmuth JR, Garfinkel PE. The treatment of anorexia nervosa in young adolescents. Child and Adolescent Psychiatric Clinics of North America, 2:154–160, 1993.

Wadworth AN, McTavish D. Zopiclone: A review of its pharmacological properties and therapeutic efficacy as an hypnotic. Drugs and Aging, 3:441–459, 1993.

Werry J. Pharmacotherapy of disruptive behavior disorders. Child and Adolescent Psychiatric Clinics of North America, 3:321–341, 1994.

Postscript

No Person Is an Island: The Current Practice of Child and Adolescent Psychopharmacology in Its Historical Context

Toward an Overview of Historical Forces in the Development of Modern Medicine

"Medicine is a science, the practice of which is an art." Those words, written by Sir William Osler about one century ago, still apply today to all of medicine and certainly to child psychiatry. The gradual shift from a predominantly theory-driven discipline principally resting on a nonverifiable system of beliefs to one that is theory based but driven by verifiable and evaluative methods can, in its broad strokes, be understood to characterize the history of medicine. Although cultural, economic, and political forces and technologic availability obviously shape the expression and pursuit of all scientific endeavors, modern medical science must also stand the test of utility. Pragmatic, effective applicability of that science toward the altruistic goal of the relief of mental and physical suffering distinguishes medicine from its intellectual cousins. The development of effective therapeutics is the cornerstone of modern medicine.

Prior to the adoption of empirical evaluative techniques that could function outside a particular construct of pathoetiology, much medical practice rested more on belief systems as to the "truth" of any one particular perspective than on any externally derived validation of that point of view. Changes in therapeutics usually arose from the substitution of one set of beliefs for another. The move from a priori certainty to empirical validation as the foundation for establishing therapeutic validity heralded the rise of modern medicine. The critical element in this gradual change (it took centuries and is not yet complete) was the demonstration and acceptance that evaluative-based methods could predict therapeutic outcome. This predictive power transcended whatever ideology drove the determination and initial application of the therapy. In short, if a treatment worked it was a "good thing." If it didn't work, it was to be discarded. Pragmatism, the operation of theory in the real world and not adherence to a particular dogma, gradually became the criterion for success in the marketplace of medical ideas.

Parallel to the development and general acceptance of the primacy of such an evaluative necessity for therapeutics, and often as an outcome of the application of the evaluative method itself, increased understanding of the psychophysiologic underpinnings of various signs and symptoms of disease and the usual or normative functioning of the body arose. These processes operated in a type of thesis-antithesis-synthesis scheme, in which better therapeutics and increased understanding of pathoetiologic processes stimulated and challenged each other. As a part of this development, many unsuccessful treatments (and often their underlying assumptions)—biologic, spiritual, or psychological—were relegated to the dustbin of history.

These changes did not occur smoothly or linearly. Applying Newton's first law (a force in one direction is met by an equal force in the opposite direction) to social processes, new applications in the treatment and understanding of various disorders were often associated with strong forces working in the opposite direction. These reactionary social forces challenged rational and empirically evaluated therapeutic methods largely by advancing mostly "irrational" and empirically unprovable alternatives. The effect of these strong counterforces was to hold back or even discredit the application of evaluative-based therapies. Furthermore, these reactionary social forces were found to occur both in society at large and within the particular medical field in which the innovation was proposed. Perhaps this is not surprising because some of these innovations would have challenged the primacy of well-established social, cultural, or institutional hierarchies.

Change, when it occurred, was also never complete, even if the innovative therapy was clearly well substantiated empirically and conferred substantial advantages, therapeutic and economic, over previously established treatments. Adherents to nonvalidated therapeutics continued to take the role of true believers and constantly raised unvalidated criticisms of the innovation. This social phenomenon can in part be understood by applying the second law of thermodynamics to social change. This law observes that when changes of state occur, heat is produced. In the social arena of medical treatments, changes of therapeutics and the challenges to established pathoetiologic understanding that arose from these changes created the heat of social friction. Thus, the outpouring of outrage, protest, and the like that accompanied the introduction of empirically validated therapeutic innovations resulted in the dissipation of large amounts of social energy to little useful end.

In one sense, the current state of affairs in the understanding and practice of child and adolescent psychiatry is undergoing one of these changes that have been so well documented in the rest of medical history. The use of demonstrably effective pharmacologic therapies for children and adolescents clearly challenges the primacy of those existing therapeutic models that derive their legitimacy mostly from a priori certainty as to their efficacy. In addition, the accompanying shift in the understanding of the pathoetiology of child and adolescent psychiatric disorders that the success of psychopharmacologic interventions supports challenges long and strongly held hypotheses and assumptions about the pathoetiology of child and adolescent psychiatric disturbances. Furthermore, the rise of any innovative and empirically validated therapy has the effect of confronting traditional and well-established social, institutional, and clinical hierarchies that have been predominantly established on less firmly substantiated foundations. As might be expected, a heat-producing clash of opposite and equal forces can be expected as the field of child and adolescent psychiatry moves toward a new synthesis.

With this predicted clash of opposite forces, comes another historically observable event. The introduction of a new and potentially effective therapeutic intervention stimulates the enthusiastic and sometimes uncritical acceptance and overapplication of that treatment, even in the absence of any compelling evidence for its efficacy. This seems to apply equally to biologic, psychological, and social interventions. Witness, for example, insulin coma, psychoanalysis for schizophrenia, and family therapy for everything. The reasons for this are undoubtably protean and range from the wish of the practitioner to "do something" to provide relief for suffering, to the less altruistic but nonetheless prevalent push for making a name or making a profit. In many cases, the clinician providing the treatment has a firmly held but misguided belief in its efficacy. This often may be the result of inadequate information about the value of the treatment or a lack of knowledge on the part of the clinician as how to evaluate its efficacy.

In many cases, such treatments become standard procedure, passed on by one uncritical practitioner to another in the worst example of the apprenticeship model of information transfer. Adherence to a particular treatment, even in the absence of validated efficacy, often begins out of deference to authority—listening to one's teacher. It is sustained, however, by the addition of the comfort that the uncritical application of a particular intervention brings to the clinician. This comfort may be based on a need to avoid ambiguity or the challenge of the unknown. Uncritical comfort with a particular treatment modality is more likely to be held by those clinicians whose training and current practice is largely made up of its application. In addition, comfort with a particular treatment modality is more likely to be held if a practitioner experiences treatment as an essential part of a belief system that explains pathoetiology and supports the theoretical viewpoint of the practitioner. To the person whose only tool is a hammer, the entire world is a nail.

The story of treatments in child and adolescent psychiatry should not be expected to differ substantially from the historical patterns of thrusts and counterthrusts that characterize all of medicine. Psychopharmacologic treatments for the psychiatric disturbances of childhood and adolescence are similarly subject to the same historical forces. The clinician should understand these forces so as to be better informed about the effects these processes have on day-to-day practice in the clinic.

Historical Overview: Forces That Shaped Child and Adolescent Psychopharmacology

A brief review of the history of child and adolescent psychopharmacology is then perhaps useful as a way of putting this activity into context and bringing it up to date. History is not a listing of firsts and successes, just as it is not memorizing the names of all the English kings and queens. Knowing only who was the ruler of England in 1701 will help one understand that society about as well as knowing who was the first investigator of methylphenidate in children will help one to understand that drug. That is not to say that this knowledge of firsts and successes in pediatric psychopharmacology is not of value—it is part of the heritage of every child and adolescent psychiatrist. We are what we are and do what we do in part because of who came before us and what they did.

However, although this is necessary knowledge, it is not sufficient. History must use this information as an investigator uses data. The interpretation of data comes from a variety of sources; data are only useful in context. Similarly, historical writing provides a context for understanding, an understanding that can be applied to the present and future as well as the past; this understanding is the goal of this chapter. I hope that this summary will not be seen as an obligatory reading at the end of a book, but as a method of raising the awareness of the participants in the process. Clinical work in the real world can lead to a new synthesis as successes and new understandings arising from the psychopharmacologic revolution in child and adolescent psychiatry are themselves critically evaluated in an ever-ongoing historical process.

Although socially sanctioned healers, parents, and other responsible and caring adults have probably always used diets, potions, pills, and powders to try to help relieve the pain and suffering of psychiatrically disturbed children and adolescents, the modern era of child and adolescent psychopharmacology can perhaps be dated, as Zrull suggests, from the early 20th century. This was the time when childhood was, if not discovered, then re-invented, and in 1906 a textbook on pediatrics written by Dr. Carr recommended that

"habit chorea or habit spasm," a psychiatric diagnosis, be treated not only with an adequate diet but also with Fowler's Solution, which contained the well-known and self-evident curative ingredients of arsenic, quinine, and strychnine. He further noted that if this was not effective, bromides could be added. Thus, in one simple stroke our intrepid Dr. Carr developed both a first-line psychopharmacotherapy for a specific child and adolescent psychiatric disorder and also established the principle of pharmacologic augmentation for treatment nonresponders.

For the perhaps more difficult to treat condition of "hysteria," the good Dr. Carr noted that the treatment of choice included the administration of aromatic spirits of ammonia and apomorphine in emetic doses. No theoretical support for this practice was offered, and, as might be expected, this procedure had not passed ethical review and subsequent assessment in a double-blind, placebo-controlled trial. At least the social and psychological treatments of their day rested on some theory, albeit unvalidated.

It is not known, but can be fairly well negatively surmised, whether these psychopharmacologic treatment recommendations arose from any systematically studied and empirically derived validity. Nor has the effect, as far as can be determined, of these suggestions been evaluated. Nevertheless, this marked one of the first references in the medical literature to psychopharmacologic treatments for mental disorders in children and adolescents. It was not until the 1930s, however, that a systematic, scientifically based psychopharmocotherapy specifically for children or adolescents began to be developed, and it was at this time that one of the most influential and yet not necessarily helpful themes regarding psychopharmacologic investigations in children and adolescents emerged.

This general trend, which dominates even today, is that pharmacologic agents used in the treatment of child and adolescent behavioral or psychiatric disorders were first studied in adult populations and flowed downward along the developmental pipeline. In many cases, the tricyclic antidepressants and antipsychotics, for example, medications used to treat psychiatric disorders in adults, were used for similar disorders in children or adolescents before sufficient age-appropriate studies had been completed to determine their efficacy or tolerability. As might be expected, in some cases these "adult treatments," as far as is now known, do not seem to be clinically indicated. In other cases, these adult treatments generally seem to be helpful, although often with some dosing modifications.

This pattern, while not optimal, is not entirely negative. Strong forces, cultural and economic, existed and still hold that make the alternative difficult if not impossible. For example, there has been and still is a strongly held yet quite irrational view among many that psychiatric disturbances in children and adolescents are solely the result of social factors. Although this may be the case in some patients, it is clearly not the case in all, and maybe not even in the majority of children and adolescents who have recognized psychiatric disorders. Following from this viewpoint, it was argued that social or psychological interventions, even in the face of splendid inefficacy, were the preferred method of "treatment." The possibility that even disorders that were primarily social or psychological in their pathoetiology could potentially be treated by pharmacologic means was dismissed out of hand, if indeed it was considered at all. This antipharmacologic argument often went further to view the use of medication for psychiatrically ill youngsters as not only useless but necessarily harmful. If no physical harm arising from the use of medications could be demonstrated, then it was argued that using medications would "ruin the transference" or some other such "necessary" part of therapeutics. At least consistency of perspective was maintained in this case, because evidence for this view was not available.

Given this social and institutional climate, it was unlikely that child and adolescent psychopharmacology could have sprung up de novo, and thus it needed to borrow from its adult counterpart. This does not mean that the development of adult psychopharmacology did not encounter similar belief systems but rather that the ability to critically challenge these perspectives was available, something that the attendant construct of the sanctity and purity of childhood would not so easily allow. After all, with due apologies to William Blake, it is psychologically easier to give an antipsychotic to a tiger than to a lamb.

Furthermore, the beginning applications of psychotropic agents from adults to children and adolescents led to two positive developments for child and adolescent psychiatry. One was the critical reconceptualization of the pathoetiology of child and adolescent psychopathology, and the second was the introduction of rigorous diagnostic schema and evaluative techniques to the study of child and adolescent therapeutics. These developments have not only improved the study and understanding of psychopharmacologic treatment for children and adolescents but have had a tremendous impact on the directions and growth of the entire field of child psychiatry.

Although the acceptance and study of child and adolescent psychopharmacology have developed apace, old viewpoints die hard and the early problem has not been solved; psychopharmacologic treatments for children and adolescents still need to be studied and developed based on the understanding of the pathoetiology and developmental features of child and adolescent psychiatric disorders. The current economic research climate, in which a great deal of psychopharmacologic research arises from or is dependent on large multinational corporations with their own economic agendas (not necessarily including children and adolescents), and current legal guidelines for prescribing medications (no requirement for appropriate studies of pharmacotropics in children and adolescents) show that the field of psychopharmacologic investigations in child and adolescent psychiatric disorders has merely moved into yet another phase, neither better nor worse than the previous one.

The resulting lag in the development of child and adolescent psychopharmacology compared with adult psychopharmacology has been noted by a number of authors. For example, as one student of this subject wrote, "If psychiatry was somewhat slow to make use of drug treatment, child psychiatry virtually dawdled." Indeed, the era of child and adolescent psychopharmacology is not usually considered to have begun prior to the pioneering studies of Bradley, whose paper, "The Behavior of Children Receiving Benzedrine," appeared in the *American Journal of Psychiatry* in 1937.

This lag was not made up quickly. Authoritative textbooks of child and adolescent psychiatry generally gave little notice to the potential clinical utility of psychotropic agents. For example, according to Rosenberg the fourth edition of Kanner's well-known text on child psychiatry, which appeared in 1972, devoted only two pages to psychopharmacologic treatment. Graham, in *Child Psychiatry: A Developmental Approach, 1986,* found space for only five pages on the topic of drugs, and the 1991 edition raised the number to six but began the section by warning that pharmacotherapy "only has a very limited place in the treatment of the psychiatric disorders of children and adolescents." Evans, in his 1985 textbook of adolescent psychiatry, devoted fewer than five pages to the use of medications, whereas analytic interventions for which no evidence of efficacy has ever been provided were blessed with about 60 pages. A more reasoned approach, although narrower in focus and intent, was the chapter by Rachel Gittleman that appeared in the 1980 textbook, *Diagnosis and Drug Treatment of Psychiatric Disorders.* Here the effect of a personal relationship between an expert in child development who was involved in child and adolescent psychopharmacologic research and an adult clinical pharmacologist provided an irresistible force that swept the available information onto the printed page.

More recent texts provide a more reasonable balance regarding the use of pharmacotropics in child and adolescent psychiatric disorders. A text published in the United States, *Child and Adolescent Psychiatry: A Comprehensive Approach,* edited by Melvin Lewis (1991), devotes a reasonable amount of its section on therapeutics to psychopharmacology, and this mode of treatment is also usually discussed under the relevant chapter headings. A similar balance is found in the well-known British text, *Child and Adolescent Psychiatry, Third Edition* (1994), edited by Michael Rutter, Eric Taylor, and Lionel Hersov, although the treatment of some classes of medications, especially the benzodiazepines, is uncharacteristically dismissive.

The arrival of the "modern era" in child and adolescent psychopharmacology may perhaps be dated from the early 1990s, and the appearance of texts and journal articles in this area followed from the recognition of the potential value of psychopharmacologic treatments and increased research activity in this field. During this period a single monograph appeared in the *Psychiatric Clinics of North America.* Edited by David Shaffer, the Professor of Child Psychiatry at Columbia University, it was devoted entirely to child and adolescent psychopharmacology. About the same time, a journal devoted to child and adolescent psychopharmacology—*The Journal of Child and Adolescent Psychopharmacology*—appeared and two volumes of the *Child and Adolescent Psychiatric Clinics of North America* dealing entirely with pediatric psychopharmacology were published. Concurrently, a number of textbooks dealing specifically with the topic of child and adolescent psychopharmacology were issued.

The period of time between the early beginnings and the arrival of more up-to-date models of child and adolescent psychopharmacology was one in which specific focused research activities were carried on by a few pioneers. Lauretta Bender, Magda Campbell, Barbara Fish, Leon Eisenberg, Keith Connor, Charles Bradley, and Rachel Gittleman-Klein, along with a number of others, began to explore the use of medications in a variety of severe psychiatric and behavioral disorders of children and adolescents. Their work, however, generally failed to reach the "authoritative tomes" of child and adolescent psychiatry, as already described.

One interesting chapter regarding the use of psychopharmacologic treatments for children and adolescents appeared during this period. The 1961 textbook *Foundations of Child Psychiatry,* edited by Emanual Miller, contained a chapter by Leon Eisenberg entitled "Psychopharmacology in Childhood: A Critique." It was the only chapter on therapeutics in the text that was presented as "a critique," although a reading of the others clearly demonstrates that the same type of critical analysis would have benefitted them enormously. In his chapter, Eisenberg summarized the psychopharmacologic knowledge available at that time and provided reasoned clinical guidelines for the use of a variety of pharmacotherapies for children and adolescents.

In addition to his erudite review, Eisenberg laid out the basic principle for the use of psychopharmacology in the psychiatric treatment of children and adolescents: "drugs can be useful agents in the management of pediatric psychiatric disorders when chosen appropriately and applied with discrimination." According to Eisenberg, and upheld by all subsequent investigators in the field, pharmacotherapy was to be an integral part of the treatment of child and adolescent psychiatric disorders. Moreover, it was obliged to meet certain standards. It could not be delivered in a haphazard manner, and treatment included criteria of specificity ("chosen appropriately") and sophisticated evaluation ("applied with discrimination"). This set of standards was of an exponentially higher order than those of all the other therapies described in Miller's text.

Further, Eisenberg went on to provide indications for using medications in psychiatrically ill children and adolescents. Drugs were to be used (1) to control symptoms not readily managed by other means and (2) to facilitate other, nonpharmacologic interventions. From its early onset, pharmacologic treatment for children and adolescents was not to be unidimensional and was not to be considered out of the entire context of necessary interventions. The complementarity of pharmacotherapy with other methods of treatment was a necessary part of the philosophy of using medications. These two fundamental features, which together made up the basis of Eisenberg's view of the practical and theoretical foundations of child and adolescent psychopharmacology, stood in stark contrast to the predominantly unidimensional models of psychotherapeutic or social interventions often favored by many practitioners at that time. Thus, from its earliest beginnings psychopharmacologic treatment of children and adolescents provided a new, inclusionary framework based on the best available scientific evidence and judged by its efficacy. The child and adolescent psychopharmacologist was, unlike many of his or her counterparts, not expected—indeed explicitly directed not to be—a "one book man."

One of the interesting and instructive features of the early period of the development of child and adolescent psychopharmacology is the emphasis on studies in the "very ill" population. Studies of various compounds, including benzedrine sulfate, dilantin sodium, and amphetamine sulfate, not only made use of the limited pharmacologic armamentarium available but applied it to those patients who were the most difficult to treat. These chronically ill patients were managed by and large in residential or hospital settings. In addition, these patients were labeled with a variety of non-standardized diagnoses, all of which did, however, identify central nervous system pathology as related to or causal of the problems. Thus, the early applications of child and adolescent psychopharmacology were in those populations deemed to be (in today's language) "treatment resistant" to the available treatment methods of their day.

The successful outcome of pharmacologic methods of treatment in a number of these severely ill patients was welcome news to their caregivers and the investigators. Indeed, the researchers may have been excused for concluding that it was their "magic bullets" that were the most significant aspect of their results. However, this perspective was not one that was generally adopted. Indeed, if anything, it could well be argued that these early psychopharmacologists played down the role of pharmacologic effects. Bradley, for example, in reporting the successful use of amphetamines in hyperactive children, concluded that the result was caused by an "improved attitude," while others, such as Bender and Cottington, writing in the *American Journal of Psychiatry* (1942), suggested "the use of the drug only as an adjunct to adequate personal psychotherapy, tutoring, and social adjustment."

From one perspective, this approach to selecting "treatment resistant" children and adolescents for the study of psychopharmacologic interventions can be seen to be a malicious onslaught on defenseless youth by controlling doctors. Although such history as paranoia perspectives always seem to have their vocal adherents, nothing could be further from the truth. The altruistic impulse and the practical necessity of providing symptom relief for this severely ill population was the foundation on which this series of investigations rested. Furthermore, the demonstration of the therapeutic efficacy of medications in this heretofore "treatment-resistant" group provided a clear challenge to the unidimensional constructs

of psychological and social interventions usually employed. This, of course, had the expected effect of raising doubts about accepted unidimensional models of pathoetiology as well. The brain became important in understanding and treating psychiatrically ill children and adolescents.

Another important aspect of these early studies was their application of the best available evaluative methodologies to the assessment of outcome in the psychopharmacologic treatment of children and adolescents. These method-based interventions borrowed techniques and perspectives from experimental psychology and adult psychopharmacology. Their use signified a radical shift in focus from the generally established frameworks for thinking about disturbed children and their treatment that were in vogue at that time. Evaluative and evidence-based rigor, it was suggested, would need to take precedence over long-standing and treatment-directing "truths." Similar criteria could now be expected from all therapies. Theory-driven models were to be exchanged for theory-based and empirically evaluated ones.

This overflow of conceptual and technical changes played an important role in the development and understanding of child and adolescent psychopathology that can, in large part, be traced to the practical issues arising from the early psychopharmacologic research. Available classification models based on presumed and theoretical pathoetiologies served as a poor basis for the scientific study of therapeutics. The development of a more "atheoretical" syndromal approach to classification in child and adolescent psychiatry seemed, therefore, to be a reasonable strategy. The child and adolescent diagnostic nomenclature found in today's *Diagnostic and Statistical Manual* owes much to this realization.

A further issue arising from this period of early child and adolescent psychopharmacologic investigations was the necessity to focus on symptoms in and of themselves as being valid targets for pharmacologic intervention. Thus, treatment studies were not and have continued to not be constrained by syndromal criteria as the single organizing focus of pharmacologic interventions. From the beginning, medications in psychiatrically ill children and adolescents were developed to target specific symptoms, and studies were designed to evaluate the differential effect of these compounds across a variety of symptom dimensions. Current-day pediatric psychopharmacologic practice reflects these origins. Medications are used both to treat recognized psychiatric syndromes and to target specific symptoms. This is a technique that adult psychopharmacologists are now once again remembering. Few, if any compounds, in the adult psychopharmacologic literature have been as intensively studied across as many discrete but possibly interrelated domains as has been methylphenidate in children.

Finally, no discussion of the lag in the development of child and adolescent psychopharmacology could be complete without a critical appraisal of just who these early investigators were. In addition to the factors of social, cultural, and dominant theories already discussed, and not without controversy, the point must be raised that many of the pioneers in this field were women—very competent and caring women, but women nonetheless. Recent historiography has sensitized us to the awareness of the often subtle (although often not so subtle) ways in which the association of female gender with various activities has resulted in a devaluing or condescending response, derived in the main from the male-dominated "establishment." Perhaps the fact that a good percentage of the pioneering investigators in the field of child and adolescent psychopharmacology were women may have kept the importance of this area from sufficient recognition. This issue, of course, cannot be clearly determined one way or the other here but should be kept in mind so as to help raise the awareness of clinicians to these gender issues when they take a hard and careful look at how we come to know the things we know.

The arrival of new pharmacologic agents in the 1950s led to a veritable boom in the activity of clinical psychopharmacologic research and treatment in adults. Some of that interest spilled over into child and adolescent psychiatry as well. However, in contrast to developments in adult psychiatry, psychopharmacologic activity as it related to children and adolescents was significantly quieter, much less organized, rather haphazardly directed, and in general less enthusiastically received. Research in child and adolescent psychopharmacology continued to be hampered by the lack of a clear and relatively atheoretical diagnostic system. In spite of this difficulty, however, the number and quality of studies increased, and a recognizable core of knowledge regarding these agents and their clinical utility in children and adolescents began to emerge.

During this period, another important outcome of the challenge of the new child and adolescent psychopharmacology to long-standing theories in child psychiatry was demonstrated. This was the story of antidepressants and the recognition of depressive disorders in children and adolescents. Prior to the introduction of antidepressant medications, the existence of childhood and adolescent depression was either unrecognized, defined as a normative transitory phenomenon, or often considered to be an expected and short-lived reaction to environmental events or the "slings and arrows" of psychological development. Earlier theory-driven models had "established" that children were not able to experience a clinical depression because they lacked the necessary level of superego development and thus were unlikely to be able to internalize guilt. Other, less restrictive viewpoints allowed for depressive states in children but considered their clinical presentation to be "masked" by externalizing behaviors, such as temper tantrums, truancy, delinquency, school refusal, and separation anxiety. Depression in adolescents was generally considered to be part of "normal adolescent turmoil" or an "understandable" psychological reaction to growing up—a type of mourning for childhood. These perspectives all had two features in common: none were based on any scientifically valid empirical information, and all were complete and cocooned tautologies in which the conclusions of the arguments were used as sufficient evidence to "prove" the assumptions on which they were based, and vice versa.

The rapidly expanding body of research into the phenomenology, epidemiology, psychology, and biology of depression in adult psychiatry that followed from the introduction of the first antidepressants percolated into the earlier age groups as well. This led to the serious empirical study of similar issues in children and adolescents, and the results of that activity revolutionized the understanding of mood disorders in children and adolescents. The influence of psychopharmacology in this process was to provide a kick start to the development and application of the scientific method to the study of depression in this population.

Although not all the individuals involved in these early paradigm shifts were trained in clinical psychopharmacology, a substantial number were familiar with the use of pharmacotherapy and were willing to consider its potential applicability to children and adolescents. These individuals also often combined skills in research methodology, which they were able to use to investigate the many questions that needed answering once the paradigm shift had begun. Cantwell, Carlson, Gittleman, and Puig-Antich in North America, and Rutter in the United Kingdom, provided the core constituents of this group. Their students also combined the study of psychopharmacology with other rigorous investigations into the entire field of child and adolescent depression.

By the early 1980s this process was not only well under way, but relatively firmly established. The publication of the monograph, *Affective Dis-*

orders in Childhood and Adolescence, edited by Dennis Cantwell and Gabrielle Carlson (1983), can be reasonably taken as the evidence that this line of study had "arrived." Similar to the process identified earlier that took place in the early years of child and adolescent psychopharmacologic investigation, the study of depression in children and adolescents opened itself up to outside viewpoints and encouraged the introduction of different disciplines in this process. This opening up or inclusion phenomenon was substantially different from the generally exclusive "school"-based practices of more traditional child and adolescent psychiatry. And this did not take long to occur. The comprehensive monograph, *Depression in Young People: Developmental and Clinical Perspectives* (1986), edited by Michael Rutter, Carroll Izard, and Peter Read, provides a convenient dating for this process.

Psychopharmacology research in child and adolescent depression has now become an impetus, training ground, and vehicle for the study of a variety of nonpharmacologically related phenomenon. Recent investigations, based on evaluative empirical research, have clarified the phenomenology, epidemiology, and clinical course of this disorder in children and adolescents. Studies relating to its optimal treatments, neurobiology, and associated psychological, family, and social aspects are under way. Hypotheses about the disorder and its treatment have been critically tested. For example, the use of tricyclics in treating child and adolescent depression has not stood up to critical investigation. Ironically, the suggestion that tricyclic antidepressants would be a useful intervention in child and adolescent depression was one of the initial driving forces in the development of scientific study in this field. Partly as a result of the influence of psychopharmacologic developments and the rigor that the study of psychopharmacology demands, the field of child and adolescent depression underwent a radical re-evaluation. Theory-driven models are now beginning to give way to theory-based models. Empirical evidence–based "proofs" that allow for the testing of the null hypothesis have begun to supplant simple belief systems based on the arguments of tautology.

The recognition of the potential efficacy of methylphenidate (synthesized in 1954) in the treatment of hyperactive children and adolescents is another example of how the effects of psychopharmacologic research in children led to substantial developments in the wider field of child and adolescent psychiatry. The activities of early investigators in this line of research identified the need for clearer diagnostic and evaluative information. This led to a search for empirically valid and reliable research tools that, once developed, were then adapted for use in clinical practice. In the United States, the newly developed Psychopharmacology Service Center of the National Institutes of Mental Health (NIMH) sponsored a conference in this area of study and provided Leon Eisenberg with the first NIMH grant (1958) to study the effect of various medications in this population.

This promising start, however, was not quickly followed up. It was not until 3 years later that the NIMH awarded another grant in child and adolescent psychopharmacology, and not until 10 years later, in the late 1960s, could the era of grant-funded studies in the general arena of child hyperactivity be said to have begun. The complex reasons for this delay involve a number of factors related to issues that arise from the technical aspects of child and adolescent psychopharmacology and to influential social, cultural, and theoretical forces. Although an improvement on the case reports or theoretical pontifications of much concurrent nonpharmacologic writings, initial psychopharmacologic studies with children and adolescents had significant methodologic shortcomings that made their results difficult to interpret. Perhaps this was a necessary developmental process. To be fair to the early investigators, the available diagnostic criteria and evaluative measures were generally unsuitable for psychopharmacology research (and, indeed, had to be created by the investigators themselves). Nevertheless, the certainty and applicability of the results of many of these early studies were less than optimal — hardly the stuff necessary to convince a clinician of the potential utility of medications.

Factors external to the field of child and adolescent psychopharmacology also played a role. Within the field of psychopharmacology itself, most attention was paid to studies in adult patients, where, as might be expected, the expertise in these types of investigations began to develop at a much faster rate than in child psychiatry. Child and adolescent psychiatrists were then put in the position of potentially needing to compete for funding against their more highly trained and methodologically sophisticated colleagues who worked with adults. It is not surprising, therefore, that the success rate of applications originating from child and adolescent psychiatrists who were, by and large, relative newcomers to the field was initially relatively low and remained so until sufficient expertise had developed from within.

Another series of external factors was possibly associated with opposition from within the discipline of child and adolescent psychiatry itself to both the use of medications as a treatment and to the shift in paradigm that the psychopharmacologic approach to research into and the pathoetiology of psychiatric disorders entailed. This type of opposition is to be expected any time a new construct is introduced, and, indeed, in child and adolescent psychiatry, although it may have delayed the development of psychopharmacology in particular, it probably served a useful role. The strength of the dominant social and psychological doctrines was such that the newer biologic models of pathoetiology that psychopharmacologic studies implied were tempered but not, in the long run, denied. This prevented the too rapid switch from one paradigm to another, and as a result the baby was not thrown out with the bathwater.

Indeed, this dialectic process in child and adolescent psychiatry had a positive effect on the development of clinical psychopharmacology in this population. For example, as discussed earlier, the claims for therapeutic efficacy of these compounds were modified by the realization that these effects occurred within the entire context of social, individual, and family interventions and that it was reasonable to look at the patient in context. The viewpoint that emerged from this was that medications could be significant and necessary components of a comprehensive treatment plan and that optimal clinical care rested on the careful integration of various treatment modalities.

Second, because many child psychiatrists, particularly those influenced by the various schools of social psychiatry, practiced in a framework that recognized the importance of other factors in a child's life—family, school, peers, etc.—the assessment and evaluations of the impact of psychopharmacologic treatments on the child's or adolescent's functioning in these areas became an important part of child and adolescent research and practice from early in the development of the discipline. As might be expected, the methodologic rigor and need for greater atheoretical diagnostic clarity affected the study and understanding of these areas in return. The outcome of this process has been to improve the study and clinical practice of both pharmacologic and nonpharmacologic interventions alike.

Furthermore, the application of the study of nonpharmacologic factors to treatment outcome with medications quickly led to the discovery that drugs had a particular role to play in specific instances. There were some aspects of a child's symptoms and functioning that they helped and others that they did not help, or even made worse. Thus medications were gradually seen to be neither the devil nor a panacea for all ills. This rather

balanced view of the role of psychopharmacology in treatment is actually a refreshing aspect of child psychiatry compared with many other medical disciplines.

In addition, the developmental perspective of clinicians who worked with psychiatrically ill children and adolescents, and their close collaboration with colleagues in pediatrics, led to the early identification of the importance of various developmental factors—physiologic, cognitive, psychological, and social — in clinical psychopharmacology. Thus, attention was paid not only to such necessary issues as age and pubertal effects on drug pharmacokinetics but also to the developmental pharmacodynamic effects of particular compounds on these multiple parameters as well, as the early studies carried out by Barbara Fish and then Magda Campbell at the Bellevue Hospital illustrate. These principles have undergone refinements but still apply today.

A further factor influencing the "delay" of the study and clinical application of psychopharmacologic treatments in children and adolescents was the level of pharmacologic sophistication held by practicing child and adolescent psychiatrists. Many of these practitioners had never been exposed in their training to even the idea of, much less the practical issues involved in, treating children and teenagers with psychotropics. In addition, these medications were relatively new and the potential short-term (let alone the long-term) effects of their use were not known. Haste may well have led to waste. The general application of psychopharmacologic treatments to regular clinical practice therefore had to wait until a critical mass of practitioners with sufficient training in psychopharmacology was actually working outside the walls of research institutions.

Furthermore, many clinicians had been trained and practiced within a narrow theoretical or therapeutic framework. Many were unable to critically evaluate their own work, the potential of other kinds of treatments, or the value of other viewpoints that differed from their own. As a result, the dominant model of believing in what one was doing actually prevented the critical review of what one did. Thus, many practicing clinicians were ill equipped to critically assess the value of new information as it became available to them. It was difficult for them to trade the certainty of their "school" for the uncertainties of critical inquiry.

This type of delay, of course, is also to be expected and in many respects is preferred to a situation in which an as-yet unproven and potentially harmful intervention is enthusiastically absorbed by clinicians. This latter course of action is only too well known in the history of psychiatry in general and medicine as a whole. For the purposes of the development of child and adolescent psychopharmacology, however, the question is whether this delay factor was reasonable or not, that is, did it last too long? Was potentially effective pharmacologic treatment of psychiatrically ill children and adolescents withheld because of inexperience or philosophical opposition?

These are questions that cannot be answered because they require an appreciation of the optimal time frame for such a historical process to have occurred. No one, except for some critics whose certainty in their estimations of what should be expected historical progress far outstrips the author's, can make such an estimation. Suffice it to say that the answer is probably both yes and no. The important lesson that this historical perspective provides for the clinician today is that reasonable delay may be necessary but that necessary delay may be unreasonable. Furthermore, as the historical record shows us, it is essential for academic child and adolescent psychiatry training programs to ensure that current and future graduates have a firm grounding in the principles and practice of psychopharmacology, and that they demonstrate the necessary critical skills to adequately evaluate the efficacy and applicability of future treatments, whatever those might be.

A further external factor in this process was the social and cultural reaction to the development of neurobiology in general and psychopharmacology in particular. Because every empirical and rational advance in science is associated with an equal and opposite mystical and irrational reaction, so too would the popular reception of medications to treat children and adolescents be expected to meet with this type of response. That this clearly occurred merely serves to illustrate the predictive value of Newton's first law when it is applied to social forces. The direction of this response became, in some instances, institutionalized and still provides a social counterweight to the psychopharmacologic treatment model.

Unfortunately, this counterweight is quite different both in degree and kind from the type of theoretical opposition to psychopharmacologic interventions that was found within the community of child and adolescent clinicians. First, this popular force has no containing boundaries. Unlike practicing clinicians, the politician, carpenter, teacher, or cleric has no need to test the validity of their belief systems in the real world of patient care. As a result, these irrational viewpoints rarely if ever are subjected to critical scrutiny and therefore have no framework that can offer feedback about the validity of their constructs. Second, if

these ideas become institutionalized, they develop what then becomes the primary purpose of their existence—the maintenance of the institution. Thus, they create a structure whose very purpose is to keep the structure alive. Once this occurs, the initial irrational reaction becomes a central tenet of faith, that is, it develops into the core of that institution's belief system. It becomes much larger than itself. It becomes the defining construct for the institution and its members. As with many belief systems, it then defines its viewpoint as "the good" and all opposing viewpoints as "the bad." In the presence of charismatic leadership or other factors, this belief system may develop fundamentalist fervor and play out its destiny in the social and political arena. The devil is a convenient construct, irregardless of how he or she is defined.

In this kind of social situation, it is difficult to steer the reasonable middle road. In the case of pharmacologic treatment of psychiatrically ill children and adolescents, the devil becomes the drug, or the doctor, or the diagnosis, or any other convenient object. Because medications are neither devil nor panacea for all ills, they stand little chance of being recognized for what they are, rather than for what they are not.

The historical lesson that these developments have taught child and adolescent psychiatry go well beyond the topic of pharmacotherapy but apply particularly well to the use of medications. Child and adolescent psychiatrists must not forget that these forces are at play and that they can become significant and sometimes destructive. Thus, the discipline as a whole must pay particular attention to the need for public education about pharmacotherapy and the need for responsible political activism to ensure that unresponsible reactionary pressures do not lead to the limiting or complete denial of effective interventions. On the contrary, the lesson suggests that proactive measures are necessary. These involve community education, development of strong and mutually beneficial links with key institutions such as schools, and a political activism that not only matches but outdoes that which arises from the irrational opposite force. There are signs that this lesson is being learned.

Finally, as the methylphenidate story also demonstrates, progress in child and adolescent psychopharmacology occurs when different disciplines bring their strengths together to study the same problem. Almost from the very beginning, and continuing today, clinical research in what is now called attention-deficit hyperactivity disorder (ADHD) is very much a collaborative venture among cognitive psychologists, neuropsychologists, neuroimagers, neurochemists, pharmacologists, and practicing clinicians. This type of critical mass and the wealth of experience, information, and skills that can be brought to focus on specific questions are very much a result of the inclusive and collaborative framework that the early studies in child and adolescent psychopharmacology demanded and still demand. Although it would be overstretching the evidence to say that this model, applied to clinical care arose from the clinical psychopharmacologic laboratory, the clinical practice and research practice of this discipline provide each other with a good potential fit.

As in the story of depression in children and adolescents already described, the pharmacologic investigations into child hyperactivity showed, over time, a thrust and counterthrust of differing findings, interpretations, and recommendations. These ranged from statements that the methylphenidate-treated child was not helped by medications but merely slowed down (interpreted in the popular press as "drugged"), to statements that stimulant medications have no positive long-term effect on academic outcome, to recommendations that stimulant use was contraindicated because specific side effects from their use had been discovered. Other studies showed quite the opposite results, and this led to the critical appraisal of study methodologies and the development of improved measurement and design. Such sophisticated issues as optimal dose and time effects, the identification and management of treatment nonresponders, and the integration of multiple methods of measurement across various separate but potentially related variables (e.g., classroom behavior, on-task activity, attention span) all arose from this healthy internal dialectic. Over time, on the weight of all available information, a reasonable consensus has emerged as to the optimal use of stimulants in children with this disorder.

This process is perhaps best illustrated by reading the classic review articles pertaining to the pharmacologic treatment of ADHD children and adolescents as they appeared over time: Everloff (1966), Barkley (1977), Aman (1980), Gittleman-Klein (1987), Wilens and Biederman (1992), and Greenhill (1995). The effects of this internal academic debate, the increasing sophistication in the design of the studies carried out, and the gradually developing evidence-based consensus regarding these compounds is well illustrated. In addition, however, the importance of directing clinical practice on the basis of the weight of empirically validated evidence and not on the strength of one report or recommendation is highlighted in this historical record. Once again, the practicing clinician is faced with the historical lessons described

earlier. The crucial issue is how is he or she going to put this into practice in the daily reality of the busy clinic.

Stories similar to those already sketched above can be found in the study of the development of every child and adolescent psychopharmacology initiative. The same trends and the same forces operate across the entire playing field. Indeed, the game is not yet over and the upcoming years will no doubt provide plenty of information, argument, counterinformation, and counterargument about many medications and their effects on the psychiatric disorders of children and adolescents. This is not, as some clinicians have expressed, a negative process. Although it is true that it may all seem a bit confusing at times, this is not only to be expected but to be positively anticipated. This apparent confusion means that the process is working and that critical evaluation of what is considered standard psychopharmacologic treatment is ongoing.

Current Issues

Currently, the place of psychopharmacology in the treatment of psychiatric disorders of children and adolescents is becoming clearer and the risks and benefits of these interventions are becoming better understood. The historical effects of social, cultural, and economic forces are still at play and will no doubt continue to influence its development. Likewise, factors internal to the discipline of child psychiatry and to the development of child and adolescent psychopharmacology are today influencing the directions of the field. A number of these factors should be identified and their role in this process recognized.

Internal to the field of child and adolescent psychopharmacology are two developments that can be expected to fundamentally influence further directions. One, the growth of research nodes, is a structural issue; the other, the limits of the borrowing paradigm, is a conceptual one. External to the field of child and adolescent psychopharmacology are the economic and structural imperatives that direct general pharmacologic research and the irrational counterthrust of social and cultural opposition to the development of effective pharmacologic treatments for this population.

Much research in child and adolescent psychiatry is currently under way. Much of it is restricted to a few centers. Thus, information about psychopharmacologic treatments tends to arise from the work of a relatively small number of investigators. Although this is probably to be expected, given the yet early development of the field and the expertise and resources that need to be available to conduct scientifically sound clinical psychopharmacologic studies, the continuation of this pattern is not necessarily advisable. Local biases creep in, even when honest and well-meaning investigators carefully try to exclude them. Set methods of "doing things" become entrenched for reasons that are not necessarily understandable. Dogmas have a way of developing into structures that are unto themselves.

The next structural step in clinical psychopharmacologic research in children and adolescents should link the expertise found in various institutions with practitioners in the wider field. This type of development would lead to research networks in which the input of primary care clinicians would be important in defining the questions to be asked and in developing appropriate methodologies by which to answer these questions. Such a model would have the consequence of enriching all of its parts. The academic nodes would benefit from fresh insights, and the reality of community-based practices and community-based clinicians would benefit from the research rigors and scientific information found in academic centers.

The potential problem of scientific safety is as much of a concern as the potential problem of limited input in future psychopharmacologic research in this population. Briefly stated, this concern identifies that much scientific research is safe, in that it by and large follows the footpath that has been marked out for it. This process tends to be reinforced by fund-granting committees and journal reviewers, who tend to reward projects or interpretations that fall within the general boundaries of what is already known or reasonably expected. This is not necessarily a "bad thing," because it puts some brakes on irresponsible research, but this process can limit the exploration of alternative hypotheses and new directions. A cautious balance between "safe" and "exploratory" research must be sought. Just how this will happen, while at the same time meeting the highest ethical guidelines, is not at all clear. This dilemma is to be expected, of course, because if it were relatively clear it would be studied as a historical (meaning from past years) process.

The second internal issue already identified was that of the limits of the borrowing paradigm. Child and adolescent psychopharmacology has been influenced, to a great degree, by developments in adult psychopharmacology. Medications found useful in adults are often studied to determine if they are also useful in children and teenagers who exhibit similar or related disturbances. Often, in the absence of age-specific research data,

these medications are used clinically without knowing if they are indeed effective or even reasonably well tolerated in children or adolescents. This is understandable, as discussed earlier, and indeed may have been absolutely necessary during the early development of child and adolescent psychopharmacologic research. It has, after all, proven to be successful in many instances. However, although this model will probably continue to prove its utility, the value of relying solely on this type of percolate-down process has major limitations.

First, it is well appreciated that from any known perspective—biologic, social, cognitive, and so on—children and adolescents are not small adults. Thus, it cannot be expected a priori that simple extrapolation downward will result in similar pharmacokinetic or pharmacodynamic effects. Second, although many psychiatric disorders well defined in adults (e.g., major depression, dysthymia, schizophrenia) are also essentially phenomenologically similar in children, the cross-sectional pathoetiologic process may not necessarily be similar in both age groups. For example, current evidence from neuroendocrine investigations shows that, whereas in some respects depressed children and adolescents show similar neuroendocrine dysregulations as adults, in many other respects they do not. This type of information suggests that the central nervous systems of children and adolescents may show different neuronal functioning than those of adults. The corollary to this is that some psychopharmacologic treatments may exert different effects in children and teens than in adults.

Third, some psychiatric disorders are clearly childhood-onset disorders that can be found in full or partial expression in adulthood. Thus psychopharmacologic treatment strategies should possibly be developed from the bottom up, rather than from the top down. The use of methylphenidate in adult attention-deficit disorder is an example of such an approach.

Occurring along with and mutually influencing the increased study of child and adolescent psychopharmacology has been the increased study of child and adolescent neural development. Current information suggests that central nervous system functioning may change or alter substantially in some brain areas over the years of child and adolescent development. These developmental central nervous system differences may be related in part to the timing of the onset of various psychiatric disorders. Following this line of reasoning, it may well be that effective psychopharmacologic interventions for phenotypically similar disturbances may differ even within the child and adolescent age group. In addition, these findings suggest that our definition of adolescence, which has heretofore been exclusively a culturally or psychologically based one, may need to be re-evaluated in light of the neurobiologic information. Simply on the basis of the incidence of some of the major mental illnesses, one could well argue that neurobiologic adolescence does not end with the teenage years but indeed continues into the mid-twenties.

Whatever the outcome of these exciting hypotheses, it is reasonable to expect that in the future child and adolescent psychopharmacology will, in addition to borrowing from adult psychopharmacology, also develop from within. While this process has to some extent begun, in the coming years much more attention should be paid to this model of pharmacologic identification and investigations. No doubt the "percolation model" will continue, but it should be enriched by the "within model" as well.

Such developments will require the effective communication between child and adolescent psychopharmacologists and basic scientists working in developmental neurobiology. Such developments will require economic support for the development of psychopharmacologic research in child and adolescent psychiatry. Currently, psychopharmacologic research is carried out, to a great extent, by multinational pharmaceutical companies, who must deal with a variety of issues at the social, economic, political, and scientific levels. In many cases investment of their resources into child and adolescent psychopharmacology is not a priority. Although one can argue without much resolution about the pros and cons of the control of research by pharmaceutical companies, the fact remains that this is the case and that many psychopharmacologic treatment studies that arrive on the table at peer-reviewed granting agencies are often turned aside with insufficient consideration. Sometimes the reviewers argue that the project should be funded by a pharmaceutical company and then complain that psychopharmacologic research is industry driven.

Widening the economic support for research into child and adolescent psychopharmacology is necessary from a variety of sources. Pharmaceutical companies need to be persuaded to consider seriously the development of psychopharmacologic research projects (using both the percolate down and the within models) in children and adolescents. In some cases, legislative directives regarding pharmaceutical funding for research (such as recent Canadian experience shows) can be helpful to the outcome of this consideration. Other funding agencies need to be convinced to take seriously the merits of child and adolescent psychopharmacologic research and not allocate their responsibility for funding this line of investigation to private industry. Some recent initiatives in industry and university cooperation could provide models for further development. University departments of psychiatry and child psychiatry should consider making psychopharmacologic research and training in this field a priority for future development. Encouraging trends in this direction have been noted at a number of premier institutions in North America. This type of support will be necessary for the further development of a rational and reasonable child and adolescent psychopharmacology.

Conclusions

The role of psychotropic agents in the treatment and management of psychiatrically ill children and adolescents is unlikely to diminish; on the contrary, it is likely to become more important over time. New compounds that at this time are undergoing early phases of development or are just now coming to market may provide significant advantages over currently available medications in terms of efficacy, tolerability, or both. Increasing sophistication in the design and measurement of medication effects may lead to a better understanding of their role in the treatment not only of the signs and symptoms of these disorders but also of the functional impairments associated with them. New models of understanding of potential pathoetiologies of many of these disorders have arisen as a result of the demonstrated efficacy of psychopharmacology treatments, and these will be put to the test.

However, as in all things therapeutic, these interventions will need to stand the test of time and empirically demonstrate their utility in the real world. Psychopharmacologic interventions are likely to remain a necessary but not sufficient form of treatment for many psychiatric disturbances in children and adolescents. The development of novel and effective medications will be the responsibility of those individuals who study their use in children and adolescents, or who economically and structurally support the development of this field. The rational use of psychopharmacologic interventions in everyday practice, however, will be the responsibility of the front-line clinician, who will need to demonstrate not only adequate knowledge about the chemistry of these compounds but also will need to understand how they can be most optimally used. It is, after all, in the clinic that the art of medicine is practiced. It is hoped that the preceding chapters have been of value in this endeavor.

SUGGESTED READINGS

Cramond WA. Lessons from the insulin story in psychiatry. Australia and New Zealand Journal of Psychiatry, 21:320–326, 1987.

Healy D. The psychopharmacological era: Notes toward a history. Journal of Psychopharmacology, 43:152–167, 1990.

Liebneau J. Medical Science and Medical Industry. Baltimore: Johns Hopkins University Press, 1987.

Parnham M, Bruinvels J. Discoveries in Pharmacology: Psycho and Neuropharmacology, Vol. 1. Amsterdam: Elsevier Press, 1983.

Swazey JP. Chlorpromazine and Psychiatry. Cambridge, MA: MIT Press, 1974.

Wiener J, Jaffe S, Goldstein G, Justice L. Historical overview of childhood and adolescent psychopharmacology. In J Wiener (ed). Diagnosis and Psychopharmacology of Childhood and Adolescent Disorders. New York: John Wiley and Sons, 1996.

Zrull JP. Pharmacotherapy. In GP Sholevar, RM Benson, BJ Blinder (eds): Emotional Disorders in Children and Adolescents: Medical and Psychological Approaches to Treatment. New York: Spectrum Publications, 1980.

Appendixes

Introduction: Scales of Clinical Utility for Child and Adolescent Psychopharmacologic Treatment

The following scales are provided for practitioner use in the routine clinical monitoring of psychopharmacologic treatment. A number of these scales have been reproduced here in full, either because they are in the public domain or because the authors' have given permission to do so. Other scales are identified, and sample items are provided. These scales are copyrighted and can be obtained by writing to the address provided.

A full listing of potentially useful measurement and monitoring instruments is both beyond the scope and purpose of this book, and is unfeasible because new instruments continue to be developed and evaluated for clinical suitability. The physician who is interested in more information about potentially useful instruments may consult listings in the public domain (Psychopharmacology Bulletin, 1985; 21:713–1111; van Riezen H, Segal M. Comparative Evaluation of Rating Scales for Clinical Psychopharmacology; Amsterdam: Elsevier, 1988; Klein R, Abikoff H, Barkley R, et al. Clinical trials in children and adolescents. In: RF Prien, DS Robinson [eds]: Clinical Evaluation of Psychotropic Drugs: Principles and Guidelines. New York: Raven Press, 1994, pp 501–546). In addition, a number of publishers and distributors may provide useful information. The three such firms listed here are not endorsed by either the author or publisher of this book but may be consulted further: Western Psychological Services, 12031 Wilshire Boulevard, Los Angeles, California, U.S.A. 90025-1251; Multi-Health Systems Inc., 65 Overlea Boulevard, Suite 210, Toronto, Ontario, Canada M4H 1P1; The Psychological Corporation, 555 Academic Court, San Antonio, Texas, U.S.A. 78204-2498.

Forms Useful
for Psychopharmacology
Clinic Operation

Psychopharmacology Consultation Request
Psychopharmacology Consultation Summary
Medication Information Form
Meducation: The Medicines
Meducation: The Symptoms
Meducation: The Side Effects
Relapse Identification

PSYCHOPHARMACOLOGY CONSULTATION REQUEST

Date: _____

Patient Name: _____ Age: _____ Sex: _____

Requesting Physician: _____ Phone: _____

Address: _____

Purpose of Consultation: _____

_____

_____

Do you wish to have the future clinical management of this patient become the primary responsibility of the consultant? **Yes** __ **No** __

If yes, why: _____

_____

_____

Primary Current or Provisional (<u>Circle One</u>) **Diagnosis:** _____

_____

Other Diagnoses: <u>Axis I</u> _____ <u>Axis II</u> _____

_____ _____

_____ _____

_____ _____

Medical Illnesses: Current or Ongoing - **Yes** __ **No** __

If yes, describe in detail: _____

_____

_____

Page 2.

Current Medications (list **all**):

Medication Name	Daily Dose	When Began	Serum Level
_____	_____	_____	_____
_____	_____	_____	_____
_____	_____	_____	_____
_____	_____	_____	_____

Comments: (outcome, side effects) _____

_____

_____

Past Medications:

Medication Name	Daily Dose	Dates	Level
_____	_____	_____	_____
_____	_____	_____	_____
_____	_____	_____	_____
_____	_____	_____	_____

Comments: (outcome, side effects) _____

_____

_____

Other important factors which you feel impact on medication management - please describe:

Family: _____

Social: _____

Individual: _____

Education: _____

Compliance: _____

PSYCHOPHARMACOLOGY CONSULTATION SUMMARY

Patient Name: _____ **Age:** _____

Assessment Date(s): _____

Presenting Problem: _____

_____

Psychiatric Diagnosis: _____

Co-morbid Diagnoses: _____

_____

Recommended Pharmacologic Treatment:

Medication Name	Daily Dose	Dose Timing	Duration
_____	_____	_____	_____
_____	_____	_____	_____
_____	_____	_____	_____
_____	_____	_____	_____

Recommended Treatment Targets and Their Evaluation:

Treatment Target	Evaluation Tool	Duration
_____	_____	_____
_____	_____	_____
_____	_____	_____
_____	_____	_____

Comments and Specific Suggestions: _____

_____

_____

_____

Re-Evaluation Suggested: **Yes** _____ , **No** _____ . If yes, when _____

Signature: _____ **Date:** _____

MEDICATION INFORMATION FORM

Patient's Name: _____   Date: _____

The information you find on this page is designed to help you take
your medication properly. If you have any questions about your
medicine, call _____ during office hours. If there
is any urgent question or you are experiencing side effects at any
time, call _____ or come to the hospital emergency
room and bring this paper with you.

Name(s) of medicine(s):

Time medication is taken and amount of medicine taken at each time
(dose):

Side effects to be aware of:

What to do if you get side effects:

Drugs (prescription and non-prescription), foods and other things
to avoid:

Other important things:

MEDUCATION: THE MEDICINES

NAME (generic & brand)				
PURPOSE (give general & specific reasons)				
DOSE (# of mg., # of tabs, # times/day)				
APPEARANCE (colour, shape, strength (mg))				
PRECAUTIONS				
SIDE EFFECTS (both possible ones & which ones you get)				
HOW TO MINIMIZE SIDE EFFECTS				
WHERE TO GET THEM AND COST				

MEDUCATION: THE SYMPTOMS

You and your nurse or doctor should identify your symptoms. The purpose of doing this is to help you monitor these symptoms and watch them improve with medication treatment. It is important to know which medications help which symptoms. You can work out with your nurse how often you need to fill in this chart of symptoms.

SYMPTOMS	DATE														

```
SCALE:  0:  NONE
        1:  MILD
        2:  MODERATE
        3:  SEVERE
        4:  WORST EVER
```

MEDUCATION: THE SIDE EFFECTS

Fill out this sheet everyday (weekdays and weekends). This will help you monitor side effects due to medication to see if they are getting worse or better over time. All possible side effects are not listed so you may need to add some on you own. See if you can determine which medication is related to each side effect by asking your nurse, pharmacist, and/or doctor.

	TUES	WED	THUR	FRI	SAT	SUN	MON
Dry Mouth							
Blurred Vision							
Constipation							
Troubles Urinating							
Tremors							
Stiffness							
Slowed Movements							
Restlessness							
Drowsiness							
Fatigue							
Insomnia							
Nausea							
Diarrhea							
Dizziness							
Poor Concentration							
Poor Memory							
Other _____							
Other _____							
SCALE: 0: NONE 1: MILD 2: MODERATE 3: SEVERE 4: WORST EVER							

RELAPSE IDENTIFICATION

Name: _____

This handout is meant to help you identify signs (things that others notice about you) and symptoms (things that you notice or feel about youself) that might mean your illness is coming back. If you and others who know you well know what to look for, if your illness does come back we will be able to help you immediately, so that you will not get so sick again.

If you or others notice one or more of the following signs and symptoms of your illness coming back, please call your doctor **immediately.** You can discuss how you are feeling with your doctor and he or she may ask to see you to determine if the illness is coming back or not. If the signs or symptoms that you or others have noticed is not the illness returning, that is good - no harm done in letting your doctor know, and no bother to anyone. If however, the signs and symptoms that you or others have noticed is the illness returning, then it is vey important for you to get help right away.

REMEMBER, IF YOU NOTICE ONE OR MORE OF THE FOLLOWING SIGNS AND SYMPTOMS, CALL YOUR DOCTOR IMMEDIATELY.

The illness is called: _____

Common Signs (what others notice about me) of the illness are:

1) _____   2) _____

3) _____   4) _____

5) _____   6) _____

7) _____   8) _____

Common Symptoms (what I notice about myself) of the illness are:

1) _____   2) _____

3) _____   4) _____

5) _____   6) _____

7) _____   8) _____

Doctor's Name: _____

Telephone Number _____

Specific Side Effect Assessments

Abnormal Involuntary Movement Scale
Extrapyramidal Symptom Rating Scale
    (ESRS)—Revised

ABNORMAL INVOLUNTARY MOVEMENT SCALE

Name: _____   Date: _____

Examination Procedure

Either before or after completing the Examination Procedure, observe the patient unobtrusively, at rest (e.g., in waiting room).

The chair to be used in this examination should be a hard, firm one without arms.

_____

1. Ask patient whether there is anything in his/her mouth (i.e., gum, candy, etc.) and if there is, to remove it.

2. Ask patient about the current condition of his/her teeth. Ask patient if he/she wears dentures. Do teeth or dentures bother patient now?

3. Ask patient whether he/she notices any movements in mouth, face, hands, or feet. If yes, ask to describe and to what extent they currently bother patient or interfere with his/her activities.

4. Have patient sit in chair with hands on knees, legs slightly apart, and feet flat on floor. (Look at entire body for movements while in this position).

5. Ask patient to sit with hands hanging unsupported. If male, betwen legs, if female and wearing a dress, hanging over knees. (Observe hands and other body areas).

6. Ask patient to open mouth. (Observe tongue at rest within mouth.) Do this twice.

7. Ask patient to protrude tongue. (Observe abnormalities of tongue movement.) Do this twice.

*8. Ask patient to tap thumb, with each finger, as rapidly as possible for 10-15 seconds; separately with right hand, then with left hand. (Observe facial and leg movements.)

9. Flex and extend patient's left and right arms (one at a time). (Note any rigidity.)

10. Ask patient to stand up. (Observe in profile. Observe all body areas again, hips included.)

*11. Ask patient to extend both arms outstretched in front with palms down. (Observe trunk, legs, and mouth.)

*12. Have patient walk a few paces, turn, and walk back to chair. (Observe hands and gait.) Do this twice.

* Activate movements

1

ABNORMAL INVOLUNTARY MOVEMENT SCALE

INSTRUCTIONS: COMPLETE EXAMINATION PROCEDURE BEFORE MAKING RATINGS.

MOVEMENT RATINGS: RATE HIGHEST SEVERITY OBSERVED. RATE MOVEMENTS
THAT OCCUR UPON ACTIVATION ONE LESS THAN THOSE
OBSERVED SPONTANEOUSLY.

---

0 = None   1 = Minimal, may be extreme normal   2 = Mild   3 = Moderate   4 = Severe

---

FACIAL AND ORAL MOVEMENTS

1.   **MUSCLES OF FACIAL EXPRESSION**   0 1 2 3 4
     e.g., movements of forehead, eyebrows, periorbital area,
     cheeks: include frowning, blinking, smiling, grimacing

2.   **LIPS AND PERIORAL AREA**   0 1 2 3 4
     e.g., puckering, pouting, smacking

3.   **JAW**   0 1 2 3 4
     e.g., biting, clenching, chewing, mouth opening, lateral
     movement

4.   **TONGUE**   0 1 2 3 4
     Rate only increase in movement both in and out of mouth,
     NOT ability to sustain movement

EXTREMITY MOVEMENTS

5.   **UPPER (arms, wrists, hands, fingers)**   0 1 2 3 4
     Include choreic movements (i.e., rapid, objectively,
     purposeless, irregular, spontaneous), athetoid movements
     (i.e., slow, irregular, complex, serpentine)
     Do NOT include tremor (i.e., repetitive, regular, rhythmic)

6.   **LOWER (legs, knees, ankles, toes)**   0 1 2 3 4
     e.g., lateral knee movement, foot tapping, heel dropping,
     foot squirming, inversion and eversion of foot.

TRUNK MOVEMENTS

7.   **NECK, SHOULDERS, HIPS**   0 1 2 3 4
     e.g., rocking, twisting, squirming, pelvic gyrations

2

ABNORMAL INVOLUNTARY MOVEMENT SCALE

INSTRUCTIONS: COMPLETE EXAMINATION PROCEDURE BEFORE MAKING RATINGS.

MOVEMENT RATINGS: RATE HIGHEST SEVERITY OBSERVED. RATE MOVEMENTS THAT OCCUR UPON ACTIVATION ONE LESS THAN THOSE OBSERVED SPONTANEOUSLY.

---

0 = None 1 = Minimal, may be extreme normal 2 = Mild 3 = Moderate 4 = Severe

---

GLOBAL JUDGEMENTS

8.   Severity of abnormal movements.   0 1 2 3 4

9.   Incapacitation due to abnormal movements.   0 1 2 3 4

10. Patient's awareness of abnormal movements.
     Rate only patient's report.

____ No awareness
____ Aware, no distress
____ Aware, mild distress
____ Aware, moderate distress
____ Aware, severe distress

DENTAL STATUS

11. Current problems with teeth and/or dentures.

____ Yes   ____ No

12. Does patient usually wear dentures?

____ Yes   ____ No

SUMMARY OF MOVEMENT RATINGS

A) Were two or more movements (items 1 - 7) rated mild?

____ Yes   ____ No

B) Was any movement (items 1 - 7) rated moderate or severe?

____ Yes   ____ No

SIGNATURE _____   DATE _____

<u>3</u>

EXTRAPYRAMIDAL SYMPTOM RATING SCALE (ESRS) - REVISED

Name: _____   Date: _____

I. PARKINSONISM, DYSTONIA AND DYSKINESIA: QUESTIONNAIRE AND BEHAVIORAL SCALE
Enquire into the status of each symptom and rate accordingly.

	Absent	Mild	Moderate	Severe
1. Impression of slowness or weakness, difficulty in carrying out routine tasks	0	1	2	3
2. Difficulty walking or with balance	0	1	2	3
3. Difficulty swallowing or talking	0	1	2	3
4. Stiffness, stiff posture	0	1	2	3
5. Cramps or pains in limbs, back or neck	0	1	2	3
6. Restless, nervous, unable to keep still	0	1	2	3
7. Tremors, shaking	0	1	2	3
8. Oculogyric crisis, abnormal sustained posture	0	1	2	3
9. Increased salivation	0	1	2	3
10. Abnormal involuntary movements (dyskinesia) of extremities or trunk	0	1	2	3
11. Abnormal involuntary movements (dyskinesia) of tongue, jaw, lips or face	0	1	2	3
12. Dizziness when standing up (especially in the morning)	0	1	2	3

Total: _____

II. PARKINSONISM: PHYSICIAN'S EXAMINATION

1. **Expressive automatic movements (facial mask/speech**
   - 0: normal
   - 1: very mild decrease in facial expressiveness
   - 2: mild decrease in facial expressiveness
   - 3: rare spontaneous smile, decrease blinking, voice slightly monotonous
   - 4: no spontaneous smile, staring gaze, low monotonous speech, mumbling
   - 5: marked facial mask, unable to frown, slurred speech
   - 6: extremely severe facial mask with untelligible speech

2. **Bradykinesia**
   - 0: normal
   - 1: global impression of slowness in movements
   - 2: definite slowness in movements
   - 3: very mild difficulty in initiating movements
   - 4: mild to moderate difficulty in initiating movements
   - 5: difficulty in starting or stopping any movement, or freezing on initiating voluntary act
   - 6: rare voluntary movement, almost completely immobile

3. **Rigidity**

   right arm _____
   left arm _____
   right leg _____
   left leg _____

   Total _____

   - 0: normal muscle tone
   - 1: very mild, barely perceptible
   - 2: mild (some resistance to passive movements)
   - 3: moderate (definite resistance to passive movements)
   - 4: moderately severe (moderate resistance but still easy to move the limb)
   - 5: severe (marked resistance with definite difficulty to move the limb)
   - 6: extremely severe (nearly frozen)

1

4. **Gait & posture**

0: normal
1: mild decrease of pendular arm movement
2: moderate decrease of pendular arm movement, normal steps
3: no pendular arm movement, head flexed, steps more or less normal
4: stiff posture (neck, back), small step (shuffling gait)
5: more marked, festination or freezing on turning
6: triple flexion, barely able to walk

5: **Tremor** (0 = none, 1 = borderline, 2 = occasional, 3 = frequent, 4 = constant)

right arm _____
left arm _____
right leg _____
left leg _____
head _____
tongue _____

Total _____

6. **Akathisia**

0: none
1: looks restless, nervous, impatient, uncomfortable
2: needs to move at least one extremity
3: often needs to move one extremity or to change position
4: moves one extremity almost constantly if sitting, or stamps feet while standing
5: unable to sit downformore than a short period of time
6: moves or walks constantly

7. **Sialorrhea**

0: absent
1: very mild
2: mild
3: moderate, impairs speech
4: moderately severe
5: severe
6: extremely severe, drooling

8. **Postural stability**

0: normal
1: hesitation when pushed but no retropulsion
2: retropulsion but recovers unaided
3: exaggerated retropulsion without falling
4: absence of postural response, would fall if not caught by examiner
5: unstable while standing, even without pushing
6: unable to stand without assistance

III. DYSTONIA: PHYSICIAN'S EXAMINATION

1. **Acute torsion dystonia:**

(0 = absent, 2 = mild, 3 = moderate, 4 = moderately severe, 5 = severe, 6 = extremely severe)

right arm _____
left arm _____
right leg _____
left leg _____
head _____
jaw _____
tongue _____
lips _____

Total _____
2

IV. DYSKINETIC MOVEMENTS: PHYSICIAN'S EXAMINATION

(0 = none, 1 = borderline, 2 = occasional, 3 = frequent, 4 = constant)

1. **Lingual movements** (slow lateral or torsion   0   1   2   3   4
   movement of tongue)

2. **Jaw movements** (lateral movement, chewing,   0   1   2   3   4
   biting, clenching)

3. **Bucco-labial movements** (puckering, pouting   0   1   2   3   4
   smoking, etc.)

4. **Truncal movements** (rocking, twisting,   0   1   2   3   4
   pelvic gyrations)

5. **Upper extremeties** (choreoethetoid movements   0   1   2   3   4
   only: arms, wrists, hands, fingers)

6. **Lower extremeties** (choreoathetoid movements   0   1   2   3   4
   only, legs, knees, ankles, toes)

7. **Other involuntary movements** (swallowing,   0   1   2   3   4
   irregular respiratoin, frowning, blinking,
   grimacing, sighing, etc.)

     Specify _____

V. CLINICAL GLOBAL IMPRESSION OF SEVERITY OF DYSKINESIA
Considering your clinical experience, how severe is the dyskinesia at this time?

0: absent	3: mild	6: marked
1: borderline	4: moderate	7: severe
2: very mild	5: moderately severe	8: extremelly severe

VI. CLINICAL GLOBAL IMPRESSION OF SEVERITY OF PARKINSONISM
Considering your clinical experience, how severe is the parkinsonism at this time?

0: absent	3: mild	6: marked
1: borderline	4: moderate	7: severe
2: very mild	5: moderately severe	8: extremelly severe

VII. STAGE OF PARKINSONISM (Hoehn & Yahr)

0:    normal
1:    unilateral involvement only, minimal or no functional impairment (stage I)
2:    bilateral or midline involvement, without impairment of balance (stage II)
3:    mildly to moderately disabling: first signs of impaired righting or postural reflex (unsteadiness as the patient turns or when he is pushed from standing equilibrium with the feet together and eyes closed), patient is physically capable of leading independent life (stage III)
4:    severely disabling: patient is still able to walk and stand unassisted but is markedly incapacitated (stage IV)
5:    confinement to bed or wheelchair (stage V)

Signature _____   Date: _____

Medication-Specific Side Effects Scales

Antidepressants (TCA and SSRI)
Benzodiazepines
Bupropion
Buspirone
Carbamazepine
Clonidine
Clozapine
Guanfacine
Light Therapy
Lithium
Monamine Oxidase Inhibitors
Naltrexone
Neuroleptics—Objective
Neuroleptics
Risperidone
Stimulants
Valproic Acid/Divalproex
Zopiclone

SIDE EFFECTS OF ANTIDEPRESSANTS

Name: _____ Date: _____

Medication: _____ Dose: _____

Circle the number which best describes how the patient has experienced <u>each</u> of the following possible side effects over the past week.

Subjective side effects	never		somewhat		constantly
Trouble sleeping	0	1	2	3	4
Heart racing	0	1	2	3	4
Heart pounding	0	1	2	3	4
Feeling dizzy	0	1	2	3	4
Feeling tense inside	0	1	2	3	4
Restlessness	0	1	2	3	4
Numbness of hands or feet	0	1	2	3	4
Tingling in hands or feet	0	1	2	3	4
Trouble keeping balance	0	1	2	3	4
Dry mouth	0	1	2	3	4
Blurred vision	0	1	2	3	4
Seeing double	0	1	2	3	4
Constipation	0	1	2	3	4
Diarrhea	0	1	2	3	4
Delays when urinating	0	1	2	3	4
Itchiness	0	1	2	3	4
Light hurting eyes	0	1	2	3	4
Nausea	0	1	2	3	4
Vomiting	0	1	2	3	4
Increased/poor appetite (circle)	0	1	2	3	4
Stomach pains	0	1	2	3	4
Drowsy	0	1	2	3	4
Leg spasms at night	0	1	2	3	4
Sweating	0	1	2	3	4
Tremor	0	1	2	3	4
Headache	0	1	2	3	4
Sexual: _____	0	1	2	3	4
Other: _____	0	1	2	3	4

<u>Objective side effects</u> (to be determined from the appropriate clinical examination)

BP sitting: _____   Pulse: _____   Weight: _____

BP standing: _____

EKG report summary: _____

Signature: _____

SIDE EFFECTS OF BENZODIAZEPINES

Name: _____   Date: _____

Medication: _____   Dose: _____

Circle the number which best describes how the patient has experienced <u>each</u> of the following possible side effects over the past week.

Subjective side effects	never		somewhat		constantly
Drowsy in morning	0	1	2	3	4
Drowsy in afternoon	0	1	2	3	4
Poor memory	0	1	2	3	4
Poor concentration	0	1	2	3	4
Unsteadiness	0	1	2	3	4
Dizziness	0	1	2	3	4
Talkative	0	1	2	3	4
Intrusive	0	1	2	3	4
Headaches	0	1	2	3	4
Upset stomach/bowels	0	1	2	3	4
Dry mouth	0	1	2	3	4
Skin rash	0	1	2	3	4
Other: _____	0	1	2	3	4
Other: _____	0	1	2	3	4

<u>Treatment Withdrawal:</u>

Rebound insomnia	0	1	2	3	4
Anxiety	0	1	2	3	4
Sweating	0	1	2	3	4
Restlessness	0	1	2	3	4
Agitation	0	1	2	3	4
Memory difficulties	0	1	2	3	4
Unusual dreams	0	1	2	3	4
Upset stomach/bowels	0	1	2	3	4
Sensitivity to light/sound	0	1	2	3	4
Loss of appetite	0	1	2	3	4
Tremor	0	1	2	3	4
Fainting spells/blackouts	0	1	2	3	4
Other: _____	0	1	2	3	4

<u>Objective side effects</u> (to be determined from the appropriate clinical examination): list and rate: 0=none; 1=mild; 2=moderate, 3=severe.

_____

_____

Signature: _____

SIDE EFFECTS OF BUPROPION

Name: _____   Date: _____
Dose: _____

Circle the number which best describes how the patient has experienced <u>each</u> of the
following possible side effects over the past week.

Subjective side effects	never		somewhat		constantly
Dry mouth	0	1	2	3	4
Constipation	0	1	2	3	4
Nausea	0	1	2	3	4
Vomiting	0	1	2	3	4
Loss of appetite	0	1	2	3	4
Weight loss	0	1	2	3	4
Headache	0	1	2	3	4
Sweating	0	1	2	3	4
Rash	0	1	2	3	4
Dizziness	0	1	2	3	4
Fainting spells	0	1	2	3	4
Blackouts	0	1	2	3	4
Seizures	0	1	2	3	4
Drowsiness	0	1	2	3	4
Insomnia	0	1	2	3	4
Tremor	0	1	2	3	4
Restlessness	0	1	2	3	4
Excitability	0	1	2	3	4
Irritability/agitation	0	1	2	3	4
Mood swings	0	1	2	3	4
Confusion	0	1	2	3	4
Disorganized thoughts	0	1	2	3	4
Racing thoughts	0	1	2	3	4
Paranoid thoughts	0	1	2	3	4
Hallucinations	0	1	2	3	4
Other: _____	0	1	2	3	4
Other: _____	0	1	2	3	4
Other: _____	0	1	2	3	4

<u>Objective side effects:</u> (to be determined from the appropriate clinical examination): list
and rate 0=none; 1=mild; 2=moderate; 3=severe.

_____

psychomotor agitation: _____   Pulse: _____
tremulousness: _____

                              Signature: _____

SIDE EFFECTS OF BUSPIRONE

Name: _____   Date: _____

Dose: _____

Circle the number which best describes how the patient has experienced <u>each</u> of the following possible side effects over the past week.

Subjective side effects	never		somewhat		constantly
Headaches	0	1	2	3	4
Drowsiness	0	1	2	3	4
Lethargy	0	1	2	3	4
Feeling faint	0	1	2	3	4
Feeling dizzy	0	1	2	3	4
Sleeplessness	0	1	2	3	4
Nausea	0	1	2	3	4
Vomiting	0	1	2	3	4
Diarrhea	0	1	2	3	4
Heart racing	0	1	2	3	4
Sweating	0	1	2	3	4
Tremor	0	1	2	3	4
Numbness of hands or feet	0	1	2	3	4
Tingling in hands or feet	0	1	2	3	4
Sadness	0	1	2	3	4
Irritable	0	1	2	3	4
Excitable	0	1	2	3	4
Confused	0	1	2	3	4
Nervous	0	1	2	3	4
Other: _____	0	1	2	3	4
Other: _____	0	1	2	3	4

<u>Objective side effects</u> (to be determined from the appropriate clinical examination)

BP sitting: _____   Pulse: _____
BP standing: _____

Signature: _____

SIDE EFFECTS OF CARBAMAZEPINE

Name: _____   Date: _____

Dose: _____

Circle the number which best describes how the patient has experienced <u>each</u> of the following possible side effects over the past week.

Subjective side effects	never		somewhat		constantly
Dry mouth	0	1	2	3	4
Drowsiness	0	1	2	3	4
Unsteady gait	0	1	2	3	4
Blurred vision	0	1	2	3	4
Double vision	0	1	2	3	4
Tremor	0	1	2	3	4
Headache	0	1	2	3	4
Feeling dizzy	0	1	2	3	4
Tinnitus	0	1	2	3	4
Skin rash	0	1	2	3	4
Nausea	0	1	2	3	4
Vomiting	0	1	2	3	4
Diarrhea	0	1	2	3	4
Constipation	0	1	2	3	4
Stomach pains	0	1	2	3	4
Decreased appetite	0	1	2	3	4
Leg cramps	0	1	2	3	4
Muscle aches	0	1	2	3	4
Fever & chills	0	1	2	3	4
Cough/cold symptoms	0	1	2	3	4
Other: _____	0	1	2	3	4
Other: _____	0	1	2	3	4

<u>Objective side effects</u> (to be determined from the appropriate clinical examination): rate as 0=none; 1=mild; 2=moderate; 3=severe.

Nystagmus: _____   Truncal ataxia: _____
Alternating movements: _____   Balance (Rt foot): _____
Diplopia: _____   Balance (Lt foot): _____
Dysarthria: _____   Other: _____ _____

BP sitting: _____   Pulse: _____   WBC: _____
BP standing: _____
Weight: _____   Signature: _____

SIDE EFFECTS OF CLONIDINE

Name: _____   Date: _____
Dose: _____

Circle the number which best describes how the patient has experienced <u>each</u> of the
following possible side effects over the past week.

Subjective side effects	never		somewhat		constantly
Dry mouth	0	1	2	3	4
Drowsiness	0	1	2	3	4
Constipation	0	1	2	3	4
Dizziness	0	1	2	3	4
Headache	0	1	2	3	4
Fatigue	0	1	2	3	4
Weakness	0	1	2	3	4
Lethargy	0	1	2	3	4
Vivid dreams/nightmares	0	1	2	3	4
Insomnia	0	1	2	3	4
Nervousness	0	1	2	3	4
Restlessness	0	1	2	3	4
Anxiety	0	1	2	3	4
Depressed mood	0	1	2	3	4
Confusion	0	1	2	3	4
Nausea	0	1	2	3	4
Vomiting	0	1	2	3	4
Rapid heart beat	0	1	2	3	4
Pounding heart	0	1	2	3	4
Weight gain	0	1	2	3	4
Fluid retention	0	1	2	3	4
Rash	0	1	2	3	4
Impotence	0	1	2	3	4
Difficulties urinating	0	1	2	3	4
other: _____	0	1	2	3	4
other: _____	0	1	2	3	4
other: _____	0	1	2	3	4

<u>Objective side effects</u> (to be determined from the appropriate clinical examination)

BP sitting: _____   Pulse: _____
BP standing: _____

Signature: _____

SIDE EFFECTS OF CLOZAPINE

Name:_____ Date: _____

Dose: _____

Circle the number which best describes how the patient has experienced <u>each</u> of the following possible side effects over the past week.

Subjective side effects	never		somewhat		constantly
Drowsiness	0	1	2	3	4
Dizziness/lightheadedness	0	1	2	3	4
Loss of balance	0	1	2	3	4
Fatigue	0	1	2	3	4
Excess salivation	0	1	2	3	4
Constipation	0	1	2	3	4
Fever	0	1	2	3	4
Rapid heart rate	0	1	2	3	4
Increased appetite	0	1	2	3	4
Nausea	0	1	2	3	4
Vomiting	0	1	2	3	4
Stomach pain/cramps	0	1	2	3	4
Dry mouth	0	1	2	3	4
Blurred vision	0	1	2	3	4
Sweating	0	1	2	3	4
Fever	0	1	2	3	4
Sore throat	0	1	2	3	4
Cough/cold symptoms	0	1	2	3	4
Blackouts	0	1	2	3	4
Lapses in memory	0	1	2	3	4
Restlessness	0	1	2	3	4
Stiffness	0	1	2	3	4
Tremor	0	1	2	3	4
Slowed movements	0	1	2	3	4
Nocturnal enuresis	0	1	2	3	4
Other: _____	0	1	2	3	4
Other: _____	0	1	2	3	4

<u>Objective Side Effects</u> (to be determined from the appropriate clinical examination): rate 0=none; 1=mild; 2=moderate; 3=severe.

_____

_____

BP sitting: _____ Pulse: _____ WBC: _____

BP standing: _____ Granulocytes:_____

Weight: _____ Signature_____

SIDE EFFECTS OF GUANFACINE

Name: _____   Date: _____

Dose: _____

Circle the number which best describes how the patient has experienced <u>each</u> of the following possible side effects over the past week.

Subjective side effects	never		somewhat		constantly
Dry mouth	0	1	2	3	4
Constipation	0	1	2	3	4
Stomach pain	0	1	2	3	4
Sedation	0	1	2	3	4
Dizziness	0	1	2	3	4
Lightheadedness	0	1	2	3	4
Fainting spells	0	1	2	3	4
Weakness	0	1	2	3	4
Nausea	0	1	2	3	4
Vomiting	0	1	2	3	4
Diarrhea	0	1	2	3	4
Bitter/unpleasant taste	0	1	2	3	4
Insomnia	0	1	2	3	4
Rapid heart beat	0	1	2	3	4
Pounding heart beat	0	1	2	3	4
Impotence	0	1	2	3	4
Other: _____	0	1	2	3	4
Other: _____	0	1	2	3	4
Other: _____	0	1	2	3	4

<u>Objective side effects</u> (to be determined from the appropriate clinical examination)

BP sitting: _____   Pulse: _____
BP standing: _____

Signature: _____

LIGHT THERAPY SIDE EFFECTS SCALE

Name: _____   Date: _____

Dose: _____

Circle the number which best describes how the patient has experienced <u>each</u> of the following possible side effects over the past week.

Subjective side effects	never		somewhat		constantly
Inner restlessness	0	1	2	3	4
Numbness of hands or feet	0	1	2	3	4
Tingling of hands or feet	0	1	2	3	4
Irritability	0	1	2	3	4
Agitation	0	1	2	3	4
Headaches	0	1	2	3	4
Diarrhea	0	1	2	3	4
Tension	0	1	2	3	4
Nausea	0	1	2	3	4
Constipation	0	1	2	3	4
Nervousness	0	1	2	3	4
Eye strain	0	1	2	3	4
Hair loss	0	1	2	3	4
Fatigue	0	1	2	3	4
Rash	0	1	2	3	4
Other: _____	0	1	2	3	4
Other: _____	0	1	2	3	4

Signature: _____

SIDE EFFECTS OF LITHIUM

Name: _____ Date: _____

Dose: _____

Circle the number which best describes how the patient has experienced each of the following possible side effects over the past week.

Subjective side effects	never		somewhat		constantly
Urinary frequency	0	1	2	3	4
Thirst	0	1	2	3	4
Dry mouth	0	1	2	3	4
Blurry vision	0	1	2	3	4
Fatigue	0	1	2	3	4
Metallic taste	0	1	2	3	4
Feeling hot/cold	0	1	2	3	4
Weight gain	0	1	2	3	4
Tremor	0	1	2	3	4
Confusion	0	1	2	3	4
Muscle weakness	0	1	2	3	4
Headache	0	1	2	3	4
Nausea	0	1	2	3	4
Vomiting	0	1	2	3	4
Diarrhea	0	1	2	3	4
Stomach pains	0	1	2	3	4
Anorexia	0	1	2	3	4
Acne	0	1	2	3	4
Itchiness	0	1	2	3	4
Folliculitis	0	1	2	3	4
Seborrhoea	0	1	2	3	4
Psoriasis	0	1	2	3	4
Rash	0	1	2	3	4
Other: _____	0	1	2	3	4
Other: _____	0	1	2	3	4

Objective side effects (to be determined from the appropriate clinical examination): rate 0=none; 1=mild; 2=moderate; 3=severe.

Goitre   0   1   2   3
Lid Lag   0   1   2   3

BP sitting: _____ Pulse: _____

BP standing: _____

Weight: _____ Signature _____

SIDE EFFECTS OF MONOAMINE OXIDASE INHIBITORS

Name: _____   Date: _____

Drug: _____   Dose: _____

Circle the number which best describes how the patient has experienced <u>each</u> of the following possible side effects over the past week.

Subjective side effects	never		somewhat		constantly
Trouble sleeping	0	1	2	3	4
Feeling dizzy	0	1	2	3	4
Feeling weak or faint	0	1	2	3	4
Feeling tense or nervous	0	1	2	3	4
Restlessness	0	1	2	3	4
Irritability	0	1	2	3	4
Heart racing	0	1	2	3	4
Heart pounding	0	1	2	3	4
Pressure in head	0	1	2	3	4
Nausea	0	1	2	3	4
Vomiting	0	1	2	3	4
Headache	0	1	2	3	4
Sweating	0	1	2	3	4
Trouble keeping balance	0	1	2	3	4
Dry mouth	0	1	2	3	4
Blurred vision	0	1	2	3	4
Constipation	0	1	2	3	4
Diarrhea	0	1	2	3	4
Abdominal fullness	0	1	2	3	4
Stomach pains	0	1	2	3	4
Delays when urinating	0	1	2	3	4
Itchiness/dry skin	0	1	2	3	4
Rash	0	1	2	3	4
Light hurting eyes	0	1	2	3	4
Increase/loss of appetite (circle)	0	1	2	3	4
Drowsy	0	1	2	3	4
Tremor	0	1	2	3	4
Sexual: _____	0	1	2	3	4
Other: _____	0	1	2	3	4

<u>Objective side effects</u> (to be determined from the appropriate clinical examination)

BP sitting: _____   Pulse: _____

BP standing: _____

Weight: _____   Signature: _____

SIDE EFFECTS OF NALTREXONE

Name: _____   Date: _____

Dose: _____

Circle the number which best describes how the patient has experienced <u>each</u> of the following possible side effects over the past week.

Subjective side effects	never		somewhat		constantly
Abdominal pain/cramps	0	1	2	3	4
Nausea	0	1	2	3	4
Vomiting	0	1	2	3	4
Constipation	0	1	2	3	4
Loss of appetite	0	1	2	3	4
Weight loss	0	1	2	3	4
Headache	0	1	2	3	4
Fatigue	0	1	2	3	4
Weakness	0	1	2	3	4
Insomnia	0	1	2	3	4
Anxiety	0	1	2	3	4
Nervousness	0	1	2	3	4
Irritability	0	1	2	3	4
Dizziness	0	1	2	3	4
Confusion	0	1	2	3	4
Aches/pains	0	1	2	3	4
Rash	0	1	2	3	4
Chills	0	1	2	3	4
Thirst	0	1	2	3	4
Other: _____	0	1	2	3	4
Other: _____	0	1	2	3	4
Other: _____	0	1	2	3	4

<u>Objective side effects</u> (to be determined from the appropriate clinical examination) - symptoms of opiate withdrawal: (drug craving, confusion, drowsiness, visual hallucinations, abdominal pain, vomiting, diarrhea, fever, chills, shallow breathing, sweating, sialorrhea, lacrimation, rhinorrhea, mydriasis, etc.): list and rate 0=none; 1=mild; 2=moderate; 3=severe.

_____

_____

Signature: _____

NEUROLEPTIC TREATMENT: OBJECTIVE SIDE EFFECT SCALE

Name: _____ Date: _____
Medication: _____ Dose: _____

Cardiovascular:
BP sitting: _____
BP standing: _____ Heart Rate: _____
EKG completed: Yes/No
EKG summary: _____
_____

Dermatologic:
Skin Rash: _____ Description: _____

[Scoring Scale: 0 = none \ 1 = mild \ 2 = moderate \ 3 = severe]

Gastrointestinal:
Nausea: _____ Vomiting: _____ Diarrhea: _____ Anorexia: _____
Weight: _____

Neurologic:
A) EXTRAPYRAMIDAL SCALE (overall examination)
    expressive automatic movements: ____
    bradykinesia: ____
    rigidity: ____
    gait and posture: ____
    tremor: ____
    akathisia: ____
    increased salivation: ____
    acute dystonia: ____
    non-acute dystonia: ____

B) EXTRAPYRAMIDAL SCALE (abnormal involuntary movements)
    lingual: ____
    jaw: ____
    bucco-labial: ____
    truncal: ____
    upper extremities: ____
    lower extremities: ____
    other involuntary: _____ ____

Signature: _____

SIDE EFFECTS OF NEUROLEPTICS

Name: _____   Date: _____

Medication: _____   Dose: _____

Circle the number which best describes how the patient has experienced <u>each</u> of the following possible side effects over the past week.

Subjective side effects	never		somewhat		constantly
Daytime drowsiness	0	1	2	3	4
Morning drowsiness	0	1	2	3	4
Fatigue	0	1	2	3	4
Constipation	0	1	2	3	4
Diarrhea	0	1	2	3	4
Stiffness	0	1	2	3	4
Slowed movements	0	1	2	3	4
Tremor	0	1	2	3	4
Twitches	0	1	2	3	4
Dizziness	0	1	2	3	4
Loss of appetite	0	1	2	3	4
Increased appetite	0	1	2	3	4
Restlessness	0	1	2	3	4
Nervousness	0	1	2	3	4
Dry mouth	0	1	2	3	4
Blurred vision	0	1	2	3	4
Itchiness	0	1	2	3	4
Skin rash	0	1	2	3	4
Fainting	0	1	2	3	4
Trouble swallowing	0	1	2	3	4
Sore throat/tongue	0	1	2	3	4
Sexual: _____	0	1	2	3	4
Other: _____	0	1	2	3	4
Other: _____	0	1	2	3	4
Other: _____	0	1	2	3	4

<u>Objective side effects</u> (to be determined from the appropriate clinical examination <u>plus</u> recorded on the Neuroleptic Treatment Objective Side Effect Scale)

BP sitting: _____   Pulse: _____   Weight: _____
BP standing: _____

Signature: _____

SIDE EFFECTS OF RISPERIDONE

Name: _____   Date: _____

Medication: _____   Dose: _____

Circle the number which best describes how the patient has experienced <u>each</u> of the following possible side effects over the past week.

Subjective side effects	never		somewhat		constantly
Daytime drowsiness	0	1	2	3	4
Morning drowsiness	0	1	2	3	4
Fatigue	0	1	2	3	4
Constipation	0	1	2	3	4
Diarrhea	0	1	2	3	4
Stiffness	0	1	2	3	4
Slowed movements	0	1	2	3	4
Tremor	0	1	2	3	4
Twitches	0	1	2	3	4
Dizziness	0	1	2	3	4
Loss of appetite	0	1	2	3	4
Increased appetite	0	1	2	3	4
Restlessness	0	1	2	3	4
Nervousness	0	1	2	3	4
Dry mouth	0	1	2	3	4
Blurred vision	0	1	2	3	4
Sexual: _____	0	1	2	3	4
Other: _____	0	1	2	3	4
Other: _____	0	1	2	3	4
Other: _____	0	1	2	3	4

<u>Objective side effects</u> (to be determined from the appropriate clinical examination <u>plus</u> recorded on the Neuroleptic Treatment Objective Side Effect Scale)

BP sitting: _____   Pulse: _____   Weight: _____

BP standing: _____

Signature: _____

SIDE EFFECTS OF STIMULANTS

Name: _____   Date: _____

Stimulant: _____   Dose: _____

Circle the number which best describes how the patient has experienced <u>each</u> of the following possible side effects over the past week.

Subjective side effects	never		somewhat		constantly
Anorexia	0	1	2	3	4
Weight loss	0	1	2	3	4
Abdominal pain	0	1	2	3	4
Dry mouth	0	1	2	3	4
Nausea	0	1	2	3	4
Vomiting	0	1	2	3	4
Fearful	0	1	2	3	4
Emotional lability	0	1	2	3	4
Irritable	0	1	2	3	4
Sadness	0	1	2	3	4
Restlessness	0	1	2	3	4
Headaches	0	1	2	3	4
Trouble sleeping	0	1	2	3	4
Drowsiness	0	1	2	3	4
Rash	0	1	2	3	4
Acne	0	1	2	3	4
Dyskinesia	0	1	2	3	4
Tics	0	1	2	3	4
Other movements	0	1	2	3	4
Other _____	0	1	2	3	4

<u>Objective side effects</u> (to be determined from the appropriate clinical examination)

BP sitting: _____   Pulse: _____
BP standing: _____

Weight: _____   Height: _____

Signature: _____

VALPROIC ACID/DIVALPROEX SIDE EFFECTS

Name: _____   Date: _____

Dose: _____

Circle the number which best describes how the patient has experienced <u>each</u> of the
following possible side effects over the past week.

Subjective side effects	never		somewhat		constantly
Tremor	0	1	2	3	4
Drowsiness	0	1	2	3	4
Unsteady gait	0	1	2	3	4
Headache	0	1	2	3	4
Dizziness	0	1	2	3	4
Double vision	0	1	2	3	4
Numbness of hands or feet	0	1	2	3	4
Tingling in hands or feet	0	1	2	3	4
Swelling of hands or feet	0	1	2	3	4
Muscle weakness	0	1	2	3	4
Nausea	0	1	2	3	4
Vomiting	0	1	2	3	4
Decreased appetite	0	1	2	3	4
Stomach pains	0	1	2	3	4
Heartburn	0	1	2	3	4
Diarrhea	0	1	2	3	4
Constipation	0	1	2	3	4
Weight gain	0	1	2	3	4
Change in taste	0	1	2	3	4
Hair loss	0	1	2	3	4
Bruising	0	1	2	3	4
Rash	0	1	2	3	4
Irregularity of periods	0	1	2	3	4
Bloated abdomen	0	1	2	3	4
Other: _____	0	1	2	3	4
Other: _____	0	1	2	3	4

<u>Objective Side Effects</u> (to be determined from the appropriate clinical examination): rate
0=none; 1=mild; 2=moderate; 3=severe.

Alternating movements: _____   Bilateral grip strength: _____
Truncal ataxia: _____   Nystagmus on lateral gaze: _____
Balance (Rt foot): _____   Dysarthria: _____
Balance (Lt foot): _____

Weight: _____

Signature: _____

SIDE EFFECTS OF ZOPICLONE

Name: _____   Date: _____

Dose: _____

Circle the number which best describes how the patient has experienced <u>each</u> of the following possible side effects over the past week.

Subjective side effects	never		somewhat		constantly
Bitter taste	0	1	2	3	4
Dry mouth	0	1	2	3	4
Morning drowsiness	0	1	2	3	4
Daytime sedation	0	1	2	3	4
Dizziness	0	1	2	3	4
Lightheadedness	0	1	2	3	4
Incoordination	0	1	2	3	4
Clumsiness	0	1	2	3	4
Nausea	0	1	2	3	4
Loss of appetite	0	1	2	3	4
Increased appetite	0	1	2	3	4
Rash	0	1	2	3	4
Nightmares	0	1	2	3	4
Vivid dreams	0	1	2	3	4

<u>Treatment Withdrawal</u>:

Rebound insomnia	0	1	2	3	4
Anxiety	0	1	2	3	4
Restlessness	0	1	2	3	4
Agitation	0	1	2	3	4
Memory difficulties	0	1	2	3	4
Unusual dreams	0	1	2	3	4
Other: _____	0	1	2	3	4
Other: _____	0	1	2	3	4
Other: _____	0	1	2	3	4

<u>Objective side effects</u> (to be determined from the appropriate clinical examination): list and rate: 0=none; 1=mild; 2=moderate, 3=severe.

_____

_____

Signature: _____

Global Assessments

Global Assessment of Functioning Scale
Children's Global Assessment Scale (C-GAS)
Overall Clinical Impression

GLOBAL ASSESSMENT OF FUNCTIONING SCALE (GAF SCALE)

Name: _____   Date: _____

Consider psychological, social, and occupational functioning on a hypothetical continuum of mental health-illness. Do not include impairment in functioning due to physical (or environmental) limitations.

Note: Use intermediate codes when appropriate, e.g., 45, 68, 72.

Code

90
|
|
|
|
81
Absent or minimal symptoms (e.g., mild anxiety before an exam), **good functioning in all areas, interested and involved in a wide range of activities, socially effective, generally satisfied with life, no more than everyday problems or concerns** (e.g., an occasional argument with family members).

80
|
|
71
If symptoms are present, they are transient and expectable reactions to psychosocial stressors (e.g., difficulty concentrating after family argument); **no more than slight impairment in social, occupational, or school functioning** (e.g., temporarily falling behind in school work).

70
|
|
61
Some mild symptoms (e.g. depressed mood and mild insomnia) **OR some difficulty in social, occupational, or school functioning** (e.g., occasional truancy, or theft within the household), **but generally functioning pretty well, has some meaningful interpersonal relationships**.

60
|
51
Moderate symptoms (e.g., flat affect and circumstantial speech, occasional panic attacks) **OR moderate difficulty in social, occupational, or school functioning** (e.g., no friends, unable to keep job).

50
|
41
Serious symptoms (e.g., suicidal ideation, severe obsessional rituals, frequent shoplifting) **OR any serious impairment in social, occupational, or school functioning** (e.g., no friends, unable to keep job).

40
|
|
|
|
|
Some impairment in reality testing or communication (e.g. speech is at times illogical, obscure, or irrelevant) **OR major impairment in several areas, such as work or school, family relations, judgment, thinking, or mood** (e.g., depressed man avoids friends, neglects family, and is unable t work; child frequently beats up younger children, is defiant at home, 31 da is failing at school).

30
|
|
21
Behaviour is considerably influenced by delusions or hallucinations OR serious impairment in communication or judgment (e.g., sometimes incoherent, acts grossly inappropriately, suicidal preoccupation) **OR inability to function in almost all areas** (e.g., stays in bed all day; no job, home or friends).

20
|
|
11
Some danger of hurting self or others (e.g., suicide attempts without clear expectation of death, frequently violent, manic excitement) **OR occasionally fails to maintain minimal personal hygiene** (e.g., smears feces) **OR gross impairment in communication** (e.g., largely incoherent or mute).

10
|
1
Persistent danger of severely hurting self or others (e.g., recurrent violence) **OR persistent inability to maintain minimal personal hygiene OR serious suicidal act with clear expectation of death.**

Signature: _____

CHILDREN'S GLOBAL ASSESSMENT SCALE (C-GAS)

Name: _____   Date: _____

Rate the subject's most impaired level of general functioning for the specified time period by selecting the **lowest** level which describes his or her functioning on a hypothetical continuum of health-illness. Use the intermediary levels (e.g., 35, 58, 62).

Rate actual functioning regardless of treatment or prognosis. The examples of behaviour provided are only illustrative and are not required for a particular rating.

100-91   **Superior functioning in all areas** (at home, at school and with peers); involved in a wide range of activities and has many interests (e.g., has hobbies or participates in extracurricular activities or belongs to an organized group such as Scouts, etc.); likeable, confident; "everyday" worries never get out of hand; doing well in school; no symptoms.

90-81   **Good functioning in all areas**; secure in family, school and, with peers; there may be transient difficulties and "everyday" worries that occasionally get out of hand (e.g., mild anxiety associated with an important exam, occasional "Blow-ups" with siblings, parents or peers).

80-71   **No more than slight impairment in functioning** at home, at school, or with peers; some disturbance of behaviour or emotional distress may be present in response to life stresses (e.g., parental separations, deaths, birth of a sib), but these are brief and interference with functioning is transient; such children are only minimally disturbing to others and are not considered deviant by those who know them.

70-61   **Some difficulty in a single area, but generally functioning pretty well** (e.g., sporadic or isolated antisocial acts, such as occasionally playing hooky or petty theft; consistent minor difficulties with school work; mood changes of brief duration; fears and anxieties which do not lead to gross avoidance behaviour; self-doubts); has some meaningful interpersonal relationships; most people who do not know the child well would not consider him/her deviant but those who do know him/her well might express concern.

60-51   **Variable functioning with sporadic difficulties or symptoms in several but not all social areas**; disturbance would be apparent to those who encounter the child in a dysfunctional setting or time but not to those who see the child in other settings.

1

50-41 **Moderate degree of interference in functioning in most social areas or severe impairment of functioning in one area**, such as might result from, for example, suicidal preoccupations and ruminations, school refusal and other forms of anxiety, obsessive rituals, major conversion symptoms, frequent anxiety attacks, poor or inappropriate social skills, frequent episodes of aggressive or other anti-social behaviour with some preservation of meaningful social relationships.

40-31 **Major impairment in functioning in several areas and unable to function in one of these areas**, i.e., disturbed at home, at school, with peers, or in the society at large, e.g., persistent aggression without clear instigation; markedly withdrawn and isolated behaviour due to either mood or thought disturbance, suicidal attempts with clear lethal intent; such children are likely to require a special schooling and/or hospitalization or withdrawal from school (but this is not a sufficient criterion for inclusion in this category).

30-21 **Unable to function in almost all areas**, e.g., stays at home, in ward or in bed all day without taking part in social activities **or** severe impairment in communications (e.g., sometimes incoherent or inappropriate).

20-11 **Needs considerable supervision** to prevent hurting others or self (e.g., frequently violent, repeated suicide attempts) **or** to maintain personal hygiene **or** gross impairment in all forms of communication, e.g., severe abnormalities in verbal and gestural communication, marked social aloofness, stupor, etc.

10-1 **Needs constant supervision** (24-hour care) due to severely aggressive or self-destructive behaviour or gross impairment in reality testing, communication, cognition, affect, or personal hygiene.

C-GAS Score _____   Rater's Signature _____

CHILDREN'S GLOBAL ASSESSMENT SCALE - For children 4-16 years of age. David Shaffer, M.D., Madelyn S. Gould, Ph.D., Hector Bird, M.D., Prudence Fisher, B.A. **Adaptation of the Adult Global Assessment Scale** (Robert L. Spitzer, M.D., Miriam Gibbon, M.S.W., Jean Endicott, Ph.D.)

2

OVERALL CLINICAL IMPRESSION

Name: _____   Date: _____

Considering your total clinical experience, what is the intensity
of disorder in the patient at this time?

     +3   Markedly Improved

     +2   Moderately Improved

     +1   Minimally Improved

      0   No Change from Baseline OR Baseline

     -1   Minimally Worse

     -2   Moderately Worse

     -3   Markedly Worse

Score: _____

                        Signature _____

Symptom Assessments

AUTISM AND MENTAL RETARDATION

The Childhood Autism Rating Scale, (Sample)
Aberrant Behavior Checklist—Community, (Sample)
Real Life Rating Scale for Autism

ANXIETY DISORDERS

State-Trait Anxiety Inventory for Children (State), (Sample)
State-Trait Anxiety Inventory for Children (Trait), (Sample)
Revised Children's Manifest Anxiety Scale (RCMAS), (Sample)
Beck Anxiety Inventory (BAI), (Sample)
Hamilton Anxiety Rating Scale
Panic Attack Diary

MOOD DISORDERS

Beck Depression Inventory (BDI), (Sample)
Self-Rating Depression Scale (SDS)
Modified Manic State Rating Scale (MMRS)
Children's Depression Inventory (CDI), (Sample)

PSYCHOTIC DISORDERS

Positive and Negative Syndrome Scale, (Sample)
Brief Psychiatric Rating Scale
Scale for the Assessment of Negative Symptoms (SANS)
Scale for the Assessment of Positive Symptoms (SAPS)

ATTENTION-DEFICIT HYPERACTIVITY DISORDER

ADHD Rating Scale
ADHD Symptoms Rating Scale
Talland Letter Cancellation Test

OBSESSIVE COMPULSIVE DISORDER

Yale Brown Obsessive Compulsive Scale (Y-BOCS)
OCD Impact Scale

OTHER USEFUL RATING SCALES OF SYMPTOMS

Hopkins Motor/Vocal Tic Scale

Motor Tic, Obsession and Compulsion and Vocal Tic Evaluation
  Scale (MOVES)

Yale Global Tic Severity Scale

Ward Scale of Impulsive Action Patterns—Outpatient

Ward Scale of Impulsive Action Patterns—Inpatient

Overt Aggression Scale (OAS)

Autism and Mental Retardation

<u>THE CHILDHOOD AUTISM RATING SCALE, (SAMPLE)</u>

<u>DIRECTIONS</u>: For each category, use the space provided below each scale for taking notes concerning the behaviors relevant to each scale. After you have finished observing the child, rate the behaviors relevant to each item of the scale. For each item, circle the number which corresponds to the statement that best describes the child. You may indicate the child is between two descriptions by using ratings of 1.5, 2.5, or 3.5. Abbreviated rating criteria are presented for each scale. See chapter 2 of the Manual for detailed rating criteria.

1.RELATING TO PEOPLE

1. **No evidence of difficulty of abnormality in relating to people.** The child's behavior is appropriate for his or her age. Some shyness, fussiness or annoyance at being told what to do may be observed, but not to an atypical degree.

1.5

2. **Mildly abnormal relationships.** The child may avoid looking the adult in the eye, avoid the adult or become fussy if interaction is forced, be excessively shy, not be as responsive to the adult as is typical, or cling to parents somewhat more than most children of the same age.

2.5

3. **Moderately abnormal relationships.** The child shows aloofness (seems unaware of adult) at times. Persistent and forceful attempts are necessary to get the child's attention at times. Minimal contact is initiated by the child.

3.5

4. **Severely abnormal relationships.** The child is consistently aloof or unaware of what the adult is doing. He or she almost never responds or initiates contact with the adult. Only the most persistent attempts to get the child's attention have any effect.

1

2. VERBAL COMMUNICATION

1. Normal verbal communication, age and situation appropriate.

1.5

2. **Mildly abnormal verbal communication.** Speech shows overall retardation. Most speech is meaningful; however, some echolalia or pronoun reversal may occur. Some peculiar words or jargon may be used occasionally.

2.5

3. **Moderately abnormal verbal communication.** Speech may be absent. When present, verbal communication may be a mixture of some meaningful speech and some peculiar speech such as jargon, echolalia or pronoun reversal. Peculiarities in meaningful speech include excessive questioning or preoccupation with particular topics.

3.5

4. **Severely abnormal verbal communication.** Meaningful speech is not used. The child may make infantile squeals, weird or animal-like sounds, complex noises approximating speech, or may show persistent, bizarre use of some recognizable words or phrases.

<u>2</u>

ABERRANT BEHAVIOR CHECKLIST - COMMUNITY, (SAMPLE)

INSTRUCTIONS

The ABC-Community rating scale is designed to be used with clients living in the community. Please note that the term *client* is used throughout to refer to the person being rated. This may be a child of school age, an adolescent, or an adult.

Please rate this client's behavior for the last four weeks. For each item, decide whether the behavior is a problem and circle the appropriate number:

>   0 = not at all a problem
>   1 = the behavior is a problem but slight in degree
>   2 = the problem is moderately serious
>   3 = the problem is severe in degree

When judging this client's behavior, please keep the following points in mind:

(a) Take relative *frequency* into account for each behavior specified. For example if the client averages more temper outbursts than most other clients you know or most others in his/her class, it is probably moderately serious (2) or severe (3) even if these occur only once or twice a week. Other behaviors, such as noncompliance, would probably have to occur more frequently to merit an extreme rating.

(b) If you have access to this information, consider the experiences of other care providers with this client. If the client has problems with others but not with you, try to take the whole picture into account.

(c) Try to consider whether a given behavior interferes with his/her *development, functioning, or relationships*. For example, body rocking or social withdrawal may not disrupt other children or adults, but it almost certainly hinders individual development or functioning.

Do not spend too much time on each item - your first reaction is usually the right one.

1.	Excessively active at home, school, work, or elsewhere	0	1	2	3
2.	Injures self on purpose	0	1	2	3
3.	Listless, sluggish, inactive	0	1	2	3
4.	Aggressive toother children or adults (verbally or physically)	0	1	2	3

1

5. Seeks isolaton from others   0   1   2   3

6. Meaningless, recurring body movements   0   1   2   3

7. Boisterous (inappropriately noisy and rough)   0   1   2   3

8. Screams inappropriately   0   1   2   3

9. Talks excessively   0   1   2   3

10. Temper tantrums/outbursts   0   1   2   3

11. Stereotyped behavior; abnormal, repetitive movements   0   1   2   3

12. Preoccupied; stares into space   0   1   2   3

13. Impulsive (acts withoug thinking)   0   1   2   3

14. Irritable and whiny   0   1   2   3

15. Restless, unable to sit still   0   1   2   3

16. Withdrawn; prefers solitary activities   0   1   2   3

17. Odd, bizarre in behavior   0   1   2   3

18. Disobedient; difficult to control   0   1   2   3

19. Yells at inappropriate times   0   1   2   3

20. Fixed facial expression; lacks emotional responsiveness   0   1   2   3

REAL LIFE RATING SCALE FOR AUTISM

Instructions:

a) Patient is to be observed in the same setting, at the same time of day, and on the same day of the week for 30 minutes. Notes may be made by the observer. The data sheet is to be completed at the end of each 30 minute observation session.

b) Coding frequency of behaviors. Each behavior is rated as follows:

> 0 = Never
> 1 = Rarely - target behavior is seen 1 - 3 times
> 2 = Frequently - target behavior is seen 4 or more times
> 3 = Almost always - target behavior is seen almost
> constantly

In scoring SCALE IV - Sensory Responses, behavior 1 should be totalled and this number subtracted from the other items (2 - 16) before computing the scale subscore. In scoring scale V - Language, items 1, 2, and 3 should be totalled and this sum subtracted from the other items (4 - 10) before computing the scale subscore.

The Overall Scale Score is determined by adding the scale subscores (I - V) together and dividing by 5.

RITVO-FREEMAN REAL LIFE RATING SCALE

Name: _____   **Date:** _____

Setting: _____   **Time:** _____

Never = 0; Rarely = 1; Frequently = 2; Almost Always = 3

SCALE I:
Sensory Motor Behaviors

1. Whirls   ____
2. Flaps   ____
3. Pacing   ____
4. Bangs/hits self ____
5. Rocks   ____
6. Toe walks   ____
7. Other   ____

         SUM I: ____
         MEAN   ____

1

SCALE II:
<u>Social Relationship to People</u>

*1. Appro. Resp. to Interaction Attempt   ____
*2. Appro. Resp. to Activities in Envir.   ____
*3. Initiates Appro. Physical Interaction   ____
 4. Ignores Interaction Attempt   ____
 5. Disturbs Others   ____
 6. Changes Activities   ____
 7. Genital Manipulation   ____
 8. Isolates Self   ____
 9. Resp. to Hugs/Being Held by Rigidity   ____

                              SUM II: ____
                              MEAN: ____

SCALE III:
<u>Affectual Reactions</u>

1. Abrupt Change   ____
2. Grimaces   ____
3. Temper Outburst/Unpred.   ____
4. Cries   ____
5. Other   ____

                    SUM III: ____
                    MEAN: ____

SCALE IV:
<u>Sensory Responses</u>

*1. Uses Objects Appro.   ____
 2. Agitated by Noise   ____
 3. Whirls/Spins Objects   ____
 4. Rubs Surfaces   ____
 5. Agitated by New Activity   ____
 6. Watches Motion Hand/Obj   ____
 7. Repetitive/Stereotypic   ____
 8. Sniffs Self or Objects   ____
 9. Lines up Objects   ____
10. Visual Detail/Scrutiny   ____
11. Destructive to Objects   ____
12. Repetitive Vocalizations   ____
13. Stares   ____
14. Covers Ears or Eyes   ____
15. Flicks   ____
16. Other   ____

                    SUM IV: ____
                    MEAN: ____

<u>2</u>

SCALE V:
<u>Language</u>

*1. Communicative Use of Language   ____
*2. Initiates or Resp. to Communication   ____
*3. Initiates Appro. Verbal Communication   ____
 4. Noncommunicative use of D. Echolalia   ____
 5. Immediate Echolalia   ____
 6. Delusions   ____
 7. Auditory Hallucination   ____
 8. Visual Hallucination   ____
 9. Noncommunicative Vocalizations   ____
10. No or Brief Resp to Comm. Attempts   ____

SUM V: ____
MEAN: ____

<u>OVERALL SCALE</u>:

SUM:

I _.__   II _.__   III _.__   IV _.__   V _.__ ÷ 5 = __.__

*   Score of Behavior is subtracted from others before computing the Mean

REAL LIFE RATING SCALE: TARGET BEHAVIORS AND DEFINITIONS

SCALE I. **SENSORY-MOTOR SCALE**
1. _Whirls_. Sits or stands in one place and spins himself around.
2. _Flaps arms, hands, fingers_. Moves arms, hands and/or fingers in an up-down, side-to-side or circular motion at least two times. He/she may utilize one or both arms and hands, one or all fingers during this activity. Fingers may be wiggled individually or in unison. May flap his arms, hands and/or fingers in front of, to the side or behind body. Frequently the child will engage in this behavior in front of eyes, in which case "Watches motion or own hands or objects" is noted in addition.
3. _Pacing_. Walks, skips or runs in a repetitive course.
4. _Bang head, hits self_. Three types of behaviors are included here:
   (1) Hits head or any part of his/her body with own hand or object
   (2) Strikes head against another object or person such as wall, table, floor, etc.
   (3) Hits any part of his body.
5. _Rocks head or body_. Sits or stands in one place and moves his body and/or head in a back-and-forth side-to side, or circular motion at least two times.
6. _Toe walks_. Child stands or walks on balls of feet or toes.
7. _Other_. Any other idiosyncratic motor behavior. Specify the behavior.

SCALE II. **SOCIAL-RELATIONSHIP TO PEOPLE SCALE**
1. _Appropriate response to interaction attempt_. Refers to gestures, facial reactions, and posture.
2. _Appropriate response to activities and events in the environment_. This encompasses a broad number of responses. Some examples are: shows interest in conversation around him, responds appropriately to noises (such as a siren, shout, object being dropped).
3. _Initiates appropriate physical interaction with others_. An appropriate affectionate or play interactions.
4. _Ignores or withdraws from interaction attempt_. Ignores or withdraws from approach or attempt to initiate interaction. This may be seen as the following: appears to be oblivious to the interaction attempt, showing no facial, physical or verbal reactions.
5. _Physically provokes or disturbs others_. Hits, pokes, kicks, bites, pushes, pinches other children or adults. Include also attempts of aggression (e.g., child swings fist to hit another person, but misses), and token aggression.

4

6. <u>Changes activities</u>. Interrupts obvious normal sequences for no apparent reason (suddenly runs to door, darts to a wall).

7. <u>Genital manipulation</u>. Touches or rubs genital area or breasts using hands, fingers or another object, such as a toy, eating utensil and the like. Child also may rub against other people or objects (e.g., rug, wall, chair).

8. <u>Isolates self from the group</u>. Sits, stands, wanders, or runs away from the group. Or may remain with the group, but not actively participate or show interest in the group's activities or conversation. Does not seek out others for conversation or gestural interaction. Also usually seen at these times may be behaviors from the solitary motor, affectual reactions, sensory responses. Categories (noncommunication, vocalizations, immediate or noncommunicative delayed or echolalia, hallucinatory or delusion any behavior). These should be noted in the appropriate categories.

9. <u>Responses to hugs/being held by rigidity</u>. Body becomes rigid and stiff and responses to a hug or being held. Does not extend arms to the person initiating the holding-hugging behavior.

SCALE III. **AFFECTUAL RESPONSE SCALE**

1. <u>Abrupt affectual changes</u>. Suddenly begins to cry, laugh, giggle, or smile without any apparent reasons or stimulus from the immediate environment.

2. <u>Grimaces</u>. Funny or strange facial expressions or movements. This may be seen while staring into a mirror.

3. <u>Temper outbursts, explosive and unpredictable behaviour</u>. Anger directed or expressed by body movement.

4. <u>Cries</u>.

5. <u>Other</u>. Any other idiosyncratic affectual behaviours observed.

SCALE IV. **SENSORY RESPONSE SCALE**

1. <u>Uses objects and toys appropriately</u>. Uses objects in the manner in which they were intended. This includes eating utensils.

2. <u>Agitated by loud/sudden noises</u>.

3. <u>Whirls or spins objects</u>.

4. <u>Rubs surfaces</u>. Uses his hand, fingers or any part of his/her body to rub against another person or object. May be a repetitive act.

5. <u>Agitated by new activities or environment</u>. Cries, becomes agitated or upset when given a new activity or as a result of a change in the environment, or change to a new environment.

6. <u>Watches motion of own hands or objects</u>. Includes finger wiggling.

7. <u>Repetitive behavior-(stereotypic actions)</u>. Repeats some behavior at least two times. Examples are: waving objects, tapping objects, repeatedly putting food in mouth, then spiting it out, picking up napkin and dropping it again.

8. <u>Sniff self or objects</u>. Smells any part of his/her body, other people or objects.

9. <u>Lines up objects</u>. Lines up, orders or arranges 2 or more objects, such as toys, or food, or furniture.

10. <u>Visual detail scrutiny</u>. Scrutinizes small details, i.e., looks at objects in front of eyes.

11. <u>Destructive to objects</u>. Throws, hits, bangs, kicks and bites objects or toys.

12. <u>Repetitive vocalizations</u>. Makes same sound at least two times - clicking of teeth.

13. <u>Stares</u>. Stares into space for at least 5 seconds.

14. <u>Covers eyes, ears</u>. Covers eye(s) and/or ear(s) with his/her hand or object.

15. <u>Flicks objects</u>. Uses fingers to flick repetitively.

16. <u>Other</u>. Any idiosyncratic sensory response - specify behavior.

SCALE V.   **LANGUAGE SCALE**

1. <u>Communication use of language</u>. Speech not directed to other people. Included here is labelling of objects.

2. <u>Initiates or responds to communication using gestures</u>. Two behaviors constitute this category:
    (a) Starts up an appropriate verbal exchange.
    (b) Verbally lets needs or desires be known. For example: "I have to go to the bathroom."

3. <u>Noncommunicate use of delayed echolalia</u>. Says words, phrases, and sentences heard in the past, with little or no relationship to current situation.

4. <u>Immediate echolalia</u>. Repeats words or phrases after hearing them. May repeat a question in part or whole instead of answering.

5. <u>Delusions</u>. Verbalized non-rational (psychotic) ideation.

6. <u>Auditory hallucinations</u>. Appears to be hearing things that are not there.

7. <u>Visual hallucinations</u>. Appears to be seeing things that are not there.

8. <u>Noncommunicative vocalizations</u>. Makes single vowel (aaaa) or consonant (mmm) sounds, or combines vowels and consonants in a non-repetitive pattern (3.g.ba na da go). Nondirected screaming and screeching is included here.

9. <u>No or brief response to communication attempts</u>. Answers briefly or not at all when others attempt conversation.

From Freeman BJ, Ritvo ER, Yokota A, Ritvo A. A scale for rating symptoms of patients with the syndrome of autism in real life settings. <u>Journal of the American Academy of Child and Adolescent Psychiatry</u>, 25:130–136, 1986. Reprinted by permission of Waverly.

6

Anxiety Disorders

<u>**STATE-TRAIT ANXIETY INVENTORY FOR CHILDREN (STATE) - (SAMPLE)**</u>

<u>**HOW-I-FEEL QUESTIONNAIRE**</u>

Name: _____   Date: _____

Age: _____

DIRECTIONS: A number of statements which boys and girls use to describe themselves are given below. Read each statement carefully and decide how you feel **RIGHT NOW**. Then put an **x** beside the word or phrase which best describes how you feel. There are no right or wrong answers. Don't spend too much time on any one statement. Remember, find the word or phrase which best describes how you feel right now, **AT THIS VERY MOMENT**.

1. I feel ... very calm ____   calm ____   not calm ____

5. I feel ... very jittery ____   jittery ____   not jittery ____

8. I feel ... very relaxed ____   relaxed ____   not relaxed ____

12. I feel ... very happy ____   happy ____   not happy ____

16. I feel ... very bothered ____   bothered ____   not bothered ____

STATE-TRAIT ANXIETY INVENTORY FOR CHILDREN (TRAIT) - (SAMPLE)

HOW-I-FEEL QUESTIONNAIRE

Name: _____   Date: _____

Age: _____

DIRECTIONS: A number of statements which boys and girls use to describe themselves are given below. Read each statement carefully and decide if **HARDLY EVER,** or **SOMETIMES,** or **OFTEN** is true for you. Then for each statement put an **x** on the line under the word that seems to describe you best. There are no right or wrong answers. Don't spend too much time on any one statement. Remember, choose the word which seems to describe how you usually feel.

	HARDLY EVER	SOMETIMES	OFTEN
1. I worry about making mistakes	__	__	__
6. I worry too much	__	__	__
11. I worry about school	__	__	__
16. My hands get sweaty	__	__	__
20. I worry about what others think of me	__	__	__

REVISED CHILDREN'S MANIFEST ANXIETY SCALE (RCMAS) - (SAMPLE)

WHAT I THINK AND FEEL

Name: _____   Today's Date: _____

Age: _____   Sex: (Circle one) - Girl Boy

School: _____   Grade: _____

Directions

Here are some sentences that tell how some people think and feel about themselves. Read each sentence carefully. Circle the word "Yes" if you think it is true about you. Circle the word "No" if you think it is not true about you. Answer every question even if some are hard to decide. Do not circle both "Yes" and "No" for the same sentence.

There are no right or wrong answers. Only you can tell us how you think and feel about yourself. Remember, after you read each sentence, ask yourself "Is it true about me?". If it is,, circle "Yes". If it is not, circle "No".

1.	I have trouble making up my mind.	Yes	No
7.	I am afraid of a lot of things.	Yes	No
13.	It is hard for me to get to sleep at night.	Yes	No
20.	I am always nice to everyone.	Yes	No
29.	I wake up scared some of the time.	Yes	No
37.	I often worry about something bad happening to me.	Yes	No

BECK ANXIETY INVENTORY (BAI) - (SAMPLE)

Name: _____   Date: _____

Age: _____   Sex: _____

Below is a list of common symptoms of anxiety. Please carefully read each item in the list. Indicate how much you have been bothered by each symptom during the PAST WEEK, INCLUDING TODAY, by placing an "**X**" in the corresponding space in the column next to each symptom.

SYMPTOMS	NOT AT ALL	MILDLY It did not bother me much.	MODERATELY It was very unpleasant but I could stand it.	SEVERELY I could barely stand it
1. Numbness or tingling.				
4. Unable to relax.				

HAMILTON ANXIETY RATING SCALE

Name: _____ Date: _____

Using the following guidelines, <u>circle</u> the most appropriate number.
0 = Not present.
1 = Mild (occurs irregularly and for short periods of time).
2 = Moderate (occurs more constantly and of longer duration, requiring considerable effort on part of patient to cope).
3 = Severe (continuous, dominates patient's life).
4 = Very severe (incapacitating).

1. **ANXIOUS MOOD**: Worries, anticipation of the worst, fearful anticipation, irritability.	0 1 2 3 4
2. **TENSION**: Feelings of tension, fatigability, startle response, moved to tears easily, trembling, feelings of restlessness, inability to relax.	0 1 2 3 4
3. **FEARS**: Of dark, of strangers, of being left alone, of animals, of traffic, of crowds.	0 1 2 3 4
4. **INSOMNIA**: Difficulty in falling asleep, broken sleep, unsatisfying sleep and fatigue on waking, dreams, nightmares, night terrors.	0 1 2 3 4
5. **INTELLECTUAL** (cognitive): Difficulty in concentration, poor memory.	0 1 2 3 4
6. **DEPRESSED MOOD**: Loss of interest, lack of pleasure in hobbies, depression, early waking, diurnal swing.	0 1 2 3 4

Psychological Total _____

7. **SOMATIC** (muscular): Pains and aches, twitching, stiffness, myoclonic jerks, grinding of teeth, unsteady voice, increased muscular tone.	0 1 2 3 4
(sensory): Tinnitus, blurring of vision, hot and cold flashes, feeling of weakness, prickling sensation.	0 1 2 3 4
8. **CARDIOVASCULAR SYMPTOMS**: Tachycardia, palpitations, pain in chest, throbbing of vessels, fainting feelings, missing beat.	0 1 2 3 4
9. **RESPIRATORY SYMPTOMS**: Pressure of constriction in chest, choking feelings, sighing and dyspnea.	0 1 2 3 4
10. **GASTROINTESTINAL SYMPTOMS**: Difficulty in swallowing, wind abdominal pain, burning sensation, abdominal fullness, nausea, vomiting, borborygmi, looseness of bowels, loss of weight, constipation.	0 1 2 3 4
11. **GENITOURINARY SYMPTOMS**: Frequency of micturition, amenorrhea, menorrhagia, development of frigidity, premature ejaculation, loss of libido, impotence.	0 1 2 3 4
12. **AUTONOMIC SYMPTOMS**: Dry mouth, flushing, pallor, tendency to sweat, giddiness, tension headache, raising of hair.	0 1 2 3 4
13. **BEHAVIOUR AT INTERVIEW**: Fidgeting, restlessness or pacing, tremor of hands, furrowed brow, strained face, sighing or rapid respiration, facial pallor, swallowing, belching, brisk tendon jerks, dilated pupils, exophthalmus.	0 1 2 3 4

Physiological Total _____

TOTAL SCORE _____

Signature: _____

From Hamilton M. The assessment of anxiety by rating. British Journal of Medical Psychology, 32:50–55, 1959. Reprinted by permission of the British Psychological Society.

PANIC ATTACK DIARY

Name: _____

DATE	ATTACK #	SEVERITY: 1 = mild 2 = severe	LENGTH: 1 = 5 minutes or less 3 = 10 minutes or more

Mood Disorders

BECK DEPRESSION INVENTORY (BDI) - (SAMPLE)

Name: _____   Date: _____

Age: _____   Sex: _____

This questionnaire consists of 21 groups of statements. After reading each group of statements carefully, circle the number (0, 1, 2 or 3) next to the one statement in each group which **best** describes the way you have been feeling the **past week, including today.** If several statements within a group seem to apply equally well, circle each one. **Be sure to read all the statements in each group before making your choice.**

1. 0   I do not feel sad.

    1   I feel sad.

    2   I am sad all the time and I can't snap out of it.

    3   I am so sad or unhappy that I can't stand it.

12. 0   I have not lost interest in other people.

    1   I am less interested in other people than I used to be.

    2   I have lost most of my interest in other people.

    3   I have lost all of my interest in other people.

SELF-RATING DEPRESSION SCALE (SDS)

Name: _____   Date: _____

Please circle the score to the right of each item which best describes how you have been feeling overall, during the past week.

Item	A little of the time	Some of the time	Good part of the time	Most of the time
1. I feel down-hearted and blue.	1	2	3	4
2. Morning is when I feel the best.	4	3	2	1
3. I have crying spells, or feel like it.	1	2	3	4
4. I have trouble sleeping at night.	1	2	3	4
5. I eat as much as I used to.	4	3	2	1
6. I still enjoy sex.	4	3	2	1
7. I notice that I am losing weight.	1	2	3	4
8. I have trouble with constipation.	1	2	3	4
9. My heart beats faster than usual.	1	2	3	4
10. I get tired for no reason.	1	2	3	4
11. My mind is as clear as it used to be.	4	3	2	1
12. I find it easy to do the things I used to.	4	3	2	1
13. I am restless and can't keep still.	1	2	3	4
14. I feel hopeful about the future.	4	3	2	1
15. I am more irritable than usual.	1	2	3	4
16. I find it easy to make decisions.	4	3	2	1
17. I feel that I am useful and needed.	4	3	2	1
18. My life is pretty full.	4	3	2	1
19. I feel that others would be better off if I were dead.	1	2	3	4
20. I still enjoy the things I used to.	4	3	2	1
Total	_____	_____	_____	_____

Signature: _____

From Zung WWK, Richards CB, Short MJ. Self-rating depression scale in an outpatient clinic. Archives of General Psychiatry, 13:508–515, 1965. Reprinted by permission of the American Medical Association.

Date: |__|__| |__|__| |__|__| Name: _____
       DD   MM   YY

Item	Operational Definition	RATINGS						Comment
		0	1	2	3	4	5	
	"is observed" - Information gleaned during interview; "is reported" - Information from staff notes and case notes; "admits" - patient's self report.	absent	slight flavor or suspicion of pathology by clinician;	clearly noticeable mild or occuring not more than twice during interview;	clearly present and occuring 3-4 times during interview;	definitely present and and frequent;	continuous and gross.	
1) Is depressed:	is observed to be sad, tearful, de-jected, unresponsive, sighing, to have retarded movements and expresses depressive thoughts.							
2) Is talking:	is observed to have a raised voice, increased rate of speaking, reluctance to allow interruptions and absence of natural pauses.	0	1	2	3	4	5	
3) Restlessness:	is observed or is reported to gesture and change posture excessively, to examine objects in room and return to place, to shift position round room.	0	1	2	3	4	5	
4) Makes threats:	is reported or is observed to use threatening language, to make threatening gestures.	0	1	2	3	4	5	
5) Has poor judgement:	is inferred to lack appreciation of effect of own behavior and to show impairment of sight into present state.	0	1	2	3	4	5	
6) Is hallucinating:	admits to hallucinatory experiences (true hallucinations appearing in external space without insight rate high, pseudo hallucinations experience in internal space and with insight rate low). If symptom present given example.	0	1	2	3	4	5	

	Operational Definition	RATINGS						Comment
		0	1	2	3	4	5	
7) Looks happy and chearful:	in interview is observed to display excessive joviality, playfulness and bonhomie	0	1	2	3	4	5	
8) Seeks out others:	reported to show sociability, e.g. keeps patients awake, distracts staff from duty, buttonholes complete strangers.	0	1	2	3	4	5	
9) Is distractable:	admits to difficult in concentration or in application, and or is observed to be distracted by immediate environment or transient thoughts.	0	1	2	3	4	5	
10) Has grandiose ideas:	admits to exaggerated ideas of ability or status, not of delusional intensity (if item 11 is rated 1 or more then score 5 for this item).	0	1	2	3	4	5	
11) Has grandiose delusions:	admits to beliefs or delusional status (false and firmly fixed which may be exalted, grandiose. egostical or of assistance). Partial delusions score low (e.g. if pushed, patient may admit of some doubt), full systematized and acted on delusions score high.	0	1	2	3	4	5	
12) Is angry:	admits to strong objection to people and situations, accompanied by signs of physical arousal, that is, in voice, complexion and posture. It gives a physical excession to anger against people or objects score 5 in this item.	0	1	2	3	4	5	
13) Is suspicious:	admits to or is observed to show (a) caution in accepting validity of overt information (this will be of non-delusional intensity), (b) simple ideas of reference. If item 14 is rated as 1 or more then score 5 on this item.	0	1	2	3	4	5	

Cont.....

Operational Definition			RATINGS				Comment
	0	1	2	3	4	5	
14) Has delusions of persecution: admits to persecutory beliefs of delusional intensity or to delusions of reference (score low for partial delusions and high for systematization of delusions and action taken by patient thereon).	0	1	2	3	4	5	
15) Is active: is reported as showing excessive activity, activity being defined as purposeful motor behaviour.	0	1	2	3	4	5	
16) Is irritable: is observed to be argumentative in interview situation or admits to excessive querulousness in responding to events.	0	1	2	3	4	5	
17) Jumps from one topic to another: this covers discursive talk which must be intelligible to the listener. If it is unintelligible score 5 on this item and rate on item 18.	0	1	2	3	4	5	
18) Shows flight of ideas: in interview is unintelligibly discursive in talk, or shows punning, rhyming and clang associations.	0	1	2	3	4	5	
19) Is careless about dress and grooming: is observed to show carelessness in the areas of cleanliness and tidiness only.	0	1	2	3	4	5	
20) Has diminished impulse control: is reported to have shown major and sudden change in the following areas of activity: spending, travel, job, making telephone calls and writing, sexual behaviour, housing, alcohol or drug intake. Also rate isolated uncharacteristic, violent responses to valid provocation.	0	1	2	3	4	5	
21) Verbalizes feelings of well-being: admits to a state of optimism, contentment, happiness and freedom from physical constraints. This does not refer to plans and assessments of abilities nor to reality testing.	0	1	2	3	4	5	
22) Makes plans: admits to increasing activity scheduled for the future, formulated definitely, rating high for increasing unrealizability in terms of the patient's intelligence, social, educational and cultural background.	0	1	2	3	4	5	

	Operational Definition	0	1	2	3	4	5	Comment
23) Demands contact:	admits to need for social contact of non-sexual nature in response to specific questioning in interview.	0	1	2	3	4	5	
24) Is sexually preoccupied:	admits to increased sexual thoughts or activity (expecially masturbation, coitus or homosexual contact). Rate high for new or increasing number of partners and for attempted sexual behavious in hospital.	0	1	2	3	4	5	
25) Is emotionally labile:	shows bipolar fluctuations in mood spontaneous or in response to interview questioning.	0	1	2	3	4	5	
26) Is religiose:	admits to increased prayer, reading of religious or philosophical books, rating high for discovery of new meanings and attempted proselytizing of staff and patient.	0	1	2	3	4	5	
27) Is disinhibited	is observed to be over free with confidential information, to allow excessive familiarity in interview situation to use swearwords, to produce noisy or offensive alimentary release or sexual provocation.	0	1	2	3	4	5	
28) Has disturbed sleep:	is reported to show disturbance of sleep especially brevity of actual sleep time. Rate 5 for observed duration of sleep of 2 hours or less and rate high for time spent out of bed during the night. Rate low for an admission that less sleep is needed than usual.	0	1	2	3	4	5	

RATINGS

TOTAL SCORE

From Blackburn IM, London JB, Ashworth OM. A new scale for measuring mania. Psychological Medicine, 7:453–458, 1977. Reprinted with permission of Cambridge University Press.

CHILDREN'S DEPRESSION INVENTORY (CDI) - (SAMPLE)

by Maria Kovacs, Ph.D.

Name: _____   **Date:** _____

Age: _____   **Sex:** _____

Kids sometimes have different feelings and ideas.

This form lists the feelings and ideas in groups. From each group of three sentences, pick one sentence that describes you best for the past two weeks. After you pick a sentence from the first group, go on to the next group.

There is no right answer or wrong answer. Just pick the sentence that best describes the way you have been recently. Put a mark like this □ next to your answer. Put the mark in the box next to the sentence that you pick.

Here is an example of how this form works. Try it. Put a mark next to the sentence that describes you **best**.

Example:
- □ I read books all the time.
- □ I read books once in a while
- □ I never read books.

When you are told to do so, tear off this top page. Then, pick the sentences that describe you best on the first page. After you finish the first page, turn to the back. Then, answer the items on that page.

Remember, pick out the sentences that describe you best in the PAST TWO WEEKS.

Sample Items:

1. □ I am sad once in a while.
   □ I am sad many times.
   □ I am sad all the time.

2. □ Nothing will ever work out for me.
   □ I am not sure if things will work out for me.
   □ Things will work out for me O.K.

3. □ I do most things O.K.
   □ I do many things wrong.
   □ I do everything wrong.

4. □ I have fun in many things.
   □ I have fun in some things.
   □ Nothing is fun at all.

5. □ I am bad all the time.
   □ I am bad many times.
   □ I am bad once in a while.

6. □ I think about bad things happening to me once in a while.
   □ I worry that bad things will happen to me.
   □ I am sure that terrible things will happen to me.

Psychotic Disorders

<u>**POSITIVE AND NEGATIVE SYNDROME SCALE - (SAMPLE)**</u>

All items use the following scoring key:

        1 = Absent
        2 = Minimal
        3 = Mild
        4 = Moderate
        5 = Moderate/Severe
        6 = Severe
        7 = Extreme

The scale is comprised of Four Sections:

        Positive Symptoms (7 items)
        Negative Symptoms (7 items)
        General Psychopathology (16 items)
        Supplementary - Aggression Risk (3 items)

An example of each Section follows.

POSITIVE SCALE (P)

P1. Delusions. Beliefs which are unfounded, unrealistic, and idiosyncratic. **Basis for rating**: thought content expressed in the interview and its influence on social relations and behavior as reported by primary care workers or family.

	Rating	Criteria
1	Absent	Definition does not apply.
2	Minimal	Questionable pathology; may be at the upper extreme of normal limits.
3	Mild	Presence of one or two delusions which are vague, uncrystallized, and not tenaciously held. Delusions do not interfere with thinking, social relations or behavior.
4	Moderate	Presence of either a kaleidoscopic array of poorly formed, unstable delusions or of a few well-formed delusions that occasionally interfere with thinking, social relations, or behavior.
5	Moderate Severe	Presence of numerous well-formed delusions that are tenaciously held and occasionally interfere with thinking, social relations, or behavior.
6	Severe	Presence of a stable set of delusions which are crystallized, possibly systematized, tenaciously held, and clearly interfere with thinking, social relations, and behavior.
7	Extreme	Presence of a stable set of delusions which are either highly systematized or very numerous, and which dominate major facets of the patient's life. This frequently results in inappropriate and irresponsible action, which may even jeopardize the safety of the patient or others.

2

NEGATIVE SCALE (N)

N1. Blunted Affect.   Diminished emotional responsiveness as characterized by a reduction in facial expression, modulation of feelings, and communicative gestures.   **Basis for rating**: observation of physical manifestations of affective tone and emotional responsiveness during the course of the interview.

	Rating	Criteria
1	Absent	Definition does not apply.
2	Minimal	Questionable pathology; may be at the upper extreme of normal limits.
3	Mild	Changes in facial expression and communicative gestures seem to be stilted, forced, artificial, or lacking in modulation.
4	Moderate	Reduced range of facial expression and few expressive gestures result in a dull appearance.
5	Moderate Severe	Affect is generally "flat", with only occasional changes in facial expression and a paucity of communicative gestures.
6	Severe	Marked flatness and deficiency of emotions exhibited most of the time. There may be unmodulated extreme affective discharges, such as excitement, rage, or inappropriate uncontrolled laughter.
7	Extreme	Changes in facial expression and evidence of communicative gestures are virtually absent. Patient seems constantly to show a barren or "wooden" expression.

GENERAL PSYCHOPATHOLOGY SCALE (G)

G1. Somatic Concern. Physical complaints or beliefs about illness or malfunctions. This may range from a vague sense of ill being to clear-cut of catastrophic physical disease. **Basis for rating:** thought content expressed in the interview.

	Rating	Criteria
1	Absent	Definition does not apply.
2	Minimal	Questionable pathology; may be at the upper extreme of normal limits.
3	Mild	Distinctly concerned about health or somatic issues, as evidenced by occasional questions and desire for reassurance.
4	Moderate	Complains about poor health or bodily malfunction, but there is no delusional conviction, and over-concern can be allayed by reassurance.
5	Moderate Severe	Patient expresses numerous or frequent complaints about physical illness or bodily malfunction, or else patient reveals one or two clear-cut delusions involving these themes but is not preoccupied by them.
6	Severe	Patient is preoccupied by one or a few clear-cut delusions about physical disease or organic malfunctino, but affect is not fully immersed in these themes, and thoughts can be diverted by the interviewer with some effort.
7	Extreme	Numerous and frequently reported somatic delusions, or only a few somatic delusions of a catastrophic nature, which totally dominate the patient's affect and thinking.

4

SUPPLEMENTARY ITEMS FOR THE AGGRESSION RISK PROFILE

S1. Anger. Subjective state of displeasure and irritation directed at others. **Basis for rating:** verbal report of angry feelings during the course of the interview and, thereupon, corresponding hostile behaviors observed during the interview or noted from reports by primary care workers or family.

	Rating	Criteria
1	Absent	Definition does not apply
2	Minimal	Questionable pathology; may be at the upper extreme of normal limits.
3	Mild	Expresses some irritation or ill feelings toward others but, otherwise, shows no emotional or behavioral signs of anger.
4	Moderate	Presents an overtly angry exterior, but temper remains under control.
5	Moderate Severe	Patient appears highly irritable, and anger is vented through frequently raised voice, occasional verbal abuse, or thinly veiled threats.
6	Severe	Patient appears highly irritable, and anger is vented through repeated verbal abuse, overt threats, or destructiveness.
7	Extreme	An explosive level of anger is evidenced by physical abuse directed or attempted at others.

BRIEF PSYCHIATRIC RATING SCALE

Name: _____   Date: _____

1. **Somatic Concern**: preoccupation with physical health,   0 1 2 3 4 5 6
   fear of physical illness, hypochondriasis.

2. **Anxiety**: worry, fear, over-concern for present or   0 1 2 3 4 5 6
   future.

3. **Emotional Withdrawal**: lack of spontaneous interaction   0 1 2 3 4 5 6
   isolation, deficiency in relating to others.

4. **Conceptual Disorganization**: thought processes   0 1 2 3 4 5 6
   confused, disconnected, disorganized, disrupted.

5. **Guilt Feelings**: self-blame, shame, remorse for   0 1 2 3 4 5 6
   past behavior.

6. **Tension**: physical and motor manifestations or   0 1 2 3 4 5 6
   nervousness, over-activation, tension.

7. **Mannerisms and Posturing**: peculiar bizarre   0 1 2 3 4 5 6
   unnatural motor behaviours (not including tics).

8. **Grandiosity**: exaggerated self-opinion, arrogance,   0 1 2 3 4 5 6
   conviction of unusual power or abilities.

9. **Depressed Mood**: sorrow, sadness, despondency,   0 1 2 3 4 5 6
   pessimism.

10. **Hostility**: animosity, contempt, belligerence,   0 1 2 3 4 5 6
    disdain for others.

11. **Suspiciousness**: mistrust, belief others harbour   0 1 2 3 4 5 6
    malicious or discriminatory intent.

12. **Hallucinatory Behaviour**: perceptions without   0 1 2 3 4 5 6
    normal external stimulus correspondence.

13. **Motor Retardation**: slowed, weakened movements or   0 1 2 3 4 5 6
    speech, reduced body tone.

14. **Unco-operativeness**: resistance, guardedness,   0 1 2 3 4 5 6
    rejection of authority.

15. **Unusual Thought Content**: unusual odd, strange   0 1 2 3 4 5 6
    bizarre thought content.

16. **Blunted Affect**: reduced emotional tone, reduction   0 1 2 3 4 5 6
    in normal intensity of feelings, flatness.

17. **Elation/Euphoria**: increased sense of well-being,   0 1 2 3 4 5 6
    euphoria, hypomania, manic and ecstatic states.

18. **Excitation**: increased rate and amount of speech   0 1 2 3 4 5 6
    and movements, excitement, delirium.

19. **Disorientation**: confusion or lack of proper   0 1 2 3 4 5 6
    association for person, place or time.

                                                        TOTAL _____

SCALE FOR THE ASSESSMENT OF NEGATIVE SYMPTOMS

0=None 1=Questionable 2=Mild 3=Moderate 4=Marked 5=Severe

AFFECTIVE FLATTENING OR BLUNTING

1   **Unchanging Facial Expression**   0 1 2 3 4 5
The patient's face appears wooden, changes less than
expected as emotional content of discourse changes.

2   **Decreased Spontaneous Movements**   0 1 2 3 4 5
The patient shows few or no spontaneous movements, does
not shift position, move extremities, etc.

3   **Paucity of Expressive Gestures**   0 1 2 3 4 5
The patient does not use hand gestures, body position,
etc., as an aid to expressing his ideas.

4   **Poor Eye Contact**   0 1 2 3 4 5
The patient avoids eye contact or "stares through"
interviewer even when speaking.

5   **Affective Nonresponsivity**   0 1 2 3 4 5
The patient fails to smile or laugh when prompted.

6   **Lack of Vocal Inflections**   0 1 2 3 4 5
The patient fails to show normal vocal emphasis patterns,
is often monotonic.

7   **Global Rating of Affective Flattening**   0 1 2 3 4 5
This rating should focus on overall severity of symptoms,
especially unresponsiveness, eye contact, facial expression,
and vocal inflections.

ALOGIA

8   **Poverty of Speech**   0 1 2 3 4 5
The patient's replies to questions are restricted in amount,
tend to be brief, concrete, and unelaborated.

9   **Poverty of Content of Speech**   0 1 2 3 4 5
The patient's replies are adequate in amount but tend to be
vague, overconcrete, or overgeneralized, and convey little
information.

10   **Blocking**   0 1 2 3 4 5
The patient indicates, either spontaneously or with prompting,
that his train of thought was interrupted.

11   **Increased Latency of Response**   0 1 2 3 4 5
The patient takes a long time to reply to questions;
prompting indicates the patient is aware of the question.

12   **Global Rating of Alogia**   0 1 2 3 4 5
The core features of alogia are poverty of speech and poverty
of content.

AVOLITION-APATHY

13   **Grooming and Hygiene**   0 1 2 3 4 5
The patient's clothes may be sloppy or soiled, and he may have
greasy hair, body odor, etc.

1

0=None   1=Questionable   2=Mild   3=Moderate   4=Marked   5=Severe

14   **Impersistence at Work or School**   0 1 2 3 4 5
The patient has difficulty seeking or maintaining employment,
completing school work, keeping house, etc. If an inpatient,
cannot persist at ward activities, such as OT, playing cards,
etc.

15   **Physical Anergia**   0 1 2 3 4 5
The patient tends to be physically inert. He may sit for hours
and does not initiate spontaneous activity.

16   **Global Rating of Avolition-Apathy**   0 1 2 3 4 5
Strong weight may be given to one or two prominent symptoms if
particularly striking.

ANHEDONIA-ASOCIALITY

17   **Recreational Interests and Activities**   0 1 2 3 4 5
The patient may have few or no interests. Both the quality
and quantity of interests should be taken into account.

18   **Sexual Activity**   0 1 2 3 4 5
The patient may show a decrease in sexual interest and
activity, or enjoyment when active.

19   **Ability to Feel Intimacy and Closeness**   0 1 2 3 4 5
The patient may display an inability to form close or intimate
relationships, especially with the opposite sex and family.

20   **Relationships with Friends and Peers**   0 1 2 3 4 5
The patient may have few or no friends and may prefer to spend
all of his time isolated.

21   **Global Rating of Anhedonia-Asociality**   0 1 2 3 4 5
This rating should reflect overall severity, taking into
account the patient's age, family status, etc.

ATTENTION

22   **Social Inattentiveness**   0 1 2 3 4 5
The patient appears uninvolved or unengaged. He may seem
"spacy".

23   **Inattentiveness During Mental Status Testing**   0 1 2 3 4 5
Tests of "serial 7s" (at least five subtractions) and
spelling "world" backwards:
Score: 2=1 error; 3=2 errors; 4=3 errors

24   **Global Rating of Attention**   0 1 2 3 4 5
This rating should assess the patient's overall concentration,
clinically and on tests.

2

SCALE FOR THE ASSESSMENT OF POSITIVE SYMPTOMS

0=None   1=Questionable   2=Mild   3=Moderate   4=Marked   5=Severe

HALLUCINATIONS

1   **Auditory Hallucinations**   0 1 2 3 4 5
    The patient reports voices, noises, or other sounds that
    no one else hears.

2   **Voices Commenting**   0 1 2 3 4 5
    The patient reports a voice which makes a running
    commentary on his behavior or thoughts.

3   **Voices Conversing**   0 1 2 3 4 5
    The patient reports hearing two or more voices conversing.

4   **Somatic or Tactile Hallucinations**   0 1 2 3 4 5
    The patient reports experiencing peculiar physical sensations
    in the body.

5   **Olfactory Hallucinations**   0 1 2 3 4 5
    The patient reports experiencing unusual smells which no
    one else notices.

6   **Visual Hallucinations**   0 1 2 3 4 5
    The patient sees shapes or people that are not actually
    present.

7   **Global Rating of Hallucinations**   0 1 2 3 4 5
    This rating should be based on the duration and severity
    of the hallucinations and their effects on the patient's life.

DELUSIONS

8   **Persecutory Delusions**   0 1 2 3 4 5
    The patient believes he is being conspired against or
    persecuted in some way.

9   **Delusions of Jealousy**   0 1 2 3 4 5
    The patient believes his *spouse is having an affair with
    someone.
    * or appropriate alternative in the case of an adolescent patient

10 **Delusions of Guilt or Sin**   0 1 2 3 4 5
    The patient believes that he has committed some terrible
    sin or done something unforgiveable.

11 **Grandiose Delusions**   0 1 2 3 4 5
    The patient believes he has special powers or abilities.

12 **Religioius Delusions**   0 1 2 3 4 5
    The patient is preoccupied with false beliefs of a religious
    nature.

13 **Somatic Delusions**   0 1 2 3 4 5
    The patient believes that somehow his body is diseased,
    abnormal, or changed.

14 **Delusions of Reference**   0 1 2 3 4 5
    The patient believes that insignificant remarks or events
    refer to him or have some special meaning.

1

0=None 1=Questionable 2=Mild 3=Moderate 4=Marked 5=Severe

15   **Delusions of Being Controlled**   0 1 2 3 4 5
     The patient feels that his feelings or actions are
     controlled by some outside force.

16   **Delusions of Mind Reading**   0 1 2 3 4 5
     The patient feels that people can read his mind or know
     his thoughts.

17   **Thought Broadcasting**   0 1 2 3 4 5
     The patient believes that his thoughts are broadcast so
     that he himself or others can hear them.

18   **Thought Insertion**   0 1 2 3 4 5
     The patient believes that thoughts that are not his own
     have been inserted into his mind.

19   **Thought Withdrawal**   0 1 2 3 4 5
     The patient believes that thoughts have been taken
     away from his mind.

20   **Global Rating of Delusions**   0 1 2 3 4 5
     This rating should be based on the duration and
     persistence of the delusions and their effect on the
     patient's life.

BIZARRE BEHAVIOR

21   **Clothing and Appearance**   0 1 2 3 4 5
     The patient dresses in an unusual manner or does other
     strange things to alter his appearance.

22   **Social and Sexual Behavior**   0 1 2 3 4 5
     The patient may do things considered inappropriate
     according to usual social norms (e.g., masturbating in
     public).

23   **Aggressive and Agitated Behavior**   0 1 2 3 4 5
     The patient may behave in an aggressive, agitated
     manner, often unpredictably.

24   **Repetitive or Stereotyped Behavior**   0 1 2 3 4 5
     The patient develops a set of repetitive action or rituals
     that he must perform over and over.

25   **Global Rating of Bizarre Behavior**   0 1 2 3 4 5
     This rating should reflect the type of behavior and the
     extent to which it deviates from social norms.

POSITIVE FORMAL THOUGHT DISORDER

26   **Derailment**   0 1 2 3 4 5
     A pattern of speech in which ideas slip off track onto
     ideas obliquely related or unrelated.

27   **Tangentiality**   0 1 2 3 4 5
     Replying to a question in an oblique or irrelevant
     manner.

0=None 1=Questionable 2=Mild 3=Moderate 4=Marked 5=Severe

28   **Incoherence**   0 1 2 3 4 5
     A pattern of speech which is essentially
     incomprehensible at times.

29   **Illogicality**   0 1 2 3 4 5
     A pattern of speech in which conclusions are reached
     which do not follow logically.

30   **Circumstantiality**
     A pattern of speech which is very indirect and delayed in
     reaching its goal idea.   0 1 2 3 4 5

31   **Pressure of Speech**   0 1 2 3 4 5
     The patient's speech is rapid and difficult to interrupt;
     the amount of speech produced is greater than that
     considered normal.

32   **Distractible Speech**   0 1 2 3 4 5
     The patient is distracted by nearby stimuli which
     interrupt his flow of speech.

33   **Clanging**   0 1 2 3 4 5
     A pattern of speech in which sounds rather than
     meaningful relationships govern word choice.

34   **Global Rating of Positive Formal Thought Disorder**   0 1 2 3 4 5
     This rating should reflect the frequency of abnormality
     and degree to which it affects the patient's ability to
     communicate.

INAPPROPRIATE AFFECT

35   <u>Inappropriate Affect</u>   0 1 2 3 4 5
     The patient's affect is inappropriate or incongruous,
     not simply flat or blunted.

<u>3</u>

Attention-Deficit Hyperactivity Disorder

ADHD RATING SCALE

Child's Name _____ Age ____ Grade _____

Completed by _____

Circle the number in the *one* column which best describes the child.

	Not at all	Just a little	Pretty much	Very much
1. Often fidgets or squirms in seat.	0	1	2	3
2. Has difficulty remaining seated.	0	1	2	3
3. Is easily distracted.	0	1	2	3
4. Has difficulty awaiting turn in groups.	0	1	2	3
5. Often blurts out answers to questions.	0	1	2	3
6. Has difficulty following instructions.	0	1	2	3
7. Has difficulty sustaining attention to tasks.	0	1	2	3
8. Often shifts from one un-completed activity to another.	0	1	2	3
9. Has difficulty playing quietly.	0	1	2	3
10. Often talks excessively.	0	1	2	3
11. Often interrupts or intrudes on others.	0	1	2	3
12. Often does not seem to listen.	0	1	2	3
13. Often loses things necessary for tasks.	0	1	2	3
14. Often engages in physically dangerous activities without considering consequences.	0	1	2	4

SCORING INSTRUCTIONS:

Parent Ratings

Total score: Sum items 1-14
Inattention-Hyperactivity:
Sum items 1-3, 6-8, 12-14
Impulsivity-Hyperactivity:
Sum items 1, 2, 4, 5, 9-11, 14.

Teacher Ratings

Total score: Sum items 1-14
Inattention-Hyperactivity:
1-3, 6-8, 12, 13.
Impulsivity-Hyperactivity:
Sum items 1, 2, 4, 5, 9-11, 14.

From "Parent and Teacher Ratings of ADHD Symptoms: Psychometric Properties in a Community Based Sample" by G. P. DuPaul, 1991, Journal of Clinical Child Psychology, 20, pp. 245–253. Copyright 1991 by Lawrence Erlbaum Associates, Inc. Reprinted by permission.

ADHD SYMPTOMS RATING SCALE

Name: _____ Date: _____

Medication: _____ Dose: _____

Category	Never				Continuously
Restless	1	2	3	4	5
Excitable	1	2	3	4	5
Inattentive	1	2	3	4	5
Difficulty concentrating	1	2	3	4	5
Disturbs others	1	2	3	4	5
Quarrelsome	1	2	3	4	5
Temper outbursts	1	2	3	4	5
Attention seeking	1	2	3	4	5
Fails to complete tasks	1	2	3	4	5
Easily distracted	1	2	3	4	5
Impulsive	1	2	3	4	5
Needs supervision	1	2	3	4	5
Trouble with others	1	2	3	4	5
Fidgety	1	2	3	4	5
Difficulty staying seated	1	2	3	4	5
On the go - "driven"	1	2	3	4	5
Disorganized	1	2	3	4	5
Speaks out of turn, interrupts others	1	2	3	4	5

Comments _____

_____

Signature: _____

TALLAND LETTER CANCELLATION TEST

Note to Clinician   If you are using this test, make sure you:

1. Read the instructions carefully and explain them to the subject to be tested.

2. Make sure that <u>only</u> 60 seconds per page make up the testing time.

3. Use the accompanying scoring key to determine the subjects omission and error percentages.

Testing Materials: 6 pages of letters
Stopwatch
Pen (unerasable)

Instructions:

<u>CAPS</u>   First sheet (starts with u r) "In this test, you are to look for the capital letters and mark each one with a slash. Go across the lines, from left to right, one after the other, marking the capital letters as quickly as you can. Try not to miss any". Show, on the last line, how to mark it, and also, if an error has been made, how to indicate it by making another slash so the mark becomes a cross. "Go ahead." Stop after 60 seconds and indicate the subject's place.

Second sheet (starts with w b) "You are going to do the same thing on this sheet as you did on the last one; mark all capital letters." "Go ahead." Stop after 60 seconds; mark where the subject ended.

<u>SPACES</u>   Third sheet (starts with O a) "This time, you are to look for the double spaces (show them on the last line), and mark the letter that precedes and the one that follows the double space" (show them on the last line). "Go as quickly as you can without missing any. Go ahead." Stop after 60 seconds; mark where the subject ended.

Fourth sheet (starts with t o) "This is another sheet on which to look for the double spaces. Mark the letters before and after the double space, just the way you did on the last page. Go ahead." Stop after 60 seconds; mark where the subject ended.

<u>BOTH</u> Fifth sheet (starts with u S) "Now you have to do both tasks at once; mark the capital letters as well as the letters before and after double spaces. Go ahead." Stop after 60 seconds; mark where the subject ended.

<u>1</u>

Sixth sheet (starts with u d) "This is a last sheet, just like the one before. Mark the capital letters and the letters before and after the double spaces. Go ahead." Stop afater 60 seconds; mark where the subject ended.

LETTER CANCELLATION TEST Scoring Information:

There are 36 letters/line, 10 of which are capital letters; there are four double spaces in each line.

To find the number of letters surveyed, count all letters u pto and including the last one marked.

> Omit = number of letters that should have been marked, but weren't.

> Commit = number of letters marked that shouldn't have been.

You might find it helpful to indicate errors in red, circling omissions and making squares around commissions.

Scoring the Test

1. Record for each sheet:

> A) # of letters or spaces crossed out (total)
> B) # of letters or spaces correctly crossed out
> C) # of letters or spaces omitted
> D) # of letters or spaces incorrectly crossed out

2. There are 6 sheets. Each task is comprised of 2 sheets. For each task compute the percent omitted using the following formula. Refer to item one above for letter definitions in the formula below.

$$\frac{\frac{C_1}{A_1} + \frac{C_2}{A_2}}{2} \times 100 = \text{Percent Omitted}$$

3. There are 6 sheets. Each task is comprised of 2 sheets. For each task compute the percentage error using the following formula. Refer to item one above for letter definitions in the formula below.

$$\frac{\frac{C_1 + D_1}{B_1} + \frac{C_2 + D_2}{B_2}}{2} \times 100 = \text{Percentage Error}$$

From Talland. Deranged Memory. Orlando: Academic Press, 1965. Reprinted by permission of Academic Press.

2

TASK ONE

urns iVpiotxorEdaq sIHeEOukT ksaQx KwkeL

IsS erunqnU krasxCBLwbIAbRxfvqbXr t tdke

cQbahUxAuiswRhxpfhik MbkPzGtZw iv H Npaa

ZnuuUa gRriicAll hEh klZgKwBqjEZ rnqcquj

srZgeNb xquh bPAiqNxfv m vDunvkiDXPrFFyg

lvstNyeLgu uAtr tovhUfACgF oi qOqvZngaDm

w McXKZgnDxIhaelQbwng cwuh dyUmphZDuog l

mwGjiynbYjlsvKrSfQuqcJ hcSm mPpAos vLr r

hvxc NOR pi aznvvybapvvL pQVsGghjlsDIRyt

h swugd aBZvpdnYq FXiicce jskOnSvPunqBMv

yg pGzZtXalHsuWxiEybzmzxFX z z rNzhctePi

Auhamjzl gasUr hF ObtestdoXzVMVj HiWfspj

tJfjR rmq xXjl NVNqRmc JdceHcX hbmjmzegly

cuyIiksFzOvboPbofbQK e ekZvNyg llmFOdi c

DyzD ku yvpWzv RPZmbnAHjHVftgpzigttmxz s

WIqB bxNMidOwAJxpxGsi syqovy rzqntara Ef

gizcnerl Ajx WpPFn jzAuuefyYcbAocqBvBZ b

dvpcdfF fQNam wnVrmiPobjIzbx tePjKYwma V

wsIwkRl BteyEpQhfrvU Usbsdzawe TD bjvhUs

hzOHqzD hvoxipPt C eJeABrgk ccBqvnubnuQx

<u>TASK ONE</u>   2

w b i L m p p   h   c g m r A f v I Z a d f j   r y c Z M e F I   w k s w X i D

c n p d t   U v l h   z h r t b v S m   x B G s F y z k b I V E E   Q c u N i k

o x k G e X t c o j W i l   r r s   r O k L z i f t x c i n   S h Z V Z y   f W

t v X L x u a l Y u   n q s s x n o r h j s G H   B z d t   D T   a b d f d B H

c   B y v x a v a q m v Z L w z F g x l l A   R r   j W p H v R   r y B v y e u

u j T b q A f w r l i n b   n a A   J c Q W p X g i W B a g G y   h e l w   g i

y   b s   q T   o z g s v o N x g r E P U m q q z Z D a R f r d o h   g t M z M

w t y   d d   o H n W   v X   i z v D l Q n B q h e y T k m o i f a v K h W z S

i d C   f j n u R f   d A i M f j j m L f r   b D p t T B m V   v d s y z c X m

w j Y y F   b d f V l p l U b   O p w o u m Q l i E H k   i F y u l b   f F v g

t z t v s n M   i d S l M p p D R j c   u v g A j i r E n   q m Y   k v A l z G

S x h m w W x o a r   z y p v y   G q e i v r O j C c J B H   m r y G   o j n U

b   h b   K t W Z o j a m q m j Q X v   c h N c   c i l D z a V r C L i y w u c

f P E j k N R   n l i W c h g o j Z   M l H   p n D j v r t e z t J z d t z   a

g C c g a   k J P b b y f   f   V X g z j s o e v   a d V u Z n n j V d J h N z

J C l f p i B Y a J z j c   S p d n d m m   f K c Q m F i o   l g c p   a L u m

q y j g U x f   D n g n f f R c   j u   I Z G   j X d Q o j v Q k u Z p d r o p

i B o e o F L   R a   v v h I f u g o y r x u   W r   R h f t r h l i v Z H t M

Q s T I x e b F w J r q   i N O o w   B b   j y w j m   k b S p h d i X e k p v

B n z   f I o b h R g i   Y z x a m f L z x h H k Y T h s z k I   j c F   q f n

TASK TWO 3

O a j l P A y   x x N f j V   d q w z l r f S W o o F y v r   s   Y G n e z b y

w   u Y S U d c a x q T j c g q g o z x g e M t W z g   V   e v N d X r u   z B

Z c n s h e K   r y W O c r Y l Z Q j m x   s g i v V f o   C x f f z z   R w c

q X c f a   v j h Y h   a E m D d f O c j j m R z m   b R a g s c S y m   z G U

y c k b C l y y k y f m b   i u q n t i n v v y x T L   L S   m M Z N Q t   h W

j   V C a v z w k t q o E i f d d l   w   t c y B a M L   d e c M M l K R g b w

d y b r   v d X g s S i g X f Y W h e   r T   W c p U n T X u j b w   z b z d j

V w j t g r u   g r k U x f   Y m   m g l M   H I C x g N u u u y Z y f e Q z l

o U s d g v o k t N Y p K c O   y L h a c n h   r   m m K Y x P h   r z Y k b c

E h g v y u q C t w s u d   j z Y k g q b A Z   c V a Y w e j Z   r   X I x y k

w g i w d o   D   Q J e o h m x n   k o b M r V r m   E f z U u k y k m V b L S

d b v z l d q e r i d   g u K w L G K j   y r c r e A k L   i V S p v T t   k Z

K L q t   X u k G f z r   k o h j w w z g y v a h a b f B E   p v N I b Y a   P

R   s l r f v l r d m e z Q p   n i a P i m N j g   I A   E w   G o r w B j T x

k g a D p   d v S N q z t q J U   t a   e w a b c r n i v   x f e N L C u K U f

L s g a n   s   E I Q f s h T e I b s c k j   d m l c z k H   s t q r i S R C e

d j e Q   n e z e d A h M w j Y   Q g l r c w S   Q g f e q s U   W z Z d m n j

y c B   b c i G L e c X G   i z c U u T p l b n   w i w c p k b P k u i t   i G

m z v t z v g n x x z   L l J h k R   j N m   D D b D h e u m O m   a t y y B T

e a   M H   m C u   m   v e a y a z k a A i B c j U d J b z A w U u k o z n b P

TASK TWO

4

t o   J x M z m K y R z l a w r   d v H t a u m E k s m e w E   z M V r b P p

x a X g p n a E Q   l b z I o m X   g u x b l q o d i j K S   x l l k T D   Q r

r v Z t y j s n i o r c y H q j y E M Y   n S   q v g A v   R i x m M   x p U e

o t r p n m   l l g y l a v e E N B Q   w F M k   u s y n I a   Z y v n z U Y p

l K b r   t A m t L A G a o c z h   p S   D b t V y v E   j h g i J h j n n d o

b O v f D   t y h v P p v o d N p e K M   t n e Z   b   A y T w r S o v d l q r

M f r j Y n S u   l a z k m V A c G N w y A p f x q a   y o u y   a   F N s s h

l   e q b   w x   s M z h l f X G h B n o j y g L Z V a w   u C f f j h S e I o

K t l r k   i z u Z q l w w a L k   w i J m j l   v q   E k r O u s V g H j T q

e k Y i N x I s m k p E t   Y K d g t e x e f h N   S q m q q G e u w   V u   v

j c R r   i a x h g R D b E j w   j z   P B   v a X j t X f s h o Z e m v m Q h

c e r E o c x   d M k c L c x o v B F A   R   g n G g   g v r D f r n l y A b t

b x x R   y r   b V G b f r y m c c p c L   W k S b J Q S o a z M q   y p l y e

h   u z h v j w u   g o   P x u   W X n l r i B q l U U p N x P v a z F N n d e

R v c   e d   R r q d x t   N j O V C u i i t L d R e   L u m s c l c j U y r o

e e U Q   f b E M a O t v v b M E F g h O e e s b Z c h   p   o b k d y n c   p

y   m g y A i w k i Q k r o n o y l o p R K   J D i M q v   c X b X r d   B l q

g a Y n U s A g v c X d i q k p H W r G q   t   f t y   y Y n m w z v M D   v x

y m D B   a b   d E h p S p   G s f h n N Q r j   n z b H D y q h l R w o p h q

p c p   g g i Y K F u n w S j   j   h r y t Y r u T d l W u i Q   b u W u b K q

<u>TASK THREE</u>   5

u S G u l x g   v z   p u Q g g W u O l j W u u   G   u j Y z R c u d E h q a w

c j H m k k l H x w g w b u q u y   L W o   T p b   P v z X U I w f d r   B c o

A b   x   b i p y m f g h i q d T Z U a w J I K   d m j w C z W O c c n   x c l

r J m k F j   v N t x t v F U f t n d k f z r A Z   S u e N   c a c G x   w m q

b N L I   n n k x o M f f a   b   J n t k G g b e t P e R w t w J   f F v v t e

t b   n   I u g z L w v W   a k i k l e N H l B i c x i s a s m b Q z   W R J c

z W k e I m i f w p r R h o   q P n Z   c   Q b m b R f b j h x o   G K c c X h

k S h Q e J h o   m K   D q n g r q B h v   d a x x L   n r K l e p u m N g C b

o   W G j r X l e L N e C o   c j v b d A   T f C d a t c a f   r j k q Q r o j

w O v u k a Y F x i n n c n I g d   H x y Q   W k h Q t   p l H j   h y g e i F

l r   W y R U   d d q z g n n o v U w A y a n w K Z m h n Q t   d   B M p a x j

t M g l n u s i   K J p   v G D Y s n   Y a T y   d T n l y s b x C u f r v y x

v g l e e K u k N r i   c W f h b t v k E o g g u u   W E   f T c W   B y c V e

f g j h m   W o Q e i O   d r j L c y o m   z K z d d w q d   A b e O A n I s K

a e s D K b f p k l k h L z s e P o X q   m m   g   Q   x i m C C N t a h u M q

p w m n Q o B R s   z y f h T   x r Q g   C z R t d p   u k S c z j O s g T p g

w p n s w f g P N b f   u n U w t v B u g   d o m w W   c L G X W a t x X n   f

q L N z   H a s b y R m   K E P y o g t T c R h e y b d q   u j   s u Y c f n v

p K F p r   r   P h o j i K y s s G j t t v y Q   f o R q P c y v e   C w f B u

P v   q V G n   e L y c   r z b B u j w D p d D d v e z O y I b X j   a g z o a

TASK THREE

u d q C g b P X F n M U i w T e j b m l t c q z Y n v e n g B s x R z t

u o r w P g j̃ Z e L l f l T q a j x R V n t l w g S a h G q f c r G A m

s u o h w n p k F x m k y r F x N Q A v i E F m l U d r t i D w h f A s

J G f o r z m y D t r M i y X y w y t f p b J E r J c F o e D t d j g c

s F g d x r c H o m b u z G x k I W s s s g R j n t B h q Q r y w N Z j

e s w q Z w I x B w h u t m M r o v m j n q w X h X y h a O g m U z M O

b G p Z q b L p k J j x n o v f s X z v w J u A e q b p A X l f H f a t

Z j I i U b k a u r t b g t l Z p q D H i u d E I Y n a i i r n n k R q

c L z y v k G i u c o d b v N C m z y s s t O y a I d t X o H u G n C m

r i k o Q j m G z u D V M k d p x o w P s g U l g w M s l Y s T m a n t

r A e x j j y q s h i C w s F P e h c Q d X x r b B Y o T u E q j h z l

l W Q E p s A V w W I c r g x m u f e a f t r x p Z m u m n R d z e o G

t h p n h c K F f o z L T Q D t m O v k e r o n w u F k J s m d i F i w

i j J u d A l h t p B a U w H r M s g o p v W d q U i t Q e m j h s f K

u i j a P t L e o l y x R r P n z P r i q w K o z h c x k t l o K J C Y

L n Q m c J k v d w m h i v z I f j w n t p L W h p a z N h u e O u Z T

Y a v j D F s c m w K n m t g z s k u b o h Z w O d s N y w Y Y n q k E

d w g Y v V R j w h o m k f z r X V c o W I k z y g C a i h f q y n R M

C e B h o f a u u t d s z x f F s D m p K s Z o v Q u s O y R j b z r S

g L k k t F Z c e C x M f k R H u A x y W h e f b c b x u s W q b r h t

Obsessive Compulsive Disorder

Yale-Brown Obsessive Compulsive Scale (Y-BOCS)

Patient's Name

Date of 1st report

Therapy

Date of this report

Instructions: Complete Y-BOCS Symptom Checklist (flip side) before administering Y-BOCS (below). In administering Y-BOCS, make specific reference to patient's principal obsessions and compulsions.

	None	Mild	Moderate	Severe	Extreme
1. TIME SPENT ON OBSESSIONS	0	1	2	3	4
2. INTERFERENCE FROM OBSESSIONS	0	1	2	3	4
3. DISTRESS OF OBSESSIONS	0	1	2	3	4
	Definitely resists				Completely yields
4. RESISTANCE	0	1	2	3	4
	Complete control	Much control	Moderate control	Little control	No control
5. CONTROL OVER OBSESSIONS	0	1	2	3	4

OBSESSION SUBTOTAL (Items 1-5)

	None	Mild	Moderate	Severe	Extreme
6. TIME SPENT ON COMPULSIONS	0	1	2	3	4
7. INTERFERENCE FROM COMPULSIONS	0	1	2	3	4
8. DISTRESS OF COMPULSIONS	0	1	2	3	4
	Definitely resists				Completely yields
9. RESISTANCE	0	1	2	3	4
	Complete control	Much control	Moderate control	Little control	No control
10. CONTROL OVER COMPULSIONS	0	1	2	3	4

COMPULSION SUBTOTAL (Items 6-10)

Total Y-BOCS Score (Items 1-10)

Y-BOCS Symptom Checklist

Instructions: Generate a *Target Symptoms List* from the attached *Y-BOCS Symptom Checklist* by asking the patient about specific obsessions and compulsions. Check all that apply. Distinguish between current and past symptoms. Mark principal symptoms with a "p." These will form the basis of the *Target Symptoms List.* Items marked "*" may or may not be OCD phenomena.

AGGRESSIVE OBSESSIONS

Current Past

____ ____ Fear might harm self
____ ____ Fear might harm others
____ ____ Violent or horrific images
____ ____ Fear of blurting out obscenities or insults
____ ____ Fear of doing something else embarrassing*
____ ____ Fear will act on unwanted impulses (eg, to stab friend)
____ ____ Fear will steal things
____ ____ Fear will harm others because not careful enough (eg, hit/run motor vehicle accident)
____ ____ Fear will be responsible for something else terrible happening (eg, fire, burglary)
____ ____ Other _____

CONTAMINATION OBSESSIONS

____ ____ Concerns or disgust with bodily waste or secretions (eg, urine, feces, saliva)
____ ____ Concern with dirt or germs
____ ____ Excessive concern with environmental contaminants (eg, asbestos, radiation, toxic waste)
____ ____ Excessive concern with household items (eg, cleansers, solvents)
____ ____ Excessive concern with animals (eg, insects)
____ ____ Bothered by sticky substances or residues
____ ____ Concerned will get ill because of contaminant
____ ____ Concerned will get others ill by spreading contaminant (Aggressive)
____ ____ No concern with consequences of contamination other than how it might feel
____ ____ Other _____

SEXUAL OBSESSIONS

____ ____ Forbidden or perverse sexual thoughts, images, or impulses
____ ____ Content involves children or incest
____ ____ Content involves homosexuality*
____ ____ Sexual behavior towards others (Aggressive)*
____ ____ Other _____

HOARDING/SAVING OBSESSIONS

(distinguish from hobbies and concern with objects of monetary or sentimental value)

____ ____ _____

RELIGIOUS OBSESSIONS (Scrupulosity)

____ ____ Concerned with sacrilege and blasphemy
____ ____ Excess concern with right/wrong, morality
____ ____ Other _____

OBSESSION WITH NEED FOR SYMMETRY OR EXACTNESS

____ ____ Accompanied by magical thinking (eg, concerned that another will have accident unless things are in the right place)
____ ____ Not accompanied by magical thinking

MISCELLANEOUS OBSESSIONS

____ ____ Need to know or remember
____ ____ Fear of saying certain things
____ ____ Fear of not saying just the right thing
____ ____ Fear of losing things
____ ____ Intrusive (nonviolent) images
____ ____ Intrusive nonsense sounds, words, or music
____ ____ Bothered by certain sounds/noises*
____ ____ Lucky/unlucky numbers
____ ____ Colors with special significance
____ ____ Superstitious fears
____ ____ Other _____

SOMATIC OBSESSIONS

Current Past

____ ____ Concern with illness or disease*
____ ____ Excessive concern with body part or aspect of appearance (eg, dysmorphophobia)*
____ ____ Other _____

CLEANING/WASHING COMPULSIONS

____ ____ Excessive or ritualized handwashing
____ ____ Excessive or ritualized showering, bathing, toothbrushing, grooming, or toilet routine
____ ____ Involves cleaning of household items or other inanimate objects
____ ____ Other measures to prevent or remove contact with contaminants
____ ____ Other _____

CHECKING COMPULSIONS

____ ____ Checking locks, stove, appliances, etc.
____ ____ Checking that did not/will not harm others
____ ____ Checking that did not/will not harm self
____ ____ Checking that nothing terrible did/will happen
____ ____ Checking that did not make mistake
____ ____ Checking tied to somatic obsessions
____ ____ Other _____

REPEATING RITUALS

____ ____ Rereading or rewriting
____ ____ Need to repeat routine activities (eg, in/out door, up/down from chair)
____ ____ Other _____

COUNTING COMPULSIONS

____ ____ _____

ORDERING/ARRANGING COMPULSIONS

____ ____ _____

HOARDING/COLLECTING COMPULSIONS

(distinguish from hobbies and concern with objects of monetary or sentimental value (eg, carefully reads junk mail, piles up old newspapers, sorts through garbage, collects useless objects))

MISCELLANEOUS COMPULSIONS

____ ____ Mental rituals (other than checking/counting)
____ ____ Excessive listmaking
____ ____ Need to tell, ask, or confess
____ ____ Need to touch, tap, or rub*
____ ____ Rituals involving blinking or staring*
____ ____ Measures (not checking) to prevent: harm to self ____; harm to others ____; terrible consequences ____
____ ____ Ritualized eating behaviors*
____ ____ Superstitious behaviors
____ ____ Trichotillomania*
____ ____ Other self-damaging or self-mutilating behaviors*
____ ____ Other _____

OCD Impact Scale
- Parent Report about Child -

Name: _____   Date: _____

Informant: _____   Clinician: _____   Week _____

Please rate how much your child's OCD (unwanted thoughts and rituals) has caused problems for him or her in the following areas over the past month. If the question does not apply (for example, he or she doesn't take Gym Class - Question 11) mark "Not at all".

In the past month, how much trouble has your child had doing the following because of his/her OCD?	Not at all	Just a Little	Pretty Much	Very Much

SCHOOL ACTIVITIES

1. Getting to school on time in the morning _____ _____ _____ _____

2. Being absent from school _____ _____ _____ _____

3. Getting to classes on time during the day _____ _____ _____ _____

4. Giving oral reports or reading out loud _____ _____ _____ _____

5. Being prepared for class, e.g., having his/her books, paper or pencils ready when needed _____ _____ _____ _____

6. Writing in class _____ _____ _____ _____

7. Taking tests or exams _____ _____ _____ _____

8. Completing assignments in class _____ _____ _____ _____

9. Doing homework _____ _____ _____ _____

10. Getting good grades _____ _____ _____ _____

11. Participating in gym or P.E. activities _____ _____ _____ _____

12. Changing or showering for gym _____ _____ _____ _____

13. Doing fun things during recess or free time _____ _____ _____ _____

14. Concentrating on his/her work _____ _____ _____ _____

15. Eating lunch with other kids _____ _____ _____ _____

16. Going to school outings or field trips _____ _____ _____ _____

Next Page ➡

In the past month, how much trouble has your child had doing the following because of his/her OCD?	Not at all	Just a Little	Pretty Much	Very Much

SOCIAL ACTIVITIES

17. Making new friends

18. Keeping friends he/she already has

19. Leaving the house

20. Talking on the phone

21. Being with a group of people he/she knows

22. Being with a group of strangers

23. Going to a friend's house during the day

24. Having a friend come to his/her house during the day

25. Spending the night at a friend's house

26. Having someone spend the night at his/her house

27. Letting someone touch or use his/her things, like toys, records, or clothes

28. Doing activities where someone else touches him/her, like playing sports, dancing, or having someone comb his/her hair

29. Going to the movies

30. Going to a sports event or ball game

31. Going shopping or trying on clothes

32. Going on a date

33. Having a boyfriend/girlfriend

34. Going to a restaurant or fast food place

35. Eating in public other than a restaurant, like on a picnic, in the park, or at a friend's house

Next Page ➡

OCD Impact Scale - Parent about Child   Page 3

In the past month, how much trouble has your child had doing the following because of his/her OCD?	Not at all	Just a Little	Pretty Much	Very Much

HOME/FAMILY ACTIVITIES

36. Getting dressed in the morning

37. Bathing or grooming (brushing his/her teeth or combing his/her hair) in the morning

38. Bathing or grooming at other times, like before going out in the evening

39. Doing chores that he/she is asked to do, like washing the dishes, taking the garbage out, or cleaning his/her room

40. Eating meals at home

41. Eating different kinds of food that he/she usually likes

42. Watching television or listening to music

43. Reading books, magazines, or newspapers for fun

44. Getting ready for bed at night

45. Sleeping at night

46. Going to the bathroom

47. Getting along with his/her brothers or sisters

48. Getting along with his/her parents

49. Visiting relatives

50. Having relatives visit

51. Going on a family vacation

52. Going to church or temple

Please list any other areas where intrusive thoughts or rituals are causing problems for your child:

53. _____

54. _____

Next Page ➡

In the past month, how much trouble has your child had doing the following because of his/her OCD?	Not at all	Just a Little	Pretty Much	Very Much
55. Overall, how much are your child's intrusive thoughts or rituals causing problems for him/her at <u>school</u>?	___	___	___	___
56. Overall, how much are your child's intrusive thoughts or rituals causing problems for him/her <u>socially</u>, that is with friends?	___	___	___	___
57. Overall, how much are your child's intrusive thoughts or rituals preventing him/her from <u>going places</u> with friends or relatives?	___	___	___	___
58. Overall, how much are your child's intrusive thoughts or rituals causing problems for your <u>family and at home</u>?	___	___	___	___

Developed by John Piacentini, Ph.D., Child and Adolescent OCD Program, UCLA-Neuropsychiatric Institute, Los Angeles, CA and Marni Jaffer, R.N., Cornell University-Westchester Division, White Plains, NY.

OCD Impact Scale
- Child and Adolescent Report -

Name: _____   Date: _____

Clinician: _____   Treatment Week: _____

> Please rate how much your OCD (unwanted thoughts and rituals) have caused problems for you in thefollowing areas over the past month. If the question does not apply to you (for example, you don't take Gym Class - Question 11) mark "Not at all".

In the past month, how much trouble have you had doing the following things because of your OCD?	Not at all	Just a Little	Pretty Much	Very Much

SCHOOL ACTIVITIES

1.	Getting to school on time in the morning	____	____	____	____
2.	Being absent from school	____	____	____	____
3.	Getting to classes on time during the day	____	____	____	____
4.	Giving oral reports or reading out loud	____	____	____	____
5.	Being prepared for class, like having my books, paper or pencils ready when needed	____	____	____	____
6.	Writing in class	____	____	____	____
7.	Taking tests or exams	____	____	____	____
8.	Completing assignments in class	____	____	____	____
9.	Doing homework	____	____	____	____
10.	Getting good grades	____	____	____	____
11.	Participating in gym or P.E. activities	____	____	____	____
12.	Changing or showering for gym	____	____	____	____
13.	Doing fun things during recess or free time	____	____	____	____
14.	Concentrating on my work	____	____	____	____
15.	Eating lunch with other kids	____	____	____	____
16.	Going to school outings or field trips	____	____	____	____

Next Page ➡

OCD Impact Scale - Child   Page 2

In the past month, how much trouble have you had doing the following things because of your OCD?	Not at all	Just a Little	Pretty Much	Very Much

SOCIAL ACTIVITIES

17. Making new friends

18. Keeping friends I already have

19. Leaving the house

20. Talking on the phone

21. Being with a group of people that I know

22. Being with a group of strangers

23. Going to a friend's house during the day

24. Having a friend come to my house during the day

25. Spending the night at a friend's house

26. Having someone spend the night at my house

27. Letting someone touch or use my things, like toys, records, or clothes

28. Doing activities where someone else touches me, like playing sports, dancing, or having someone comb my hair

29. Going to the movies

30. Going to a sports event or ball game

31. Going shopping or trying on clothes

32. Going on a date

33. Having a boyfriend/girlfriend

34. Going to a restaurant or fast food place

35. Eating in public other than a restaurant, like on a picnic, in the park, or at a friend's house

Next Page ➡

OCD Impact Scale - Child   Page 3

In the past month, how much trouble have you had doing the following things because of your OCD?	Not at all	Just a Little	Pretty Much	Very Much

HOME/FAMILY ACTIVITIES

36. Getting dressed in the morning

37. Bathing or grooming (brushing my teeth or combing my hair) in the morning

38. Bathing or grooming at other times, like before going out in the evening

39. Doing chores that I am asked to do, like washing the dishes, taking the garbage out, or cleaning my room

40. Eating meals at home

41. Eating different kinds of food that I usually like

42. Watching television or listening to music

43. Reading books, magazines, or newspapers for fun

44. Getting ready for bed at night

45. Sleeping at night

46. Going to the bathroom

47. Getting along with my brothers or sisters

48. Getting along with my parents

49. Visiting relatives

50. Having relatives visit

51. Going on a family vacation

52. Going to church or temple

Please list any other areas where your intrusive thoughts or rituals are causing problems for you:

53. _____

54. _____

Next Page ➡

OCD Impact Scale - Child   Page 4

	Not at all	Just a Little	Pretty Much	Very Much

GLOBAL ITEMS

55. Overall, how much is your OCD (intrusive thoughts or rituals) causing problems for you at <u>school</u>?

56. Overall, how much is your OCD (intrusive thoughts or rituals) causing problems for you <u>socially</u>, that is with friends?

57. Overall, how much is your OCD (intrusive thoughts or rituals) preventing you from <u>going places</u> with friends or relatives?

58. Overall, how much is your OCD (intrusive thoughts or rituals) causing problems for you with your <u>family and at home</u>?

Developed by John Piacentini, Ph.D., Child and Adolescent OCD Program, UCLA-Neuropsychiatric Institute, Los Angeles, CA and Marni Jaffer, R.N., Cornell University-Westchester Division, White Plains, NY.

Other Useful Rating Scales of Symptoms

MEASUREMENT OF TIC SEVERITY

HOPKINS MOTOR/VOCAL TIC SCALE

Name: _____

Date: _____

Assessment	Motor	Vocal
Parent	____	____
Physician	____	____
Overall	____	____

For each tic listed below, place a mark on the line that would best describe its severity over the past week.

MOTOR

<u>Head</u>   None   Mild   Moderate   Moderately   Severe
                                                                  Severe

    eye blinking   [_____]

    face _____   [_____]

    _____   [_____]

    _____   [_____]

<u>Neck</u> _____   [_____]

<u>Shoulder</u> _____   [_____]

<u>Extremities</u>
    arm _____   [_____]

    fingers _____   [_____]

    legs _____   [_____]

    _____   [_____]

    _____   [_____]

VOCAL _____   [_____]

    _____   [_____]

    _____   [_____]

    _____   [_____]

On the line below place a mark which would describe how symptoms are today compared to the worst they have ever been or when totally absent.

    [_____]
No Symptoms   **Worst Ever**

Compare with previous (p. 467) generation [3-27-97]

From Walkup JT, Rosenberg LA, Brown J, Singer HS. The validity of instruments measuring tic severity in Tourette's syndrome. <u>Journal of the American Academy of Child and Adolescent Psychiatry</u>, 31:472, 1992. Reprinted by permission of Dr. Walkup and the Journal of the American Academy of Child and Adolescent Psychiatry.

MOVE SURVEY

Answer the questions below for the past ___ week(s)	NEVER	SOMETIMES	OFTEN	ALWAYS
1. I make noises (like grunts) that I can't stop.				
2. Parts of my body jerk again and again, that I can't control.				
3. I have bad ideas over and over, that I can't stop.				
4. I have to do things in certain order or certain ways (like touching things)				
5. Words come out that I can't stop or control.				
6. At times I have the same jerk or twitch over and over.				
7. Certain bad words or thoughts keep going through my mind.				
8. I have to do exactly the opposite of what I'm told.				
9. The same unpleasant or silly thought or picture goes through my mind.				
10. I can't control all my movements.				
11. I have to do several movements over and over again, in the same order.				
12. Bad or swear works come out that I don't mean to say.				
13. I feel pressure to talk, shout or scream.				
14. I have ideas that bother me (like germs or like cutting myself).				
15. I do certain things (like jumping or clapping) over and over.				
16. I have habits or movements that come out more when I'm nervous.				
17. I have to repeat things that I hear other people say.				
18. I have to do things I see other people do.				
19. I have to make bad gestures (like the finger).				
20. I have to repeat words or phrases over and over.				

Motor tic, Obsession and compulsion, and Vocal tic Evaluation Scale (MOVES)
Reprinted with permission: Mary Ann Liebert, Inc. Publishers

YALE GLOBAL TIC SEVERITY SCALE

A. *Instructions*

This clinical rating scale is designed to rate the overall severity of tic symptoms across a range of dimensions (number, frequency, intensity, complexity, and interference). Use of the YGTSS requires the rater to have clinical experience with Tourette's syndrome patients. The final rating is based on all available information and reflects the clinician's overall impression for each of the items to be rated.

The style of the interview is semistructured. The interviewer should first complete the Tic Inventory (a list of motor and phonic tics present during the past week, as reported by the parent/patient, and observed during the evaluation). It is then best to proceed with questions based on each of the individual items, using the content of the anchor points as a guide.

B. *Tic Inventory*

1. *Description of Motor Tics:* (Check motor tics present during past week)

   a. *Simple Motor Tics:* (Rapid, Darting, "Meaningless"):
   ___ Eye blinking
   ___ Eye movements
   ___ Nose movements
   ___ Mouth movements
   ___ Facial grimace
   ___ Head jerks/movements
   ___ Shoulder shrugs
   ___ Arm movements
   ___ Hand movements
   ___ Abdominal tensing
   ___ Leg or foot or toe movements
   ___ Other_____

   _____

   b. *Complex Motor Tics:* (Slower, "Purposeful"):
   ___ Eye gestures or movements
   ___ Mouth movements
   ___ Facial movements or expressions
   ___ Head gestures or movements
   ___ Shoulder gestures
   ___ Arm or hand gestures
   ___ Writing tics
   ___ Dystonic postures
   ___ Bending or gyrating
   ___ Rotating
   ___ Leg or foot or toe movements
   ___ Tic-related compulsive behaviors (touching, tapping, grooming, evening-up)
   ___ Copropraxia
   ___ Self abusive behavior (describe) _____
   ___ Paroxysms of tics (displays),
       duration ___ seconds
   ___ Disinhibited behavior (describe)* _____
   ___ Other_____

   _____

   ___ Describe any orchestrated patterns or sequences of motor tic behaviors _____

2. *Description of Phonic Tic Symptoms:* (Check phonic tics present over the past week)

   a. *Simple Phonic Symptoms:* (Fast, "Meaningless" Sounds): Sounds, noises: (circle: coughing, throat clearing, sniffing, grunting, whistling, animal or bird noises)
   Other (list) _____

   b. *Complex Phonic Symptoms:* (Language: Words, Phrases, Statements):
   ___ Syllables: (list) _____
   ___ Words: (list) _____
   ___ Coprolalia: (list) _____
   ___ Echolalia _____
   ___ Palalalia _____
   ___ Blocking _____
   ___ Speech atypicalities: (describe) _____
   ___ Disinhibited speech: (describe)*_____
   ___ Describe any orchestrated patterns or sequences of phonic tic behaviors _____

C. *Ordinal Scales* (Rate motor and phonic tics separately unless otherwise indicated).

a. *Number:* Motor Score: [ ] Phonic Score: [ ]
Score Description (Anchor Point)
0   None
1   Single tic
2   Multiple discrete tics (2–5)
3   Multiple discrete tics (>5)
4   Multiple discrete tics plus at least one orchestrated pattern of multiple simultaneous or sequential tics where it is difficult to distinguish discrete tics.
5   Multiple discrete tics plus several (>2) orchestrated patterns of multiple simultaneous or sequential tics where it is difficult to distinguish discrete tics.

b. *Frequency:* Motor Score: [ ] Phonic Score: [ ]
Score Description (Anchor Point)
0   *None,* no evidence of specific tic behaviors.
1   *Rarely,* specific tic behaviors have been present during previous week. These behaviors occur infrequently, often not on a daily basis. If bouts of tics occur, they are brief and uncommon.
2   *Occasionally,* specific tic behaviors are usually present on a daily basis, but there are long tic-free intervals during the day. Bouts of tics may occur on occasion and are not sustained for more than a few minutes at a time.
3   *Frequently,* specific tic behaviors are present on a daily basis. Tic-free intervals as long as 3 hours are not uncommon. Bouts of tics occur regularly but may be limited to a single setting.
4   *Almost always,* specific tic behaviors are present virtually every waking hour of every day, and periods of sustained tic behaviors occur regularly. Bouts of tics are common and are not limited to a single setting.
5   *Always,* specific tic behaviors are present virtually all the time. Tic-free intervals are difficult to identify and do not last more than 5 to 10 minutes at most.

*Do not include this item in rating the ordinal scales.

c. *Intensity:* Motor Score: [ ]   Phonic Score: [ ]

Score   Description (Anchor Point)

0   *Absent*

1   *Minimal intensity,* tics not visible or audible (based solely on patient's private experience) or tics are less forceful than comparable voluntary actions and are typically not noticed because of their intensity.

2   *Mild intensity,* tics are not more forceful than comparable voluntary actions or utterances and are typically not noticed because of their intensity.

3   *Moderate intensity,* tics are more forceful than comparable voluntary actions but are not outside the range of normal expression for comparable voluntary actions or utterances. They may call attention to the individual because of their forceful character.

4   *Marked intensity,* tics are more forceful than comparable voluntary actions or utterances and typically have an "exaggerated" character. Such tics frequently call attention to the individual because of their forceful and exaggerated character.

5   *Severe intensity,* tics are extremely forceful and exaggerated in expression. These tics call attention to the individual and may result in risk of physical injury (accidental, provoked, or self-inflicted) because of their forceful expression.

d. *Complexity:* Motor Score:[ ]   Phonic Score: [ ]

Score   Description (Anchor Point)

0   *None,* if present, all tics are clearly "simple" (sudden, brief, purposeless) in character.

1   *Borderline,* some tics are not clearly "simple" in character.

2   *Mild,* some tics are clearly "complex" (purposive in appearance) and mimic brief "automatic" behaviors, such as grooming, syllables or brief meaningful utterances such as "ah huh," "hi," that could be readily camouflaged.

3   *Moderate,* some tics are more "complex" (more purposive and sustained in appearance) and may occur in orchestrated bouts that would be difficult to camouflage but could be rationalized or "explained" as normal behavior or speech (picking, tapping, saying "you bet" or "honey," brief echolalia).

4   *Marked,* some tics are very "complex" in character and tend to occur in sustained orchestrated bouts that would be difficult to camouflage and could not be easily rationalized as normal behavior or speech because of their duration and/or their unusual, inappropriate, bizarre, or obscene character (a lengthy facial contortion, touching genitals, echolalia, speech atypicalities, longer bouts of saying "what do you mean" repeatedly, or saying "fu" or "sh").

5   *Severe,* some tics involve lengthy bouts of orchestrated behavior or speech that would be impossible to camouflage or successfully rationalize as normal because of their duration and/or extremely unusual, inappropriate, bizarre, or obscene character (lengthy displays or utterances often involving copropraxia, self-abusive behavior, or coprolalia).

e. *Interference:* Motor Score: [ ]   Phonic Score: [ ]

Score   Description (Anchor Point)

0   *None.*

1   *Minimal,* when tics are present, they do not interrupt the flow of behavior or speech.

2   *Mild,* when tics are present, they occasionally interrupt the flow of behavior or speech.

3   *Moderate,* when tics are presnt, they frequently interrupt the flow of behavior or speech.

4   *Marked,* when tics are present, they frequently interrupt the flow of behavior or speech, and they occasionally disrupt intended action or communication.

5   *Severe,* when tics are present, they frequently disrupt intended action or communication.

f. *Impairment:* Overall Impairment: [ ] (Rate Overall Impairment for Motor and Phonic Tics):

Score   Description (Anchor Point)

0   *None*

10   *Minimal,* tics associated with subtle difficulties in self-esteem, family life, social acceptance, or school or job functioning (infrequent upset or concern about tics vis à vis the future; periodic, slight increase in family tensions because of tics; friends or acquaintances may occasionally notice or comment about tics in an upsetting way).

20   *Mild,* tics associated with minor difficulties in self-esteem, family life, social acceptance, or school or job functioning.

30   *Moderate,* tics associated with some clear problems in self-esteem, family life, social acceptance, or school or job functioning (episodes of dysphoria, periodic distress and upheaval in the family, frequent teasing by peers or episodic social avoidance, periodic interference in school or job performance because of tics).

40   *Marked,* tics associated with major difficulties in self-esteem, family life, social acceptance, or school or job functioning.

50   *Severe,* tics associated with extreme difficulties in self-esteem, family life, social acceptance, or school or job functioning (severe depression with suicidal ideation, disruption of the family [separation/divorce, residential placement], disruption of social ties—severely restricted life because of social stigma and social avoidance, removal from school or loss of job).

D. *Score Sheet.*

Name _____   Date _____

DOB _____   Sex _____

Sources of Information _____

Raters _____

Motor Tics:

Number	[ ]	
Frequency	[ ]	
Intensity	[ ]	
Complexity	[ ]	
Interference	[ ]	
Total Motor Tic Score	[ ]	

Phonic Tics:

Number	[ ]	
Frequency	[ ]	
Intensity	[ ]	
Complexity	[ ]	
Interference	[ ]	
Total Phonic Tic Score	[ ]	

Overall Impairment Rating   [ ]

Global Severity Score
(Motor + Phonic + Impairment)   [ ]

From Leckman JF, Riddle MA, Hardin MT, Ort SI, Swartz KL, Stevenson J, Cohen DJ. The Yale Global Tic Severity Scale. *Journal of the American Academy of Child and Adolescent Psychiatry,* 1989, 28, 4:566–573. Reprinted by permission of Waverly and Dr. Leckman.

WARD SCALE OF IMPULSIVE ACTION PATTERNS

OUTPATIENT SCALE

Name: _____   Date: _____

ITEMS	Not present 0	Slight 1	Mild 2	Moderate 3	Marked 4
SCALE OF IMPULSIVE ACTION 1) Inability to tolerate frustration or delay gratification (e.g., temper tantrums).	0	1	2	3	4
2) Demanding and/or un-reasonable requests of staff (unpredicated demands which exceed expectable behaviour).	0	1	2	3	4
3) Any drug/alcohol use.	0	1	2	3	4
4) Self-mutilation (wrist cutting, scratching, head banging).	0	1	2	3	4
5) Suicidal threat.	0	1	2	3	4
6) Suicidal gesture.	0	1	2	3	4
7) Assaultiveness towards others.	0	1	2	3	4
8) Assaultiveness threat (e.g., verbal intimidation).	0	1	2	3	4
9) Destruction of property.	0	1	2	3	4
10) Inappropriate or symptomatic sexual behaviour (e.g., ego dysstonic), promiscuity, includes provocative dress or behaviour in office).	0	1	2	3	4
11) Antisocial behaviour (disruptive, inciting others).	0	1	2	3	4
12) Manipulative behaviour.	0	1	2	3	4

SIGNATURE: _____

From Soloff PH, George A, Nathan RS, Schulz PM, Ulrich RF, Perel JM. Progress in Pharmacotherapy of borderline disorders: A double-blind study of amitriptyline, haloperidol, and placebo. Arch Gen Psychiatry 1986; 43:691–697. Reprinted by permission of the American Medical Association.

WARD SCALE OF IMPULSIVE ACTION PATTERNS

INPATIENT SCALE

Name: _____   Date: _____

ITEMS	Not present 0	Slight 1	Mild 2	Moderate 3	Marked 4
1) Inability to tolerate frustration or delay gratification (e.g., temper tantrums, unable to wait one's turn, share T.V., pool table with others)	0	1	2	3	4
2) Demanding and/or un-reasonable requests of staff (unpredicated demands which exceed expectable behaviour, e.g., demands to go on walk when restricted to unit).	0	1	2	3	4
3) Drug/alcohol use on ward or attempted smuggling.	0	1	2	3	4
4) Self-mutilation (wrist cutting, scratching, head banging).	0	1	2	3	4
5) Suicidal threat.	0	1	2	3	4
6) Suicidal gesture.	0	1	2	3	4
7) Assaultiveness towards others.	0	1	2	3	4
8) Assaultiveness threat (e.g., verbal intimidation).	0	1	2	3	4
9) Destruction of ward property.	0	1	2	3	4
10) Sexual behaviour on ward (verbally or physically provocative, teasing, physical contact with others including open erotic display with visitors).	0	1	2	3	4
11) Antisocial behaviour (disruptive, inciting others, practical jokes, disregard of ward rules, management problem).	0	1	2	3	4
12) Manipulative behaviour (e.g., threatening to sign out if not placated, "acting out" to get attention, somatizing, attempted but half-hearted elopement).	0	1	2	3	4

SIGNATURE: _____

From Soloff PH, George A, Nathan RS, Schulz PM, Ulrich RF, Perel JM. Progress in Pharmacotherapy of borderline disorders: A double-blind study of amitriptyline, haloperidol, and placebo. Arch Gen Psychiatry 1986; 43:691–697. Reprinted by permission of the American Medical Association.

OVERT AGGRESSION SCALE (OAS)

IDENTIFYING DATA

Name of Patient	Name of Rater
Sex of Patient: 1 Male 2 Female	Date / / (mo/da/yr) Shift: 1 Night 2 Day 3 Evening
_____ No agressive incident(s) (verbal or physical) against self, others or objects during the shift. (check here)	

AGGRESSIVE BEHAVIOR (check all that apply)

VERBAL AGGRESSION	PHYSICAL AGGRESSION AGAINST SELF
___ Makes loud noises, shouts angrily ___ Yells mild personal insults, e.g., "You're stupid!" ___ Curses viciously, uses foul language in anger, makes moderate threats to others or self ___ Makes clear threats of violence toward others or self, (I'm going to kill you.) or requests to help to control self	___ Picks or scratches skin, hits self, pulls hair, (with no or minor injury only) ___ Bangs head, hits fist into objects, throws self onto floor or into objects, (hurts self without serious injury) ___ Small cuts or bruises, minor burns ___ Mutilates self, makes deep cuts, bites that bleed, internal injury, fracture, loss of consciousness, loss of teeth.
PHYSICAL AGGRESSION AGAINST OBJECTS	**PHYSICAL AGGRESSION AGAINST OTHER PEOPLE**
___ Slams door, scatters clothing, makes a mess ___ Throws objects down, kicks furniture without breaking it, marks the wall ___ Break objects, smashes windows ___ Sets fires, throws objects dangerously	___ Makes threatening gesture, swings at people, grabs at clothes ___ Strikes, kicks, pushes, pulls hair (without injury to them) ___ Attacks others causing mild-moderate physical injury (bruises, sprain, welts) ___ Attacks others causing severe injury (broken bones, deep lacerations, internal injury
Time incident began: ___ ___ : ___ ___ am/pm	Duration of incident: ___ ___ : ___ ___ (hours/minutes)

INTERVENTION (check all that apply)

___ None ___ Talking to patient ___ Closer observation ___ Holding patient	___ Immediate medication given by mouth ___ Immediate medication given by injection ___ Isolation without seclusion (time out) ___ Seclusion	___ Use of restraints ___ Injury requires immediate medical treatment for patient ___ Injury requires immediate treatment for other person

COMMENTS

WEIGHTED SCORES: OVERT AGGRESSION SCALE

Verbal Aggression
____ Makes loud noises, shouts angrily. **(1)**
____ Yells mild personal insults, eg, "You're stupid!" **(2)**
____ Curses viciously, uses foul language in anger, makes moderate
      threats to others or self. **(3)**
____ Makes clear threats of violence toward others or self,
      (I'm going to kill you) or requests help to control self. **(4)**

Physical Aggression Against Objects
____ Slams door, scatters clothing, makes a mess. **(2)**
____ Throws objects down, kicks furniture without breaking it,
      marks the wall. **(3)**
____ Breaks objects, smashes windows. **(4)**
____ Sets fires, throws objects dangerously. **(5)**

Physical Aggression Against Self
____ Picks or scratches skin, hits self on arms or body, pinches
      self, pulls hair (with no or minor injury only). **(3)**
____ Bangs head, hits fist into objects, throws self onto floor   ▯
      into objects (hurts self without serious injury). **(4)**
____ Small cuts or bruises, minor burns. **(5)**
____ Mutilates self, makes deep cuts, bites that bleed, internal
      injury, fracture, loss of consciousness, loss of teeth. **(6)**

Physical Aggression Against Others
____ Makes threatening gestures, swings at people, grabs at
      clothes. **(3)**
____ Strikes, kicks, pushes, pulls hair (without injury to them). **(4)**
____ Attacks others causing mild-moderate physical injury
      (bruises, sprain, welts). **(5)**
____ Attacks others causing severe physical injury (broken bones,
      deep lacerations, internal injury). **(6)**

Interventions
____ Talking to patient. **(1)**
____ Closer observation. **(2)**
____ Holding patient. **(3)**
____ Isolation without seclusion. **(3)**
____ Immediate medication given by mouth. **(4)**
____ Immediate medication given by injection. **(4)**
____ Seclusion **(5)**
____ Use of restraints. **(5)**

*Numbers following behaviors or interventions indicate "weighted"
score.*

From Yudofsky SC, Silver JM, Jackson W, Endicott J, Williams D. The overt aggression scale for the objective rating of verbal and physical aggression. American Journal of Psychiatry, 143:35–39, 1986. Copyright 1986, the American Psychiatric Association. Reprinted by permission.

Functioning Assessments

Social Adjustment Inventory for Children and Adolescents (SAICA)
Autonomous Functioning Checklist
School and Social Disability Scale
Sickness Impact Profile—Adolescent Version
Duke Social Support and Stress Scale
Duke Health Profile
Academic Performance Rating Scale
Multigrade Inventory for Teachers

SAICA

Name: _____   Date: _____

ASK PARENTS AND CHILDREN

<u>Note</u>: *Time period assess is the CURRENT GRADE IN SCHOOL (including the previous summer for out of school behavior) unless too little time (1-2 months) has been spent in or too little information is available on the current grade. In such instances, the preceding school year should be included in the assessment.*

DATE AT BEGINNING OF ASSESSMENT PERIOD:

MONTH   YEAR

DATE AT END OF ASSESSMENT PERIOD:

MONTH   YEAR

SCHOOL AND TEACHER INFORMATION
Ask about current year and prior year. Record information on teacher form.
    a. What school do you go to? Where is that located?

    For children grades k-6
    b. What is the name of your teacher this year?

    For children 7-12
    c. Who is the teacher who knows you best? What does s/he teach?

A. SCHOOL FUNCTIONING

1. How are you doing in school? What subjects do you have? What kind of grades do you get?
Please rate academic subjects on the following scale:

	Above Average	Average	Below Average	Failing
a. READING/ENGLISH	1	2	3	4
b. ARITHMETIC/MATH	1	2	3	4
List additional subjects and review ratings				
c. _____	1	2	3	4
d. _____	1	2	3	4
e. _____	1	2	3	4

2. Are there different reading and arithmetic groups in your class at school? Which group are you in?
Review ratings (specify academic 'track' or group) If discrepancies exist make notes but CODE FOR HIGHEST ACHIEVEMENT

X Not applicable

1 Above Average

2 Average

3 Below Average

4 Far below average

3. How do you feel about school? Do you enjoy school? Do you like your teachers? Do your teachers like you?... How much? What about the other kids? Do you get along well with them?

	Positive	More Positive Than Negative	More Negative Than Positive	Negative
a. ATTITUDE TOWARDS SCHOOL WORK	1	2	3	4
b. ATTITUDE TOWARDS TEACHERS	1	2	3	4
c. TEACHER'S ATTITUDE TOWARDS CHILD	1	2	3	4
d. RELATIONSHIPS WITH OTHER STUDENTS	1	2	3	4

4. Do you have problems or do you get into trouble at school? How about for *(list)*: Is that more than the other kids? How much of a problem is it? *[Note: Ask mother if teacher reported]*

	Not a Problem	Mild Problem	Moderate Problem	Severe Problem
a. Not paying attention or listening	1	2	3	4
b. Not doing as well as you can/ not working up to your ability	1	2	3	4
c. Being noisy; bothering other kids/ being disruptive in class	1	2	3	4
d. Being too shy/ not participating/ being introverted	1	2	3	4
e. Getting into fights/ being assaultive	1	2	3	4
f. Being left out/ excluded by others	1	2	3	4
g. Damaging school or other people's property	1	2	3	4
h. Getting very upset/ having difficulty accepting mistakes or criticism	1	2	3	4
i. Giving up too easily/ being defeated/not trying	1	2	3	4
j. Always wanting to be noticed/ the center of attention	1	2	3	4
k. Being overly anxious to please/ concerned with rules	1	2	3	4
GLOBAL RATING OF SCHOOL BEHAVIOR PROBLEMS *Interviewer rate according to chronicity and seriousness of consequences*	1	2	3	4

2

B. Spare Time Activities

1. What kinds of things do you like to do in your free time? How about *(list)*? Do you like doing that a lots... How much do you do that?

	Very Involved	Pretty Involved	Not Very Involved	Not at All Involved
a. Collecting/ making things	1	2	3	4
b. Sports/ physical activities	1	2	3	4
c. Reading/ looking at books	1	2	3	4
d. Listening to music	1	2	3	4
e. Playing musical instruments	1	2	3	4
f. Playing with toys, games, etc.	1	2	3	4
g. Extra curricular school, church, or community activities	1	2	3	4
h. Jobs/chores	1	2	3	4
i. Other constructive activity Specify:_____	1	2	3	4
GLOBAL RATING OF SPARE TIME ACTIVITIES	1	2	3	4

GLOBAL RATING OF SPARE TIME ACTIVITIES
Interviewer rate according to amount of time spent, interest in, and age appropriate quality of spare time activities

2. During the school year, how much TV do you usually watch every week? After school? After supper? On Saturday?

1 7 or fewer hours per week

2 8-14 hours per week

3 15-21 hours per week

4 22-35 hours per week

5 More than 35 hours per week

3. Do you spend free time mostly alone or mostly with other kids? More with others than alone, or more alone than with others?

1 Mostly with others

2 More with others than alone

3 More alone than with others

4 Mostly alone

3

4. Do you have any problems in your free time?
How about *(list)*:... How much of a problem is that?

	Not a Problem	Mild Problem	Moderate Problem	Severe Problem
a. Being bored	1	2	3	4
b. Not liking/ having trouble playing or working along	1	2	3	4
c. Hanging out (e.g. downtown, arcades)	1	2	3	4
d. Not being interested in anything much/ being indifferent to most activities	1	2	3	4
e. Spending a lot of time daydreaming,/ in fantasy	1	2	3	4
f. Getting into mischief/destroying things	1	2	3	4
GLOBAL RATING OF SPARE TIME PROBLEMS *Interviewer rate according to chronicity and seriousness of consequences*	1	2	3	4

C. Peer Relations

1. How do you get along with other kids? Do you make friends easily? Are kids always calling you to do things? Would you say you're popular? Do you have a best friend? Do you have a group of friends? Have you stayed friends with the same kids for a long time? Are you the kind of kid that other kids follow or are you more likely to do what the others are doing?...How true is that?

	Very True	Pretty True	Not Very True	Not At All True
a. Makes new friends easily	1	2	3	4
b. Is popular with others	1	2	3	4
c. Has one or two special friends	1	2	3	4
d. Has a steady group of friends	1	2	3	4
e. Is a leader	1	2	3	4

Very Active	Pretty Active	Not Very Active	Not At All Active
1	2	3	4

GLOBAL RATING OF ACTIVITY WITH PEERS
Interviewer rate according to interests in, time spent, and positive involvement with peers

4

2. Do you ever have any problems with other children? How about *(list):* Is that more than other kids?...How much of a problem is it?

	Not a Problem	Mild Problem	Moderate Problem	Severe Problem
a. Being shy with other kids	1	2	3	4
b. Being teased/ bullied by other kids	1	2	3	4
c. Bullying other kids	1	2	3	4
d. Having trouble keeping friends	1	2	3	4
e. Wanting to be with grownups	1	2	3	4
f. Wanting to be with older kids	1	2	3	4
g. Wanting to be with younger kids	1	2	3	4
h. Wanting to be with girls/boys (opposite sex)	1	2	3	4
i. Doing things because other kids are doing them even if you may get into trouble	1	2	3	4
j. Hanging out with other kids who get into trouble	1	2	3	4
GLOBAL RATING OF PEER PROBLEMS *Interviewer rate according to chronicity and seriousness of consequences*	1	2	3	4

NOTE: For children approximately 12 years or older

3. Do you have friends who are girls /boys? Do you go to school dances or boy-girl parties? Do you have a girlfriend/boyfriend? Do you go out alone with girls/boys?... How true is that?

	Very True	Pretty True	Not Very True	Not At All True
a. Has friends of opposite sex	1	2	3	4
b. Attends school dances/ boy-girl parties	1	2	3	4
c. Has a girlfriend/boyfriend	1	2	3	4
d. Dates	1	2	3	4

	Very Active	Pretty Active	Not Very Active	Not At All Active
GLOBAL RATING OF BOY-GIRL RELATIONSHIPS *Interviewer rate according to interests in, time spent, and positive involvement with opposite sex*	1	2	3	4

5

4. Do you have problems in your relationships with girls/boys? How about with *(list)*: Is that more than other kids?... How much of a problem is it?

	Not a Problem	Mild Problem	Moderate Problem	Severe Problem
a. Going steady *(fused relationship)*	1	2	3	4
b. Having sex with many different boys/ girls *(promiscuity)*	1	2	3	4
c. Avoiding boys/girls	1	2	3	4
d. Having trouble establishing relationships with girls/ boys	1	2	3	4
GLOBAL RATING OF PROBLEMS WITH OPPOSITE SEX *Interviewer rate according to chronicity and seriousness of consequences*	1	2	3	4

D. Current Home Behavior

Determine the applicability of the following items and consider the ages of siblings, etc. In your ratings.

1. How well do you get along with your brother(s) and/or sister(s)? Do you play with them or do things with them? Are you friendly/affectionate toward them? Do you talk with them?...How true is that?

	Very True	Pretty True	Not Very True	Not At All True	NA
a. Plays or does things with them	1	2	3	4	X
b. Is friendly toward/ affectionate with them	1	2	3	4	X
c. Talks with them	1	2	3	4	X

	Very Active	Pretty Active	Not Very Active	Not At All Active	NA
GLOBAL RATING OF SIBLING RELATIONSHIPS *Interviewer rate according to age appropriate positive involvement with siblings*	1	2	3	4	X

6

2. Do you have any problems with your brother(s) and/or sister(s)? How about *(list)*: Is that more than other kids?...How much of a problem is it?

	Not a Problem	Mild Problem	Moderate Problem	Severe Problem	NA
a. Avoiding (contact) with sibling(s)	1	2	3	4	X
b. Scapegoating/ bullying sibling(s)	1	2	3	4	X
c. Injurying sibling(s)	1	2	3	4	X
d. Being avoided by sibling(s)	1	2	3	4	X
e Being scapegoated/ bullied by sibling(s)	1	2	3	4	X
f. Being injured by sibling(s)	1	2	3	4	X
GLOBAL RATING OF PROBLEMS WITH SIBLINGS	1	2	3	4	X

GLOBAL RATING OF PROBLEMS WITH SIBLINGS
Interviewer rate according to chronicity and seriousness of events

3. How well do you get along with your mother? Do you do things with her? Are you friendly and affectionate toward her? Do you talk with her? How true is that?

	Very True	Pretty True	Not Very True	Not At All True	NA
a. Does things with mother	1	2	3	4	X
b. Is friendly/ affectionate toward mother	1	2	3	4	X
c. Talks with mother	1	2	3	4	X

	Very Active	Pretty Active	Not Very Active	Not At All Active	NA
GLOBAL RATING OF RELATIONSHIP WITH MOTHER	1	2	3	4	X

GLOBAL RATING OF RELATIONSHIP WITH MOTHER
Interviewer rate according to age-appropriate positive involvement with mother

7

4. How well do you get along with your father? Do you do things with him? Are you friendly and affectionate toward him? Do you talk with him? How true is that?

	Very True	Pretty True	Not Very True	Not At All True	NA
a. Does things with father	1	2	3	4	X
b. Is friendly/ affectionate toward father	1	2	3	4	X
c. Talks with father	1	2	3	4	X

	Very Active	Pretty Active	Not Very Active	Not At All Active	NA
GLOBAL RATING OF RELATIONSHIP WITH FATHER	1	2	3	4	X

GLOBAL RATING OF RELATIONSHIP WITH FATHER
Interviewer rate according to age- appropriate positive involvement with father

5. Do you have problems with things that your parents ask you to do? For example, when they ask you to do chores or come home at a particular time, what happens? How about *(list)*: Is that more than for other kids?... How much of problem is it?

	Not a Problem	Mild Problem	Moderate Problem	Severe Problem
a. Strong negative reaction or refusal to do chores or honor restrictions	1	2	3	4
b. Dangerous irresponsibility around the house (e.g. leaves stove on)	1	2	3	4
c. Damages home or family property	1	2	3	4
d. Physically threatens or attacks parents	1	2	3	4
GLOBAL RATING OF PROBLEMS WITH PARENTS	1	2	3	4

GLOBAL RATING OF PROBLEMS WITH PARENTS
Interviewer rate according to chronicity and seriousness of events

Reprinted with the permission of Karen John, 11 Berkeley Place, Camden Road, Bath, BA1 5JH, England.

8

AUTONOMOUS FUNCTIONING CHECKLIST

Name: _____   Date: _____

Grade in School:_____   Informant: _____
                                    (Mother, father, guardian, other)

Instructions

The purpose of this checklist is to learn about what your teenager does every day. There are no "right" or "wrong" things for your teenager to do, since teenagers of different ages do many different things. These questions are simply for the purpose of getting an idea of your teenager's daily activity.

When you answer these questions, first, read the question and think about whether or not it describes what you see or have seen your teenager do. You should answer the questions according to what you know your teenager does or does not do rather than what you **believe** or **think** he or she **could** do or **could not** do.

Second, tell us how the question describes what your teenager does by choosing one of the alternatives "0", "1", "2", "3", or "4" from the scale and circling that number in the space to the right of the item. Here is how to use the rating scale with a sample question.

0	1	2	3	4
does not do	does only rarely	does about half the time there is an opportunity	does most of the time there is an opportunity	does every time there is an opportunity

Sample Item. Pick up trash in the yard.   0 1 2 3 4

0 - Circle "0" if you have never seen your teenager to this, even if he or she may never have had an opportunity. (For example mark "0" if your teenager has never done it, even if you live in an apartment and do not have a yard.)

1 - Circle "1" if you have seen your teenager to this when there has been a chance, but if there have been many more times that he or she has not done it.

2 - Circle "2" if your teenager does this about half the time there is a chance, but if he or she does not it readily or comfortably.

3 - Circle "3" if there are more times that your teenager does this than does not do it, given the chance, and if he or she does it readily.

4 - Circle "4" if your teenager does this whenever there is a chance and if he or she does it readily.

<u>1</u>

Your teenager will not have had the chance to participate in some of the activities the questions described. These items should be answered as "does not do", even though you may feel that your teenager would do it if given the chance. Please circle "0" for questions that describe activities your teenager has **never had the chance** to do.

Some questions describe things that your teenager may do with help from others. Answer these questions after you think about who has the most responsibility for completing the activity. For example, your teenager may cook the family meals and may be helped by other family members who set the table or chop vegetables. If your teenager is the family member with the most responsibility for cooking every meal that the family eats together, your answer would be "4", which stands for "does every time there is an opportunity." On the other hand, if your teenager helps other family members by doing jobs that they tell him or her to do, and never has the most responsibility for fixing dinner, your answer would be "0", for "does not do."

0	1	2	3	4
does not do	does only rarely	does about half the time there is an opportunity	does most of the time there is an opportunity	does every time there is an opportunity

My teenager:

1. Keeps own personal items and belongings in order (e.g., makes bed, puts away own clothing and belongings). 0 1 2 3 4

2. Prepares food that does not require cooking for himself/herself (e.g., cereal, sandwich). 0 1 2 3 4

3. Care for his/her own clothing (e.g., laundry simple repair, shoe cleaning). 0 1 2 3 4

4. Travels to and from daily activities (e.g., rides bike or walks, takes bus, arranges for transportation, drives car). 0 1 2 3 4

5. Prepares food that requires cooking for himself/herself (e.g., hamburger, soup). 0 1 2 3 4

6. Performs simple first aid or medical care for himself/herself (e.g., bandages, takes own temperature). 0 1 2 3 4

7. Purchases his/her own clothing and personal items that are used on a daily basis (e.g., underwear, toiletries). 0 1 2 3 4

0	1	2	3	4
does not do	does only rarely	does about half the time there is an opportunity	does most of the time there is an opportunity	does every time there is an opportunity

My teenager:

8. Performs minor repair and maintenace in his/her own environment (e.g., changes light bulbs, hangs pictures).   0 1 2 3 4

9. Shops for and purchases his/her own groceries.   0 1 2 3 4

10. Responds to his/her own medical emergency by calling parent.   0 1 2 3 4

11. Responds to his/her own medical emergency by calling doctor or hospital.   0 1 2 3 4

12. Does designated household maintenance chores involving family living areas (e.g., cleans, takes out trash, does simple yard work).   0 1 2 3 4

13. Performs routine daily personal care for another family member (e.g., dresses, feeds).   0 1 2 3 4

14. Keeps personal items and belongings of another family member in order (e.g., makes bed, puts away clothing and belongings).   0 1 2 3 4

15. Prepares meals for other family member(s).   0 1 2 3 4

16. Transports (or arranges for transport of) another family member to and from daily activities.   0 1 2 3 4

17. Purchases clothing and personal items (that are used on a daily basis) for other family members.   0 1 2 3 4

18. Shops for and purchases family groceries.   0 1 2 3 4

19. Performs minor repairs and maintenance in family living areas (e.g., changes light bulbs, hangs pictures).   0 1 2 3 4

20. Repairs and maintains (or makes arrangement for repair and maintenance of) major household needs (e.g., plumbing, yard work, electrical wiring).   0 1 2 3 4

<u>3</u>

0	1	2	3	4
does not do	does only rarely	does about half the time there is an opportunity	does most of the time there is an opportunity	does every time there is an opportunity

My teenager:

21. Responds to household emergency (e.g. stove fire, plumbing problem) by calling parent or neighbour).   0 1 2 3 4

22. Responds to household emergency (e.g., stove fire, plumbing problem) by calling fire department, using fire extinguisher, or calling repair service or shutting off water.   0 1 2 3 4

23. Uses the telephone directories.   0 1 2 3 4

24. Carries out transactions with sales people (e.g., listens to information, asks questions, gives payment, receives change).   0 1 2 3 4

25. Uses postal services (e.g., uses postage, mails letters, packages).   0 1 2 3 4

26. Uses bank (e.g., fills out deposit or withdrawal slips, uses passbook).   0 1 2 3 4

27. Uses travel-related services for short trips (e.g., taxi, bus, subway).   0 1 2 3 4

28. Uses travel-related services for long trips (e.g., airline, train, bus).   0 1 2 3 4

29. Uses library services (e.g., checks out books or uses photocopy machine).   0 1 2 3 4

30. Maintains and uses his/her own savings account.   0 1 2 3 4

31. Maintains and uses his/her own checking or charge account.   0 1 2 3 4

32. Maintains adequate personal care and grooming (e.g., bathes, trims fingernails and toenails when needed).   0 1 2 3 4

33. Maintains his/her routine general health and fitness (e.g., adequate eating, sleeping and exercise habits).   0 1 2 3 4

<u>4</u>

0	1	2	3	4
does not do	does only rarely	does about half the time there is an opportunity	does most of the time there is an opportunity	does every time there is an opportunity

My teenager:

34. Selects clothing that is suited to weather (e.g., raincoat if raining, warm clothes in winter). 0 1 2 3 4

35. Plans and initiates activity for himself/herself everyday unscheduled free time (e.g., chooses to watch television or work on a hobby if bored). 0 1 2 3 4

36. Plans activity for his/her long-term free time (e.g., makes plans for summer vacation, mid-semester vacation). 0 1 2 3 4

37. Initiates friendships with peers (e.g., plans or attends parties, outings, games, club meetings). 0 1 2 3 4

38. Meets nonacademic social obligations or commitments (e.g., keeps appointments for family and peer related social events arranged by self or others). 0 1 2 3 4

39. Meets academic obligations and commitments (e.g., completes homework assignments on time, brings necessary supplies to class). 0 1 2 3 4

40. Plans transportation to and from special activities (e.g., arranges for rides with friends or family or plans car or bus route and schedule. 0 1 2 3 4

41. Manages his/her own budget from allowance or income (e.g., saves money for large purchases, pays for routine expenses throughout week without running out of money). 0 1 2 3 4

42. Makes long-term educational and/or career plans (e.g., selects courses, investigates colleges or technical schools). 0 1 2 3 4

5

0	1	2	3	4
does not do	does only rarely	does about half the time there is an opportunity	does most of the time there is an opportunity	does every time there is an opportunity

When my teenager is free to choose how he/she will spend his/her unscheduled free time, he/she chooses to:

43. Listen to music (e.g., radio or stereo).   0 1 2 3 4

44. Read for relaxation (e.g., books or newspapers).   0 1 2 3 4

45. Play games or puzzles (e.g., cards, crossword puzzles, jigsaw puzzles, computer games).   0 1 2 3 4

46. Write letters to friends, relatives, acquaintances.   0 1 2 3 4

47. Work on or take lessons in crafts or hobbies (e.g., cooking, collections, pet care, sewing, model building, car repair).   0 1 2 3 4

48. Practice or take lessons that involve a trained artistic or academic skill (e.g., piano, or other musical instrument, ballet, singing, creative writing, foreign language).   0 1 2 3 4

49. Go to movies, rock concerts, dances   0 1 2 3 4

50. Go to plays, theatre, lectures.   0 1 2 3 4

51. Pursue activities that are related to his/her career interest(s) (e.g., runs a business, works on a computer, practises piano for professional preparation).   0 1 2 3 4

52. Go for walks.   0 1 2 3 4

53. Go shopping, or spend time at shopping centres or in shopping areas.   0 1 2 3 4

54. Attend club meetings or other organized social group meetings.   0 1 2 3 4

55. Work for pay (e.g., baby-sit, play in a band do yard work, walk dogs, work at a part-time job, deliver papers.   0 1 2 3 4

0	1	2	3	4
does not do	does only rarely	does about half the time there is an opportunity	does most of the time there is an opportunity	does every time there is an opportunity

When my teenager is free to choose how he/she will spend his/her unscheduled free time, he/she chooses to:

56. Clean and/or maintain living environment or belongings (e.g., clean house, wash or repair clothes, wash car, make household repairs).   0 1 2 3 4

57. Work on school work (e.g., spend extra time on homework, make special preparations for class projects, spend time in library).   0 1 2 3 4

58. Spend time with family (e.g., work on family projects, have discussions or casual conversations, attend family gatherings such as picnics or parties).   0 1 2 3 4

On these final items please check "Yes" or "No" in response to each description. Check "Yes" if the description fits your teenager. Check "No" if it does not.

My teenager:

		<u>Yes</u>	<u>No</u>
59.	Has casual friendships with teenagers of the opposite sex.	____	____
60.	Has close friendships with teenagers of the opposite sex.	____	____
61.	Has casual friendships with adults outside the family (e.g., teachers, neighbours, coaches, scout leaders).	____	____
62.	Has close friendships with adults outside the family, (e.g., teachers, neighbours, coaches, scout leaders).	____	____
63.	Has casual friendships with younger children.	____	____
64.	Has close friendships with younger children.	____	____
65.	Is active in casual/recreational groups of teenage friends.	____	____
66.	Has many friendships.	____	____

	Yes	No

My teenager:

67. Is active in one or more organized extracurricular group (e.g., French club, student
council, sports team). ____ ____

68. Has leadership position in one or more organized
extracurricular group (e.g., president of
student council, captain of sports team). ____ ____

69. Has close friendship with adult member of the
extended family (e.g., uncle, aunt, grandparent). ____ ____

70. Works or has worked either for pay or volunteer
in an area of particular career interest. ____ ____

71. Works or has worked to earn money by providing
a service on a regular scheduled basis (e.g.,
contracts for yard work, dog walking, baby-
sitting). ____ ____

72. Works or has worked to earn money by using a
special skill (e.g., musical performance,
typing, tutoring). ____ ____

73. Works or has worked to earn money in a self- or
peer-run organization or business. ____ ____

74. Works or has worked to earn money fundraising
for an organization or charity (e.g., scouts
church groups, political organizations). ____ ____

75. Does or has done volunteer work without pay for a
service, a school or political organization, a
social agency, a club, a church, or a hospital. ____ ____

76. Participates or has participated in prevocational
(career) or vocational (career) classes or
training (e.g., any technical training or career
development class). ____ ____

77. Has explored career interest by visiting work
sites or interviewing people in that job or ____ ____

78. Has spent time reading, researching, or
"finding out" about a career that particularly
interests him/her. ____ ____

8

<u>Comments</u>:

If you have any additional information about your teenager's everyday independent or self-sufficient behaviour, use the space below to write your comments.

Thank you.

Bradley Hospital, 1988 Version
Carl B. Feinstein, M.D., Associate Director, Department of Psychiatry, Kennedy Krieger Institute,707 North Broadway, Baltimore, Maryland, U.S.A., (410) 550-9000. Reprinted by permission.

<u>9</u>

SCHOOL AND SOCIAL DISABILITY SCALE

Evaluate the overall school and social functioning of the patient according to the following scale:

1. No complaints, normal activities.

2. Symptoms mild but do not interfere with normal school, work or social activities.

3. Symptoms interfere with normal activities in minor ways.

4. Symptoms interfere with normal school, work or social activities markedly, but they are not prevented or radically changed.

5. Symptoms radically change or prevent normal school, work or social activities.

Score: _____

Signature:_____

Reprinted with the permission of Dr. S. Kutcher, Department of Psychiatry, Dalhousie University, Queen Elizabeth II Health Sciences Centre, 1763 Robie Street, Suite 4018, Halifax, Nova Scotia, Canada. B3H 3G2.

SICKNESS IMPACT PROFILE: ADOLESCENT VERSION

Name: _____   Date: _____

Introduction

On the next few pages are statements which describe things people often do when they are not well.

As you read them, think of yourself **AS YOU ARE DOING NOW**.
- If a statement describes you **AS YOU ARE DOING NOW**, mark the box under "Yes". (Yes, this statement describes me today).
- However, if a statement does not describe you **AS YOU ARE DOING NOW**, or does not apply to you, mark the box under "No". (No, this statement does not describe me today, or does not apply to me).

For Example

"I am not doing any of the shopping that I would usually do"
- If you have not been doing any shopping for some time, and still are not doing any shopping now, check "Yes". (Yes, this statement describes me as I am doing now).
- If you are doing your shopping as usual check "No". (No, this statement does not describe me now, or does not apply to me.)

Read and respond to the statements in the order listed. Some of the statements will differ only in a few words, so please read each one carefully. While you may wish to go back to change a response, your first answer is usually best. Please do not read ahead in the questionnaire. Please mark your answers by placing an "X" in the appropriate box like this. ☐   Thank you for your time and help.

How would you describe your present health?
☐ very good   ☐ good   ☐ fair   ☐ poor   ☐ very poor

How would you describe your present quality of life (how things are going for you generally)?
☐ very good   ☐ good   ☐ fair   ☐ poor   ☐ very poor

A. **These statements describe your sleep and rest**.

		Yes	No
1.	I spend much of the day lying down in order to rest.	☐	☐
2.	I sit for much of the day.	☐	☐
3.	I am sleeping or dozing much of the time - day & night.	☐	☐
4.	I lie down more often than my friends during the day in order to rest.	☐	☐
5.	I sit around half asleep.	☐	☐
6.	I sleep less at night, for example, I wake up easily, I do not fall asleep for a long time, I keep waking up.	☐	☐
7.	I sleep or doze more during the day.	☐	☐

1

B. **These statements describe your daily work around the house.**

		Yes	No
1.	I only do work that I need to do around the house for short periods of time or I rest often.	☐	☐
2.	I am doing less of the daily household chores that I would usually do.	☐	☐
3.	I am not doing any of the daily household chores that I would usually do.	☐	☐
4.	I am not doing any of the shopping that I would usually do.	☐	☐
5.	I am not doing any of the cleaning that I would usually do.	☐	☐
6.	I am not doing any of the clothes washing that I would usually do.	☐	☐

C. **These statements describe your contact with your family and friends.**

		Yes	No
1.	I am going out less to visit people.	☐	☐
2.	I am not going out to visit people at all.	☐	☐
3.	I show less interest in other people's problems, for example, I do not listen when they tell me about their problems.	☐	☐
4.	I am often irritable with those around me, for example I snap at people or criticize easily.	☐	☐
5.	I show less affection.	☐	☐
6.	I take part in fewer social activities than I used to, for example, I go to fewer parties or social events.	☐	☐
7.	I am cutting down the length of visits to friends.	☐	☐
8.	I avoid having visitors.	☐	☐
9.	My sexual activity is decreased.	☐	☐
10.	I talk less with those around me.	☐	☐
11.	I make demands on other people that they find irritating, for example, I insist that they do things for me, or tell them how to do things.	☐	☐
12.	I stay alone much of the time.	☐	☐
13.	I am disagreeable with my family, for example, I act spitefully or stubbornly.	☐	☐
14.	I frequently get angry with my family, for example, I hit them, scream or throw things at them.	☐	☐
15.	I isolate myself as much as I can from the rest of my family.	☐	☐
16.	I refuse contact with my family, for example, I turn away from them.	☐	☐
17.	I am not joking with my family members as I usually do.	☐	☐

D. **These statements describe your feelings.**

		Yes	No
1.	I am confused and start to do more than one thing at a time.	☐	☐
2.	I have more minor accidents, for example, I drop things, I trip and fall or bump into things.	☐	☐
3.	I react slowly to things that are said or done.	☐	☐

	Yes	No
4. I do not finish things I start.	☐	☐
5. I have difficulty reasoning and solving problems, for example, making plans, making decisions, learning new things.	☐	☐
6. I sometimes get confused, for example, I do not know where I am, who is around, or what day it is.	☐	☐
7. I forget a lot, for example, things that happened recently, where I put things, or to keep appointments.	☐	☐
8. I do not keep my attention on any activity for long.	☐	☐
9. I make more mistakes than usual.	☐	☐
10. I have difficulty doing things which involve thought and concentration, for example, paying attention in school or at my job.	☐	☐

E. **These statements are about how you talk to other people and write.**

	Yes	No
1. I am having trouble writing or typing.	☐	☐
2. I am having trouble talking to people.	☐	☐
3. I am not comfortable in most social situations like parties.	☐	☐
4. I speak with difficulty, for example, I get stuck for words, I stutter, I stammer, I slur my words.	☐	☐
5. I do not speak clearly when I am under stress.	☐	☐

F. **The following statements describe the activities you usually do in your spare time for relaxation, entertainment or just to pass the time.**

	Yes	No
1. I spend shorter periods of time on my hobbies and recreation than usually.	☐	☐
2. I am going out and enjoying myself less often.	☐	☐
3. I am cutting down on some of my usual inactive pastimes, for example, I watch less TV, play cards less, or read less.	☐	☐
4. I am not doing any of my usual inactive pastimes, for example, I watch less TV, play cards, or read less.	☐	☐
5. I am doing more inactive pastimes in place of my other usual active activities, for example, I watch TV instead of going for a walk.	☐	☐
6. I am taking part in fewer activities with my friends.	☐	☐
7. I am cutting down on some of my usual physical recreation or more active pastimes.	☐	☐
8. I am not doing any of my usual physical recreation or more active pastimes.	☐	☐

** Now please look through this questionnaire and make sure that you have read every question. Thank you once again for your help.

Adapted by Dr. S. Kutcher, Queen Elizabeth II Health Sciences Centre, Dalhousie University, from Sickness Impact Profile, Dr. G. Awad, Clarke Institute of Psychiatry, University of Toronto.

3

DUKE SOCIAL SUPPORT AND STRESS SCALE (DUSOCS)

I. People Who Give Personal Support

[A *supportive* person is one who is helpful, will listen to you or who will back you up when you are in trouble.]

> Instructions: Please look at the following list and decide how much each person (or group of persons) is supportive for you at this time in your life. Check (✓) your answer.

A. Family Members

	This person is supportive now:			There is No Such Person
	None	Some	A Lot	
1. Your wife, husband, or significant other person	____	____	____	____
2. Your children or grandchildren	____	____	____	____
3. Your parents or grandparents	____	____	____	____
4. Your brothers or sisters	____	____	____	____
5. Your other blood relatives	____	____	____	____
6. Your relatives by marriage (for example: in-laws, ex-wife, ex-husband)	____	____	____	____

B. Non-family Members

	None	Some	A Lot	No Such Person
7. Your neighbors	____	____	____	____
8. Your co-workers	____	____	____	____
9. Your church members	____	____	____	____
10. Your other friends	____	____	____	____

C. Special Supportive Person

	Yes	No
11. Do you have one particular person whom you trust and to whom you can go with personal difficulties?	____	____

12. If you answered "yes", which of the above types of person is he or she? (for example: child, parent, neighbor) _____

(over)

DUSOCS *(continued)*

II. People Who Cause Personal **Stress**

[A person who *stresses* you is one who causes problems for you or makes your life more difficult.]

> Instructions: Please look at the following list and decide how much each person (or group of persons) is a stress for you at this time in your life. Check (✔) your answer.

A. Family Members

	I feel stressed by this person now:			There is No Such Person
	None	Some	A Lot	
1. Your wife, husband, or significant other person	_____	_____	_____	_____
2. Your children or grandchildren...............	_____	_____	_____	_____
3. Your parents or grandparents...............	_____	_____	_____	_____
4. Your brothers or sisters....................	_____	_____	_____	_____
5. Your other blood relatives.................	_____	_____	_____	_____
6. Your relatives by marriage (for example: in-laws, ex-wife, ex-husband)....	_____	_____	_____	_____

B. Non-family Members

7. Your neighbors.........................	_____	_____	_____	_____
8. Your co-workers........................	_____	_____	_____	_____
9. Your church members...................	_____	_____	_____	_____
10. Your other friends......................	_____	_____	_____	_____

C. Most Stressful Person

	Yes	No
11. Is there one particular person who is causing you the most personal stress now?	_____	_____

12. If you answered "yes", which of the above types of person is he or she? (for example: child, parent, neighbor) _____

Date Today: _____   Date of Birth: _____   Female: ___   Male: ___   ID Number: _____

DUKE HEALTH PROFILE (The DUKE)

Copyright ● 1989 and 1994 by the Department of Community and Family Medicine,
Duke University Medical Center, Durham, N.C., U.S.A.

INSTRUCTIONS:

Here are a number of questions about your health and feelings. Please read each question carefully and check (√) your best answer. You should answer the questions in your own way. There are no right or wrong answers. (Please ignore the small scoring numbers next to each blank.)

	Yes, describes me exactly	Somewhat describes me	No, doesn't describe me at all
1. I like who I am	12	11	10
2. I am not an easy person to get along with	20	21	22
3. I am basically a healthy person	32	31	30
4. I give up too easily	40	41	42
5. I have difficulty concentrating	50	51	52
6. I am happy with my family relationships	62	61	60
7. I am comfortable being around people	72	71	70

TODAY would you have any physical trouble or difficulty:

	None	Some	A Lot
8. Walking up a flight of stairs	82	81	80
9. Running the length of a football field	92	91	90

DURING THE PAST WEEK: How much trouble have you had with:

	None	Some	A Lot
10. Sleeping	102	101	100
11. Hurting or aching in any part of your body ..	112	111	110
12. Getting tired easily	122	121	120
13. Feeling depressed or sad	132	131	130
14. Nervousness	142	141	140

DURING THE PAST WEEK: How often did you:

	None	Some	A Lot
15. Socialize with other people (talk or visit with friends or relatives)	150	151	152
16. Take part in social, religious, or recreation activities (meetings, church, movies, sports, parties)	160	161	162

DURING THE PAST WEEK: How often did you:

	None	1-4 Days	5-7 Days
17. Stay in your home, a nursing home, or hospital because of sickness, injury, or other health problem	172	171	170

SCORING THE DUKE HEALTH PROFILE*

Copyright* 1994 by the Department of Community and Family Medicine
Duke University Medical Center, Durham, N.C., U.S.A.
(Revised October 1994)

Item		Raw Score	
8	=	_____	**PHYSICAL HEALTH SCORE**
9	=	_____	
10	=	_____	
11	=	_____	
12	=	_____	
Sum	=	_____ × 10 =	

Item		Raw Score	
1	=	_____	**MENTAL HEALTH SCORE**
4	=	_____	
5	=	_____	
13	=	_____	
14	=	_____	
Sum	=	_____ × 10 =	

Item		Raw Score	
2	=	_____	**SOCIAL HEALTH SCORE**
6	=	_____	
7	=	_____	
15	=	_____	
16	=	_____	
Sum	=	_____ × 10 =	

GENERAL HEALTH SCORE

Physical Health score = _____
Mental Health score = _____
Social Health score = _____
Sum = _____ ÷ 3 =

PERCEIVED HEALTH SCORE

Item		Raw Score	
3	=	_____ × 50 =	

Item		Raw Score	**SELF-ESTEEM SCORE**
1	=	_____	
2	=	_____	
4	=	_____	
6	=	_____	
7	=	_____	
Sum	=	_____ × 10 =	

To calculate the scores in this column the raw scores
must be revised as follows:
If 0, change to 2; if 2, change to 0; if 1, no change.

Item		Raw Score		Revised	
2	=	_____	→	_____	**ANXIETY SCORE**
5	=	_____	→	_____	
7	=	_____	→	_____	
10	=	_____	→	_____	
12	=	_____	→	_____	
14	=	_____	→	_____	
		Sum	=	_____ × 8.333 =	

Item		Raw Score		Revised	
4	=	_____	→	_____	**DEPRESSION SCORE**
5	=	_____	→	_____	
10	=	_____	→	_____	
12	=	_____	→	_____	
13	=	_____	→	_____	
		Sum	=	_____ × 10 =	

Item		Raw Score		Revised	
4	=	_____	→	_____	**ANXIETY-DEPRESSION**
5	=	_____	→	_____	**(DUKE-AD) SCORE**
7	=	_____	→	_____	
10	=	_____	→	_____	
12	=	_____	→	_____	
13	=	_____	→	_____	
14	=	_____	→	_____	
		Sum	=	_____ × 7.143 =	

PAIN SCORE

Item		Raw Score		Revised	
11	=	_____	→	_____ × 50 =	

DISABILITY SCORE

Item		Raw Score		Revised	
17	=	_____	→	_____ × 50 =	

*Raw Score = last digit of the numeral adjacent to the blank checked by the respondent for each item. For example, if the second blank is checked for item 10 (blank numeral = 101), then the raw score is "1", because 1 is the last digit of 101.

Final Score is calculated from the raw scores as shown and entered into the box for each scale. For physical health, mental health, social health, general health, self-esteem, and perceived health, 100 indicates the best health status, and 0 indicates the worst health status. For anxiety, depression, anxiety-depression, pain, and disability, 100 indicates the worst health status and 0 indicates the best health status.

Missing Values: If one or more responses is missing within one of the eleven scales, a score cannot be calculated for that particular scale.

ACADEMIC PERFORMANCE RATING SCALE

Student _____   Date _____

Age _____ Grade _____   **Teacher** _____

For each of the below items, please estimate the above student's performance over the *past week*. For each item, please circle *one* choice only.

1. Estimate the percentage of written math work **completed** (regardless of accuracy) relative to classmates.	0-49% 1	50-69% 2	70-79% 3	80-89% 4	90-100% 5
2. Estimate the percentage of written language arts work **completed** (regardless of accuracy) relative to classmates.	0-49% 1	50-69% 2	70-79% 3	80-89% 4	90-100% 5
3. Estimate the **accuracy** of completed written math work (i.e., percent correct of work done).	0-49% 1	50-69% 2	70-79% 3	80-89% 4	90-100% 5
4. Estimate the **accuracy** of completed written arts language work (i.e., percent correct of work done).	0-49% 1	50-69% 2	70-79% 3	80-89% 4	90-100% 5
5. How consistent has the quality of this child's academic work been over the past week?	Consistently poor 1	More poor than successful 2	Variable 3	More successful than poor 4	Consistently successful 5
6. How frequently does the student accurately follow teacher instructions and/or class discussion during large-group (e.g., whole class) instruction?	Never 1	Rarely 2	Sometimes 3	Often 4	Very often 5
7. How frequently does the student accurately follow teacher instructions and/or class discussion during small-group (e.g., reading group) instruction?	Never 1	Rarely 2	Sometimes 3	Often 4	Very often 5
8. How quickly does this child learn new material (i.e., pick up novel concepts)?	Very slowly 1	Slowly 2	Average 3	Quickly 4	Very quickly 5
9. What is the quality or neatness of this child's handwriting?	Poor 1	Fair 2	Average 3	Above average 4	Excellent 5
10. What is the quality of this child's reading skills?	Poor 1	Fair 2	Average 3	Above average 4	Excellent 5

11. What is the quality of this child's speaking skills?	Poor	Fair	Average	Above average	Excellent
	1	2	3	4	5

12. How often does the child complete written work in a careless, hasty fashion?	Never	Rarely	Sometimes	Often	Very often
	1	2	3	4	5

13. How frequently does the child take more time to complete work than his/her classmates?	Never	Rarely	Sometimes	Often	Very often
	1	2	3	4	5

14. How often is the child able to pay attention without you prompting him/her?	Never	Rarely	Sometimes	Often	Very often
	1	2	3	4	5

15. How frequently does this child require your assistance to accurately complete his/her work?	Never	Rarely	Sometimes	Often	Very often
	1	2	3	4	5

16. How often does the child begin written work prior understanding the directions?	Never	Rarely	Sometimes	Often	Very often
	1	2	3	4	5

17. How frequently does this child have difficulty recalling material from a previous day's lesson?	Never	Rarely	Sometimes	Often	Very often
	1	2	3	4	5

18. How often does the child appear to be staring excessively or "spaced out"?	Never	Rarely	Sometimes	Often	Very often
	1	2	3	4	5

19. How often does the child appear withdrawn or tend to lack an emotional response in a social situation?	Never	Rarely	Sometimes	Often	Very often
	1	2	3	4	5

SCORING INSTRUCTIONS: ACADEMIC PERFORMANCE RATING SCALE

Total score: Sum items 1-19 with the following items reverse-keyed: 12, 13, 15, 16, 17, 18, 19.
Learning Ability: Sum items 3-5, 8, 10, 11, 15, 17 with items 15 & 17 reverse-keyed.
Impulse Control: Sum items 6, 7, 9, 12, 14, 16 with items 12 & 16 reverse-keyed.
Academic Performance: Sum items 1-7, 13, 14 with item 13 reverse-keyed.
Social Withdrawal: Sum items 13, 15, 17-19 with all items reverse-keyed.

MULTIGRADE INVENTORY FOR TEACHERS

Name: _____   Date: _____

Within the class, this child's reading level is:

                    Highest - 1
                    High   - 2
                    Middle - 3
                    Low   - 4
                    Lowest - 5

Mastery, at his/her current grade level of the following academic skills:

Reading/Language Arts	Superior	Above Average	Average	Below Average	Poorest - Lowest 1-2 in class
Decoding	1	2	3	4	5
Comprehension	1	2	3	4	5
Written Expression	1	2	3	4	5
Handwriting	1	2	3	4	5

Math

Arithmetic Processes	1	2	3	4	5
Arithmetic Reasoning	1	2	3	4	5

At approximately what placement level is this student for the following subjects:

(Please check appropriate boxes. Please do not leave any boxes blank)

	Honors Accelerated	Above Average	Average	Below Average	Remedial	Special Education	Not Applicable
Reading	1	2	3	4	5	6	7
English Language Arts	1	2	3	4	5	6	7
Math	1	2	3	4	5	6	7

Signature _____

Index

Note: Page numbers in *italics* refer to illustrations; page numbers followed by t refer to tables.